Pharmacology
I, II, III, IV

Subcourses
MD0804, MD0805, MD0806, MD0807

Edition 100

Pharmacology
I, II, III, IV

Subcourses
MD0804, MD0805, MD0806, MD0807

Edition 100

Pharmacology I, II, III, IV: Subcourses MD0804, MD0805, MD0806, MD0807; Edition 100

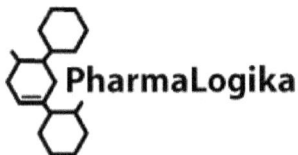
PharmaLogika

PharmaLogika, Inc.
PO Box 461
Willow Springs, NC 27592

www.pharmalogika.com

Author / Editor: Mindy J. Allport-Settle

Published by PharmaLogika, Inc.

Printed in the United States of America. First Printing.

ISBN 0-9830719-5-0
ISBN-13 978-0-9830719-5-2

Contents

LIST OF TABLES

Pharmacology II

ANNEX-- Drug Pronunciation Guide.. A-1

LIST OF ILLUSTRATIONS

Pharmacology III

LIST OF ILLUSTRATIONS

Pharmacology IV

Overview

About this Book

The United States Army is recognized internationally as the standard for complete, efficient and effective adult education. The Army has a tradition of pioneering training systems (including computer-based training) that then transition into the corporate sector. This manual has been continuously tested and updated to successfully educate every member of the modern United States Army. The needs of the instructor, the student, and the Army are perfectly balanced. This is the model all educators strive to follow when developing and delivering training programs.

Included Documents and Features

Pharmacology I

1. Professional References in Pharmacy
2. Anatomy, Physiology, and Pathology Important to Pharmacology
3. Introduction to Pharmacology
4. Local Anesthetic Agents
5. The Central Nervous System
6. Agents Used During Surgery
7. Sedative and Hypnotic Agents
8. Anticonvulsant Agents
9. Psychotherapeutic Agents
10. Central Nervous System (CNS) Stimulants
11. Narcotic Agents

Pharmacology II

1. Dermatological Agents
2. The Human Muscular System

3. Skeletal Muscle Relaxants

4. Analgesic, Anti-Inflammatory, and Antigout Agents

5. Review of Ocular and Auditory Anatomy and Physiology

6. Review of the Autonomic Nervous System

7. Adrenergic Agents

8. Adrenergic Blocking Agents

9. Cholinergic Agents

10. Cholinergic Blocking Agents (Anticholinergic Agents)

Pharmacology III

1. The Respiratory System and Respiratory System Drugs

2. The Human Cardiovascular and Lymphatic Systems

3. Cardiac Drugs

4. Vasodilator Drugs

5. Drugs Acting on the Hematopoietic System

6. The Human Urogenital Systems

7. Antihypertensive Agents

8. Diuretic and Antidiuretic Agents

9. Toxicology and Poison Control

Pharmacology IV

1. The Human Digestive System

2. Antacids and Digestants

3. Emitics, Antiemetics, and Antidiarrheals

4. Cathartics

5. Fluid and Electrolyte Therapy

6. Review of the Endocrine System

7. Thyroid, Antithyroid, and Parathyroid Preparations

8. Reproductive Hormones and Oral Contraceptives

9. Adrenocortical Hormones

10. Insulin and the Oral Hypoglycemic Agents

11. Oxytocics and Ergot Alkaloids

Orientation

Pharmacology

Pharmacology (from the Greek *pharmakon*, "poison" in classic Greek; "drug" in modern Greek; and *-logia*, "study of") is the branch of medicine and biology concerned with the study of drug action.[1] More specifically, it is the study of the interactions that occur between a living organism and chemicals that affect normal or abnormal biochemical function. If substances have medicinal properties, they are considered pharmaceuticals. The field encompasses drug composition and properties, interactions, toxicology, therapy, and medical applications and antipathogenic capabilities. The two main areas of pharmacology are pharmacodynamics and pharmacokinetics. The former studies the effects of the drugs on biological systems, and the latter the effects of biological systems on the drugs. In broad terms, pharmacodynamics discusses the interactions of chemicals with biological receptors, and pharmacokinetics discusses the absorption, distribution, metabolism, and excretion of chemicals from the biological systems. Pharmacology is not synonymous with pharmacy and the two terms are frequently confused. Pharmacology deals with how drugs interact within biological systems to affect function. It is the study of drugs, of the reactions of the body and drug on each other, the sources of drugs, their nature, and their properties. In contrast, pharmacy is a biomedical science concerned with preparation, dispensing, dosage, and the safe and effective use of medicines.

Dioscorides' De Materia Medica is often said to be the oldest and most valuable work in the history of pharmacology.[2] The origins of clinical pharmacology date back to the Middle Ages in Avicenna's The Canon of Medicine, Peter of Spain's Commentary on Isaac, and John of St Amand's Commentary on the Antedotary of Nicholas.[3] Clinical pharmacology owes much of its foundation to the work

---

[1] Vallance P, Smart TG (January 2006). "The future of pharmacology." British journal of pharmacology 147 Suppl 1: S304–7. doi:10.1038/sj.bjp.0706454. PMC 1760753. PMID 16402118.
http://www.pubmedcentral.nih.gov/articlerender.fcgi?tool=pmcentrez&artid=1760753.
[2] Gulsel M. Kavalali (2003). "Urtica: therapeutic and nutritional aspects of stinging nettles." CRC Press. p.15. ISBN 041530833X
[3] Brater DC, Daly WJ (May 2000). "Clinical pharmacology in the Middle Ages: principles that presage the 21st century." Clin. Pharmacol. Ther. 67 (5): 447–50. doi:10.1067/mcp.2000.106465. PMID 10824622.

of William Withering.[4] Pharmacology as a scientific discipline did not further advance until the mid-19th century amid the great biomedical resurgence of that period.[5] Before the second half of the nineteenth century, the remarkable potency and specificity of the actions of drugs such as morphine, quinine and digitalis were explained vaguely and with reference to extraordinary chemical powers and affinities to certain organs or tissues.[6] The first pharmacology department was set up by Rudolf Buchheim in 1847, in recognition of the need to understand how therapeutic drugs and poisons produced their effects.[7]

Early pharmacologists focused on natural substances, mainly plant extracts. Pharmacology developed in the 19th century as a biomedical science that applied the principles of scientific experimentation to therapeutic contexts.[8]

Divisions of Pharmacology

Clinical Pharmacology   Effects of medication on humans and animals studied in the field.

Neuropharmacology   Effects of medication on nervous system functioning.

Psychopharmacology   Effects of medication on the brain; observing changed behaviors of the body and read the effect of drugs on the brain.

Pharmacogenetics   Clinical testing of genetic variation that gives rise to differing response to drugs.

Pharmacogenomics   Application of genomic technologies to new drug discovery and further characterization of older drugs.

---

[4] Mannfred A. Hollinger (2003)."Introduction to pharmacology." CRC Press. p.4. ISBN 0415280338

[5] Rang HP (January 2006). "The receptor concept: pharmacology's big idea." Br. J. Pharmacol. 147 Suppl 1: S9–16. doi:10.1038/sj.bjp.0706457. PMC 1760743. PMID 16402126.
http://www.pubmedcentral.nih.gov/articlerender.fcgi?tool=pmcentrez&artid=1760743.

[6] Maehle AH, Prüll CR, Halliwell RF (August 2002). "The emergence of the drug receptor theory." Nat Rev Drug Discov 1 (8): 637–41. doi:10.1038/nrd875. PMID 12402503.

[7] Rang HP (January 2006). "The receptor concept: pharmacology's big idea." Br. J. Pharmacol. 147 Suppl 1: S9–16. doi:10.1038/sj.bjp.0706457. PMC 1760743. PMID 16402126.
http://www.pubmedcentral.nih.gov/articlerender.fcgi?tool=pmcentrez&artid=1760743.

[8] Rang, H.P.; M.M. Dale, J.M. Ritter, R.J. Flower (2007). Pharmacology. China: Elsevier. ISBN 0-443-06911-5.

Divisions of Pharmacology

Pharmacoepidemiology   Study of effects of drugs in large numbers of people.

Toxicology   Study of harmful or toxic effects of drugs.

**Theoretical
Pharmacology**   Study of metrics in Pharmacology.

Posology   How medicines are dosed. It also depends upon various factors like age, climate, weight, sex, and so on.

Pharmacognosy   A branch of pharmacology dealing especially with the composition, use, and development of medicinal substances of biological origin and especially medicinal substances obtained from plants also known as deriving medicines from plants.

**Behavioral
Pharmacology**   Behavioral pharmacology, also referred to as psychopharmacology, is a interdisciplinary field which studies behavioral effects of psychoactive drugs. It incorporates approaches and techniques from neuropharmacology, animal behavior and behavioral neuroscience, and is interested in the behavioral and neurobiological mechanisms of action of psychoactive drugs. Another goal of behavioral pharmacology is to develop animal behavioral models to screen chemical compounds with therapeutic potentials. People in this field (called behavioral pharmacologists) typically use small animals (e.g. rodents) to study psychotherapeutic drugs such as antipsychotics, antidepressants and anxiolytics, and drugs of abuse such as nicotine, cocaine, methamphetamine, etc.

Scientific Background

The study of chemicals requires intimate knowledge of the biological system affected. With the knowledge of cell biology and biochemistry increasing, the field of pharmacology has also changed substantially. It has become possible, through molecular analysis of receptors, to design chemicals that act on specific cellular signaling or metabolic pathways by affecting sites directly on cell-surface receptors (which modulate and mediate cellular signaling pathways controlling cellular function).

A chemical has, from the pharmacological point-of-view, various properties. Pharmacokinetics describes the effect of the body on the chemical (e.g. half-life and volume of distribution), and pharmacodynamics describes the chemical's effect on the body (desired or toxic).

When describing the pharmacokinetic properties of a chemical, pharmacologists are often interested in LADME:

- **Liberation** - disintegration (for solid oral forms {breaking down into smaller particles}), dispersal and dissolution

- **Absorption** - How is the medication absorbed (through the skin, the intestine, the oral mucosa)?

- **Distribution** - How does it spread through the organism?

- **Metabolism** - Is the medication converted chemically inside the body, and into which substances. Are these active? Could they be toxic?

- **Excretion** - How is the medication eliminated (through the bile, urine, breath, skin)?

Medication is said to have a narrow or wide therapeutic index or therapeutic window. This describes the ratio of desired effect to toxic effect. A compound with a narrow therapeutic index (close to one) exerts its desired effect at a dose close to its toxic dose. A compound with a wide therapeutic index (greater than five) exerts its desired effect at a dose substantially below its toxic dose. Those with a narrow margin are more difficult to dose and administer, and may require therapeutic drug monitoring (examples are warfarin, some antiepileptics, aminoglycoside antibiotics). Most anti-cancer drugs have a narrow therapeutic margin: toxic side-effects are almost always encountered at doses used to kill tumors.

Medicine Development and Safety Testing

Development of medication is a vital concern to medicine, but also has strong economical and political implications. To protect the consumer and prevent abuse, many governments regulate the manufacture, sale, and administration of medication. In the United States, the main body that regulates pharmaceuticals is the Food and Drug Administration and they enforce standards set by the United States Pharmacopoeia. In the European Union, the main body that regulates pharmaceuticals is the EMEA and they enforce standards set by the European Pharmacopoeia.

The metabolic stability and the reactivity of a library of candidate drug compounds have to be assessed for drug metabolism and toxicological studies. Many methods have been proposed for quantitative predictions in drug metabolism; one example of a recent computational method is SPORCalc.[9] If the chemical structure of a medicinal compound is altered slightly, this could slightly or dramatically alter the medicinal properties of the compound depending on the level of alteration as it relates to the structural composition of the substrate or receptor site on which it exerts its medicinal effect, a concept referred to as the structural activity relationship (SAR). This means that when a useful activity has been identified, chemists will make many similar compounds called analogues, in an attempt to maximize the desired medicinal effect(s) of the compound. This development phase can take anywhere from a few years to a decade or more and is very expensive.[10]

These new analogues need to be developed. It needs to be determined how safe the medicine is for human consumption, its stability in the human body and the best form for delivery to the desired organ system, like tablet or aerosol. After extensive testing, which can take up to 6 years, the new medicine is ready for marketing and selling.[11]

As a result of the long time required to develop analogues and test a new medicine and the fact that of every 5000 potential new medicines typically only one will ever reach the open market, this is an expensive way of doing things, costing millions of dollars. To recoup this outlay pharmaceutical companies may do a number of things:[12]

- Carefully research the demand for their potential new product before spending an outlay of company funds.

[9] James Smith; Viktor Stein (2009). "SPORCalc: A development of a database analysis that provides putative metabolic enzyme reactions for ligand-based drug design." Computational Biology and Chemistry 33 (2): 149–159. doi:10.1016/j.compbiolchem.2008.11.002. PMID 19157988.
[10] Newton, David; Alasdair Thorpe, Chris Otter (2004). Revise A2 Chemistry. Heinemann Educational Publishers. pp. 1. ISBN 0-435-58347-6.
[11] Newton, David; Alasdair Thorpe, Chris Otter (2004). Revise A2 Chemistry. Heinemann Educational Publishers. pp. 1. ISBN 0-435-58347-6.
[12] Newton, David; Alasdair Thorpe, Chris Otter (2004). Revise A2 Chemistry. Heinemann Educational Publishers. pp. 1. ISBN 0-435-58347-6.

- Obtain a patent on the new medicine preventing other companies from producing that medicine for a certain allocation of time.

Drug Legislation and Safety

In the United States, the Food and Drug Administration (FDA) is responsible for creating guidelines for the approval and use of drugs. The FDA requires that all approved drugs fulfill two requirements:

1. The drug must be found to be effective against the disease for which it is seeking approval.

2. The drug must meet safety criteria by being subject to extensive animal and controlled human testing.

Gaining FDA approval usually takes several years to attain. Testing done on animals must be extensive and must include several species to help in the evaluation of both the effectiveness and toxicity of the drug. The dosage of any drug approved for use is intended to fall within a range in which the drug produces a therapeutic effect or desired outcome.[13]

The safety and effectiveness of prescription drugs in the U.S. is regulated by the federal Prescription Drug Marketing Act of 1987.

The Medicines and Healthcare products Regulatory Agency (MHRA) has a similar role in the UK.

Army Medical Command

The U.S. Army Medical Command (MEDCOM) is a major command of the U.S. Army that provides command and control of the Army's fixed-facility medical, dental, and veterinary treatment facilities, providing preventive care, medical research and development and training institutions.

Structure and Subordinate Commands

MEDCOM is divided into Regional Medical Commands that oversee day-to-day operations in military treatment facilities, exercising command and control over the medical treatment facilities in their regions. There are currently five of these regional commands:

- Europe Regional Medical Command

---

[13] Nagle, Hinter; Barbara Nagle (2005). Pharmacology: An Introduction. Boston: McGraw Hill. ISBN 0-07-312275-0.

- Southern Regional Medical Command

- Northern Regional Medical Command

- Pacific Regional Medical Command

- Western Regional Medical Command.

Additional subordinate commands of MEDCOM include:

- Army Medical Department Center & School (AMEDDC&S)

- U.S. Army Public Health Command (Provisional), (known as the U.S. Army Center for Health Promotion & Preventive Medicine prior to 1 October 2009 {USACHPPM or CHPPM})

- U.S. Army Medical Research and Materiel Command (USAMRMC)

- Warrior Transition Command (WTC)

- U.S. Army Dental Command (DENCOM)

Operations

In Garrison (Peacetime)

MEDCOM maintains day-to-day health care for soldiers, retired soldiers and the families of both. Despite the wide range of responsibilities involved in providing health care in traditional settings as well as on the battlefield, the Army Medical Department's quality of care compares very favorably with that of civilian health organizations, when measured by civilian standards. Many Army medical facilities report on their own quality-of-care standards on their individual Internet sites.

Deployments

When Army field hospitals deploy, most clinical professional and support personnel come from MEDCOM's fixed facilities. In addition to support of combat operations, deployments can be for humanitarian assistance, peacekeeping, and other stability and support operations. Under the Professional Officer Filler System (PROFIS), up to 26 percent of MEDCOM physicians and 43 percent of MEDCOM nurses are sent to field units during a full deployment. To replace PROFIS losses, Reserve units and Individual Mobilization Augmentees (non-unit reservists) are mobilized to work in medical treatment facilities. The department also provides trained medical specialists to the Army's combat medical units, which are assigned directly to combatant commanders.

Many Army Reserve and Army National Guard units deploy in support of the Army Medical Department. The Army depends heavily on its Reserve component for medical support—about 63 percent of the Army's medical forces are in the Reserve component.

Army Medical Department

The Army Medical Department of the U.S. Army (AMEDD) comprises the Army's six medical Special Branches (or "Corps") of officers and medical enlisted soldiers. It was established as the "Army Hospital" in July 1775 to coordinate the medical care required by the Continental Army during the Revolutionary War. The AMEDD is led by the Surgeon General of the U.S. Army, a lieutenant general.

The AMEDD is the U.S. Army's healthcare organization, not a U.S. Army command. The AMEDD is found in all three components of the Army: the Active Army, the U.S. Army Reserve, and the Army National Guard. Its headquarters are at Fort Sam Houston, San Antonio, Texas, which hosts·the AMEDD Center and School. Equal numbers of AMEDD senior leaders can be found in Washington D.C., divided between the Pentagon and the Walter Reed Army Medical Center (WRAMC).

The Academy of Health Sciences, under the Army Medical Department Center & School, provides training to the officers and enlisted soldiers of the AMEDD. As a result of BRAC 2005, enlisted medical training was transferred to the new Medical Education and Training Campus, consolidating most military enlisted medical training at Fort Sam Houston.[14]

Medical Special Branches

- Medical Corps (MC)

- Nurse Corps (AN)

- Dental Corps (DC)

- Veterinary Corps (VC)

---

[14] U.S. Army Medical Department AMEDD Center and School Portal available on the Internet at: http://www.cs.amedd.army.mil/. Additional information specific to the Fort Sam Houston consolidation is available n the Internet at: http://www.aetc.af.mil/shared/media/document/AFD-071026-035.pdf

- Medical Service Corps (MS)

- Medical Specialist Corps (AMSC)

United States Army Training and Doctrine Command

Established 1 July 1973, the United States Army Training and Doctrine Command (TRADOC) is an army command of the United States Army headquartered at Fort Monroe, Virginia. It is charged with overseeing training of Army forces, the development of operational doctrine, and the development and procurement of new weapons systems. TRADOC operates 33 schools and centers at 16 Army installations. TRADOC schools conduct 2,734 courses (81 directly in support of mobilization) and 373 language courses. The 2,734 courses include 503,164 seats for 434,424 soldiers; 34,675 other-service personnel; 7,824 international soldiers; and 26,241 civilians.[15]

TRADOC MissionThe official mission statement for TRADOC states:

> TRADOC develops the Army's Soldiers and Civilian leaders and designs, develops and integrates capabilities, concepts and doctrine in order to build a campaign-capable, expeditionary Army in support of joint warfighting capability through Army Force Generation (ARFORGEN).[16]

TRADOC is the official command component that is responsible for training and developing the United States Army.

TRADOC History

TRADOC was established as a major U.S. Army command on 1 July 1973. The new command, along with the U.S. Army Forces Command (FORSCOM), was created from the Continental Army Command (CONARC) located at Fort Monroe, VA. That action was the major innovation in the Army's post-Vietnam reorganization, in the face of realization that CONARC's obligations and span of control were too broad for efficient focus. The new organization functionally realigned the major Army commands in the continental United States. CONARC, and Headquarters, U.S. Army Combat Developments Command (CDC), situated at Fort Belvoir, VA, were discontinued, with TRADOC and FORSCOM at Fort Belvoir assuming the realigned missions. TRADOC assumed the combat developments mission from CDC, took over the

---

[15] TRADOC fact sheet available at: http://www.tradoc.army.mil/about.htm
[16] TRADOC commander on ARFORGEN, and the US Army available at: http://www.tradoc.army.mil/about.htm

individual training mission formerly the responsibility of CONARC, and assumed command from CONARC of the major Army installations in the United States housing Army training center and Army branch schools. FORSCOM assumed CONARC's operational responsibility for the command and readiness of all divisions and corps in the continental U.S. and for the installations where they were based.

Joined under TRADOC, the major Army missions of individual training and combat developments each had its own lineage. The individual training responsibility had belonged, during World War II, to Headquarters Army Ground Forces (AGF). In 1946 numbered Army areas were established in the U.S. under AGF command. At that time, the AGF moved from Washington, D.C. to Fort Monroe, VA. In March 1948, the AGR was replaced at Fort Monroe with the new Office, Chief of Army Field Forces (OCAFF). OCAFF, however, did not command the training establishment. That function was exercised by Headquarters, Department of the Army through the numbered Armies to the corps, division, and Army Training Centers. In February 1955, HQ Continental Army Command (CONARC) replaced OCAFF, assuming its missions as well as the training missions from DA. In January, HQ CONARC was redesignated U.S. Continental Army Command. Combat developments emerged as a formal Army mission in the early 1950s, and OCAFF assumed that role in 1952. In 1955, CONARC assumed the mission. In 1962, HQ U.S. Army Combat Development Command (CDC) was established to bring the combat developments function under one major Army command.[17]

TRADOC Priorities

1. Leader Development

2. Initial Military Training

3. Concepts and Capabilities Integration

4. Human Capital Enterprise

5. Army Training and Learning Concept

6. Doctrine

---

[17] TRADOC history available at: http://www.tradoc.army.mil/about.htm

Pharmacology I

Subcourse MD0804

This page intentionally left blank.

U. S. ARMY MEDICAL DEPARTMENT CENTER AND SCHOOL
FORT SAM HOUSTON, TEXAS 78234

PHARMACOLOGY I

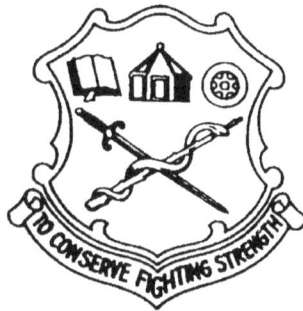

TO CONSERVE FIGHTING STRENGTH

SUBCOURSE MD0804

EDITION 100

DEVELOPMENT

This subcourse is approved for resident and correspondence course instruction. It reflects the current thought of the Academy of Health Sciences and conforms to printed Department of the Army doctrine as closely as currently possible. Development and progress render such doctrine continuously subject to change.

The instructional systems specialist for the revision of this version of the subcourse was: Mr. John Arreguin; AMEDDC&S, ATTN: MCCS-HCP, 3151 Scott Road, Fort Sam Houston, TX 78234; DSN 471-8958; john.arreguin@amedd.army.mil.

The subject matter expert responsible for the revision of this version of the subcourse was: MSG Karen K. Reynolds, MCCS-HCP, Pharmacy Branch, Department of Clinical Support Services.

ADMINISTRATION

Students who desire credit hours for this correspondence subcourse must meet eligibility requirements and must enroll through the Nonresident Instruction Branch of the U.S. Army Medical Department Center and School (AMEDDC&S).

Application for enrollment should be made at the Internet website: http://www.atrrs.army.mil. You can access the course catalog in the upper right corner. Enter School Code 555 for medical correspondence courses. Copy down the course number and title. To apply for enrollment, return to the main ATRRS screen and scroll down the right side for ATRRS Channels. Click on SELF DEVELOPMENT to open the application and then follow the on screen instructions.

In general, eligible personnel include enlisted personnel of all components of the U.S. Army who hold an AMEDD MOS or MOS 18D. Officer personnel, members of other branches of the Armed Forces, and civilian employees will be considered eligible based upon their AOC, NEC, AFSC or Job Series which will verify job relevance. Applicants who wish to be considered for a waiver should submit justification to the Nonresident Instruction Branch at e-mail address: accp@amedd.army.mil.

For comments or questions regarding enrollment, student records, or shipments, contact the Nonresident Instruction Branch at DSN 471-5877, commercial (210) 221-5877, toll-free 1-800-344-2380; fax: 210-221-4012 or DSN 471-4012, e-mail accp@amedd.army.mil, or write to:

NONRESIDENT INSTRUCTION BRANCH
AMEDDC&S
ATTN: MCCS-HSN
2105 11TH STREET SUITE 4191
FORT SAM HOUSTON TX 78234-5064

TABLE OF CONTENTS

LIST OF FIGURES

LIST OF TABLES

CORRESPONDENCE COURSE OF THE
U.S. ARMY MEDICAL DEPARTMENT CENTER AND SCHOOL

SUBCOURSE MD08O4

Pharmacology I

INTRODUCTION

A patient who visits a physician or physician extender frequently receives a
prescription for a medication. That prescription is brought to the pharmacy to be filled.
The patient expects professional attention at the pharmacy. Part of that expectation
involves any caution or warning the patient should heed while taking the medication.

In your role you will serve as a source of drug information. Patients and friends
will ask you specific questions concerning the use of prescription and over-the-counter
medications. You must know the trade and generic names of literally hundreds of
medications. Furthermore, you must know the cautions and warnings associated with
many agents.

How are you to know this information about drugs? Certainly you have had
instruction which presented the basics of anatomy, physiology, and pharmacology. This
instruction has given you a sound foundation for learning more in these areas. This
subcourse will present instruction in anatomy, physiology, and pharmacology. The
material in anatomy and physiology is included to refresh your memory or to give you
additional information so you can better understand the pharmacology material.

This subcourse is not intended to be used as an authoritative source of drug
information. As you know, new drugs are constantly being discovered and new uses for
existing drugs are being found through research. Therefore, you must rely upon this
subcourse to review concepts or to learn new information. You are then to use other
sources (see lesson 1 of this subcourse) to gain new information as it is discovered.

Subcourse Components:

This subcourse consists of 11 lessons and an examination. The lessons are:

Lesson 1.   Professional References in Pharmacy.

Lesson 2.   Anatomy, Physiology, and Pathology Important to Pharmacology.

Lesson 3.   Introduction to Pharmacology.

Lesson 4.   Local Anesthetic Agents.

Credit Awarded:

Upon successful completion of this subcourse, you will be awarded 14 credit hours.

Lesson Materials Furnished:

Lesson materials provided include this booklet, an examination answer sheet, and an envelope. Answer sheets are not provided for individual lessons in this subcourse because you are to grade your own lessons. Exercises and solutions for all lessons are contained in this booklet. You must furnish a #2 pencil.

Procedures for Subcourse Completion:

You are encouraged to complete the subcourse lesson by lesson. When you have completed all of the lessons to your satisfaction, fill out the examination answer sheet and mail it to the AMEDDC&S along with the Student Comment Sheet in the envelope provided. *Be sure that your social security number is on all correspondence sent to the AMEDDC&S.* You will be notified by return mail of the examination results. Your grade on the exam will be your rating for the subcourse.

Study Suggestions:

Here are some suggestions that may be helpful to you in completing this subcourse:

Read and study each lesson carefully.

Complete the subcourse lesson by lesson. After completing each lesson, work the exercises at the end of the lesson, marking your answers in this booklet.

After completing each set of lesson exercises, compare your answers with those on the solution sheet which follows the exercises. If you have answered an exercise incorrectly, check the reference cited after the answer on the solution sheet to determine why your response was not the correct one.

As you successfully complete each lesson, go on to the next. When you have completed all of the lessons, complete the examination. Mark your answers in this booklet; then transfer your responses to the examination answer sheet using a #2 pencil.

Student Comment Sheet:

Be sure to provide us with your suggestions and criticisms by filling out the Student Comment Sheet (found at the back of this booklet) and returning it to us with your examination answer sheet. Please review this comment sheet before studying this subcourse. In this way, you will help us to improve the quality of this subcourse.

LESSON ASSIGNMENT

LESSON 1   Professional References in Pharmacy.

TEXT ASSIGNMENT   Paragraphs 1-1 through 1-6.

LESSON OBJECTIVES   After completing this lesson, you should be able to:

1-1. Given a description of a reference used in a pharmacy and a list of pharmacy references, select the particular reference being described.

1-2. Given a description of a situation requiring the use of a pharmacy reference and a list of pharmacy references, select the reference most likely to contain the information required in that situation.

SUGGESTION   After studying the assignment, complete the exercises at the end of this lesson. These exercises will help you to achieve the lesson objectives.

LESSON 1

PROFESSIONAL REFERENCES IN PHARMACY

Section I. GENERAL

1-1. CONSIDERATIONS INVOLVED IN SELECTING A REFERENCE

a.   At this point, you may already possess a strong background in pharmacology. However, if you do not take steps to maintain and expand your knowledge in pharmacology, you will quickly find yourself out-of-date in terms of drugs and drug therapy. Furthermore, no individual knows everything about every drug used in medicine. What happens when a drug-related question arises? What sources of drug information should be readily available in the pharmacy? Which reference should be consulted to find the answer to a specific question? These questions will be examined in this lesson.

b.   This lesson does not attempt to every available pharmaceutical reference. Instead, this lesson will focus on some references that are commonly used in the practical of pharmacy.

c.   Some references, by design, are tailored to meet the needs of those persons who have strong backgrounds in pharmacy, physiology, and/or medicine. Therefore, you should carefully select references that are written to a level comparable to your background and experience. An individual who lacks a technical background can become frustrated when reading a highly technical reference.

1-2. HUMAN SOURCES

Use human sources of information. Most health care professionals are more than willing to share their knowledge and experience. Carefully identify those professionals who are willing to instruct you and/or answer your questions. Also, you should be willing to share your knowledge and experience with others.

Section II. PHARMACEUTICAL JOURNALS

1-3. OVERVIEW

a.   Journals serve as excellent sources of drug information. For the most part, the information contained in journals is up-to-date. Journals reflect the state of the art of that discipline at that point in time.

b.   Some journals are designed to be read by many members of the medical community. Other journals are specifically written to meet the needs of the individuals who are directly involved with the field of pharmacy. Further, some journals are especially written for pharmacy personnel, who work in hospitals, while others are designed for those who work in retail.

c.   As you know, there are many journals written for people who work in the medical field. Some journals are designed to be read by the members of many medical disciplines, while other journals focus on a particular job specialty (that is, nursing, pharmacy, or medical technology). Many journals are written to meet the needs of those in pharmacy practice. Some of these journals are especially written for pharmacy personnel who work in an inpatient setting, while other journals are designed for those who work in an outpatient environment.

d.   To meet your individual needs, you should become familiar with some frequently used pharmacy journals, the type of information each contains, and the particular group(s) for whom the journal is written.

e.   As you read a journal, do not limit yourself to the main articles. Letters to the editor, advertisements, and job announcements also provide information, which can be very helpful. For example, these parts of a journal can provide up-to-date information on new products, changes in old products, as well as short- and long-term trends in the state of the art of pharmacy practice.

1-4. SPECIFIC JOURNALS

a.   **The American Journal of Health-Systems Pharmacists**. The American Journal of Health-Systems Pharmacists (AJHP) is an official publication of the American Society of Health-Systems Pharmacists. It is published on a twice monthly basis. As the name implies, this journal is tailored to pharmacy personnel who practice in a hospital setting. The AJHP can be read and understood by almost all-medical personnel who have a background in pharmacy. The AJHP contains information on drug therapy, new and innovative pharmacy practices, and other topics of particular interest to hospital pharmacy personnel.

b.   **Hospital Pharmacy.** This journal is a monthly publication of the L. B. Lippincott Company. Although designed for hospital pharmacists, the journal's contents can be read and understood by medical personnel who have a background in pharmacy. Hospital Pharmacy contains information on innovative pharmacy procedures (that is, unit dose), drug therapies, and other topics of general interest. One section, "Medication Error Reports," provides a constant reminder of the types of medication errors that occur in a hospital.

c.   **The American Journal of Intravenous Therapy.** The McMahon Publishing Company on a bimonthly basis publishes this journal. The journal is tailored toward those persons directly involved with the preparation and/or administration of intravenous products. Therefore, it is particularly useful to the pharmacy personnel who work in the unit-dose/sterile product area. Experienced sterile product prepares should be able to read and understand this journal. Articles in this journal focus on the theoretical and practical considerations of intravenous therapy.

    d.   **American Pharmacy.** This journal is the official publication of the American Pharmaceutical Society. It is published on a monthly basis. It is especially designed for pharmacists who work in an outpatient environment, although the journal contains useful information for all pharmacy personnel. Articles in American Pharmacy cover a variety of pharmacy-related topics. For example, changes in drug laws, changes in drug therapies, and perspectives on the various aspects of health-care management are found in the journal

    e.   **Clinical Pharmacology and Therapeutics.** This journal is the official publication of the American Society for Clinical Pharmacology and Therapeutics and the American Society for Pharmacology and Experimental Therapeutics. As the name implies, the journal is designed to communicate up-to-date drug information and research related to pharmacology to those medical personnel who have an in-depth background in pharmacology, therapeutics, and the basic sciences.

    f.   **The Journal of Clinical Pharmacology.** This journal is the official publication of the American College of Clinical Pharmacology. This publication is designed for those medical personnel who have an excellent background in pharmacology, therapeutics, and the basic sciences. Articles focus on clinical research pertaining to pharmacology.

Section III. PHARMACEUTICAL TEXTS

1-5. OVERVIEW

    As with journals, many texts are available to pharmacy personnel. Some texts require a certain amount of background knowledge in physiology, anatomy, and/or pharmacology. It is important for you to recognize your background strengths and weaknesses before you begin to search for a text to answer a particular question. You should also be familiar with the subjects discussed in each of these texts. Being able to identify a text on your knowledge level, which can provide you with the answer you are seeking, can pay dividends in terms of saved time and reduced frustration.

1-6. SPECIFIC TEXTS

    a.   **The Physicians' Desk Reference.** The Physicians' Desk Reference (PDR) is published on an annual basis by the Medical Economics Company. The drug manufacturers, whose products are listed in the reference, prepare the information contained in the PDR. For the most part, the drug monographs in the PDR come directly from the package inserts for the drugs. The publisher supplies periodic supplements to the text. The PDR is written primarily for physicians; however, many medical personnel have the background to use the reference. The PDR is divided into the following nine areas:

(1)   The Manufacturers' Index. This section supplies information (that is, address and telephone number) on the manufacturers who supplied prescribing information for the PDR.

(2)   The Product Name Index. This section provides an alphabetical listing of the drug products by trade name and the page number where the drug product information may be located.

(3)   The Product Classification Index. This section of the PDR provides an alphabetical listing of the drug products by their therapeutic classifications. Page numbers for locating the drug products are provided for quick reference.

(4)   The Generic and Chemical Name Index. In this section, the products are categorized under generic and chemical name headings according to their principal components.

(5)   The Product Identification Section. This section of the PDR provides a pictorial display (by manufacturer) of capsules, tablets, and containers. This area can be used to identify products that one does not immediately recognize by appearance.

(6)   The Product Information Section. Manufacturer lists this alphabetical arrangement of over 2,500 pharmaceuticals. The drug products are fully described in the following areas: common names, generic compositions, chemical names, composition, action and uses, administration and dosage, contraindications, precautions, side effects, supplied, and other information concerning use.

(7)   The Diagnostic Product Information Section. The PDR focuses on the descriptions of diagnostic products. This section of PDR focuses on the descriptions of diagnostic products. The products are listed alphabetically.

(8)   The Poison Control Centers Section. This section contains a list of poison control centers and their emergency telephone numbers.

(9)   The Guide to Management of Drug Overdose Section. This section is located on the inside back cover of the PDR. The aim of this section is to provide the physician with useful information on the management of drug overdoses. Of course, any individual who is suspected to have ingested an overdose of medication should be taken to the nearest medical treatment facility for prompt attention and treatment.

b.   **Remington's Pharmaceutical Sciences.** Mack Publishing Company publishes this text. Although written for pharmacists, who work in any pharmacy setting, the reference can be read, understood, and used by other medical/pharmacy personnel. Remington's deals with the theory and practice of the art of pharmacy. It provides essential information about drugs. Furthermore, the text is especially useful as an information source for the compounding of extemporaneous products.

    c.   **The Pharmacological Basis of Therapeutics**. Louis Goodman and Alfred Gilman wrote this text. This reference is written for medical personnel who have a strong background in physiology and pharmacology. Indeed, it is <u>not</u> written for a reader who has a weak or limited background in the sciences. The clinical application of drug knowledge is the aim of the text. The book is divided into major sections based upon therapeutic categories. Sections are subdivided into chapters that focus on specific drug uses. Each chapter has an excellent overview of the therapeutic area and a discussion of considerations pertinent to the topic being examined.

    d.   **American Medical Association Drug Evaluations.** The American Medical Association (AMA) Department of Drugs prepares this text. The book is written on a level that can be read and understood by medical personnel who have a good background in physiology and pharmacology. American Medical Association Drug Evaluations is divided into sections based upon therapeutic classifications. Each chapter has an introductory statement that discusses considerations involved with that therapeutic category. Further, each chapter contains informative monographs on drugs pertinent to that category. Dosage information is provided under each drug monograph.

    e.   **Drug Interactions**. Philip D. Hansten wrote this text. It is written for the health-care provider who is concerned about drug interactions and/or the effects upon clinical laboratory tests by specific agents. Section one of the book is divided into chapters based upon drug interactions of particular therapeutic categories. Section two deals with the impact of certain medications upon specific clinical laboratory test results.

    f.   **Dorland's Illustrated Medical Dictionary**. W. B. Saunders Company publishes this reference. This medical dictionary is a useful reference for all medical personnel. In particular, the dictionary can be used by pharmacy personnel whenever unfamiliar medical terms are encountered.

    g.   **Handbook of Injectable Drugs**. This book was written by Lawrence A. Trissel. It is especially tailored to meet the needs of pharmacy personnel who are directly involved with the preparation of intravenous admixtures. The text is easily used; however, care should be exercised when using the charts provided in the reference. The drugs listed are limited to injectable products. For each drug, a monograph is provided which includes information on drug concentration, stability, pH, dosage, compatibility, and incompatibility.

    h.   **The American Hospital Formulary Service**. The American Hospital Formulary Service (AHFS) is a two-volume collection of drug monographs published by the American Society of Health-Systems Pharmacists. The AHFS is designed to be used by all pharmacy personnel. It is divided into sections based upon therapeutic categories. A general statement pertaining to the therapeutic category is included at the beginning of each individual section. Individual drug monographs that present information on drug chemistry, dosage, and preparations follow this general statement. Information on the drug monographs is kept current by periodic supplements to the AHFS.

      i.   **The American Drug Index**. Norman Billups writes the American Drug Index (ADI). The book is designed to provide information to all medical personnel in general and to pharmacy personnel in particular. The monographs contained in the ADI are listed in alphabetical order. Both trade and generic names are provided. The monographs in the ADI do not provide information on actions and dosage. Instead, specific information (that is, manufacturer, amount of each ingredient present in the dosage form and the use of the drug) is provided for each product listed.

      j.   **Pharmaceutical Calculations.** Mitchell J. Stoklosa wrote this reference. It was designed for use as a calculation text. Although it is not a pharmacology text, it is useful to rely on such a reference when questions on dosage calculations arise. Periodic review of calculation concepts is helpful to all pharmacy personnel.

      k.   **Facts and Comparisons**. Facts and Comparisons, Inc wrote this reference. It is designed to be used by most medical personnel in general and by pharmacy personnel in particular. Facts and Comparisons are organized into twelve main chapters by drug use. Drugs and/or drug products are listed together in such a way as to provide rapid comparisons between drugs or products that are similar in use or content. Individual drug monographs provide comprehensive information on drug actions, contraindications, warnings and precautions, drug interactions, adverse reactions, over-dosage, and administration and dosage. The publisher provides monthly updates of this loose-leaf text. These updates ensure that the most recent information on new products and developments in drug therapy are available to the reader. Moreover, the publisher has available a slide-tape presentation which provides information on the use of the reference.

      l.   **Handbook of Poisoning: Diagnosis and Treatment**. This text was written by Dr. Robert H. Dreisbach and published by Lange Medical Publications. This reference provides a concise summary of the diagnosis and treatment of many poisons. The book is divided into chapters that discuss such topics as general considerations (that is, prevention and management), agricultural poisons, industrial hazards, household hazards, medicinal poisons, and animal and plant hazards. Information on first-aid measures is found on the front and back covers of the text.

      m.   **The United States Pharmacopoeia and The National Formulary**. The United States Pharmacopoeia and The National Formulary reference contains standards and tests for quality, purity, strength, packaging, and labeling of drugs in the United States. This reference is designed to be used by researchers and pharmacists who are concerned about the standards that have been established for drugs. The United States Pharmacopoeia and The National Formulary reference has information that is useful for personnel who are involved in both inpatient and outpatient pharmacy practice. Annual supplements to the reference ensure that it contains the latest information on the state of the art of pharmacy.

n. **United States Pharmacopoeia Dispensing Information**. The United States Pharmacopoeia Convention, Inc publishes the United States Pharmacopoeia Dispensing Information annual publication. This reference is designed to be used by individuals who dispense drugs and by persons who administer drugs after the drugs have been prescribed. The following information about a drug is discussed in the text: category of use, precautions to use, (that is, drug interactions and medical warnings), drug preparation immediately prior to administration, side effects with an indication of their significance, guidelines for patient consultation on safe and effective use of the drug, dosing information, and requirements for packaging and storage. One section, "Advice for the Patient," provides guidelines for patient use of the drug. These guidelines are written in lay terms. Bimonthly updates keep the information in the United States Pharmacopeial Dispensing Information current.

Section IV. ELECTRONIC DRUG INFORMATION SERVICES

1-7. OVERVIEW

As with journals and texts, electronic forms of drug information are now available to pharmacy personnel. Most of the reference texts discussed previously are available on CD-ROM for single or network use. Some examples are Facts and Comparisons, the PDR, and Clinical Pharmacology. The advantages of this form of information include easy access to information and timely updates (monthly, quarterly, semiannually). Micromedex® is another information system available as a subscription at most military pharmacies. Micromedex® provides drug information monographs, drug identification (Identidex®), poison information (Poisindex®), material safety data sheets, Martindale's Extra Pharmacopeoia, AfterCare Notes®, as well as many other options. The majority of these systems are user friendly and easy to use with minimal orientation.

The most current information about drug use, even prior to approval by the Food and Drug Administration, is available in medical journals. Medical journals are accessed through on-line searches such as Medline® and Grateful Med®. Many U.S. medical teaching institutions and major medical centers offer search capabilities via the Internet or through their respective medical libraries. The use of on-line information services often requires a thorough orientation to perform a good search.

Continue with Exercises

EXERCISES, LESSON 1

INSTRUCTIONS: Answer the following exercises by marking the lettered response that best answers the exercise, by completing the incomplete statement, or by writing the answer in the space provided at the end of the exercise.

After you have completed all of these exercises, turn to "Solutions to Exercises" at the end of the lesson and check your answers. For each exercise answered incorrectly, reread the material referenced with the solution.

1. A friend has brought several capsules for you to identify; however, at first glance you are unable to name the particular medication. Select, references below, the reference you would use to identify the capsule.

    a.   The Physicians' Desk Reference.

    b.   Dorland's Illustrated Medical Dictionary.

    c.   The United States Pharmacopoeia and the National Formulary.

    d.   America Medical Association Drug Evaluations.

2. Select, from the list below, the reference that deals with the theory and practice of the art of pharmacy. It is especially useful as an information source for the extemporaneous compounding of products.

    a.   The Pharmacological Basis of Therapeutics.

    b.   The United States Pharmacopoeia Dispensing Information.

    c.   The American Hospital Formulary Service.

    d.   Remington's Pharmaceutical Sciences.

3. Select, from the list below, the journal that focuses on the sterile products/unit-dose area of the hospital pharmacy.

    a.   The American Journal of Health-Systems Pharmacists.

    b.   Hospital Pharmacy.

    c.   The American Journal of Intravenous Therapy.

    d.   American Pharmacy.

4. Select, from the references below, the journal tailored to meet the needs of pharmacy personnel whose practice is in a hospital setting. This journal contains information on drug therapy and new and innovative pharmacy practices.

    a. The American Journal of Intravenous Therapy.

    b. The American Journal of Health-Systems Pharmacists.

    c. The Journal of Clinical Pharmacology.

    d. American Pharmacy.

5. Select, from the list below, the journal that primarily contains articles related to clinical research in pharmacology.

    a. The Journal of Clinical Pharmacology.

    b. American Pharmacy

    c. The Pharmacological Basis of Therapeutics.

    d. Hospital Pharmacy.

6. Select, from the list below, the journal that is tailored to meet the needs of pharmacists who work in an outpatient pharmacy environment.

    a. The Journal of Clinical Pharmacology.

    b. Clinical Pharmacology and Therapeutics.

    c. The Physicians' Desk Reference.

    d. American Pharmacy.

7. You have a question pertaining to the effect upon a particular laboratory test by a specific medication. From the list below, select the reference most likely to provide you the information you need.

    a. America Medical Association Drug Evaluation.

    b. Drug Interactions.

    c. Handbook on Injectable Drugs.

    d. Remington's Pharmaceutical Sciences.

8. During your reading of a journal article, you encounter the word "retroinfection." From the references below, select the reference you would use to find the meaning of that term.

    a. Dorland's Illustrated Medical Dictionary.

    b. America Medical Association Drug Evaluations.

    c. Remington's Pharmaceutical Sciences.

    d. Handbook on Injectable Drugs.

9. A friend of yours is concerned about the safety of his children. It seems that he believes he has many poisonous plants and chemicals in his home. From the list below, select the reference most likely to give him the information he needs to make a

    a. Facts and Comparisons.

    b. The American Hospital Formulary Service.

    c. Handbook of Poisoning: Diagnosis and Treatment.

    d. The American Drug Index.

10. Select, from the list below, the reference that contains a section, which provides pharmacy personnel with specific information that should be communicated to the patient concerning the use of a particular drug.

    a.   The American Drug Index.

    b.   Handbook of Poisoning: Diagnosis and Treatment.

    c.   The Pharmacological Basis of Therapeutics.

    d.   The United States Pharmacopeia Dispensing Information.

Check Your Answers on Next Page

SOLUTIONS TO EXERCISES, LESSON 1

1. a   <u>The Physicians' Desk Reference.</u> (para 1-6a)

2. d   <u>Remington's Pharmaceutical Sciences</u>. (para 1-6b)

3. c   <u>The American Journal of Intravenous Therapy</u>. (para 1-4c)

4. b   <u>The American Journal of Health-Systems Pharmacists</u>. (para 1-4a)

5. a   <u>The Journal of Clinical Pharmacology</u>. (para 1-4f)

6. d   <u>American Pharmacy</u>. (para 1-4d)

7. b   <u>Drug Interactions</u>. (para 1-6e)

8. a   <u>Dorland's Illustrated Medical Dictionary</u>. (para 1-6f)

9. c   <u>Handbook of Poisoning: Diagnosis and Treatment.</u> (para 1-6l)

10. d   The United States Pharmacopoeia Dispensing Information. (para 1-6n)

End of Lesson 1

LESSON ASSIGNMENT

LESSON 2   Anatomy, Physiology, and Pathology Important
                               to Pharmacology.

TEXT ASSIGNMENT   Paragraphs 2-1 through 2-20.

LESSON OBJECTIVES   After completing this lesson, you should be able to:

2-1.   Given a term pertaining to anatomy, physiology
       or pathology and a group of definitions, select
       the definition of that term.

2-2.   Given the name of a system of the body and a
       group of functions, select the function of that
       system.

2-3.   Given the name of a structural component of a
       cell and a group of descriptions, select the
       most appropriate description of that structure.

2-4.   Given the name of a type of tissue and a group
       of descriptions, select the most appropriate
       description of that type of tissue.

2-5.   Select from a list of functions the function of
       the skin.

2-6.   Given the name or type of a disease of the skin
       and a group of descriptions, select the best
       description of that particular disease.

2-7.   Given a cause of disease and a group of
       statements discussing various causes of
       disease, select the statement that best
       describes that cause.

SUGGESTION   After studying the assignment, complete the exercises
                               at the end of this lesson. These exercises will help
                               you to achieve the lesson objectives.

LESSON 2

ANATOMY, PHYSIOLOGY, AND PATHOLOGY IMPORTANT TO PHARMACOLOGY

Section I. PRINCIPLES OF ANATOMY AND PHYSIOLOGY

2-1. ANATOMY AND PHYSIOLOGY

a.   Anatomy is the study of the structure of the body. Often, you may be more interested in functions of the body. Functions include digestion, respiration, circulation, and reproduction. Physiology is the study of the functions of the body.

b.   The body is a chemical and physical machine. As such, it is subject to certain laws. These are sometimes called natural laws. Each part of the body is engineered to do a particular job. These jobs are functions. For each job or body function, there is a particular structure engineered to do it.

c.   In order to read and understand basic concepts in pharmacology, you must be familiar with certain topics in anatomy, physiology, and pathology. It is not the intent of this subcourse to discuss these areas in detail. Instead, the content of this lesson should give you the knowledge required to complete this subcourse. If you want, you can read texts and references that discuss these areas in detail.

2-2. ORGANIZATION OF THE HUMAN BODY

The human body is organized into cells, tissues, organs, organ systems, and the total organism.

a.   Cells are the smallest living unit of body construction.

b.   A tissue is a grouping of like cells working together. Examples are muscle tissue and nervous tissue.

c.   An organ is a structure composed of several different tissues performing a particular function. Examples include the lungs and the heart.

d.   Organ systems are groups of organs, which together perform an overall function. Examples are the respiratory system and the digestive system.

e.   The total organism is the individual human being. You are a total organism.

2-3. SYSTEMS OF THE BODY

A system is a combination of parts or organs, which, in association, perform some particular function. The systems of the body are as follows:

a. **Integumentary.** Covers and protects the body from drying, injury, and infection, and has functions of sensation, temperature regulation, and excretion.

b. **Skeletal.** Provides a framework for the body, supports the organs, and furnishes a place of attachment for muscles.

c. **Muscular.** Provides the force for the motion and propulsion of the body.

d. **Respiratory.** Absorbs oxygen from the air and gives off the carbon dioxide produced by the body tissues.

e. **Cardiovascular.** Functions in the transportation of blood throughout the body.

f. **Lymphatic (System of Vessels and Glands).** Returns protein and fluid to the blood from the various body tissues; also furnishes the body with protective mechanisms against pathogenic organisms.

g. **Gastrointestinal**. Digests and absorbs food substances and excretes waste products.

h. **Genitourinary.** Excretes and transports urine (urinary), and elaborates and transports reproductive cells and sex hormones (reproductive).

i. **Nervous and Special Senses**. Gives the body awareness of its environment, and enable it to react to that environment.

j. **Endocrine.** Manufactures hormones, which are active in the control of much of the body activity and behavior.

Section II. CELLS

2-4. INTRODUCTION

Each of the 100 trillion cells in a human being is a living structure that is capable of surviving indefinitely. In most instances, the cell can reproduce itself provided its surrounding fluids remain intact. To understand the function of the various organs and other structures of the human body, it is essential that you first understand the basic organization of the cell and the functions of its component parts.

2-5. STRUCTURAL COMPONENTS OF A CELL

The cell was once viewed as a bag of fluid, enzymes, and chemicals. Now, we understand that the cell is an extremely complex living the entity. With the advent of electron microscopy in the early 1940's, several distinct cellular structures called organelles were clearly recognized. A typical animal cell contains several types of these organelles (Figure 2-1). Each organelle has an important role in the functioning of the cell. It is important for you to become familiar with these organelles.

a. **Cell Membrane.** (Animal cells do not have cell walls; they have cell membranes only. Plant cells have both cell walls and cell membranes.)

(1) Practically all the structures within the cell, as well as the cell itself, are lined with a porous, elastic membrane. The cell membrane is composed primarily of lipids (fats) and proteins that are arranged in layers at right angles to each other (Figure 2-1).

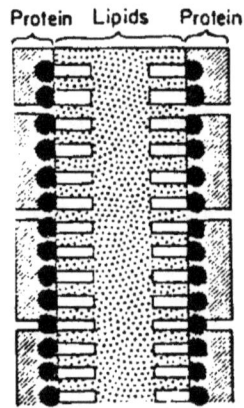

Figure 2-1. Diagram of a cell membrane.

(2) The lipids of the cell wall are composed of two portions: a long hydrocarbon chain (that is insoluble in water) and a glycerol-phosphate head (that is soluble in water). The long chains are in the center of the protein and the glycerol-phosphate group is attached to the end of the protein.

(3) The cell membrane contains many pores. It is through these pores that lipid-insoluble particles, such as water and urea, pass between the interior and the exterior of the cell. Diffusion experiments have shown that particles up to approximately 8-Angstrom units in diameter pass through the pores freely.

(4) The main function of the cell membrane is to regulate the flow of substances into and out of the cell. This regulation of flow is accomplished by the membrane's selective permeability. That is, only certain substances may pass through

the pores. This is important, since the cell must obtain the nutrients for its growth from the extracellular fluid (fluid outside the cell) and discard waste products back into the extracellular fluid.

b. **Cytoplasm (Figure 2-2).** Cytoplasm is the fluid or semifluid contained inside the cell membrane, but outside the nucleus. The cytoplasm functions as a medium to contain many substances, such as fats, glucose, proteins, water, and electrolytes. The clear portion of the cytoplasm is called hyaloplasm. Located within the cytoplasm are the organelles that perform highly specialized functions in the cell.

c. **Nucleus (Figure 2-2).** The nucleus is the control center for the cell. It controls the reproduction of the cell as well as the chemical reactions that occur within the cell. The nucleus contains large amounts of deoxyribonucleic acid (DNA). The DNA is responsible for controlling the characteristics of the protein enzymes of the cytoplasm, and thus, it controls cytoplasmic activities. The DNA is also responsible for controlling the hereditary characteristics of individuals.

d. **Mitochondria (Figure 2-2).** The mitochondria may be called the power house" of the cell. The mitochondria are the site of cell respiratory activity. The mitochondria are found in the cytoplasm. They are usually located near energy requiring structures (that is, nodes of nerves, contracting ligaments of muscles, active transport mechanisms in membranes and ribosomes). Their numbers depend on the amount of energy required by the cell to perform its function. Several infoldings of the inner unit membrane form shelves on which practically all of the oxidative enzymes of the cell are said to be absorbed. When nutrients and oxygen meet these enzymes, they combine to form carbon dioxide, water, and energy. The liberated energy is used to synthesize ATP (adenosine triphosphate). This ATP then diffuses throughout the cell and releases its energy whenever it is needed for cellular functions.

e. **Lysosomes (Figure 2-2).** Lysosomes may be called the digestive organs of the cell. Lysosomes are surrounded by a membrane and contain digestive (hydrolytic) enzymes. When this membrane ruptures, it releases the digestive enzymes that will break down particles or molecules located near the ruptured area. For example, they surround pinocyticle vesicles containing food particles and digest them. If a sufficient number of lysosomes rupture, the entire cell may be digested. When the lysosomes function properly, products of digestion can be used by the cell.

f. **Nucleoli (Figure 2-2).** In the nucleus of many cells, there may be one or more structures called nucleoli. The nucleoli do not have a limiting membrane, as do most organelles. These structures are primarily aggregate of loosely bound granules composed mainly of ribonucleic acid (RNA). Hereditary units called genes are thought to synthesize and store in the nucleolus. This stored RNA diffuses into the cytoplasm where it controls cytoplasmic function. Therefore, the main functions of the nucleolus are the synthesis of RNA and the storage of RNA.

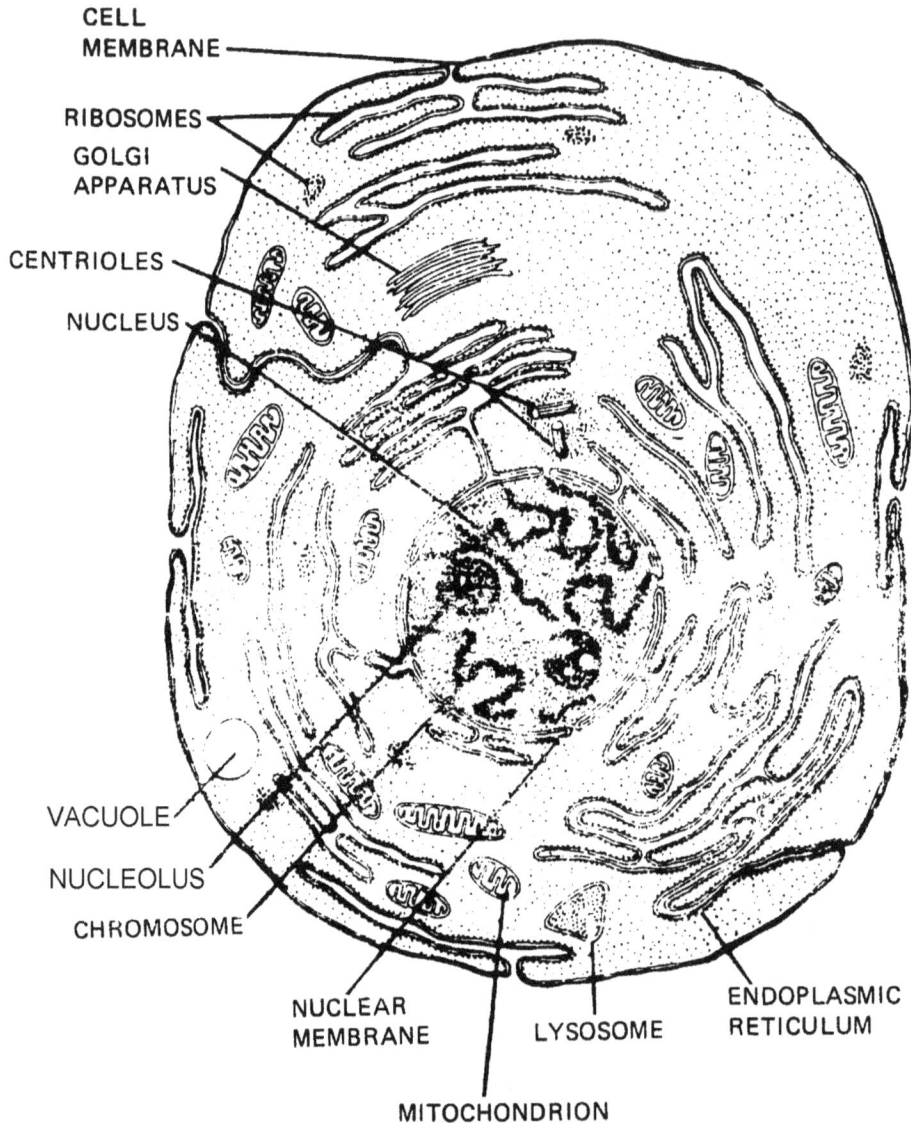

Figure 2-2. Diagram of the cell.

g. **Endoplasmic Reticulum (Figure 2-2).** The endoplasmic reticulum is a network of tubules and vesicles (saclike structures) in the cytoplasm. The inside of the tubules and vesicles is filled with endoplasmic matrix, a fluid medium, which is different from the fluid outside the endoplasmic reticulum. In the matrix, there are enzyme systems. The first function of the endoplasmic reticulum is to use these enzymes to synthesize various substances (that is, lipids). The endoplasmic reticulum is connected to the nuclear membrane and, in some cases, it is connected directly through small openings to the exterior of the cell. A second function of the endoplasmic reticulum is to transport various substances, through the vast network of tubules, from one part of the cell to another area of the cell. A third function of the endoplasmic reticulum is to store various substances within the cell.

      h. **Ribosomes (Figure 2-2).** Ribosomes are small particles that are usually attached to the endoplasmic reticulum. Ribosomes are the site of protein synthesis and are referred to as "protein factories" of the cell. Ribosome is composed mainly of ribonucleic acid (RNA).

2-6. PINOCYTOSIS

      Pinocytosis is the engulfing of small particles or fluids by the cell. That is, when these substances meet the cell membrane, they cause the membrane to form a channel. At the end of this channel, small vesicles form. These vesicles contain the substance and some extracellular fluid. The vesicle then breaks away from the rest of the membrane and migrates toward the center of the cell. Figure 2-3 illustrates the process of pinocytosis.

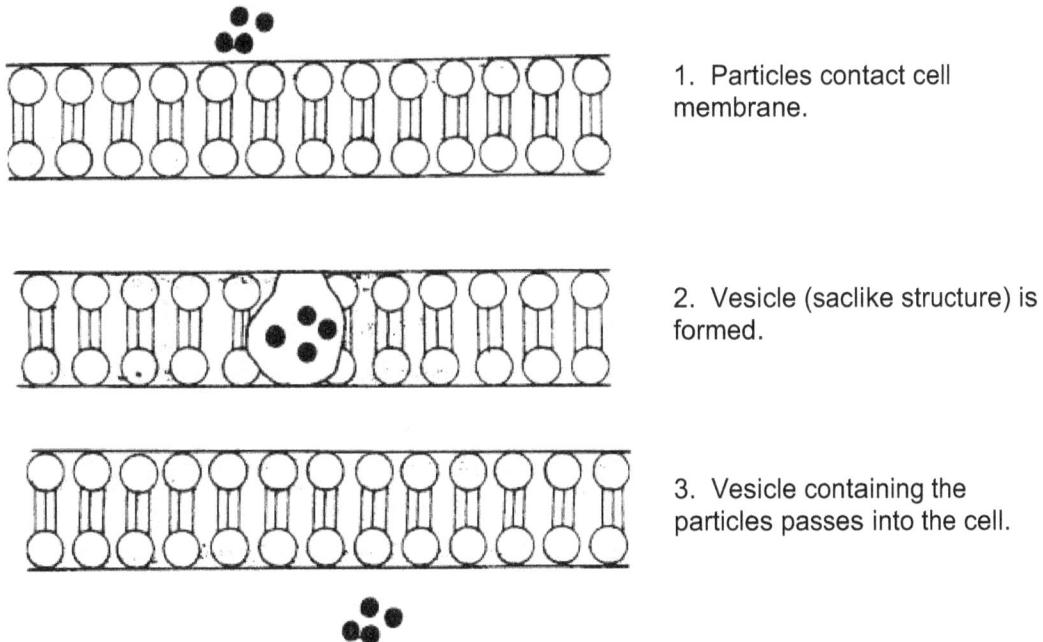

1. Particles contact cell membrane.

2. Vesicle (saclike structure) is formed.

3. Vesicle containing the particles passes into the cell.

Figure 2-3. Pinocytosis.

2-7. PHAGOCYTOSIS

Phagocytosis is the engulfing of solid particles by a cell. For example, bacteria could be surrounded and ingested by a cell. The mechanism of phagocytosis is similar to that of pinocytosis. However, in phagocytosis, the cell acts to surround the particle with the cell membrane and form a vesicle (sac) containing the particle and cytoplasm. Then, the vesicle breaks away from the cell wall and moves toward the center of the cell. Figure 2-4 illustrates phagocytosis.

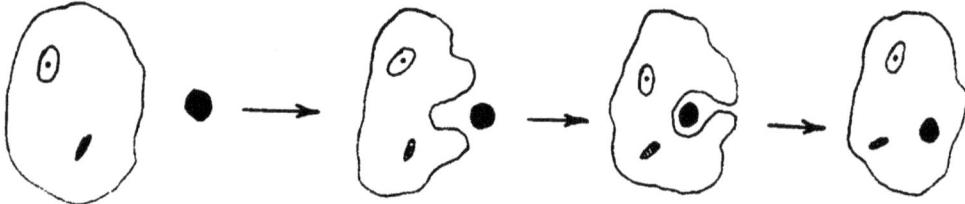

Figure 2-4. Phagocytosis.

Section III. TISSUE

2-8. DEFINITION OF TISSUE

A tissue is composed of a group of cells, which are the same or similar in nature. For example, liver cells are bound together into a tissue called liver, and bone cells are bound together with a large amount of lime salts to form bony tissue. The various tissues of the body have different characteristics because the cells that make up these tissues are different both in structure and in function.

2-9. TYPES OF TISSUE

There are four primary tissues as follows: epithelial, connective, muscular, and nervous.

a. **Epithelial (Figure 2-5).** This tissue covers the outer surface of the body and forms the lining of the intestinal and respiratory systems. A special form called endothelium lines the heart and blood vessels. As serous membranes, it lines the cavities of the abdomen, the chest, and the heart, and covers the organs that lie in these cavities. Epithelial tissue forms the glands and parts of the sense organs. According to its location, this tissue has different functions. As the skin, it protects underlying structures; in the small intestine, it absorbs; in the lungs, it is a highly permeable membrane; in glands, it secretes; and in the kidneys and liver, it both secretes and excretes. There are three types of epithelial tissue based on the shape of the cells. These are squamous (flat), cuboidal, and columnar. These cells are further designated as simple if they are arranged in a <u>single</u> layer, or <u>stratified</u> if arranged in layers.

a.   **b.**   **c.**

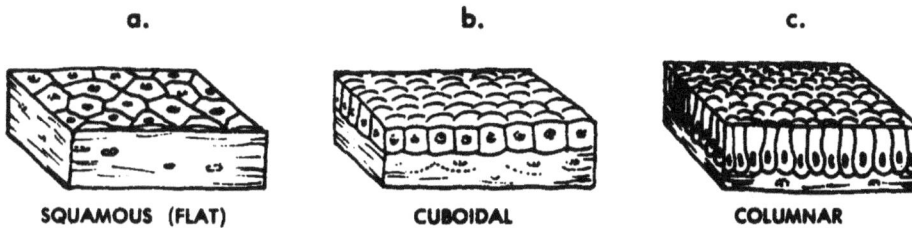

SQUAMOUS (FLAT)   CUBOIDAL   COLUMNAR

Figure 2-5. Epithelial tissue.

   b.   **Connective (Figure 2-6).** This tissue is widely distributed throughout the body. It binds other tissues together and supports them, forms the framework of the body, and repairs other tissues by replacing dead cells. Principal types of connective tissue are osseous (bony), cartilaginous, fibrous, elastic, and fatty. <u>Areolar</u> tissue, which lies under the skin and serves to fill many of the sharp corners and small spaces of the body, is a mixed type composed of fibrous, elastic, and fatty connective tissue.

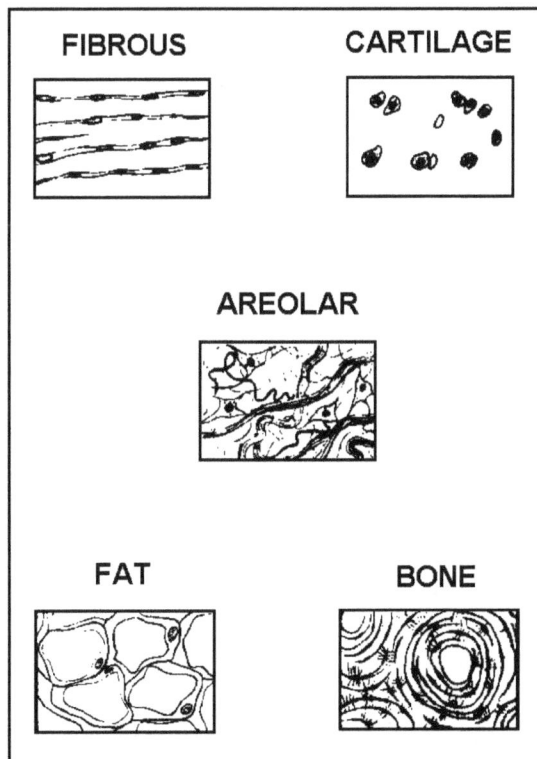

FIBROUS   CARTILAGE

AREOLAR

FAT   BONE

Figure 2-6. Connective tissue.

c. **Muscular (Figure 2-7).** This tissue is of three kinds: voluntary (striated), involuntary (smooth), and cardiac.

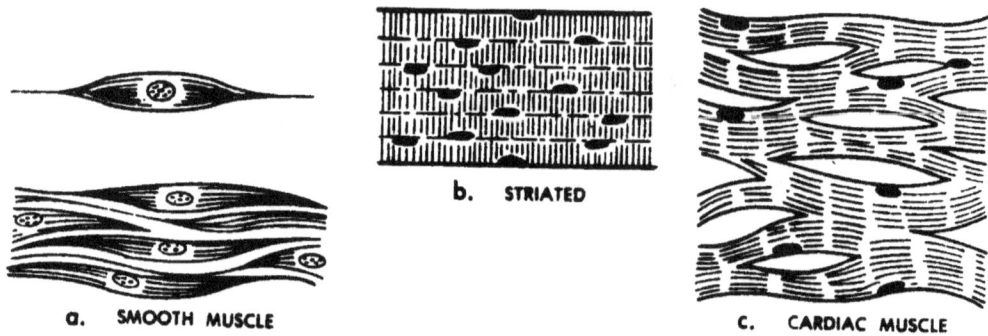

Figure 2-7. Muscle tissue.

d. **Nervous (Figure 2-8).** This tissue is made up of nerve cells (neurons) and supporting structure of nervous tissue (neuroglia).

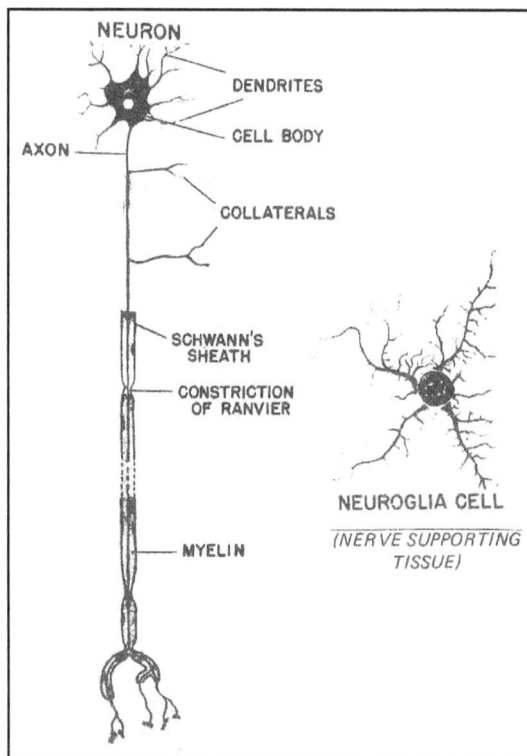

Figure 2-8. Neuron and neuroglia.

Section IV. SKIN

2-10. DESCRIPTION OF SKIN

The skin is a tough, elastic structure covering the entire body (Figure 2-9). It is made up of two principal layers, the epidermis or cuticle and the dermis or true skin. The epidermis, which overlies the dermis, is itself composed of a superficial layer and an inner layer. The superficial or horny layer consists of dead cells that are constantly being worn off. These are replaced from the living cells that form the inner layer. The dermis is the thicker part of the skin, and consists of connective tissue containing blood vessels, nerve endings, sweat glands, sebaceous glands, and hair follicles. The dermis is held in place by a layer of areolar connective tissue.

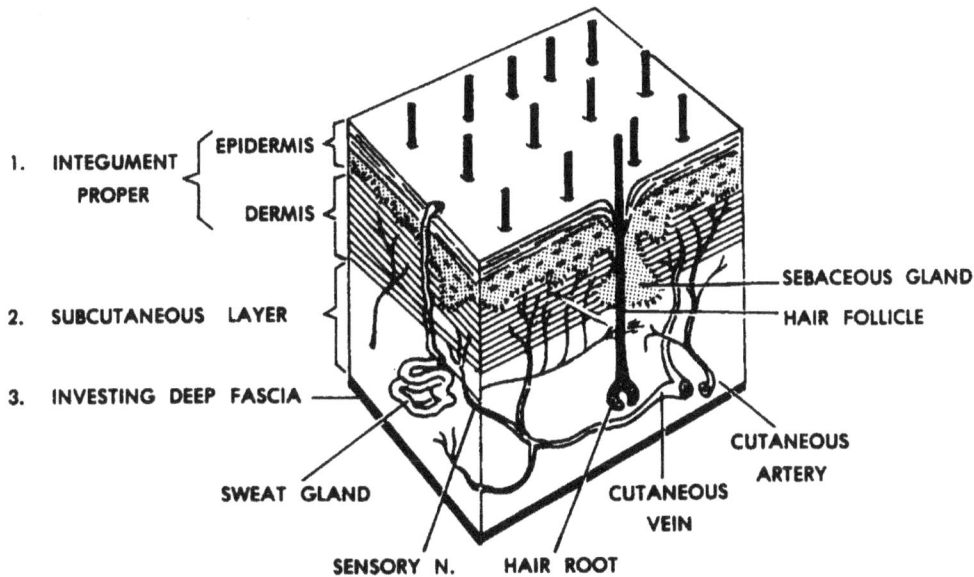

Figure 2-9. Structure of the skin (cross section).

2-11. FUNCTIONS OF THE SKIN

a. **Protection.** The skin protects underlying structures by acting as a mechanical barrier. When the skin is broken, bacteria may invade the body through the opening.

b. **Regulation of Body Temperature**. The skin regulates the body temperature by controlling heat loss in two ways:

(1)   The blood vessels in the skin change in size; they dilate and bring warm blood to the surface to increase heat loss, and they constrict to decrease heat loss.

(2)   The skin produces sweat which, when it evaporates, cools the body surface.

c.   **Sensory Perception**. The skin acts as an organ of perception. It contains sensory nerve endings which are specialized to detect heat, cold) pressure (touch), and pain.

d.   **Excretion**. The excretion of waste products through the skin is a function of the sweat glands that open by a duct onto the skin surface. The opening is called a pore. These glands are distributed in large numbers over the body and secrete an average of a quart of perspiration each day; although, the amount varies considerably, depending on the temperature and humidity of the atmosphere, and the amount of exercise performed by the individual. Perspiration is continuous, but it may be so slow and the sweat may evaporate so quickly that it is imperceptible. Sweat consists chiefly of water (99 percent), with small quantities of salts and organic materials which are waste products. Skin also secretes a thick substance, sebum. This material is the product of the sebaceous glands, and its purpose is to lubricate the skin and keep it soft and pliable.

e.   **Absorption**. Although not one of its normal functions, the skin is capable of absorbing water and other substances. Physicians take advantage of this fact by prescribing local application of certain drugs.

2-12. APPENDAGES OF THE SKIN

The appendages of the skin include the glands (sweat and sebaceous), the hair, and the nails. Each hair consists of a shaft (the portion projecting from the surface) and a root (the part implanted in the skin); each hair root is implanted in an involution of the epidermis called the hair follicle. A fingernail or toenail grows from a nail bed. If the bed is destroyed, the nail will no longer grow.

2-13. DISEASES OF THE SKIN

a.   **General**. Diseases of the skin make up a large portion of the physician's practice, whether in civilian life or in the Army. A specialist in diseases of the skin is called a dermatologist. Descriptive terms used in dermatology are:

(1)   Bulla--large blister filled with serous fluid.

(2)   Excoriation--superficial discontinuity or scratch.

(3)   Induration--hardness.

(4)   Lesion--any localized abnormality.

(5)   Macula--small, flat discoloration or freckle.

(6)   Papule--small, elevated lesion.

(7)   Pruritis--intense itching.

(8)   Pustule--vesicle containing pus.

(9)   Squamous--scaly.

(10) Vesicle--small blister.

b.   **Virus Infections**. Virus infections of the skin include the follows:

(1)   Verruca vulparis. Verruca vulparis is the common wart.

(2)   Herpes simplex. This is often called a fever blister, or cold sore.

(3)   Herpes zoster. Herpes zoster is a painful infection commonly known as shingles.

c.   **Bacterial Infections**. Bacterial infections of the skin include the following:

(1)   Furuncle (also called "boil.") This is an acute, inflammatory lesion produced by the infection of a hair follicle or a skin gland by staphylococci bacteria. The lesion begins as a pustule. As the pustule enlarges, the skin becomes reddened, tense, and shiny. Pain and tenderness develop. The furuncle rapidly matures (comes to a head), and usually ruptures spontaneously, discharging pus. The treatment is heat, and incision and drainage. Under certain circumstances, antibiotics, such as penicillin, are indicated.

(2)   Carbuncle. A lesion that resembles the furuncle, since it has the same cause and early course, but carbuncles are larger, and produce fever and leukocytosis (elevated white cell count in the blood). When a carbuncle ruptures, pus is discharged through several openings in the skin. The treatment consists of surgical drainage of the carbuncle and penicillin.

(3)   Cellulitis. An acute, deep-spreading inflammation of the skin and subcutaneous tissues. Streptococcic infections tend to spread more than staphylococcic infections, because they produce an enzyme which breaks down the wall the body tries to form around the infection. The skin becomes red, tender, and swollen. The patient has fever. The infection may spread through lymph vessels, producing red streaks on the skin. It may enter the bloodstream and be carried through the body (septicemia or blood poisoning).

d.   **Fungal Infections**. Fungal infections are among the most common of all diseases. In order for the fungi to produce skin infection, certain favorable conditions are required. Some of these conditions are: lack of cleanliness; excessive moisture, usually due to perspiration; and irritation of the skin, usually because of tight clothing.

(1) Dermatophvtosis pedis. Dermatophvtosis pedis (also called tinea pedis and athlete's foot) may be recognized by the presence of superficial fissures between and toes, and vesicles on the sides and beneath under the toes. If secondary bacterial infection occurs, pustules appear, and ulceration may result.

(2) Dermatophvtosis (tinea) corporis, capitis, and cruris. These fungous infections are commonly called ringworm. Dermatophytosis (or tinea) cruris is also called "jock itch." The diagnosis of ringworm is made by the presence of a few (usually not over two or three) circular, ring-like, red, scaling lesions, clearing at the center, with advancing vesicular margins. Tinea cruris is distinguished by its location on the upper surface of the thighs. Excessive perspiration and friction from clothing are important contributing factors. Therefore, an important part of the treatment consists of exposing the involved parts to the air as much as possible.

e. **Arthropod Infestations and Infections.** The arthropods are many-celled animals with outer skeletons but without backbones, and include such organisms as crayfish, spiders, mites, ticks, centipedes, and insects (lice, mosquitoes).

(1) Pediculosis. Pediculosis is an infestation of the skin with lice.

(a) Diagnosis of louse infestation. Lice have a habit of living in the clothes and bedding of patients and coming out only at the night to feed. This fact must be taken into account when examining a patient suspected of being infested. The small louse bites may be quite difficult to locate in the absence of the louse, although the patient has usually scratched the skin in the area very vigorously, leaving scratch marks.

(b) Treatment. Pediculosis is treat by application of gamma benzene hexachloride (Lindane®).

(2) Scabies. Scabies is a disease caused by a very small mite that burrows into the skin. The infection often begins between the fingers, and spreads to the body, especially the lower abdomen, buttocks, and genitalia. The mite causes much itching (especially at night), and there is abrasion of the skin from scratching. Secondary infection by bacteria may occur, with the formation of pustules. The abrasions and pustules often obscure the typical lesions of scabies, which are threadlike, twisted lesions with a small raised area at one end. All washable clothing should be thoroughly laundered, and other clothing dry-cleaned.

f. **Allergic Conditions**. In allergic conditions, the patient is sensitive to certain foreign substances that may contact his skin, or be introduced into his body in the food he eats or the air he breathes. A first contact is necessary to produce the sensitization, following which the patient reacts to contact with the foreign substances in an abnormal manner. Some substances can provoke an allergic reaction in anyone contacting them.

Others appear to produce allergy only in certain individuals who have a constitutional or inherited predisposition to allergy.

(1) Urticaria. Urticaria (commonly called hives) is an allergic condition which results in the formation of wheals (rounded or irregular shaped, transitory elevations of the skin). Urticaria is usually caused by eating a substance to which the patient has been sensitized, but may also be caused by a local allergen such as poison ivy; or it might have a psychogenic origin. It is usually associated with much itching and may cover the whole body. Often it is difficult to determine the cause, and the disease may constantly reoccur.

(2) Contact dermatitis. Contact dermatitis (dermatitis venenata) is due to sensitization of the skin by direct contact with a sensitizing substance. The development depends on how much of the substance is contacted, and how often. Why sensitivity occurs is not known. At the beginning, the skin is reddened in the contacted area, then raised lesions appear, and then blisters. The lesions may spread over the body. The vesicles may become infected by bacteria, and pustules appear. There is marked itching. The patient may carry the sensitizing substance to other skin areas by his hands. The sensitizing substance may be almost anything. Examples include: poison ivy, medicines, clothes, and soaps. A painstaking and thorough search is necessary to find and remove the allergen. Treatment includes removal of the allergen, mild bland applications, and antihistaminics in some cases.

h. **Other Conditions**.

(1) Psoriasis. Psoriasis is a chronic, recurrent disease of the skin, characterized by reddish, rounded lesions that are covered by silvery scales. When a scale is removed, it leaves a small bleeding point. The disease tends to begin on the elbows, knees, or scalp, and to spread over the whole body.

(2) Acne vulgaris. Acne vulgaris is a chronic inflammation of the sebaceous glands (oil glands) of the skin, which usually develops during adolescence. Lesions develop rapidly and in crops, located mostly on the face, sometimes on the sternal region, the shoulders, and the back. The lesions may cause considerable scarring on healing. Treatment includes good personal hygiene to help prevent secondary infections, dietary measures, antibiotics, and various skin lotions.

2-14. SIGNS AND SYMPTOMS OF SKIN DISEASE

a. **Pruritis (Itching).** The most common, most annoying, and least specific symptom encountered in dermatologic conditions is pruritis. Among the causes of itching may be included infectious agents, allergic conditions, neuroses, parasitic infestations, dryness of the skin, anoxia of the skin, and chronic irritation of the skin. The actual pathological change responsible for this symptom takes place in minute nerve endings in the skin. The exact change is not known, but these endings become increasingly sensitive to the various causative agents, and itching will appear more easily.

b. **Pain**. Pain is not seen very often in skin disorders, although there may be a burning sensation associated with indurating lesions.

c. **Edema.** Edema is the collection of fluid in the tissues of the dermis. This is usually localized at least to a particular area of the body. When individual lesions take the form of a small area of swelling with associated pruritis, the eruption is called urticaria. The edema may be extensive, involving either the face or part of an extremity. When the edema involves the face, the eyes may be forced shut by the swollen tissues. Edema is seen in numerous systemic disorders, but there are usually enough other symptoms of the underlying disease to prevent confusion with a skin reaction to an allergen.

d. **Scales**. The upper layer of the epidermis may accelerate the production of keratinized (horny) cells, and these will begin to flake off following minimal trauma. These flakes of dry, dead tissue are called scales. Many lesions show scaling as the disease kills additional layers of the epidermis. Occasionally the scales may take characteristic shapes because of plugging pores in the skin.

e. **Weeping**. Weeping is the oozing of fluid from the surface of a lesion. This occurs whenever sufficient layers of epidermis have been destroyed and removed so that the capillary beds of the dermis are near the surface. Weeping is serious because of its tendency to macerate (soften) the lesions and the surrounding skin. As the healthy tissue breaks down, the disease spreads more easily. Weeping is frequently seen in body creases and must be guarded against. The use of powders to dry weeping lesions is the first step in the successful therapy of such conditions.

f. **Scaling and Weeping**. There may be a combination of scaling and weeping. This will result in the formation of a crust over the lesion. Any blood, pus, or other exudate from the lesion may add to this crust. The raw surface of the lesion will be protected by this crust, but the fluid collecting under it will be an excellent growth medium for bacteria, thus adding infection to the existing problems. Crusts may be a cause of itching, and frequently they will be ripped off by the patient, either on purpose or accidentally while scratching.

g. **Fissures**. Fissures are small cracks in the skin. These are very common and occur when there is an excessive drying of the skin. The corners of the mouth are common sites for this condition. Fissure may also be seen in areas of lichenification (places where the tissue has become thickened from continuous irritation). Fissures are open portals of entry for bacteria.

h. **Fever**. Fever is usually seen in infectious diseases, but it may also be present in cases of allergy. This is not a common concern to the dermatologist, because disease limited to the skin will not cause fever.

2-15. TREATMENT

a. **Symptomatic**. Many forms of treatment are available for disorders of the skin. Frequently, treatment is instituted merely to relieve the distressing symptoms and may have no effect on the course of the disease. The antipruritic (anti-itch) medications are of this type. Both lotions and powders are used and are effective in a fair percentage of cases. Systemic antipruritics are not very effective but are of some use in systemic diseases that have itching at some stage. Antihistamines are used primarily in allergic reactions, and they are extremely effective in relieving the itching as well as in suppressing the skin lesions.

b. **Drugs**.

(1) Antibiotics. Antibiotics may be used topically when there is an infection in the skin, either primary or secondary. The infection should always be present before the antibiotic is used. The prophylactic (preventive) use of topical antibiotics is dangerous because these drugs have a higher than usual incidence of sensitivity reactions when used in this manner.

(2) Steroids. The numerous synthetic steroid preparations have been of great assistance to the dermatologist. Many diseases will be controlled by steroids after all other means of treatment have failed. Steroids usually are given systemically, and they may cause serious consequences; therefore, steroids are normally used only after other means of therapy have failed. The topical use of steroids, however, is effective and safe because negligible quantities are absorbed, even through raw lesions.

(3) Antipyretics. Aspirin and acetaminophen are the most effective agents available for reducing temperatures.

Section V. NATURE AND CAUSES OF DISEASE

2-16. DEFINITION OF DISEASE

Disease can be defined as a derangement of the normal functioning of one or more of the body processes. This interference with the normal body functions either prevents them from taking place, or causes them to act in an abnormal manner. For example, a tumor may obstruct the flow of intestinal contents, or bacteria may cause irritation or inflammation. In the following text, consideration will be given to those factors which are responsible for interference with the normal body functions, in other words, the etiology (causes) of disease.

2-17. CAUSES OF DISEASE

There are nine major causes of disease (a through i below). Frequently a disease may be produced by a combination of these causes, or the same disease may be caused by different factors in different patients, or the cause may be unknown (j below).

a. **Prenatal Influences**. By this is meant those factors which may operate before birth to produce disease in the offspring; factors may be manifested at birth (congenital disease) or may not become obvious until later in life.

(1) Heredity. Among prenatal factors, one influence is heredity. A disease may be genetically transmitted from a parent to offspring. The parents who transmit the disease to their offspring may or may not have the disease themselves. Examples of some hereditary diseases are hemophilia and congenital dislocation of the hip.

(2) Congenital influence. Diseases affecting the mother while she is pregnant with the baby may adversely affect the offspring. For example, some diseases may be transmitted directly to the baby via the bloodstream, as is often seen in the case of syphilis in the mother. Alternatively, the pregnant woman may have a disease such as German measles, which interferes with the normal development of the child in the uterus (in utero), although, the child does not acquire the disease. Malnutrition in the mother could result in a poorly nourished baby, which could also interfere with the normal development of the child.

(3) Mechanical. Purely mechanical factors are also felt to be responsible for some abnormalities present at birth. Abnormal positioning of the baby in utero is felt to be occasionally responsible for wryneck; torsion or twisting of the umbilical cord would limit the blood and food supply to the baby, and dire results could occur. Any defect or disease present at the time of birth is called a congenital disease or condition. Injuries or effects sustained during the process of being born may be included here.

b. **Parasites**. Parasites are organisms that live on or within the body of the man or any other living organism, and at the expense of the one parasitized. Parasites may live on the surface of the skin (ectoparasites), or they may enter the body through the skin, the respiratory tract, the gastrointestinal tract, or the genitourinary tract where they may enter the bloodstream and be carried to distant parts of the body. If they live inside the body, but outside the cells, they are called extracellular endoparasites; if they enter the body's cells, they are called intracellular endoparasites. They all cause disease by interfering with the tissue and organ functions; they accomplish this by elaborating toxins, or poisons; by causing inflammation, or irritation; by producing enzymes which destroy tissue; and by causing mechanical blockage of function.

(1) Viruses. These are the smallest agents known to produce disease; whether they are living organisms or complex chemical compounds is not known. They are known to be intracellular endoparasites that cause such common diseases in man

as poliomyelitis, common cold, influenza, measles, mumps, chickenpox, smallpox, hepatitis, encephalitis, warts, rabies, yellow fever, and lymphogranuloma venereum.

(2) Rickettsiae. These organisms are larger than viruses, but are still very small intracellular endoparasites. These organisms are transmitted to man by mites, ticks, fleas or lice, and they produce Rocky Mountain spotted fever, typhus (epidemic and endemic), scrub typhus (tsutsugamushi fever), Q fever, and Rickettsialpox.

(3) Bacteria. Bacteria are minute, one-celled, organisms that may occur alone or in large groups called colonies. Significant bacteria can be divided by their shape into three main groups.

(a) Cocci. Cocci are round, one-celled bacteria. The primary members of this group are staphylococci, which group themselves in clusters; streptococci, which arrange themselves in chains; and diplococci, which arrange themselves in pairs. All are pyogenic (produce pus).

(b) Bacilli. Bacilli are rod-shaped; however, they vary from straight to irregular-curved and branched shapes. They cause such common diseases as typhoid fever, diphtheria, tuberculosis, and leprosy.

(c) Spirochetes. Spirochetes are spiral-shaped and can move or twist. Spirilla and Treponema pallidum are examples. The latter causes syphilis.

(4) Fungi. These extracellular endoparasites or ectoparasites are larger and higher in the scale of plant life than are the bacteria. They include the yeast and molds, and produce infections of the skin such as ringworm, and infections of the mucous membranes such as thrush. Some attack internal organs, especially the lungs and central nervous system, very often with disastrous results.

(5) Protozoa. These are one-celled animal parasites (either extracellular or intracellular) that cause such common diseases as malaria and amoebic dysentery.

(6) Metazoa. These many-celled, larger animals include the helminthes (worms) such as the ascaris, the hookworm, the pinworm, the tapeworms, and the flukes, as well as the arthropods (mites, lice, and so forth.).

c. **Intoxicants.** Intoxication is the process of taking any chemical substance that causes disease or injury into the body. Many substances are very useful in small amounts, and do not cause intoxication; but the same substances may be very toxic in larger amounts, and result in severe illness or death.

d. **Trauma.** Trauma may be defined as injury sustained by the body as the result of a physical agent or force. The physical agents that may produce trauma or injury of the body are:

(1) Light. In excessive amounts, light can cause temporary blindness.

(2) Heat. Excessive heat can cause burns of the body, heat cramps, heat exhaustion, or heatstroke.

(3) Cold. Cold is absence or deficiency of heat. Exposure to low temperatures can result in frostbite and other cold injury.

(4) Electricity. One can sustain burns, electric shock, or both when exposed to this agent.

(5) Ionizing radiation. Excessive exposure to x-rays or to radioactive elements can produce burns, radiation sickness, malignancies, cataracts of the eye, and genetic changes.

(6) Mechanical forces. These agents produce contusions, abrasions, lacerations, fractures, sprains, and strains.

(7) Sound. Exposure to excessive noise can cause temporary or permanent deafness to certain wavelengths.

e. **Circulatory Disturbances.** Any interference with the blood flow to a portion of the body results in a circulatory disturbance.

(1) Ischemia. A decrease in the normal diameter of an artery supplying a portion of the body results in a decrease in the amount of blood that flows to the part. The area becomes more pale and colder than normal, and is said to be ischemic.

(2) Thrombosis. Whenever a vessel wall becomes diseased, the blood tends to collect at the diseased or injured site and form a thrombus (clot). The presence of an intravascular blood clot is called thrombosis.

(3) Embolism. Portions of a thrombus may break loose, and then travel freely in the bloodstream until stopped by a vessel too small for the particle to pass through; or foreign particles, such as air bubbles or fat globules, may be introduced into the bloodstream and travel freely until stopped by a smaller vessel. These foreign particles are known as emboli. The process of obstruction or occlusion of a blood vessel by a transported foreign material is known as embolism.

(4) Gangrene. When an extremity or portion thereof loses its arterial blood supply as the result of thrombosis, embolism, trauma, or from any other cause, a

massive area of the tissue dies, and is said to have undergone gangrene, or to have become gangrenous.

(5) Infarction. Death of the tissue of an organ or portion thereof as the result of the loss of its blood supply is known as infarction. The necrotic (dead) area itself is called an infarct.

(6) Hemorrhage. This is the loss of blood.

f. **Neuropsychiatric Disturbances**.

(1) Organic disorders. Injury or disease of the nervous system tissue may result in the loss of the nerve supply to a particular part of the body. Therefore, because of loss of enervation, secondary changes in the tissue occur, such as atrophy. In addition, the normal functions may become paralyzed, and there may be loss of sensation and other changes.

(2) Functional disorders. Disturbances of the mind or psyche may produce neuroses, psychoses, or character and behavior disorders. Such disturbances may or may not be inherited; the environment, childhood experiences, and many other factors have a bearing on the production of psychiatric disturbances.

g. **Mechanical Disturbances**. Certain static mechanical abnormalities may result in disease within the body. For example, volvulus or twisting of the intestine on itself, torsion of the spermatic cord, strangulation of a hernia, and intussusception, are all often on a purely mechanical basis.

h. **Disorders of Metabolism, Growth, or Nutrition**. Metabolism has to do with the total chemical cycle of converting substances into forms that are usable to the body. Metabolism occurs in two phases.

(1) Anabolism. In anabolism, foodstuffs are broke down (digested) and reconverted into compounds which can be utilized as energy, or as building blocks for new tissue cells and substances. In anabolism, living tissue is manufactured from nonliving substances. This results in growth or replenishment.

(2) Catabolism. Catabolism is the breaking down of the body's complex substances by wear, tear, and age into waste products of simpler composition for elimination. Metabolism and growth then are dependent on the body's receiving enough of the proper foodstuffs in order to supply its needs, in other words, on proper nutrition. Metabolism and growth are further regulated by the vitamins and hormones. The hormones are supplied by the ductless glands of the body (the pituitary, thyroid, parathyroid, pancreas, adrenals, and gonads), and any disorder of these glands will profoundly disturb growth and metabolism. The vitamins are supplied by the diet; if the diet or nutrition is unsatisfactory, disturbances in growth and metabolism can result also. Therefore, metabolism, growth, and nutrition are closely related to one another.

i.   **Neoplasms**. Normally, the body grows by multiplication of its cells. At first, in the embryo, these cells are all alike or undifferentiated. However, as they multiply, they come under the influence of certain factors and take on different forms and different functions to make up the different tissues, organs, and systems of the body (that is, they become differentiated). This growth and differentiation is a slow, methodical, controlled process. However, some cells may not differentiate entirely, but for some unknown reasons, retain varying degrees of undifferentiation, break free of their growth control, and form a new growth (neoplasm) or tumor. Tumors cause disease by interfering with the function of normal cells, tissues, and organs. They may cause pressure on an organ so that its normal cells are destroyed or its blood supply is shut off. A tumor may fill the cavity of an organ so that the organ wall cannot contract properly. The tumor may also use up the nutritive materials taken into the body so that there is not enough for the normal tissues. Tumors are of two types: benign and malignant.

(1)   <u>Benign</u>. These are more slowly growing, the cells are more differentiated, the tumor is well separated from the surrounding tissues by its capsule, and can usually be completely removed surgically.

(2)   <u>Malignant.</u> These are more rapidly growing with very little growth control, and the cells are more primitive or undifferentiated. The cells of the tumor infiltrate or grow between the normal tissue cells, and are much more difficult to remove surgically. Because of this, the malignant tumor tends to recur and tends to metastasize or spread via the blood and the lymph vessels. The common term for malignant tumors is <u>cancer</u>. The medical profession speaks of <u>carcinoma</u> when the malignant tumor arises from tissue that covers the surface of the body, lines a hollow structure, or forms glands, and <u>sarcoma</u> when the malignant tumor arises from any other tissue in the body such as fatty, muscular, bony, or fibrous tissue.

j.   **Idiopathic (Unknown) Causes**. There are many diseases of known etiology. The affected organ and effective treatment are often known, however, the cause and the mechanism through which the disease disrupts the body's functions remain unknown.

Section VI. TREATMENT OF DISEASE AND INJURY

2-18. INTRODUCTION

Patients who have disease or injury must be properly diagnosed and treated. The physician is responsible for these functions; however, the physician may delegate the accomplishment of some of the treatments to other members of the Army Medical Department (that is, physicians' assistants and physical therapists). In general, all types of treatment may be classified as either preventive or corrective.

2-19. PREVENTIVE TREATMENT

Preventive treatment includes all measures used to prevent disease.

a.   Preventive procedures include sanitary measures such as cleanliness, proper waste disposal, inspection of food and food handlers, isolation diseased individuals, aseptic surgical technique, and the use insecticides of and rodenticides to control vectors of disease.

b.   Another preventive measure is immunization. Active immunity is the result of a direct introduction into the individual's body of an antigenic preparation (frequently bacteria or viruses) so that an individual produces his own antibodies that defend him against the particular antigen introduced. Passive immunity is produced by injecting serum-containing antibodies into an individual. This blood serum may be from animals or humans in which the antibodies were produced by an active immunity process.

c.   A third preventive measure consists of preventive psychiatry and mental health work, in which the individual or his environment is manipulated in a manner to prevent excessive mental stress.

2-20. CORRECTIVE/SYMPTOMATIC TREATMENT

People who have some disease or condition want to receive prompt medical treatment. Many people believe that the use of prescribed medications is the only way to ensure that a disease or condition will be cured or improved. The use of drugs does have an important role in the treatment of disease; however, other treatment methods are available. For example, rest, radiotherapy, and physical therapy are very useful in the treatment of certain conditions. In many cases, various treatment methods are used to benefit the patient.

a.   Rest prevents overwork of a diseased organ and includes more than freedom from physical work; a patient must have mental rest also.

b.   Diet is of extreme importance both in the prevention of disease and in medical care. An adequate intake of proteins, carbohydrates, fats, vitamins, and minerals is necessary in the treatment of all patients. Patients with fever generally require increased amounts of all dietary constituents. Patients with certain diseases require diets in which the various dietary constituents are carefully controlled. One example of a special diet of this type is that for diabetes mellitus, in which the amounts of protein, fat, and carbohydrates must be individually regulated.

c.   Nursing care is another essential part of medical care. In addition to doing technical procedures such as administering drugs, nursing service personnel watch for the appearance of changes in the patient's condition. Frequently the personalities of such personnel will be an important factor in promoting the patient's morale, securing his cooperation, and fostering in him a desire to get well.

d. Drugs are substances used in the treatment of disease. They are used to relieve the unpleasant effects of disease and to eradicate the disease. Drugs may be administered externally and internally.

e. Radiotherapy is the use of x-rays, radium, and radioactive isotopes in the treatment of disease.

f. Occupational therapy is treatment that provides a patient with activity to keep his mind and body occupied. It is also used to help the patient regain muscular coordination and control of specific parts of the body.

g. Physical therapy is the treatment of disease by physical means. Various agents used in physical therapy are light, heat, cold, electricity, water, massage, and exercise.

h. Psychotherapy is treatment by various means, which may include the use of drugs, to lessen or rectify abnormal mental conditions. Surgery performed for the same purpose is called psychosurgery.

i. Surgery is the treatment of disease by manual operation or corrective apparatus. It includes the removal of diseased tissue or organs and the repair of injured structures.

Continue with Exercises

EXERCISES, LESSON 2

INSTRUCTIONS: Answer the following exercises by marking the lettered response that best answers the exercise, by completing the incomplete statement, or by writing the answer in the space provided at the end of the exercise.

After you have completed all of these exercises, turn to "Solutions to Exercises" at the end of the lesson and check your answers. For each exercise answered incorrectly, reread the material referenced with the solution.

1. From the definition below, select the definition of the term anatomy.

   a. The study of the functions of the body.

   b. The study of the chemical substances in the body.

   c. The study of the structures of the body.

   d. The study of the systems of the body.

2. From the definitions below, select the definition of the term tissue.

   a. A grouping of like cells working together.

   b. The smallest living unit of body construction.

   c. A group of organs working together.

   d. A group of cells that have nothing in common.

3. From the functions below, select the function of the lymphatic system.

   a. Protects the body from drying.

   b. Returns proteins and fluid from the various body tissues to the blood.

   c. Manufactures hormones.

   d. Provides nutrients to the various limbs of the body.

4. From the descriptions below, select the best description of the cytoplasm.

    a. Organelles that perform highly specialized functions in the cell.

    b. A jelly-like substance that coats the outside of the cell membrane.

    c. The part of the cell which manufactures RNA and DNA.

    d. The fluid or semifluid contained inside the cell membrane, but outside the nucleus.

5. From the descriptions below, select the best description of the mitochondria.

    a. The organelle of the cell responsible for producing DNA.

    b. The site of cell respiratory activity.

    c. The part of the cell which is responsible for producing RNA.

    d. The organelle responsible for monitoring the flow of water into the cell.

6. From the definitions below, select the definition of pinocytosis.

    a. A vesicle which engulfs and destroys the cell.

    b. The organelle responsible for producing extracellular fluid.

    c. The production of fluids by the cell.

    d. The engulfing of small particles or fluids by the cell.

7. From the descriptions below, select the description of connective tissue.

    a. The tissue that binds other tissues together and supports other tissues.

    b. The tissue that covers the outer layer of the body.

    c. The tissue that forms the glands and the sense organs of the body.

    d. The tissue that covers the organs in the abdomen.

8. From the list of function below, select the function of the skin.

    a. Controls the size of the patient.

    b. Produces chemicals for body growth.

    c. Prevents perspiration on hot days.

    d. Detects heat, cold, pressure, and pain.

9. Select, from the group of descriptions below, the best description of pediculosis.

    a. An infestation of the skin with fungus.

    b. An infection of the skin with bacteria.

    c. An infestation of the skin with lice.

    d. An infection of the skin with ringworm.

10. Select, from the group of descriptions below, the best description of scabies.

    a. A disease caused by a very small mite, which burrows into the skin.

    b. A disease caused by small bacteria, which includes the skin.

    c. A disease characterized by itching and fungal growth.

    d. A disease characterized by the growth of bacteria on the skin.

11. Select, from the descriptions below, the best description of a furuncle.

    a. An acute inflammatory lesion produced by the infection of a hair follicle or skin gland by streptococci bacteria.

    b. An acute, inflammatory lesion produced by the infection of a hair follicle or skin gland by staphylococci bacteria.

    c. An acute lesion produced by an infection of a hair follicle by fungal organisms.

    d. An acute, inflammatory lesion produced by the infection of a hair follicle by allergens.

12. Select, from the definitions below, the meaning of the term pruritis.

    a. A chronic, recurrent disease characterized by reddish, rounded lesions.

    b. A chronic inflammation of the sebaceous glands of the skin.

    c. A parasitic infestation of the skin caused by lice.

    d. Itching.

13. Select, from the descriptions below, a description of edema.

    a. A collection of fluid in the tissues, resulting in swelling.

    b. A raised area of the skin characterized by cellulitis.

    c. A collection of protein in injured tissues resulting in bleeding.

    d. A collection of raised swellings on the skin characterized by itching and discoloration.

14. From the definitions below, select the definition of the term disease.

    a. A condition characterized by functioning of certain glands.

    b. A derangement of the normal functioning of one or more body processes.

    c. A dysfunction of the body caused by lack of exercise.

    d. A dysfunction of the systems of the body characterized by lowered blood sugar.

15. Select, from the descriptions below, the description of physical therapy.

    a. The use of drugs to treat disease of mental origin.

    b. The treatment of disease by the administration of antibodies.

    c. The treatment of disease by such methods of heat, light, and cold.

    d. The treatment of disease by the removal of diseased organs or tissues.

Check Your Answers on Next Page

SOLUTIONS TO EXERCISES, LESSON 2

1. c The study of the structure of the body. (para 2-1)

2. a A grouping of cells working together. (para 2-2b)

3. b Returns protein and fluid from the various body tissues to the blood. (para 2-3f)

4. d The fluid or semifluid contained inside the cell membrane, but outside the nucleus. (para 2-5b)

5. b The site of cell respiratory activity. (para 2-5d)

6. d The engulfing of small particles or fluids by the cell. (para 2-6)

7. a The tissue that binds other tissues together and supports other tissues. (para 2-9b)

8. d Detects heats, colds, pressure, and pain. (para 2-11c)

9. c An infestation of the skin with lice. (para 2-13e(1))

10. a A disease caused by a very small mite which burrows into the skin. (para 2-13e(2))

11. b An acute, inflammatory lesion produced by the infection of a hair follicle or skin gland by staphylococci bacteria. (para 2-13c(1))

12. d Itching. (para 2-14a)

13. a A collection of fluid in the tissues resulting in swelling. (para 2-14c)

14. b A derangement of the normal functioning of one or more body processes. (para 2-16)

15. c The treatment of disease by such methods of heat, light, and cold. (para 2-20g)

End of Lesson 2

LESSON ASSIGNMENT

LESSON 3	Introduction to Pharmacology.
TEXT ASSIGNMENT	Paragraphs 3-1--3-15.
LESSON OBJECTIVES	After completing this lesson, you should be able to:

3-1. Given a pharmacological term and several definitions, select the definition of that term.

3-2. Given a source of drugs and a list of names of drugs, select the drug that is derived from that source of drugs.

3-3. From a group of statements, select the use(s) of drugs.

3-4. Given a factor that influences drug dosage and a group of statements, select the statement that best describes how that factor influences drug dosage.

3-5. Given a particular route of administration and several statements, select the statement that best describes that route of administration.

3-6. Given a type of adverse reaction to a drug and several statements, select the statement that best describes that type of adverse reaction.

3-7. Given a factor that influences drug action and a group of statements, select the statement that best describes how that factor influences drug action.

3-8. Given one of the following factors that influence drug absorption: water solubility, fat solubility, and transport mechanisms, and several statements, select the statement that best describes how that factor influences drug absorption.

3-9.   From a group of statements, select the statement that best contrasts passive transport with active transport.

3-10. Given a group of statements, select the statement that best describes the Receptor Site Theory of the mechanism of drug action.

3-11. Given a group of statements, select the statement that best contrasts competitive antagonists with physiological antagonists.

3-12. From a group of statements, select the statement that best describes the importance of structure activity relationships.

SUGGESTIONS   After completing the assignment, complete the exercises at the end of this lesson. These exercises will help you to achieve the lesson objectives.

LESSON 3

INTRODUCTION TO PHARMACOLOGY

Section I. TERMS AND DEFINITIONS IMPORTANT IN PHARMACOLOGY

3-1. GENERAL

a.   It is important for you to be familiar with some terms and definitions frequently used in the study of drugs. Although the terms and definitions presented here are basic, they will provide you with a sound background for gaining additional knowledge, and understanding as you read the text of this subcourse.

b.   The terms and definitions provided in this section do not include all the medical terms used in this subcourse. Whenever possible, the meaning of a fairly difficult and unfamiliar term will be written in parentheses ( ) after that term. In the event you encounter a term you do not understand, you should use a quality medical dictionary (that is, Dorland's Illustrated Medical Dictionary) to learn the meaning of that term.

c.   No attempt is made in this subcourse to address the pronunciation of terms and drug names. If you desire assistance in this area, you should seek the services of someone who works with drugs on a frequent basis. "Pharmacists, pharmacy technicians, nurses, physicians, and other medical personnel are well-qualified to help you to learn the pronunciation of drug names."

3-2. TERMS AND DEFINITIONS

a.   **Drug**. A drug may be broadly defined as any substance or group of substances, which affects living tissue. However, the term may be specifically defined as any substance used to prevent, diagnose, or treat disease or to prevent pregnancy.

b.   **Pharmacology.** Pharmacology is the study of the actions and effects of drugs on living systems and their therapeutic uses.

c.   **Bioavailability**. Bioavailability refers to the amount of drug that is available to the target tissue after the drug has been administered. In other words, it is the amount of the drug available to produce the desired effect.

d.   **Pharmacognosy.** Pharmacognosy is the study of the characteristics of natural drugs.

e. **Toxicology**. Toxicology is the science of poisons. Toxicology includes the origin, chemical properties, toxic actions, detection, and proper antidotal therapy of poisons.

f. **Posology**. Posology is the science of dosage. It deals with the amount of drug necessary to produce a desired physiological, therapeutic, or prophylactic effect.

(1) Usual recommended dose. The usual recommended dose is the amount of drug that will ordinarily produce the effect for which the drug is intended. In addition to the usual recommended dose, the usual dosage range is indicated for many drugs in the United States pharmacopoeia/National Formulary. The usual dose range provides a guide in deciding whether the prescriber should be consulted about the correctness of the prescribed dose.

(2) Minimum dose. The minimum dose is considered the smallest dose of drug that produces the therapeutic effect.

(3) Maximum dose. The maximum dose is considered the largest dose of a drug that can be safely administered.

(4) Toxic dose. The toxic dose of a drug is considered the amount of a drug that will produce noxious (harmful) effects.

(5) Lethal dose. The lethal dose of a drug is the amount of substance that will cause death. You will often see the term "LD50" in association with lethal dose. LD50 means that 50 percent (or 1/2) of the animals given that amount of drug died. The LD50 of a drug should be used as a guide, rather than an absolute number.

(6) Single dose. The single dose of a drug is the amount of that substance to be taken at one time.

(7) Daily dose. The daily dose of a drug is the amount of that substance to be taken in a 24-hour period. The daily dose of a drug is into several individual doses.

(8) Maintenance dose. The maintenance dose of a drug is the amount of that substance taken to maintain or continue a desired therapeutic effect. Some drugs must be taken on a daily basis in order to maintain the desired therapeutic effect. For example, drugs used to treat high blood pressure often must be take daily to maintain a lowered blood pressure.

(9) Loading dose. The first dose given of a drug to achieve maintenance drug levels quickly. Drugs that are given only one or two times a day may take two or three days to reach a maximum effect. To overcome this time, a loading dose is given to achieve the levels associated with the maximum effect more quickly. Loading doses are often used in very sick patients.

Section II. INTRODUCTION TO DRUGS

3-3. SOURCES OF DRUGS

Drugs today are obtained from several sources. Some sources of drugs are discussed below. Some drugs are listed under the sources. The specific drugs mentioned are not the only drugs obtained from that source.

a. **Plants**. For thousands of years, plants have served as sources of drugs. Ephedrine, a drug used to treat nasal congestion, was used by the Chinese long before western man visited the Orient. Belladonna (or Deadly Nightshade), the source of atropine and scopolamine was used in the Middle Ages. Its name means "beautiful woman" in Italian. A solution obtained by soaking the belladonna plant in water caused the pupils of the eye to dilate and appear black. These were symbols of beauty at the time. Belladonna was a favorite poison. Opium, a product obtained from the poppy plant, is mentioned in early Greek mythology as a sleep producer.

b. **Animals**. Animals provide us with large supplies of natural products like hormones. Insulin, used in the treatment of diabetes mellitus, used to be obtained from the pancreas of pork, beef, and even fish. Heparin, a potent anticoagulant, is obtained from the intestinal and lung mucosa of beef and hogs.

c. **Minerals**. Minerals, such as iron and iodine, are essential for normal growth and development. An old remedy for pallor (a very pale complexion) was the water used to cool horseshoes in the blacksmith shop. This water contained small amounts of iron in solution.

d. **Microorganisms**. You are probably aware of the fact that microbes can cause disease and/or death. Fortunately, some microorganisms can be used to produce antibiotics. These antibiotics can be used to kill or stop the growth of other microbes. Furthermore, chemically treated or killed microorganisms can be used to produce vaccines.

e. **Synthetics**. Most drugs today are synthetically made. Examples of synthetically produced drugs are aspirin and the sulfa drugs.

3-4. USES FOR DRUGS

Drugs have many uses. In today's society, the legitimate--and not so legitimate--use of drugs is wide seen. Listed and briefly discussed below are the major uses and some representative examples of drugs:

a. **To Maintain Health**. Vitamins and minerals are used and abused in the pursuit of good health.

b. **To Reverse a Disease Process.** Antibiotics and chemotherapeutic (anticancer) agents are commonly used in medicine today. Ideally we would like these agents to cure the patient.

c. **To Relieve Symptoms.** Drugs that act to relieve symptoms do not cure the patient. Instead, they help to make the patient more comfortable in order for the patient to work or function. Since only symptoms are being relieved, the body is expected to remedy the problem.

d. **To Prevent Disease.** Vaccines and toxoids are used to prevent disease. In the 1950's, many parents kept their children at home in fear of the dreaded polio disease. Today, the only time most parents think of polio is when they take their children for their periodic (and necessary) vaccinations for this still-present threat. Further, any military veteran can quickly testify to the fact that vaccinations are an essential part of the introduction to military life.

e. **To Prevent Pregnancy**. The old saying that an ounce of prevention is better and cheaper than a pound of cure is most applicable here. The birth control "pill" or oral contraceptives and spermacidal agents in the form of creams, jellies, and suppositories are the drugs currently being used to prevent pregnancy.

Section III. CONSIDERATIONS OF DRUG THERAPY

3-5. FACTORS WHICH INFLUENCE DRUG DOSAGE EFFECTS

Many factors influence how a dose of a particular drug will affect a patient. Since not all patients are the same size, weight, age, and sex, it would be wise to consider how these factors might influence how much drug a person should receive and the effect(s) that drug might have on the patient. The usual recommended adult dose of medication, as found in standard references, is based on the assumption that the patient is a "normal" adult. Such a "normal" (or average) adult is said to be 5 feet 9 inches (173 centimeters) tall and weigh 154 pounds (70 kilograms). However, many people do not fit into this category. Therefore, the following factors should be considered when patients receive drugs:

a. **Weight.** Obese (overweight) patients may require more medication than thin patients may because the drug has more tissue to which it can go. The dosage of many drugs is calculated on a weight basis. For example, a person might be prescribed a drug that has a dosage of 5 milligrams of drug per pound of patient body weight.

b. **Surface Area.** A person's height and weight are related to the total surface area of his body. The "normal" (average) adult has a body surface area of approximately 1.73 square meters. A nomogram (see Subcourse MD0802, Pharmaceutical Calculations) is used to determine the surface area of a patient. The dosage of certain drugs (for example, the anticancer drugs) is determined by the patient's body surface area.

   c.   **Age**. As a rule, the very young and the elderly require less than the normal adult dose of most medications. Part of this requirement for less medication is due to the altered metabolism of the drug. Since body enzyme systems greatly influence drug metabolism, considering the differences in these enzyme systems based upon age is important. In the infant, some enzyme systems are not yet fully developed. On the other hand, the enzyme systems of the elderly may not function as well as in the past. Although several formulas are available for calculating a child's dose of medication, the two most accepted methods are those based upon the patient's weight (that is, milligrams per kilogram of body weight) or body surface area (that is, milligrams per square meter of surface area).

   d.   **Sex.** Physiological differences between the sexes may influence the dose or the requirement for drugs. Since females have proportionately more fat tissue than males, drugs, which have a high affinity (likeness) for fat, may require larger doses in females. Moreover, estrogen and testosterone, two sex hormones, can affect the patient's rate of metabolism which can, in turn, influence the rate at which a drug is metabolized, absorbed, or excreted from the body. The requirement for iron is much higher in the female than in the male, because of the loss of blood in each menstrual cycle.

   e.   **Genetic Factors**. Various racial and ethnic groups have differences in some metabolic and enzyme systems which can affect the utilization of drugs.

   f.   **Physical Condition of the Patient**. The physical condition of the patient influences how a particular drug might act. Consequently, the weak or debilitated patient might require smaller doses of some medications. Patients who are in extreme pain may require larger doses of analgesic agents than those patients who are in less pain.

   g.   **Psychological Condition of the Patient.** The patient's attitude about his disease or treatment can influence the effectiveness of a drug. It has been shown that patients receiving placebo tablets (tablets that contain no active ingredient) sometimes have the same side effects as the patients who were taking tablets of the same appearance that did contain the drug. In some cases, both types of patients (those taking the placebo and those taking the drug) recovered at the same time.

   h.   **Tolerance**. The therapeutic effects of some drugs are lessened in individuals after the drugs have been used for long periods. Thus, an individual who has used such a drug for a long time needs larger doses of the drug than he did when he first began to take it in order to obtain the same effect. This effect is called tolerance. Persons who use opium, heroin, cocaine, amphetamines, and barbiturates develop a tolerance to these substances. Cross-tolerance occurs when the use of one drug causes a tolerance to another drug. Alcoholics, barbiturate addicts, and narcotic addicts develop a cross-tolerance to sedatives and anesthetics.

i.   **Time of Administration.** The time when a drug is administered is important. Some orally administered medications should be taken before meals (that is, on an empty stomach) to increase the amount of drug absorbed into the system. Other oral medications (that is, those that cause irritation to the gastrointestinal tract) should be taken after meals on a full stomach.

j.   **Drug Interaction.**

The interaction between two or more drugs may influence the overall effectiveness of each of the drugs.

(1)   Synergism. Synergism is the joint action of drugs. That is, their combined effects are greater than the sum of their independent effects. Concurrent administration (giving both drugs at the same time) of synergists may require that the dose of each drug be lowered. In the case of synergism, 1 + 1 = 2 1/2. Synergism may be beneficial or harmful. Beneficial effects may be obtained when combining two potentially toxic drugs to achieve the desired therapeutic effect without causing harm to the patient. Harmful effects may occur when alcohol and some depressants are combined.

(2)   Additive. In an additive drug interaction, the combined effects are equal to the sum of the independent effects of the drugs. In the case of the additive effect, 1 + 1 = 2.

(3)   Antagonism. Antagonism is the canceling effect of one drug upon another. A sedative administered with a stimulant may antagonize or cancel the effects of the stimulant. Of course, the degree of antagonism varies from complete cancellation of the effect to varying degrees of reduced effectiveness.

k.   **Routes of Administration.** Drugs may be given to patients using a variety of methods. Some drugs are only effective if they are given in a particular dosage form. Other drugs are administered in forms that enhance or decrease their effect or localize the drug effects.

(1)   Oral. Most drugs available today can be administered by mouth (orally). Drugs can be orally administered in the form of tablets, capsules, powders, solutions, or suspensions. Drugs administered by the oral route are usually taken for their systemic effect. These medications must pass through the stomach and be absorbed in the intestinal tract. Orally administered medications are usually easy to take and are usually less expensive than other dosage forms.

(2)   Sublingual/buccal. The sublingual/buccal route of administration is closely related to the oral route; however, in the sublingual/buccal route the dosage

form is not swallowed. The tablet is to be dissolved under the tongue (sublingual) or in the pouch of the cheek (buccal). The drugs administered in this manner are rapidly absorbed and have the advantage of bypassing the gastrointestinal tract. Nitroglycerin, for heart patients, in tablet form is more likely the most frequently administered sublingual drug.

(3) Rectal. Drugs administered by the rectal route may have a local effect (as for hemorrhoids) or a systemic effect (as in the prevention of nausea and vomiting). The rectal route is convenient to use in pediatric patients (children) or in patients who are unconscious or vomiting. The amount of drug absorbed in the rectal route is usually less than if the drug were administered orally. The absorption of drugs administered rectally is unpredictable and can vary among patients.

(4) Vaginal/urethral. Drugs administered using the vaginal/urethral route are used for their local effect. That is, they are usually given to treat an infection or other pathological condition. Drugs administered in this route should not be irritating since systemic absorption may occur.

(5) Inhalation. Drugs administered by inhalation have either may a local or systemic effect. Anesthetics, like nitrous oxide, are inhaled and exert their effect after absorption into the circulatory system. Sprays for nasal congestion have their effect on the tissue in the nose and do not necessarily enter the general circulation.

(6) Topical. The topical route is probably the oldest route of administration. Topical medications are applied directly upon the skin. As long as the skin is intact (not broken or cut), drugs applied in this manner exert a local effect. The base (vehicle) used to carry the ingredients in the local preparation can influence the action of the drug. For example, dimethylsulfoxide (DMSO) will readily penetrate the skin and carry the active ingredient along with it.

(7) Parenteral. The term parenteral literally means to avoid the gut (gastrointestinal tract). Thus, parenterals are injectable drugs that enter the body directly and are not required to be absorbed in the gastrointestinal tract before they show their effect. Parenteral routes of administration usually have a more rapid onset of action (show their effects more quickly) than other routes of administration. Parenteral products must be sterile (free from living microbes). The parenteral route of administration does have its disadvantages: it hurts, it is not a convenient route, and once administered the injected drug cannot be retrieved.

(a) Intravenous (IV). The injection of a drug directly into the patient's veins is the most rapid route of administration. This type of parenteral route results in the most rapid onset of action.

(b) Intraarterial. In this parenteral route, the drug is injected directly into the patient's arteries. This route is not frequently used.

(c)   Intrathecal. The intrathecal route involves the administration of a drug directly into the spine (subarachnoid space) as in spinal anesthesia. The intrathecal route is used because the blood-brain barrier often precludes or slows the entrance of drugs into the central nervous system.

(d)   Intramuscular (IM). The intramuscular route is used when drugs are injected deeply into muscle tissue. If the drug is in aqueous (water) solution, absorption is rapid. However, if the drug is in an oily liquid or in the form of a suspension, it can prolong the release of the drug.

(e)   Intradermal (ID). In this route, the drug is injected into the (top few layers) of the skin. Ideally, the drug is placed within the dermis. The intradermal route is used almost exclusively for diagnostic agents.

(f)   Subcutaneous (Sub-Q/SC). This route involves the injection of the drug under the skin into the fatty layer, but not into the muscle. Absorption of the drug is rapid. Insulin is normally administered subcutaneously.

3-6.   TYPES OF ADVERSE REACTIONS TO DRUGS

A patient will sometimes have an adverse reaction to a drug. Adverse reactions can have a direct toxic effect on various systems of the body or the adverse reactions can occur in the form of milder side effects.

a.   **Direct Toxicity**.

(1)   In general terms, toxicity refers to the poison-like effects certain substances can produce in the body. Fortunately, most drugs do not produce toxic effects in most patients. However, when some drugs are administered to a patient over prolonged periods or when some drugs are given in high dosages, direct toxic effects can result. Direct toxicity may involve one or more of the body's systems. Certain parts of the body (that is, bone marrow) produce red and white blood cells. If a toxic accumulation of a substance affects these parts of the body, blood dyscrasias (the formation of malformed or destroyed white or red blood cells) may occur.

(2)   The liver has as one of its main functions the detoxification of chemical substances when they are absorbed. If these substances damage the liver significantly, its ability to detoxify them if greatly affected. Of course, if these substances are not detoxified, the concentration of the substance in the body (that is, blood stream) constantly increases. Thus, hepatotoxicity (the destruction of the cells of the liver) can result in the accumulation of toxic products to the point that other body systems are affected.

(3)   The kidneys are responsible for eliminating water-soluble toxic products (that is, waste products from cellular respiration) from the bloodstream. If nephrotoxicity

(damage to the kidneys) results, the accumulation of these toxic products can result in death.

(4) Toxic effects may not be limited to the person who is taking the drug. In the past, it has been demonstrated that some drugs will cross the placental barrier and enter the circulatory system of the fetus. Some drugs can exert serious effects on the developing fetus. For example, the fetus may abort or be born with any number of mental or physical defects. Since few mothers are willing to subject themselves and their unborn children to drug testing, the effects of most drugs on the fetus are unknown. Most of what is known about teratogenicity, fetal malformations, has been learned either from experimental studies with animals or from the unfortunate experiences of some mothers. The fetus is particularly susceptible to the adverse effects of medications during the first three months after conception (the first trimester). Unfortunately, many women do not realize they are pregnant until they are well into their first trimester.

b. **Allergic Reactions**. A few individuals may be allergic, or hypersensitive, to a drug. This allergy may arise because of a prior contact with a particular substance called an allergen (it may even be the drug itself). This acquiring of an allergy is called sensitization. You should understand that the symptoms of an allergy are not related to the ordinary effects of the drug. Allergic reactions to a drug may range from a mildly irritated skin rash to anaphylaxis (a fatal shock). It has been shown that penicillin, a widely prescribed antibiotic, produces varying types of allergic reactions in from 1 to 10 percent of the patients who are administered the drug.

c. **Side Effects**. Most drugs do not produce only one single effect. Instead, they may produce several physiological responses at the same time. For example, antihistamines, drugs frequently used for their anti-allergic action tend to produce drowsiness. In this case, drowsiness is a side effect of the antihistamines. With some drugs, the side effects are so worrisome and inconvenient that the patient may stop taking the medication.

d. **Drug Dependence.** All drugs have the potential of producing dependence, the need to have that drug. There are two major types of dependence: psychological and physiological.

(1) Psychological dependence may occur after a patient has been taking a medication for a long time. With psychological dependence, the patient becomes so convinced that he needs the drug (in order to continue to lead an improved life) that he will go to great lengths to ensure that he receives the medication. Patients habituated to amphetamines may demonstrate this type of dependence. Psychological dependence is very difficult to treat.

(2) With physiological dependence, the patient's body develops a real need for the drug over a long period. Since there is a physiological need for the drug, the body reacts by going through withdrawal symptoms (that is, tremors, nausea, vomiting,

and convulsions) if the drug is suddenly withheld. The patient habituated to narcotics and barbiturates have physiological dependence.

Section IV. FACTORS WHICH INFLUENCE DRUG ACTION

3-7. INTRODUCTION TO PHARMACOKINETICS

Pharmacokinetics deals with the absorption, distribution, metabolism (biotransformation), and excretion of drugs. Any time a drug is administered, these factors will directly affect the amount of drug that will arrive at the site where the drug acts. The amount of drug at the site of action will determine both the intensity of drug action and the length of time the drug will show its effect(s).

3-8. ABSORPTION OF DRUGS

Absorption involves the uptake of the drug by the body. Three factors affect the absorption of a drug: its water solubility, its fat solubility, and the transport mechanisms of the body. It is imperative that you understand that all drugs must be in solution before they can be absorbed.

3-9. FACTORS WHICH AFFECT ABSORPTION

a. **Water Solubility**. All body fluids are water based. Therefore, a drug must be soluble in water in order to be absorbed. Dissolution of the drug in aqueous (water) solution is dependent 6n the pH of the solution and the disintegration of the drug.

(1) Disintegration. Disintegration (Figure 3-1) increases the surface area of a drug. The speed at which a dosage form disintegrates is dependent upon the type of solid dosage form and the manufacturing process used to make that dosage form. The solid dosage form could be a tablet, suppository, capsule, powder, or suspension. Take a tablet for example. The manufacturer may add starch to the tablet in order to make it swell when it is added to water. The tablet may be a sublingual tablet that is made to rapidly dissolve in the mouth. On the other hand, the manufacturer may compress the contents of the tablet under great pressure so that it will slowly dissolve. Further, an enteric coating may be applied to the tablet so that it will dissolve in the intestine. In the case of some capsules, "tiny time capsules" systematically dissolve during a period and prolong the effect of the drug.

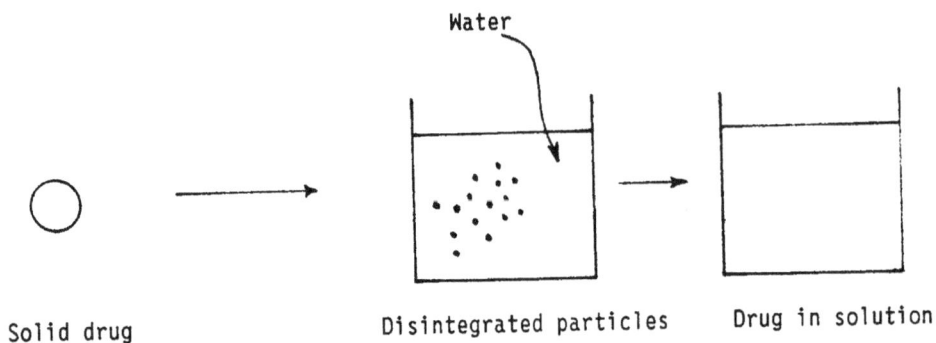

Figure 3-1. Dissolution of a drug.

(2) pH. The relative acidity or basicity of the fluids into which a drug is placed will affect how rapidly the drug will dissolve. The pH of the stomach can be as low as 1.0 (very acidic), the pH of the small intestine can range from 6.9 to 7.4 (slightly acidic to slightly basic), while the pH of the plasma is approximately 7 4 (slightly basic). Weakly acidic drugs (that is, aspirin) are more soluble in a basic or alkaline solution like the small intestine (pH above 7.4). Weakly basic drugs, such as tetracycline hydrochloride, are more soluble in an acidic solution like the stomach (pH below 7.0).

(3) Ionization. Ionization is the process whereby a substance breaks down into positively and negatively charged particles (Figure 3-2).

(a) For example, when hydrochloric acid ionizes, it forms hydrogen ions (H+) and chloride ions (Cl-).

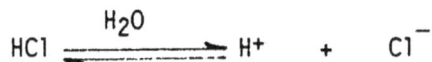

$$HCl \xrightleftharpoons{H_2O} H^+ + Cl^-$$

Figure 3-2.   The ionization of hydrochloric acid.

(b) Equilibrium is established based on the chemical nature of each drug. That is, a certain percentage of the drug ionizes, while the rest remains as the compound. In summary, dosage forms must go into solution. A solid dosage form must disintegrate and dissolve before it can be absorbed. A suspension dosage form has already been partially dissolved; the drug particles must dissolve before absorption can occur. A solution dosage form contains a drug that has already been dissolved; thus, no disintegration or dissolution is required before absorption can occur.

b. **Fat Solubility**. In the last area, the topic of water solubility was discussed. For instance, a drug is in solution. What other factors must it overcome in order to be absorbed? One is fat solubility. Almost without exception, all body membranes are lipid (fatty) in nature. Membranes separate even the various water compartments of the body. These membranes are selectively permeable. That is, these membranes will only allow certain materials to pass through them. In particular, the membranes favor the absorption of <u>unionized</u> particles (particles which have neither a positive nor a negative charge).

    c. **Transport Mechanisms**. The body either in an active or in a passive way can absorb drugs.

        (1) <u>Passive transport.</u> Passive transport (diffusion) follows a concentration gradient. That is, if there is a high concentration of a substance on one side of the barrier and a low concentration of that substance on the other side of the barrier, nature tries to balance the two concentrations so that one is equal to the other. The two concentrations can be equalized in one of two ways. One way is for the <u>liquid</u> containing the substance to move from the side with fewer particles to the side with more particles. This process, called osmosis, will ultimately result in the two sides having the same concentration. The second option is for the drug <u>particles</u> to move from the side of higher concentration to the side of the lower concentration. This process, called diffusion, will also ultimately result in the two sides having the same concentration. Most drugs are absorbed in this manner of diffusion. With diffusion, the drug particles move from the side of higher concentration through the cell membrane into the side of lower concentration.

        (2) <u>Active transport</u>.

            (a) A ride in a roller coaster would give you a background to understand this section on active transport. You have probably observed that a roller coaster car does not have an engine. Common sense would tell you that the car does not need an engine to go <u>down</u> the hills, but <u>up</u> those hills--that is a different story. You have probably observed that a mechanism exists for pulling the car up the hill.

            (b) Active transport works in much the same way. Proteins (in the cells) make up the linings of the cells. Some of these proteins have a particular affinity (attraction) for a selected drug. When the drug molecule meets the cell wall, the protein called a "carrier molecule" attaches itself to the drug, carries it across the cell membrane, and releases the drug on the other side. The drug then enters the circulation and is distributed throughout the body. Active transport can move against a concentration gradient to move a substance to a place of higher concentration. Vitamin B-12 is an example. Very little of this vitamin can pass through the intestinal wall of the gut by diffusion; however, a carrier molecule, often called "intrinsic factor" transports the vitamin across the gut. Once in circulation, the vitamin is stored in the liver. The concentration of drug in the liver is several hundred times higher than in circulation. Therefore1 if a drug is unionized, water soluble, and fat-soluble, it may pass through the cells of the gut if taken orally. Once in circulation, the drug must pass through the fatty layer of the individual cell in order to have an effect. So, even injected medications have some of the same problems as oral medications.

        (3) <u>Illustration of concepts</u>. Perhaps some insight can be gained about this whole topic of drug transport mechanisms if a diagram depicting the concepts is shown and discussed. Figure 3-3 is provided for this purpose. In the figure, several concepts are illustrated:

A--Drug A is an undissolved drug. It is not in solution and it cannot be absorbed.

B--B is a molecule of a drug in solution. It is unionized and can be absorbed.

C--C is a molecule of a drug attached to a "carrier molecule" at the cell wall.

D--D is an ion of a drug. It cannot be absorbed since the fatty layer repels it.

E--E is a molecule of a drug. It is in circulation and will be carried away.

F--F is a molecule of the drug that is being released into circulation by a carrier molecule.

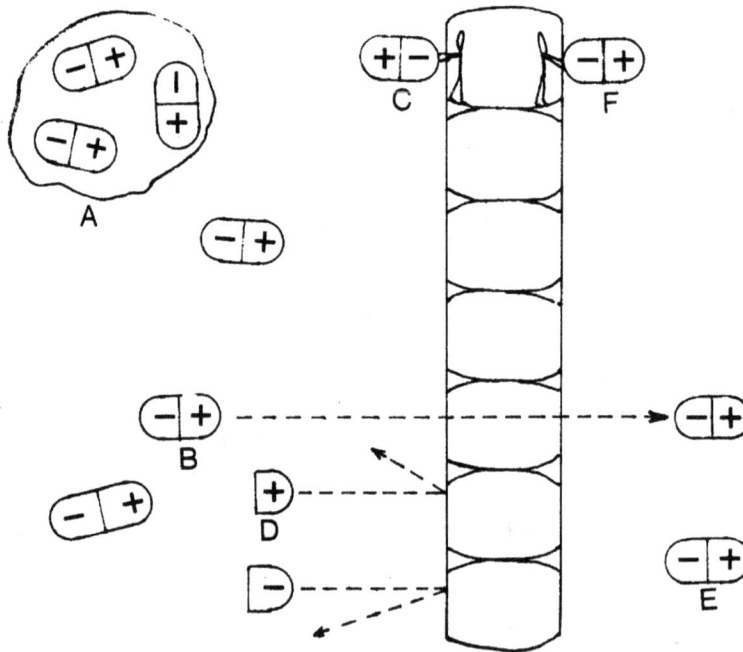

Figure 3-3. Illustration of drug transport concepts.

NOTE: Passive transport or diffusion has absorbed Molecule B. Once it has been absorbed, the circulating blood will carry it away. Consequently, the concentration of the drug will always remain higher in the gut and diffusion will continue. As the unionized particles are absorbed, the ionized particles will attach to each other to form more unionized drug. This occurs because the drug has equilibrium established between the ionized and unionized form; as the unionized form is removed, the balance shifts make up for the loss. Molecules C and F are being moved by active transport. They must also be unionized and fat soluble; however, their transport does not rely on differences in concentration. This transport process also accounts for the absorption of a drug by the individual cells within the body.

3-10. DISTRIBUTION OF DRUGS

a. Once the drug is absorbed, it enters the circulation and is carried throughout the body. The location in the body where the drug goes varies from drug to drug. The drug may be stored in bone or fat, bound to the proteins in the blood plasma, or circulate freely as the unbound drug. The drug will find its way into many organs. Finally, some of the drug will reach the target tissue where it can cause the effect for which it was administered. An equilibrium will be established between the circulating unbound drug and each area of the body.

b. The distribution of a drug in the body happens in a very systematic manner. Figure 3-4 demonstrates the concept of distribution.

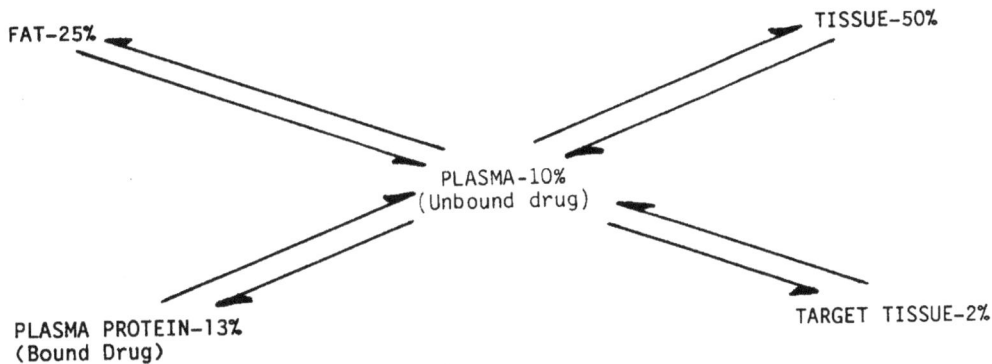

FAT–25%

TISSUE–50%

PLASMA–10%
(Unbound drug)

PLASMA PROTEIN–13%
(Bound Drug)

TARGET TISSUE–2%

Figure 3-4. Drug distribution within the body.

Assume that 100 micrograms (100 mcg) of a drug have been absorbed and is distributed based on the percentages noted in Figure 3-4. Of the 100 micrograms absorbed, only two micrograms of the drug will arrive at the target tissue to give the desired pharmacological effect. If two micrograms is enough drugs to produce the desired pharmacological effect, the desired effect will be obtained. However, if the amount of drug required to produce the effect is four micrograms, the desired pharmacological effect will not be obtained. The dose of the drug can be increased so that 200 milligrams of the drug can be absorbed, thus providing the amount of drug needed to give the desired pharmacological effect. However, doubling the dose may present problems. Doubling the dose would also double the amount of drug in the other areas of the body. Perhaps this increased dosage may produce some response by another body organ. For example, the patient may become nauseous, vomit, lose his hair, or go into convulsions. These are side effects of the drug. Thus, it is important to remember that the whole body must be taken into account when a drug is administered. If the problem of the side effects cannot be resolved, the drug may not be released for use.

NOTE: Another areas of concern in the distribution of drugs are those that crosses the placental barrier. Drugs may actively or passively cross the placental barrier and enter the fetal circulation. The enzyme systems of the developing fetus may not be able to adequately metabolize the drug. Toxic effects can result. At this time, it is virtually impossible to predict whether a drug will pass the placental barrier.

3-11. METABOLISM (BIOTRANSFORMATION)

The process of drug absorption and distribution is dynamic. That is, it is continually changing. Even as the drug is being distributed, the individual cells of the body begin to chemically change or alter the drug. This metabolic process of changing the drug is called metabolism or biotransformation. While many cells of the body will be involved in this process, the liver is the organ primarily responsible for this biotransformation. The liver changes drugs to make them more water-soluble so that they may be more easily excreted from the body. During the process of metabolism, a drug may be rendered inactive, converted from an inactive form to an active one, or be made more toxic. The liver may oxidize, reduce, hydrolyze, or conjugate (bind with a protein) the drug. The kidney will also play an active role in conjugating drugs.

3-12. BIOAVAILABILITY

a. The term bioavailability was defined in the first portion of this subcourse. In Figure 3-4, all 100 micrograms of the drug was available to the system, since it was absorbed. The amount of drug originally administered to the patient was not stated. That amount of administered drug could have ranged from 100 micrograms to 1000 milligrams or more. From the reading, you should have noted that absorption is not an easy process, and that any number of things can interfere with the process.

b. The controversy concerning generic drugs deserves consideration at this point. For example, switching a patient from one generic brand of ampicillin to another brand of ampicillin could cause some problems for some patients. Thus, one company's generic brand of a drug might not be able to be absorbed as quickly as another company's generic brand of the same drug. With other drugs and some patients the switch from one company's drug to another company's drug is of little consequence.

c. Drugs that present the most problems in terms of bioavailability are oral solids. That is because oral solids must disintegrate, dissolve, be water soluble, be fat soluble, unionize, and pass through the drastic pH changes from the stomach to the small intestine.

3-13. EXCRETION

a. Excretion is the process of eliminating a drug or its metabolites from the body. The major organ of excretion is the kidney. Secondary routes of excretion are hepatic (liver), through the bile into the feces, lungs, saliva, sweat, and breast milk.

b. The inability of a patient to excrete drugs and other waste can be life threatening. The elimination of drugs through sweat, saliva, and the lungs is of minor interest in this subcourse. Of course, the excretion of drugs in breast milk is of concern to mothers who breast-feed their infants. As a rule, drugs that are weakly basic are more likely to be excreted in breast milk, because the milk is slightly acidic; therefore, the basic drugs are more soluble in breast milk.

c. Patients who have limited liver and kidney function usually require lower doses of medication. This is because more of the drug tends to stay in the body.

3-14. MECHANISMS OF DRUG ACTION

a. **Receptor Site Theory**. A drug that finally enters a cell may produce an effect. It is able to produce this effect by a variety of complex biochemical processes. Most of the processes can be simplified into one explanation of the mechanism of drug action known as the receptor-site or "lock and key" theory. This theory states that a drug (the key) combines with a receptor-site (the lock) to produce a pharmacological effect. Drugs that will fit into the receptor-site are said to have an "affinity" for that receptor-site. Only drugs that fit into the receptor-site will produce a pharmacological response. Figure 3-5 visually represents the receptor-site theory.

b. **Chemical Structure Activity Relationship**. As a review, drug molecules have specific chemical structures. The chemical structure of a drug will determine if a drug molecule (the key) will fit into the receptor-site (the lock) and produce a pharmacological effect. For example, whether the hydroxyl (OH-) group is on the left or right side of the molecule or is at a 520 angle with the molecule can determine whether the "key" will fit the "lock." This is referred to as chemical structure activity relationship. From this, we can say that drugs that are similar in composition and chemical structure may have similar effects. The chemical structure of a drug can be altered with no effect upon the pharmacological effect the drug produces. However, the change in the chemical structure of the drug molecule can increase or decrease its side effects. Further, the modification of a drug molecule can influence its pharmacological actions. Therefore, the modification of a drug's molecular structure can result in the formation of a drug that can produce a desired pharmacological effect with a significantly lower dose and with an accompanying decrease in undesired side effects.

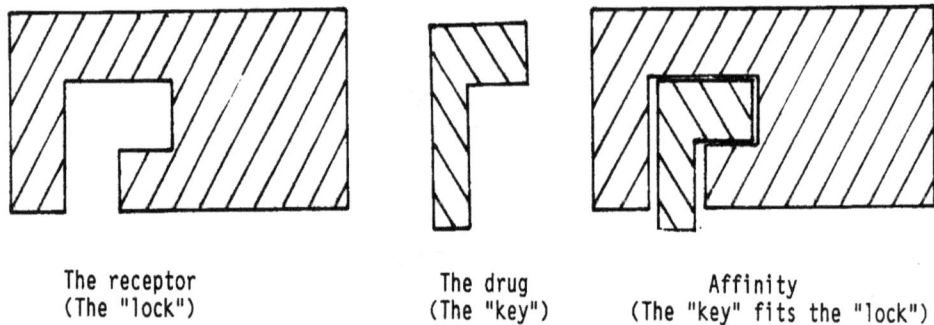

| The receptor (The "lock") | The drug (The "key") | Affinity (The "key" fits the "lock") |

Figure 3-5.   The receptor-site theory.

c. **Antagonists**. Antagonists are drugs that will or reverse block the action of other drugs. There are two types of antagonists: competitive and physiological.

(1)   Competitive antagonists. Competitive antagonists combine with the receptor-site and prevent another drug from combining with the receptor-site. A competitive antagonist does not displace a drug at the receptor-site. Figure 3-6 illustrates the concept of a competitive antagonist.

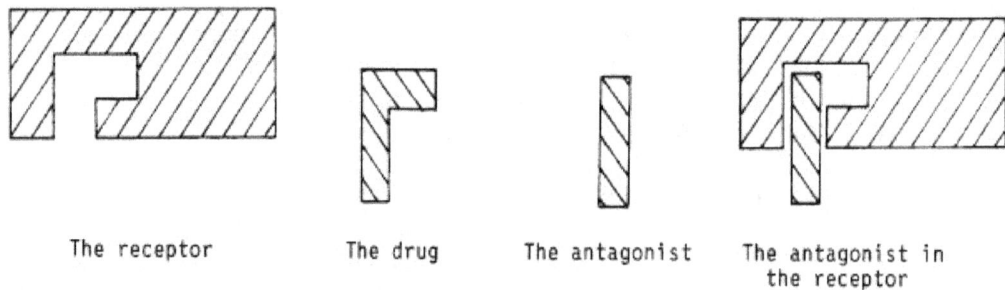

The receptor   The drug   The antagonist   The antagonist in the receptor

Figure 3-6. A competitive antagonist.

(2)   Physiological antagonists. Physiological antagonists reverse the action of the drug by acting on a different receptor-site to cause a different physiological effect.

3-15. DRUG EFFICACY

a. Drug efficacy refers to the effectiveness of a drug. Drug efficacy is measured by the clinical response of the patient. A drug is considered to have a high degree of efficacy, if it achieves desired clinical results.

b. Laboratory tests may be used to determine the amount of drug that has been absorbed. The amount of drug absorbed may be used to predict a patient's response. However, since people respond differently to the same dose of the same drug, merely knowing the amount of drug absorbed does not always indicate the response of an individual patient.

c. A general rule is that as the dose of a drug is increased, a greater effect is seen in the patient until a maximum desired effect is reached. If more drug is administered after the maximum point is reached, the side effects will normally increase. Figure 3-7 illustrates this principle.

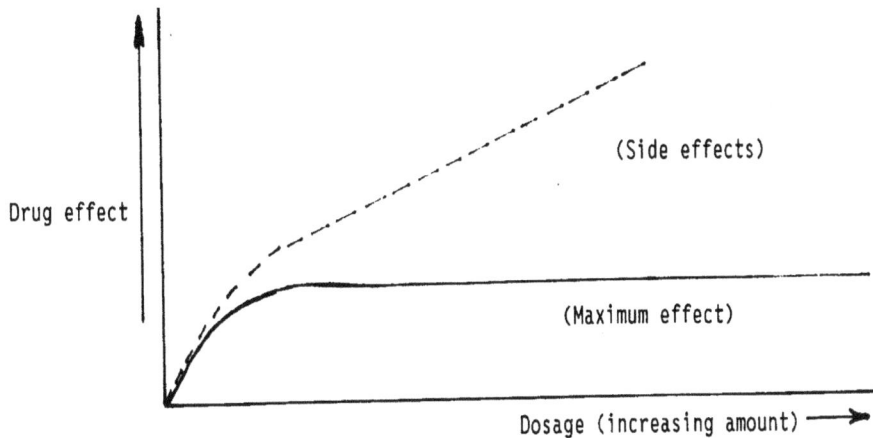

Figure 3-7. Relationship between dosage and drug effect.

Continue with Exercises

EXERCISES, LESSON 3

INSTRUCTIONS: Answer the following exercises by marking the lettered response that best answers the question, by completing the incomplete statement, or by writing the answer in the space provided at the end of the exercise.

After you have completed all of these exercises, turn to "Solutions to Exercises" at the end of the lesson and check your answers. For each exercise answered incorrectly, reread the material referenced with the solution.

    1.   From the definitions below, select the definition of the term drug.

        a.   A substance that is used to cure all diseases.

        b.   A substance used to prevent, diagnose, or treat disease or to prevent pregnancy.

        c.   A substance that can only be purchased at a drugstore.

        d.   A substance that occurs naturally and cannot cause any toxic reactions.

    2.   From the definitions below, select the definition of the term toxicology.

        a.   The science of chemicals.

        b.   The science of drugs.

        c.   The science of poisons.

        d.   The science of dosage.

    3.   Select the drug that is derived from an animal source.

        a.   Belladonna.

        b.   Heparin.

        c.   Iron.

        d.   Aspirin.

4. Select the statement that best describes a use of drugs.

    a. To produce anxiety or tension.

    b. To relieve the symptoms of a disease or condition.

    c. To cure diabetes.

    d. Both a and b.

    e. Both b and c.

5. Select the statement that best describes how the physical condition of a patient might influence the amount of drug required to obtain a specific effect.

    a. Debilitated patients always require the same amount of drug as a healthy person.

    b. The physical condition of a patient never influences the required dose of a drug.

    c. The weak patient might require smaller doses of a drug to achieve an effect.

    d. Patients in extreme pain usually require smaller doses of analgesic agents rather than patients who are in less pain.

6. Select the statement that best describes drug dependence.

    a. Drug dependence occurs whenever a patient takes a particular drug for a long period.

    b. Drug dependence is said to occur when the patient has either a physiological or psychological need for a drug.

    c. Drug dependence occurs when a patient's body requires a drug, but cannot tolerate its harmful effects.

    d. Drug dependence can only occur with certain types of drugs (like narcotics).

7.   Select, from the list below, the definition of the term synergism.

    a.   Synergism occurs when one drug lives off another drug.

    b.   Synergism occurs when the combined effect of two drugs is greater than the sum of their independent effects.

    c.   Synergism occurs when the combined effects of two drugs are equal to the sum of the independent effects of the drugs.

    d.   Synergism occurs when one drug's effects cancel the effects of another drug.

8.   Select the route of administration in which the dosage form is placed in the mouth but not swallowed.

    a.   Parenteral.

    b.   Rectal.

    c.   Sublingual/Buccal.

    d.   Oral.

9.   Select the statement that best describes the sublingual/buccal route of administration.

    a.   In this route of administration, the drug is swallowed and very quickly absorbed by the patient.

    b.   In this route of administration, the drugs are absorbed only after being taken into the gastrointestinal tract.

    c.   In this route of administration, the drug is absorbed without passing through the gastrointestinal tract.

    d.   In this route of administration, the drug is applied directly to the skin.

10.   From the statements below, select the statement that best describes how fat solubility influences drug absorption.

        a.   Since all body fluids are fat based, a drug must be soluble in fat in order to be absorbed and demonstrate its effect.

        b.   Since body membranes are lipids in nature, a drug that will pass through lipid material will be absorbed much more quickly than ionized drug particles.

        c.   The body cannot absorb a fat-soluble drug, because it is unionized.

        d.   All fat-soluble drugs must be converted into water-soluble substances before they can be absorbed.

11.   From the list below, select the definition of the term metabolism.

        a.   The chemical process of producing a drug.

        b.   The metabolic process of changing a drug.

        c.   The process of transforming a living life form.

        d.   The modification of complex substances to make them powerless.

12.   From the list below, select the definition of the term excretion.

        a.   The process of placing a drug or its metabolites into the body.

        b.   The process of metabolically changing a drug or its metabolites.

        c.   The process of eliminating a drug or its metabolites from the body.

        d.   The process of concentrating a drug and removing it from the patient's gastrointestinal tract.

13.   From the descriptions below, select the description that best describes the Receptor-Site Theory of the mechanism of drug action.

    a.   A drug (the lock) combines with a receptor-site (the key) to produce a pharmacological effect.

    b.   A drug (the key) combines with a receptor-site (the lock) to produce a pharmacological effect.

    c.   A drug (the receptor-site) combines with cell components (the lock) to produce a pharmacological effect.

    d.   A drug (the lock) combines with a receptor-site in the intestine to produce an essential effect.

14.   Select the statement that best contrasts passive transport with active transport.

    a.   Active transport occurs when molecules of the drug move from an area of high concentration to an area of low concentration, while passive transport occurs when a "carrier molecule" carries a drug molecule across a cell membrane.

    b.   Passive transport occurs in comatose patients whose cells are unable to actively absorb drugs through the normal processes.

    c.   Passive transport occurs when molecules of a drug move from an area of high concentration to an area of low concentration, while active transport occurs when a "carrier molecule" carries a drug molecule across a cell membrane.

    d.   Passive transport occurs when a "carrier molecule" carries drug molecules from an area of low concentration to an area of high concentration, while passive transport involves the movement of blood plasma from a low concentration to a high concentration.

15.   From a group below, select the description that best describes the importance of structure activity relationships.

      a.   Drugs that are similar in composition and structure may have similar effects.

      b.   Drugs that are not similar are ineffective.

      c.   Drugs that are active generally have similar structures.

      d.   Drugs that are similar in effect generally have the same trade name.

16.   Select the statement that best contrasts competitive antagonist with physiological antagonists.

      a.   Competitive antagonists combine with the receptor-site and prevent another drug from combining with the receptor-site, while physiological antagonists reverse the action of a drug by acting on a different receptor-site to cause different physiological reaction.

      b.   Competitive antagonists produce pharmacological effects by producing a physiological effect different from the drug, while physiological antagonists physiologically compete for a spot on the receptor-site.

      c.   Competitive antagonists combine with the receptor-site and remove the drug from the site, while physiological antagonists physically compete for the receptor-site.

      d.   Physiological antagonists physically remove drug molecules from the receptor-site, while competitive antagonists compete for the receptor-site.

Check Your Answers on Next Page

SOLUTIONS TO EXERCISES, LESSON 3

1. b A substance used to prevent, diagnose, or treat disease or to prevent pregnancy. (para 3-2a)

2. c The science of poisons. (para 3-2e)

3. b Heparin. (para 3-3b)

4. b To relieve the symptoms of a disease or condition. (para 3-4c)

5. c The weak patient may require smaller doses of a drug to achieve an effect. (para 3-5f)

6. b Drug dependence is said to occur when the patient has either a physiological or psychological need for a drug. (para 3-6)

7. b Synergism occurs when the combined effect of two drugs is greater than the sum of their independent effects. (para 3-5j(1))

8. c Sublingual/Buccal. (para 3-5k(2))

9. c In this route of administration the drug is absorbed without passing through the gastrointestinal tract. (para 3-5k(2))

10. b Since body membranes are lipid in nature, a drug that will pass through lipid material will be absorbed much more quickly than ionized drug particles. (para 3-9b)

11. b The metabolic process of changing a drug. (para 3-11)

12. c The process of eliminating a drug or its metabolites from the body. (para 3-13a)

13. b A drug (the key) combines with a receptor-site (the lock) to produce a pharmacological effect. (para 3-14a)

14. c Passive transport occurs when molecules of a drug move from an area of high concentration to an area of low concentration, while active transport occurs when a "carrier molecule" carries a drug molecule across a cell membrane. (para 3-9c(1) and (2))

15. a Drugs that are similar in composition and structure may have similar effects. (para 3-14b)

16. a Competitive antagonists combine with the receptor-site and prevent another drug from combining with the receptor-site, while physiological antagonists reverse the action of a drug by acting on a different receptor-site to cause a different physiological reaction. (para 3-14c(1) and (2))

End of Lesson 3

LESSON ASSIGNMENT

LESSON 4	Local Anesthetic Agents.
TEXT ASSIGNMENT	Paragraphs 4-1--4-8.
LESSON OBJECTIVES	After completing this lesson, you should be able to:

4-1. Given one of the following terms: local anesthetic, local infiltration, topical block, surface anesthesia, nerve block, peridural, and spinal anesthesia, and a group of statements, select the meaning of that term.

4-2. From a group of statements, select the statement that best describes the mechanism of action for local anesthetics.

4-3. Given a group of statements, select the statement that best describes why vasoconstrictors are used in conjunction with local anesthetics.

4-4. From a group of statements, select the caution and warning associated with the use of a local anesthetic combined with a vasoconstrictor.

4-5. Given a group of statements, select the statement that best describes why hyaluronidase (Wydase®) is used in conjunction with local anesthetics.

4-6. Given a group of statements, select the statement that describes a caution and warning associated with the use of local anesthetics.

4-7. From a list of toxicities, select the toxicity associated with the use of local anesthetics.

4-8. Given the trade name of a local anesthetic agent and a list of generic names, match the trade name of the agent with its generic name.

4-9. Given the trade and/or generic name of a local anesthetic agent and a group of possible uses or cautions and warnings, select the clinical use or caution and warning associated with that agent.

SUGGESTION

After completing the assignment, complete the exercises at the end of this lesson. These exercises will help you to achieve the lesson objectives.

LESSON 4

LOCAL ANESTHETIC AGENTS

Section I. BACKGROUND INFORMATION

4-1. BACKGROUND INFORMATION

In order to understand what a local anesthetic is and how it is used, you need to study/review the following definitions:

a. **Local Anesthetic**. A local anesthetic is an agent that interrupts pain impulses in a specific region of the body without a loss of patient consciousness. Normally, the process is completely reversible--the agent does not produce any residual effect on the nerve fiber.

b. **Local Infiltration (Local Anesthesia)**. Local infiltration occurs when the nerve endings in the skin and subcutaneous tissues are blocked by direct contact with a local anesthetic, which is injected into the tissue. Local infiltration is used primarily for surgical procedures involving a small area of tissue (for example, suturing a cut).

c. **Topical Block**. A topical block is accomplished by applying the anesthetic agent to mucous membrane surfaces and in that way blocking the nerve terminals in the mucosa. This technique is often used during examination procedures involving the respiratory tract. The anesthetic agent is rapidly absorbed into the bloodstream. For topical application (that is, to the skin), the local anesthetic is always used <u>without</u> epinephrine. The topical block easily anesthetizes the surface of the cornea (of the eye) and the oral mucosa.

d. **Surface Anesthesia**. This type of anesthesia is accomplished by the application of a local anesthetic to skin or mucous membranes. Surface anesthesia is used to relieve itching, burning, and surface pain (for example, as seen in minor sunburns).

e. **Nerve Block**. In this type of anesthesia, a local anesthetic is injected around a nerve that leads to the operative site. Usually more concentrated forms of local anesthetic solutions are used for this type of anesthesia.

f. **Peridural Anesthesia**. This type of anesthesia is accomplished by injecting a local anesthetic into the peridural space. The peridural space is one of the coverings of the spinal cord.

g. **Spinal Anesthesia**. In spinal anesthesia, the local anesthetic is injected into the subarachnoid space of the spinal cord.

4-2. MECHANISM OF ACTION OF THE LOCAL ANESTHETICS

a.   The nerve fiber is a long cylinder surrounded by a semipermeable (allows only some substances to pass) membrane. This membrane is made up of proteins and lipids (fats). Some of the proteins apparently act as channels, or pores, for the passage of sodium and potassium ions through the membrane.

b.   The movement of nerve impulses along a nerve fiber is associated with a change in the permeability of the membrane. The pores widen, and sodium ions (Na+) move to the inside of the fiber. At the same time, potassium ions (K+) diffuse out through other pores (see Figure 4-1). The entire process is called depolarization. Immediately after the nerve impulse has passed, the pores again become smaller. Sodium ions (Na+) are now "pumped" out of the fiber. At the same time, potassium ions are actively transported into the fiber. The nerve membrane is then ready to conduct another impulse.

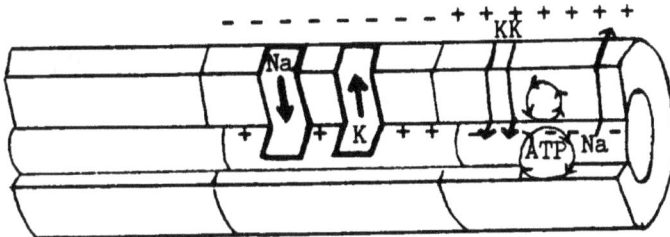

Figure 4-1. Mechanism of nerve impulse transmission.

c.   Local anesthetics block depolarization of the nerve membrane. That is, to make the conduction of the nerve impulse impossible.

d.   The local anesthetic effect lasts as long as the agent maintains a certain critical concentration in the nerve membrane. There is a potential problem: the local concentration needed to prevent conduction of the nerve impulse is much greater than the tolerable blood level. *TO AVOID A SYSTEMIC TOXIC REACTION TO THE LOCAL ANESTHETIC, THE SMALLEST AMOUNT OF THE MOST DILUTE SOLUTION THAT WILL EFFECTIVELY BLOCK THE PAIN SHOULD BE ADMINISTERED.*

4-3. THE USE OF VASOCONSTRICTORS IN CONJUNCTION NITH LOCAL ANESTHETICS

a.   **Indications.** Vasoconstrictors (like epinephrine) are sometimes used in conjunction with local anesthetics. Vasoconstrictors are used to prolong the duration of action of local anesthetics. Vasoconstrictors also help to control bleeding. Furthermore, the vasoconstrictor delays the absorption of the local anesthetic by reducing the blood flow to the affected area. This results in a reduction of the toxic effects of the local anesthetic, since the rate of absorption keeps pace with the rate the local anesthetic is metabolized by the body. Vasoconstrictors are of no value in delaying the absorption of the local anesthetic from mucous membranes (that is, topical blocks).

    b. **Cautions and Warnings of the Combination**.

        (1) It should be recognized that the injection of epinephrine-containing solutions in or around fingers, toes, and the penis is not recommended.

        (2) Freshly prepared combinations of vasoconstrictors and local anesthetics are more effective than commercially premixed epinephrine-containing local anesthetic solutions. This is because a very low pH is required to stabilize the epinephrine in these mixtures. In general, the content of one part epinephrine to 200,000 parts of the local anesthetic agent (is optimum) will minimize the side effects inherent with epinephrine. Great care must be taken in calculating this dilution. Small, precisely calibrated syringes should be used in the mixing process. It should be noted that the standard solution of epinephrine supplied is a 1:1000 (1 to 1000) concentration in each glass ampule. This means that 1 milliliter of the 1:1000 epinephrine solution contains 1 milligram of epinephrine. In preparing a 1:200,000 dilution, epinephrine should be added to a local anesthetic solution on a ratio of 0.1 milliliter-20 milliliters of local anesthetic solution. This does not apply to subarachnoid injections, in which a higher concentration of epinephrine is required.

4-4. ANOTHER AGENT WHICH CAN AFFECT THE ACTIONS OF LOCAL ANESTHETICS

    Hyaluronidase (Wydase®) is sometimes used in conjunction with local anesthetics. Hyaluronidase is an enzyme that breaks down the material that binds cells together. Thus, when hyaluronidase is combined with local anesthetic, greater infiltration (movement) of the local anesthetic in the tissues is made possible.

4-5. CAUTIONS AND WARNINGS ASSOCIATED WITH LOCAL ANESTHETICS

    a. Precautions should be taken against the danger of confusing the various agents with one another or mistaking different concentrations of the same drug.

    b. In order to avoid intravascular (into the veins) injection, aspiration in several planes with the plunger of the syringe should always be done before injecting the anesthetic solution into the tissues.

    c. The instillation of local anesthetic agents into the trachea and bronchi leads to immediate absorption, which soon reach blood levels comparable to those reached by straight intravenous injection.

    d. A previously punctured vial of local anesthetic solution should never be re-autoclaved.

e. Discolored local anesthetic solutions should be immediately thrown away.

4-6. TOXICITIES OF LOCAL ANESTHETICS

Essentially all systemic toxic reactions associated with local anesthetics are the result of over-dosage leading to high blood levels of the agent given. Therefore, <u>to avoid a systemic toxic reaction to a local anesthetic, the smallest amount of the most dilute solution that effectively blocks pain should be administered</u>.

a. **Hypersensitivity**. Some patients are hypersensitive (allergic) to some local anesthetics. Although such allergies are very rare, a careful patient history should be taken in an attempt to identify the presence of an allergy. There are two basic types of local anesthetics (the amide type and the ester type). A patient who is allergic to one type may or may not be allergic to the other type.

b. **Central Nervous System Toxicities.** Local anesthetics, if absorbed systematically in excessive amounts, can cause central nervous system (CNS) excitement or, if absorbed in even higher amounts, can cause CNS depression.

(1) <u>Excitement</u>. Tremors, shivering, and convulsions characterize the CNS excitement.

(2) <u>Depression</u>. The CNS depression is characterized by respiratory depression and, if enough drug is absorbed, respiratory arrest.

c. **Cardiovascular Toxicities**. Local anesthetics if absorbed systematically in excessive amounts can cause depression of the cardiovascular system. Hypotension and a certain type of abnormal heartbeat (atrioventricular block) characterize such depression. These may ultimately result in both cardiac and respiratory arrest.

Section II. LOCAL ANESTHETICS AND THEIR CLINICAL USES

4-7. EXAMPLES OF LOCAL ANESTHETICS

The local anesthetics you may encounter in a hospital or fields setting are described below. The discussion does not cover every fact known about the use of a particular drug. Therefore, you are encouraged to read references or to ask knowledgeable personnel your specific questions concerning points not presented in this subcourse.

a. **Lidocaine Hydrochloride (Xylocaine®).**

(1) Clinical uses. Lidocaine is used as a local anesthetic for infiltrations, nerve blocks, spinal anesthesia, topical anesthesia, and for caudal and epidural anesthesia. It has a rapid onset of action and its effects last from 75 to 150 minutes. It has also been used as a cardiac depressant (anti arrhythmic).

NOTE: Refer to Table 4-1 for an overview of the clinical uses of various local anesthetics.

	Ophthalmic Topical	Topical	Infiltration	Nerve Block	Spinal	Epidural and Caudal
1. Cocaine	X	X				
2. Procaine			X	X	X	
3. Chloroprocaine			X	X		X
4. Tetracaine	X	X			X	
5. Proparacaine	X					
6. Benzocaine		X				
7. Lidocaine		X	X	X	X	X
8. Mepivacaine			X	X		X
9. Prilocaine			X	X		X
10. Bupivacaine			X	X		X
11. Bupivacaine	X	X			X	
12. Dichlorotetra-fluorethane *		X				
13. Ethyl chloride *		X				

*Surface anesthetics for application to the skin.

Table 4-1. An overview of the clinical uses of various local anesthetics.

(2) <u>Forms available</u>. Lidocaine is available in injection form (various percentage concentrations), jelly form, and in cream form.

b. **Mepivacaine (Carbocaine®).**

(1) <u>Clinical uses</u>. Mepivacaine is pharmacologically and chemically related to lidocaine. It is used for infiltration, nerve block, peridural, and regional anesthesia. The duration of action for this drug is from 2 to 2 1/2 hours.

(2) <u>Forms available.</u> Mepivacaine is available in injection form.

c. **Prilocaine (Citanes®).**

(1) <u>Clinical uses</u>. Prilocaine is pharmacologically similar to both lidocaine and mepivacaine. It is used for infiltration, nerve block, peridural, and regional anesthesia. This drug is less toxic than lidocaine because it is metabolized and excreted faster than lidocaine.

(2) <u>Forms available.</u> Prilocaine is available in injection form.

d. **Bipivacaine (Marcaine®).**

(1) <u>Clinical uses</u>. Bipivacaine is pharmacologically related to lidocaine. It is used for infiltration, nerve block, and epidural anesthesia.

(2) <u>Forms available.</u> Procaine is available in injection form.

e. **Dibucaine (Nupercainal®, Nupercaine®).**

(1) <u>Clinical uses</u>. Dibucaine is used for spinal and topical anesthesia. It is the most potent local anesthetic. It is one of the most toxic and longest-acting local anesthetics.

(2) <u>Forms available</u>. Dibucaine is available in cream, spray, suppository, ointment, and injection forms.

f. **Procaine (Novocaine®).**

(1) <u>Clinical uses</u>. Procaine is used for infiltration, nerve block, and spinal anesthesia. Procaine is not applied topically. Its duration of action is approximately 1 hour. It is a fairly safe local anesthetic to use since it is metabolized quickly.

(2) <u>Forms available.</u> Procaine is available in injection form.

g. **Chloroprocaine (Nesacaine®, Nesacaine-C®).**

(1) <u>Clinical uses.</u> Chloroprocaine is pharmacologically similar to procaine. Chloroprocaine is used for infiltration, nerve block, caudal, and epidural anesthesia.

(2) <u>Forms available.</u> Chloroprocaine is available in injection form.

h. **Tetracaine (Pontocaine®).**

(1) <u>Clinical uses.</u> Tetracaine is used for topical, nerve block, infiltration, spinal, and caudal anesthesia. Its onset of action is 15 minutes.

(2) <u>Forms available.</u> Pontocaine is available in injection, cream, ointment, and injectable forms.

i. **Proparacaine (Alcaine®, Ophthetic®).**

(1) <u>Clinical uses.</u> Proparacaine is used primarily to produce anesthesia when applied to the eye. It has a rapid onset of action (20 seconds) and its duration of action is approximately 15 minutes.

(2) <u>Forms available.</u> Proparacaine is supplied in solution form.

j. **Benzocaine (Americaine®).**

(1) <u>Clinical uses.</u> Bezocaine is used for topical anesthesia of the mucous membranes and skin. It is used in many over-the-counter spray preparations for the treatment of sunburn and itching.

(2) <u>Forms available.</u> Benzocaine is available in solution, ointment, and spray forms.

k. **Cocaine.**

(1) <u>Clinical uses</u>. Cocaine is applied to produce local anesthesia with intensive vasoconstriction on mucous membranes. It is applied to procedure anesthesia in the nose, throat, ear, and in bronchoscopy (a procedure in which an instrument is used to inspect the bronchi).

(2) Forms available. Cocaine is supplied in the form of a white powder. Cocaine solution must be compounded. It is a Schedule II controlled substance.

4-8. LOCAL ANESTHETICS USED FOR TOPICAL APPLICATION ONLY

a. **Dichlorotetrafluorethane (Freon®)**

(1) <u>Clinical uses</u>. Dichlorotetrafluorethane is a nonflammable and non-explosive agent for topical anesthesia of the skin. It is especially useful for localized minor surgical procedures. This agent should not be sprayed on the skin for a period that exceeds 45 seconds.

(2) <u>Forms available.</u> Dichlorotetrafluorethane is available in a spray form.

b. **Ethyl Chloride**.

(1) <u>Clinical uses.</u> This agent is used for topical anesthesia of the skin.

(2) Forms available. Ethyl chloride is available in a spray form.

Continue with Exercises

EXERCISES, LESSON 4

INSTRUCTIONS: Answer the following exercises by marking the lettered response that best answers the question, by completing the incomplete statement, or by writing the answer in the space provided at the end of the exercise.

After you have completed all of these exercises, turn to "Solutions to Exercises" at the end of the lesson and check your answers. For each exercise answered incorrectly, reread the material referenced with the solution.

1. Which of the following statements best defines the term local infiltration?

    a.   A type of anesthesia achieved by applying the anesthetic agent to the surface of mucous membranes to block nerve transmissions.

    b.   A type of anesthesia achieved when the nerve endings in the skin and subcutaneous tissues are blocked by direct contact with a local anesthetic that is injected into the tissue.

    c.   A type of anesthesia accomplished by injecting a nerve that leads to the operative site.

    d.   A type of anesthesia accomplished by injecting a local anesthetic into the peridural space.

2. Which of the following statements best describes the mechanism of action of local anesthetics?

    a.   Local anesthetics destroy the nerve tissue so that electrical impulses cannot be carried.

    b.   Local anesthetics greatly increase the number of electrical impulses being transmitted so that pain cannot be felt in that particular area.

    c.   Local anesthetics block depolarization of the nerve membrane so that the conduction of the nerve impulse is impossible.

    d.   Local anesthetics remove both potassium and sodium ions from the nerve tissue so that polarity in the nerve cannot be accomplished; therefore, the impulses are not allowed to move past a certain point in the tissue.

3. Why is hyaluronidase (Wydase®) used in conjunction with local anesthetics?

    a. Hyaluronidase concentrates the local anesthetic in a particular area in order that its effects might be prolonged.

    b. Hyaluronidase neutralizes the local anesthetic so that undesired adverse effects are greatly reduced.

    c. Hyaluronidase is an enzyme that acts to tenderize the tissue and make the nerves more sensitive to the effects of the local anesthetic.

    d. Hyaluronidase increases the movement of the local anesthetic through the tissue.

4. Select the caution(s) and warning(s) associated with the use of local anesthetics.

    a. When a local anesthetic is to be injected, the plunger should be aspirated in several planes to ensure the drug is not being injected into a vein.

    b. Discolored solutions of local anesthetic should be thrown away.

    c. A previously used vial of local anesthetic solution should never be reautoclaved.

    d. All the above.

5. Select the toxicity(ies) associated with the use of local anesthetics.

    a. Large amounts of systemically absorbed local anesthetics can cause depression of the cardiovascular system.

    b. Local anesthetics, even when given in small amounts, cause tremors, shivering, and convulsions.

    c. Local anesthetics cause respiratory depression.

    d. Local anesthetics tend to produce hypersensitive reactions in most people.

INSTRUCTIONS: In Exercises 6-9, match the trade and generic names of the local anesthetics.

6. Tetracaine _____   a. Americaine®

7. Mepivacaine _____   b. Freon®

8. Dichlorotetrafluorethane _____   c. Pontocaine®

9. Benzocaine _____   d. Carbocaine®

10. Select the clinical use of ethyl chloride.

    a.   Used to produce anesthesia when applied to the eye.

    b.   Used for topical anesthesia of the skin.

    c.   Used for infiltration and caudal anesthesia.

    d.   Used to produce anesthesia in mucous membranes procedures.

11. What is the clinical use of proparacaine?

    a.   Used to produce topical anesthesia on the skin.

    b.   Used to produce both anesthesia and vasoconstriction when applied to certain tissues.

    c.   Used in nerve block, spinal, and caudal anesthesia.

    d.   Used to produce anesthesia in the eye.

12. What is the clinical use of bupivacaine (Marcaine®)?

    a.   Used to produce anesthesia when applied to the eye.

    b.   Used to produce infiltration, nerve block, and epidural anesthesia.

    c.   Used to produce anesthesia when applied to the skin or mucous membranes.

    d.   Used to produce anesthesia in a localized area when applied topically (that is, bronchoscopy).

13. Select the caution and warning associated with the use of procaine (Novocaine®).

   a. The drug should not be applied topically.

   b. The drug should not be used for infiltration anesthesia.

   c. The drug should not be used to produce spinal anesthesia.

   d. The drug should not be used to produce nerve block anesthesia.

Check Your Answers on Next Page

SOLUTIONS TO EXERCISES, LESSON 4

1. b   A type of anesthesia achieved when the nerve endings in the skin and subcutaneous tissues are blocked by direct contact with a local anesthetic that is injected into the tissue. (para 4-1b)

2. c   Local anesthetics block depolarization of the nerve membrane so that the conduction of the nerve impulse is impossible. (para 4-2)

3. d   Hyaluronidase increases the movement of the local anesthetic through the tissue. (para 4-4)

4. d   All of the above. (para 4-5b, d, and e)

5. a   Large amounts of systemically absorbed local anesthetics can cause depression of the cardiovascular system. (para 4-6c)

6. c   Pontocaine®. (para 4-7h)

7. d   Carbocaine®. (para 4-7b)

8. b   Freon®. (para 4-8a)

9. a   Americaine®. (para 4-7j)

10. b   Used for topical anesthesia of the skin. (para 4-8b)

11. d   Used to produce anesthesia in the eye. (para 4-7i)

12. b   Used to produce infiltration, nerve block, and epidural anesthesia. (para 4-7d)

13. a   The drug should not be applied topically. (para 4-7f)

End of Lesson 4

LESSON ASSIGNMENT

LESSON 5	The Central Nervous System.
TEXT ASSIGNMENT	Paragraphs 5-1--5-15.
LESSON OBJECTIVES	After completing this lesson, you should be able to:

5-1.   Given a list of types of tissue, select the two types of nervous tissues.

5-2.   From a list of functions, select the function(s) for which nervous tissues are specialized.

5-3.   Given one of the following terms: neuron, dendrite, or axon, and a group of definitions, select the definition of that term.

5-4.   Given the shape, diameter, or function of a type of neuron and a list of types of neurons, select the type of neuron described.

5-5.   Given a group of statements, select the statement that best describes the neuromuscular junction.

5-6.   Given a group of statements, select the statement that best describes the function of a neurotransmitter.

5-7.   From a list of chemical substances, select the substance(s) which is/are neurotransmitter(s).

5-8.   Given a list of names, select the names of the three major divisions of the human nervous system.

5-9.   Given a list of names, select the names of the two major subdivisions of the central nervous system.

5-10. From a list of functions, select the function(s) of the cerebrospinal fluid.

5-11. Given the name of one of the major subdivisions of the human brain and a list of functions, select the function(s) of that part.

5-12. Given a list of functions, select the function of the meninges surrounding the brain and spinal cord.

SUGGESTION

After completing the assignment, complete the exercises at the end of this lesson. These exercises will help you to achieve the lesson objectives.

LESSON 5

THE CENTRAL NERVOUS SYSTEM

Section I. BASIC CONCEPTS OF THE NERVOUS SYSTEM

5-1. TYPES OF NERVOUS TISSUES

There are two types of nervous tissues--the neurons (nerve cells) and glia (neuroglia). The neuron is the basic structural unit of the nervous system. The glia are cells of supporting tissue for the nervous system. There are several different types of glia, but their general function is support (physical, nutritive, and so forth.).

5-2. SPECIALIZATION

Nervous tissues are specialized to:

a.   Receive stimuli. Cells receiving stimuli are said to be "irritable" (as are all living cells somewhat).

b.   Transmit information.

c.   "Store" information.

Section II. THE NEURON AND ITS "CONNECTIONS"

5-3. DEFINITION OF A NEURON

A neuron (Figure 5-1) is a nerve cell body and all of its branches.

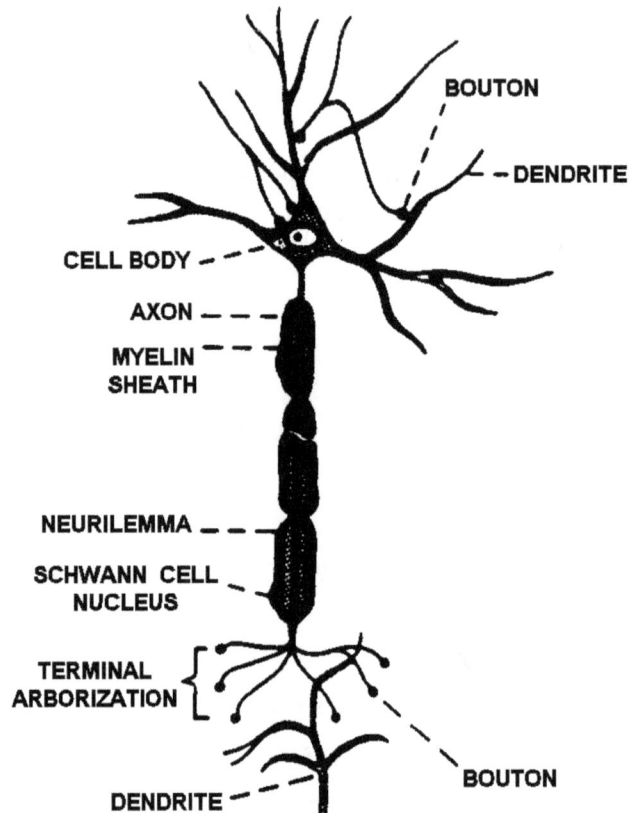

Figure 5-1. A neuron.

5-4. TYPES OF NEURON BRANCHES

There are two types of neuron branches--dendrites and axons.

   a.   **Dendrite.** A dendrite is a neuron process that carries impulses toward the cell body. Each neuron may have one or more dendrites. Dendrites receive information and transmit (carry) it to the cell body.

   b.   **Axon.** An axon is a neuron branch that transmits information from the cell body to the next unit. Each neuron has only one axon.

c. **Information Transmission**. Information is carried as electrical impulses along the length of the neuron.

d. **Coverings**. Some neuron processes have a covering that is a series of Schwann cells, interrupted by nodes (thin spots). This gives the neuron branch the appearance of links of sausages. The Schwann cells produce a lipid (fatty) material called <u>myelin</u>. This myelin acts as an electrical insulator during the transmission of impulses.

5-5. TYPES OF NEURONS

Neurons may be identified according to shape, diameter of their branches, or function.

a. **According to Shape**. A <u>pole</u> is the point where a neuron branch meets the cell body. To determine the type according to shape, count the number of poles.

(1) <u>Multipolar neurons</u>. Multipolar neurons have more than two poles (one axon and two or more dendrites).

(2) <u>Bipolar neurons</u>. Bipolar neurons have two poles (one axon and one dendrite).

(3) <u>Unipolar neurons</u>. Unipolar neurons have a single process that branches into a T-shape. One arm is an axon; the other is a dendrite.

b. **According to Diameter (Thickness) of Branches**. Neurons may be rated according to the thickness of myelin surrounding the axon. In order of decreasing thickness, they are rated A (thickest), B, and C (thinnest). The thickness affects the rate at which impulses are transmitted. The thickest carry the impulses the fastest. The thinnest carry the impulses the slowest.

c. **According to Function**.

(1) <u>Sensory neurons</u>. In sensory neurons, impulses are transmitted from receptor organs (for pain, vision, hearing, and so forth) to the central nervous system (CNS). Sensory neurons are also known as afferent neurons.

(2) <u>Motor neurons</u>. In motor neurons, impulses are transmitted from the central nervous system to muscles and glands (effector organs). Motor neurons may be called efferent neurons.

(3) <u>Interneurons</u>. Interneurons transmit information from one neuron to another. Interneurons connect sensory neurons with motor neurons.

(4) Others. There are other, more specialized types of neurons found in the body (for example, central nervous system).

5-6. NEURON "CONNECTIONS"

A neuron may "connect" either with another neuron or with a muscle fiber. A phrase used to describe such "connections" is "continuity without contact." Neurons do not actually touch. There is just enough space to prevent the electrical transmission from crossing from the first neuron to the next. This space is called the synaptic cleft. Information is transferred across the synaptic cleft by chemicals called neurotransmitters. Neurotransmitters are manufactured and stored on only one side of the cleft. Because of this, information flows in only one direction across the cleft.

a. **The Synapse**. A synapse (Figure 5-2) is a "connection" between two neurons.

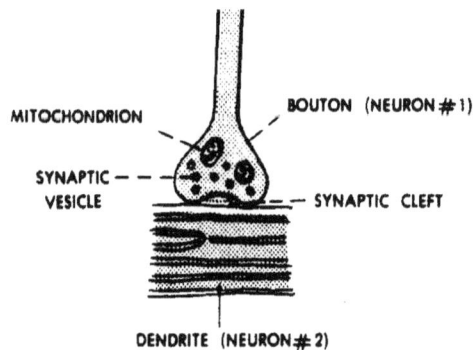

Figure 5-2. A synapse.

(1) First neuron. An axon terminates in tiny branches. At the end of each branch is found a terminal knob. Synaptic vesicles (bundles of neurotransmitters) are located within each terminal knob. That portion of the terminal knob that faces the synaptic cleft is thickened and is called the presynaptic membrane. This is the membrane through that neurotransmitters pass to enter the synaptic cleft.

(2) Synaptic cleft. The synaptic cleft is the space between the terminal knob of the first neuron and the dendrite or cell body of the second neuron.

(3) Second neuron. The terminal knob of the first neuron lies near a site on a dendrite or the cell body of the second neuron. The membrane at this site on the second neuron is known as the postsynaptic membrane. Within the second neuron is a chemical that inactivates the used neurotransmitter.

b. **The Neuromuscular Junction**. A neuromuscular junction (Figure 5-3) is a "connection" between the terminal of a motor neuron and a muscle fiber. The neuromuscular junction has an organization identical to a synapse. However, the knob is much larger. The postsynaptic membrane is also larger and has foldings to increase its surface area.

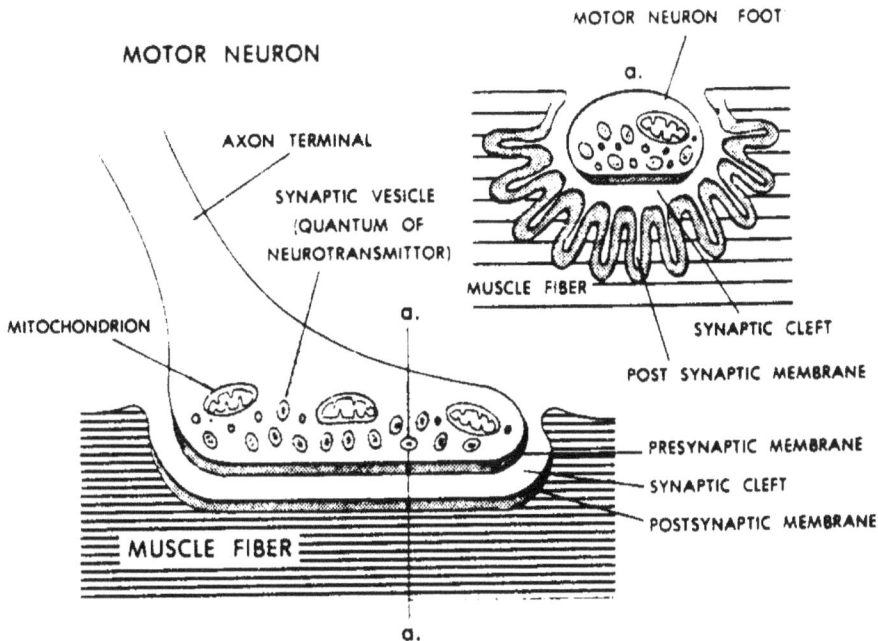

Figure 5-3. A neuromuscular junction.

    (1)   Motor neuron. The axon of a motor neuron ends as it reaches a skeletal muscle fiber. At this point, it has a terminal knob. Within this knob are synaptic vesicles (bundles of neurotransmitters). The presynaptic membrane lines the surface of the terminal knob and lies close to the muscle fiber.

    (2)   Synaptic cleft. The synaptic cleft is a space between the terminal knob of the motor neuron and the membrane of the muscle fiber.

    (3)   Muscle fiber. The terminal knob of the motor neuron protrudes into the surface of the muscle fiber. The membrane lining the synaptic space has foldings and is called the postsynaptic membrane. Beneath the postsynaptic membrane is a chemical that inactivates the used neurotransmitter.

5-7. PROCESS OF NEUROTRANSMISSION

    a.   The dendrites receive the impulse and transfer it to the nucleus. The nucleus will then cause a change in the permeability of the membrane surrounding the axon. Potassium, which is normally present in high concentrations within the axon, will diffuse out. Sodium, which is usually present in high concentrations outside the axon, will rush into the axon. This exchange of potassium and sodium is called depolarization. As these electrolytes change positions, an electrical charge is set up and the impulses will travel down the axon until it reaches the terminal bulbs. When the impulse reaches the terminal bulbs, it will cause a release of neurotransmitters stored there into the synaptic cleft. Once in the synaptic cleft, the neurotransmitters will diffuse across the synapse to the dendrite of the postsynaptic neuron causing it to depolarize (see Figure 5-4).

b.   Once the postsynaptic neuron has depolarized, the neurotransmitters must be removed from the synaptic cleft to prevent further depolarization. This is accomplished by two means. The neurotransmitter is either reabsorbed into the terminal bulb or an enzyme destroys it. This process ends the impulse.

c.   Before the neuron can depolarize again, the electrolyte sodium and potassium must resume their original positions. The sodium pump theory states that before the neuron can depolarize again the sodium is pumped out and the potassium is pumped back in (repolarized).

5-8. NEUROTRANSMITTERS

A neurotransmitter is a chemical substance that aids in the transmission of an impulse across the synapse. An impulse will cause the release of a neurotransmitter, which is synthesized and stored in terminal bulbs of the axon. The neurotransmitter will diffuse across the synaptic cleft and Initiate an impulse in the postsynaptic nerve. The neurotransmitter reacts with a receptor-site on the postsynaptic nerve initiating an impulse. The neurotransmitter must be removed from the synaptic cleft to stop the impulse.

a.   **Acetylcholine.** Acetylcholine (Ach) is destroyed by acetylcholinesterase (AchE) in the synaptic cleft.

b.   **Norepinephrine.** Norepinephrine (NE) is removed from the synaptic cleft by:

(1)   Reabsorption (reuptake) into the terminal knob.

(2)   Destroyed by catechol-o-methyl transferase (COMT).

(3)   Destroyed by monoamine oxidase (MAO).

(4)   Dilution by diffusion out of the junctional cleft.

5-9. THE ALL OR NONE LAW

This law states that if a stimulus is strong enough to cause a nerve impulse, it will cause the entire fiber to depolarize and not just part of it.

Section III. THE HUMAN CENTRAL NERVOUS SYSTEM

5-10. GENERAL COMMENTS

The human nervous system is divided into three major divisions: the central nervous system (CNS), the autonomic nervous system (ANS), and the peripheral nervous system (PNS). The central nervous system is composed of the brain and spinal cord. Both the peripheral nervous system and the autonomic nervous system carry information to and from the central nervous system. The central nervous system is so named because of its anatomical location along the central axis of the body and because it is central in function. If we use a computer analogy to understand that it is central in function, the CNS would be the central processing unit and the other two parts of the nervous system would supply inputs and transmit outputs. Figure 5-4 shows the central nervous system.

    a. **Major Subdivisions of the Central Nervous System.** The major subdivisions of the central nervous system are the brain and spinal cord.

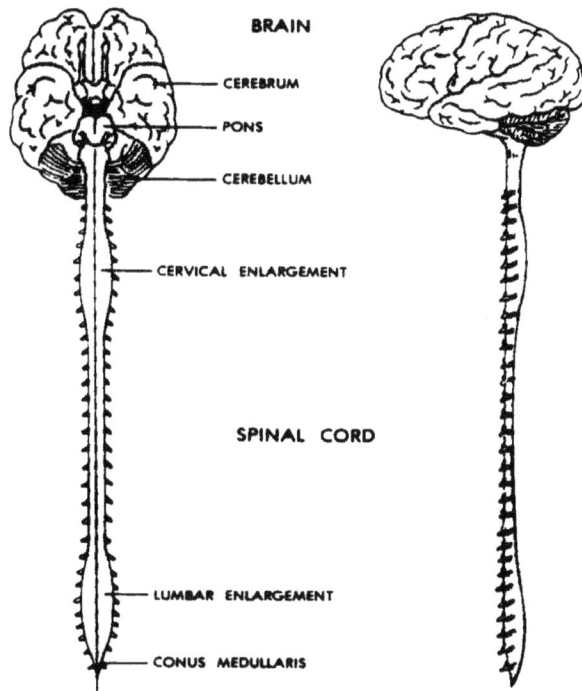

Figure 5-4. The central nervous system (CNS).

    b. **Coverings of the Central Nervous System.** Bone and fibrous tissues cover the parts of the central nervous system. These coverings help to protect the delicate tissue of the CNS.

c. **Cerebrospinal Fluid**. The cerebrospinal fluid (CSF) is a liquid that is thought to serve as a cushion and circulatory vehicle within the central nervous system.

5-11. THE HUMAN BRAIN

The human brain has three major subdivisions: brainstem, cerebellum, and the cerebrum. The central nervous system is first formed as a simple tube like structure in the embryo. The concentration of nervous tissues at one end of the human embryo to produce the brain and head is referred to as cephalization. When the embryo is about four weeks old, it is possible to identify the early forms of the brainstem, cerebellum, and the cerebrum, as well as the spinal cord. As development continues, the brain is located within the cranium in the cranial cavity. See Figure 5-5 for illustrations of the adult brain.

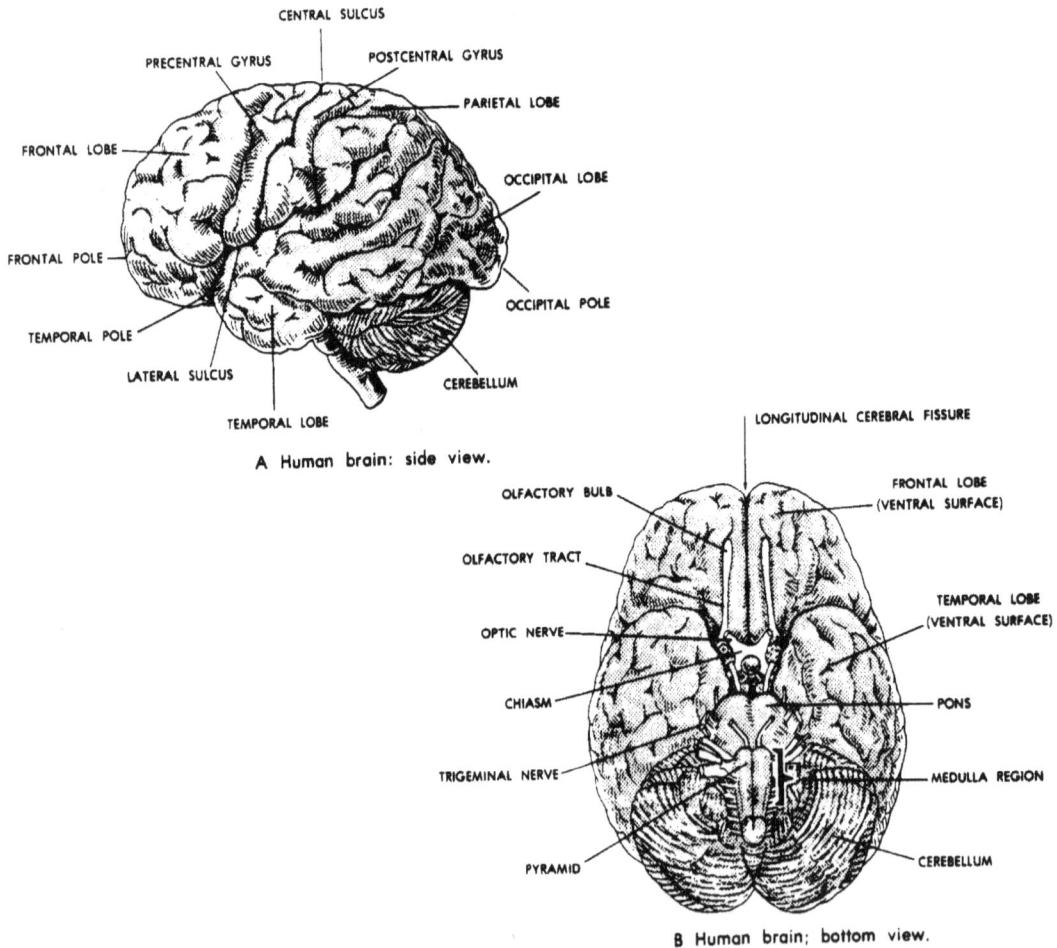

A Human brain: side view.

B Human brain: bottom view.

Figure 5-5. Human brain: A side view, B bottom view.

a. **The Brainstem**. The term brainstem refers to that part of the brain that would remain after the removal of the cerebrum and the cerebellum. The brainstem is the basal portion (portion of the base) of the brain. The brainstem can be divided as follows:

FOREBRAINSTEM   thalamus

MIDBRAINSTEM   corpora quadrigemina

HINDBRAINSTEM   pons
                                 medulla

(1)   The brainstem is continuous with the spinal cord. Together, the brainstem and the spinal cord are sometimes known as the neuraxis.

(2)   The brainstem provides major relays and controls for passing information up or down the neuraxis.

(3)   The 12 pairs of cranial nerves connect at the sides of the brainstem.

b. **Cerebellum**. The cerebellum is the spherical mass of nervous tissue attached to and covering the hindbrainstem. It has a narrow central part called the vermis and right and left cerebellar hemispheres.

(1)   Peduncles. The peduncles is a stemlike connecting part. The cerebellum is connected to the brainstem with three pairs of peduncles.

(2)   General shape and construction. A cross section of the cerebellum reveals that the outer cortex is composed of gray matter (cell bodies of neurons), with many folds and sulci (shallow grooves). More centrally located is the white matter (myelinated processes of neurons).

(3)   Function. The cerebellum is the primary coordinator/integrator of motor actions of the body.

c. **Cerebrum**. The cerebrum consists of two very much-enlarged hemispheres connected to each other by a special structure called the corpus callosum. Each cerebral hemisphere is connected to the brainstem by a cerebral peduncle. The surface of each cerebral hemisphere is subdivided into areas known as lobes. Each lobe is named according to the cranial bone under which it lies: frontal, parietal, occipital, and temporal.

(1)   The cerebral cortex is the gray outer layer of each hemisphere. Deeper within the cerebral hemispheres the tissue is white. The "gray matter" represents cell bodies of neurons. The "white matter" represents the axons.

(2)   The areas of the cortex are associated with groups of related functions.

(a)   For example, centers of speech and hearing are located along the lateral sulcus, at the side of each hemisphere.

(b)   Vision is centered at the rear in the area known as the occipital lobe.

(c)   Sensory and motor functions are located along the central sulcus, which separates the frontal and parental lobes of each hemisphere. The motor areas are located along the front side of the central sulcus, in the frontal lobe. The sensory areas are located along the rear side of the central sulcus in the parietal lobe.

d.   **Ventricles**. Within the brain, there are interconnected hollow spaces filled with cerebrospinal fluid (CSF). These hollow spaces are known as ventricles. The right and left lateral ventricles are found in the cerebral hemispheres. The third ventricle is located in the forebrainstem. The fourth ventricle is in the hindbrainstem. The fourth ventricle is continuous with the narrow central canal of the spinal cord.

5-12. THE HUMAN SPINAL CORD

a.   **Location and Extent**. Referring to Figure 5-6, you can see that the typical vertebra has a large opening called the vertebral (or spinal) foramen. Together, these foramina form the vertebral (spinal) canal for the entire vertebral column. The spinal cord, located within the spinal canal, is continuous with the brainstem. The spinal cord travels the length from the foramen magnum at the base of the skull to the junction of the first and second lumbar vertebrae.

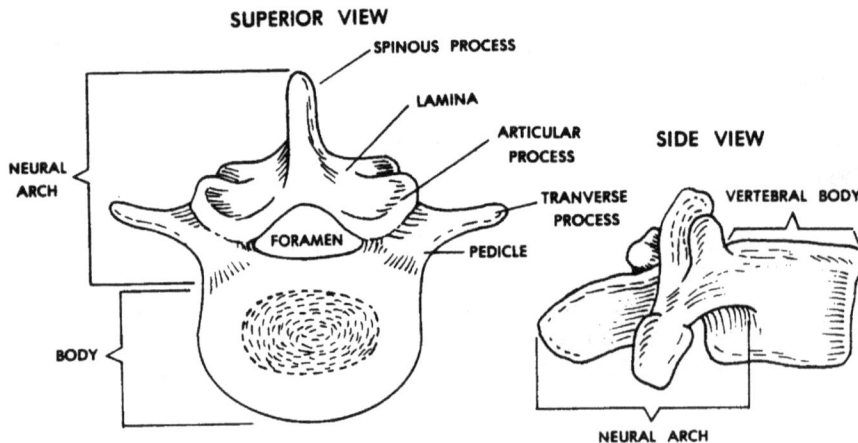

Figure 5-6. The spinal column.

(1) <u>Enlargements.</u> The spinal cord has two enlargements. One is the cervical enlargement, associated with nerves for the upper members. The other is the lumbosacral enlargement, associated with nerves for the lower members.

(2) <u>Spinal nerves</u>. A nerve is a bundle of neuron branches that carry impulses to and from the CNS. Those nerves arising from the spinal cord are spinal nerves. There are 31 pairs of spinal nerves.

b. **A Cross Section of the Spinal Cord (Figure 5-7)**. The spinal cord is a continuous structure that runs through the vertebral canal down to the lumbar region of the column. It is composed of a mass of a central gray matter (cell bodies of neurons) surrounded by peripheral white matter (myelinated branches of neurons). The gray and white matter are thus considered columns of material. However, in cross section, this effect of <u>columns</u> is lost.

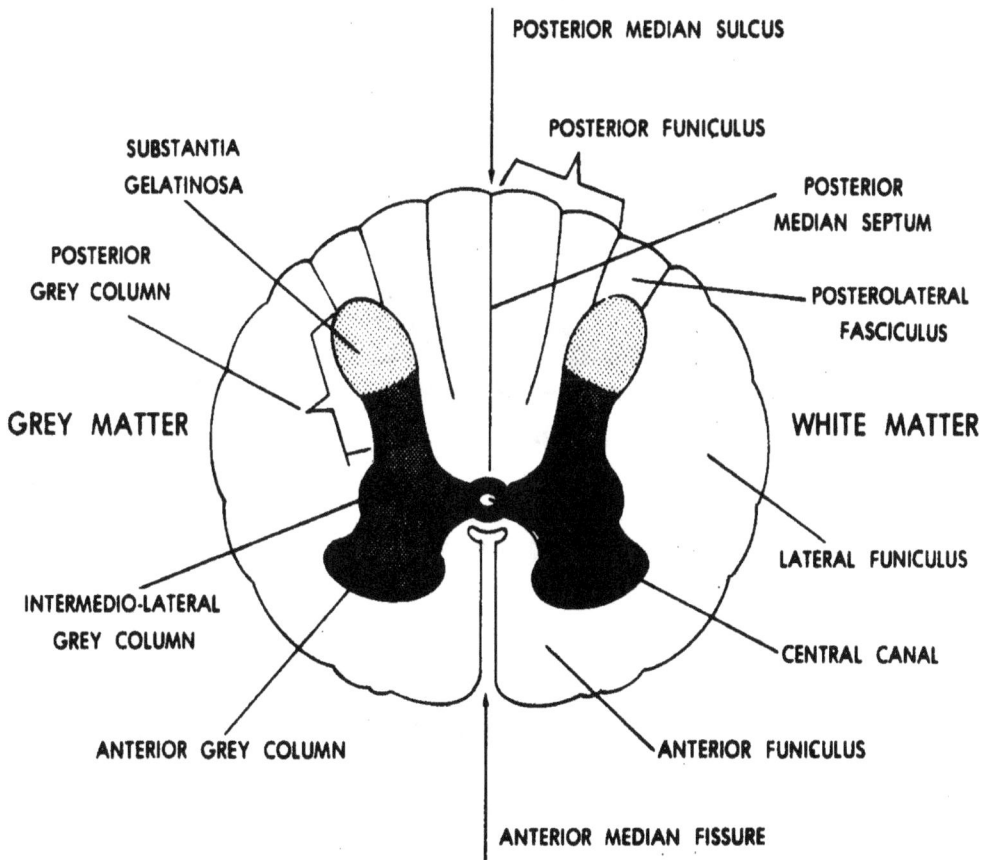

Figure 5-7. A cross section of the spinal cord.

5-13. COVERINGS OF THE CENTRAL NERVOUS SYSTEM

The coverings of the central nervous center (CNS) are skeletal and fibrous.

a. **Skeletal Coverings**.

(1) <u>Brain</u>. The bones of the cranium form a spherical case around the brain. The cranial cavity is the space enclosed by the bones of the cranium.

(2) <u>Spinal cord</u>. The vertebrae, with the vertebral foramina, form a cylindrical case around the spinal cord. The overall skeletal structure is the vertebral column (spine). The vertebral (spinal) canal is the space enclosed by the foramina of the vertebrae.

b. **Meninges (Fibrous Membranes)**. The brain and spinal cord have three different membranes called meninges surrounding them (Figure 5-8). These coverings provide protection.

(1) <u>Dura mater</u>. The dura mater is a tough outer covering for the CNS. Beneath the dura mater is the subdural space, which contains a thin film of fluid.

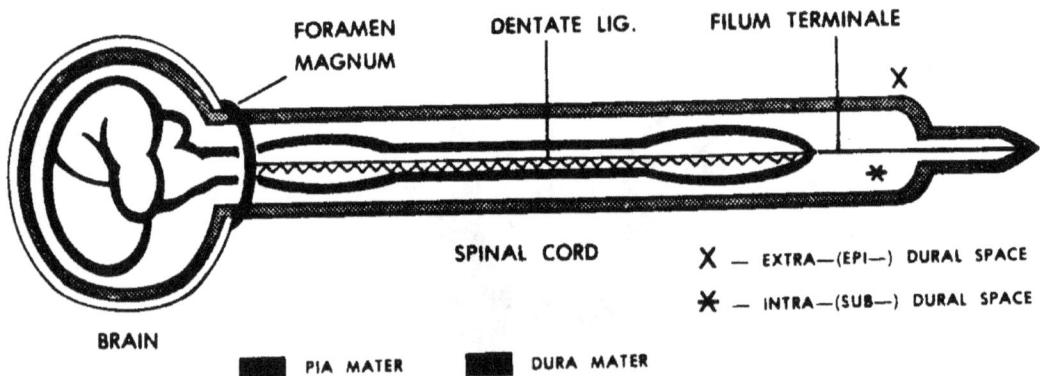

Figure 5-8. The meninges, as seen in side view of the CNS.

(2) <u>Arachnoid mater</u>. To the inner side of the dura mater and subdural space is a fine membranous layer called the arachnoid mater. It has fine spider-web type threads that extend inward through the subarachnoid space to the pia mater. The subarachnoid space is filled with cerebrospinal fluid (CSF).

ARACHNOID = Spiderlike

(3) <u>Pia mater</u>. The pia mater is a delicate membrane applied directly to the surface of the brain and the spinal cord. It carries a network of blood vessels to supply the nervous tissues of the CNS.

5-14. BLOOD SUPPLY TO THE CNS

a. **Blood Supply of the Brain**. The paired internal carotid arteries and the paired vertebral arteries supply blood rich in oxygen to the brain. Branches of these arteries join to form a circle under the base of the brain. This is called the cerebral circle (of Willis). From this circle, numerous branches supply specific areas of the brain.

(1) A single branch is often the only supply to that particular part of the brain. Such an artery is called an end artery. If it fails to supply blood to that specific area, the area will die (as in a stroke).

(2) The veins and venous sinuses of the brain drain into the paired internal jugular veins. These veins carry blood back toward the heart.

b. **Blood Supply of the Spinal Cord**. The blood supply of the spinal cord is by way of combination of three longitudinal arteries running along its length and reinforced by segmental arteries from the sides.

5-15. CEREBROSPINAL FLUID

A clear fluid called cerebrospinal fluid (CSF) is found in the cavities of the central nervous system. Cerebrospinal fluid is found in the ventricles of the brain, the subarachnoid space, and the central canal of the spinal cord. Cerebrospinal fluid and its associated structures make up the circulatory system for the CNS.

a. **Choroid Plexuses**. Choroid plexuses are special collections of arterial capillaries found in the roofs of the third and fourth ventricles of the brain. The choroid plexuses continuously produce CSF from the plasma of the blood.

b. **Path of the Cerebrospinal Fluid Flow**. Blood flows through the arterial capillaries of the choroid plexuses. As the choroid plexuses produce CSF, it flows into all four ventricles. Cerebrospinal fluid from the lateral ventricles flows into the third ventricle, through the cerebral aqueduct then into the fourth ventricle. By passing through three small holes in the roof of the fourth ventricle, CSF enters the subarachnoid space. From the subarachnoid space, the CSF is transported through the arachnoid villi (granulations) into the venous sinuses. Thus, the CSF is formed from arterial blood and returned to the venous blood.

Continue with Exercises

EXERCISES, LESSON 5

INSTRUCTIONS: Answer the following exercises by marking the lettered response that best answers the exercise, by completing the incomplete statement, or by writing the answer in the space provided at the end of the exercise.

 After you have completed all of these exercises, turn to "Solutions to Exercises" at the end of the lesson and check your answers. For each exercise answered incorrectly, reread the material referenced with the solution.

1. Which of the following is/are a type of nervous tissue?

 a. Neurons.

 b. Axons.

 c. Dendrites.

 d. Glia.

2. Select the function(s) for which nervous tissues are specialized.

 a. To transmit information.

 b. To "store" information.

 c. To receive stimuli.

 d. All the above.

3. A neuron is defined as _____.

 a. A process that carries impulses toward the cell body.

 b. A branch that transmits information from the cell body to the next unit.

 c. A nerve cell body and all of its branches.

 d. A nerve process that has two or more poles.

4. A dendrite is defined as _____.

    a. A neuron process that carries impulses toward the cell body.

    b. A neuron branch that transmits information from the cell body to the next unit.

    c. A neuron that has two poles.

    d. A nerve cell body and all of its branches.

5. From the statement below, select the type of neuron that is being described:

In this type of neuron, impulses are transmitted from the central nervous system to muscles and glands.

    a. Sensory neurons.

    b. Interneurons.

    c. Afferent neurons.

    d. Motor neurons.

6. Which of the following statements best describe the neuromuscular junctions?

    a. A connection between two neurons.

    b. A connection that relays information from muscle tissue to the brain.

    c. A connection between the terminal knob of a motor neuron and a muscle fiber.

    d. A connection which joins two neurons.

7. Which of the following substances is a neurotransmitter?

    a. Sodium chloride.

    b. Norepinephrine.

    c. Acetylcholinesterase.

    d. Catechol-o-methyl transferase (COMT).

8. Select the names of the three major subdivisions of the human nervous system.

    a. The central nervous system, brain, and spinal cord.

    b. The autonomic nervous system, the peripheral nervous system, and the central nervous system.

    c. The peripheral nervous system, the brain, and the spinal cord.

    d. The autonomic nervous system, the peripheral nervous system, and the codaptive nervous system.

9. What is the function of the meninges surrounding the brain and spinal cord?

    a. They carry nervous impulses into the brain and spinal cord.

    b. They prevent nerve impulses from injuring delicate tissue.

    c. They direct nerve impulses to the proper places in the brain.

    d. They provide protection for the brain and spinal cord.

10. What is the function of the cerebrum of the human brain?

    a. It serves as the primary coordinator/integrator of motor actions in the body.

    b. It serves as the center of speech, hearing, and vision.

    c. It provides major relays and controls for passing information up or down the neuraxis.

    d. It protects the cerebellum.

Check Your Answers on Next Page

SOLUTIONS TO EXERCISES, LESSON 5

1. a Neurons. (para 5-1)
    d Glia.

2. d All the above. (para 5-2a, b, and c)

3. c A nerve cell body and all of its branches. (para 5-3)

4. a A neuron process that carries impulses toward the cell body. (para 5-4a)

5. d Motor neurons. (para 5-5c(2))

6. c A connection between the terminal knob of a motor neuron and a muscle fiber. (para 5-6b)

7. b Norepinephrine. (para 5-8b)

8. b The autonomic nervous system, the peripheral nervous system, and the central nervous system. (para 5-10)

9. d They provide protection for the brain and spinal cord. (para 5-13b)

10. b It serves as the center of speech, hearing, and vision. (para 5-11c(2))

End of Lesson 5

LESSON ASSIGNMENT

LESSON 6   Agents Used During Surgery.

TEXT ASSIGNMENT   Paragraphs 6-1--6-10.

LESSON OBJECTIVES   After completing this lesson, you should be able to:

6-1.   Given a group of definitions, select the definition of the term general anesthetic.

6-2.   Given a list, select the types of general anesthetic.

6-3.   Given a type of medication used during surgery and a list of drugs, select the drug that belongs to that category of general anesthetics.

6-4.   Given the name of an agent used during surgery and a list of uses, side effects, and/or cautions and warnings, select the use, side effect, or caution and warning associated with that agent.

SUGGESTION   After studying the assignment, complete the exercises at the end of this lesson. These exercises will help you to achieve the lesson objectives.

LESSON 6

AGENTS USED DURING SURGERY

Section I. GENERAL ANESTHETIC AGENTS

6-1. INTRODUCTION

a. Have you ever undergone surgery? If you have, you can readily appreciate the importance of drugs used during surgery. This group of agents is widely used. The agents within the group differ widely in their uses and indications. This lesson will focus on this group of drugs with the intent of giving you a background in this important area.

b. In days gone by, various substances (that is, whiskey) were used to "put the patient to sleep" during surgery. As surgical procedures became increasingly sophisticated, the need for better anesthetic agents became more apparent. Today, general anesthetic agents comprise an important group of pharmacological agents. Their use promotes patient welfare. This section of the subcourse will discuss this important group of agents.

6-2. DEFINITION

A general anesthetic is an agent that depresses the central nervous system reversibly, producing loss of consciousness, analgesia, and muscle relaxation, with minimal depression of the patient's vital functions. That is, a general anesthetic agent places the patient in a state of anesthesia in which his muscles are relaxed and he feels no pain. Later, after the procedure has been completed, the patient can regain consciousness and recuperate.

6-3. MECHANISM OF ACTION OF GENERAL ANESTHETICS

It is known that the general anesthetic agents depress the central nervous system. Precisely how this depression occurs is unknown. Several theories attempt to explain this depression. One-theory states the agents affect lipid (fat) structures in the brain in order to produce the central nervous system depression. If you desire a detailed discussion of the various theories, you should consult a pharmacology text.

6-4. TYPES OF GENERAL ANESTHETIC AGENTS

There are two broad types of general anesthetics: The inhalation agents and the intravenous agents. It is not the purpose of this subcourse to provide a complete listing or a detailed discussion of the agents that are presented. If you desire additional information on these agents, you should consult a pharmacology text.

a. **Inhalation Agents**. Inhalation anesthetic agents are gases or volatile liquids. These substances are often mixed with oxygen and the patient is allowed to breathe the mixture. After a period, a sufficient level of the anesthetic agent is obtained in the blood and anesthesia is produced. In general, anesthesia can be well controlled with these agents because the concentration of the agent in the blood can be increased or decreased easily by either increasing or decreasing the concentration of the agent in the air the patient is breathing. It is relatively uncommon for a patient to have an allergic reaction to one of the inhalation general anesthetic agents. However, the side effects of some of these agents can be quite serious. There is rapid recovery for the patient when this type of agent is used. That is, when the patient is no longer allowed to breathe the agent, the depression of the central nervous system quickly disappears.

(1) Nitrous oxide. Nitrous oxide is a gas supplied in blue metal cylinders. Nitrous oxide is commonly referred to as laughing gas. Although nitrous oxide is a safe general anesthetic, it is relatively weak in terms of producing anesthesia and muscle relaxation. Consequently, nitrous oxide is often used in conjunction with other agents. Nitrous oxide is often used in dental surgery and in obstetrical practice during delivery.

(2) Halothane (Fluothane®). Halothane is a volatile liquid inhalation anesthetic. It is one of the most widely used general anesthetics. Since halothane does not produce potent analgesia and muscle relaxation, other agents are sometimes administered with halothane on an as-needed basis. Halothane has popularity because it is nonexplosive, rapid acting, pleasant smelling, and is compatible with other drugs.

(3) Enflurane (Erthrane®. Enflurane is a volatile liquid inhalation anesthetic with many of the properties of halothane. It produces greater muscle relaxation than halothane, but like halothane, it is a poor analgesic.

b. **Intravenous Agents**. Intravenous general anesthetics are sterile solutions intended to be administered into the patient's circulatory system. Intravenous anesthetic agents do produce loss of consciousness; however, most of these agents lack the ability to produce complete analgesia. In general, the level of anesthesia is more difficult to control with intravenous anesthetics than with inhalation anesthetics.

(1) Thiopental sodium (Pentothal®) Thiopental sodium is an ultrashort acting barbiturate. That is, this agent acts very quickly to produce anesthesia. Sometimes this agent is used alone for minor surgical procedures. In other cases, the drug is used to initiate anesthesia. Then, other anesthetic agents are used to maintain the anesthesia. Thiopental sodium is a NOTE Q item. That is, it is a controlled substance.

(2) Fentanyl (Sublimaze®) and droperidol (Innovar®). This agent is an intravenously administered product, which combines the narcotic analgesic effect of fentanyl with the sedative and antiemetic effects of droperidol. This agent produces a semiconscious state in the patient, and it is used in types of surgery in which the surgeon needs the cooperation of the patient. Innovar is usually used in combination

with nitrous oxide because of its slow induction. Innovar may also be used for various diagnostic procedures. This product is a controlled substance (Note R item).

(3)   Ketamine (Ketalar®) is a nonbarbiturate anesthetic that can be administered either intravenously or intramuscularly. Ketamine produces a dissociative type anesthesia in which the patient becomes detached mentally from the environment. Ketamine may be used for induction anesthesia or for diagnostic or minor surgical procedures in children.

Section II. OTHER AGENTS USED DURING SURGERY

6-5. INTRODUCTION

No single anesthetic agent is capable of producing the deep levels of analgesia and skeletal muscle relaxation required during all types of surgery. Consequently, other drugs that have certain desired effects are administered along with the general anesthetic being used. Five major categories of these agents will be presented in this subcourse. They are analgesic agents, drying agents, skeletal muscle relaxants, sedative and hypnotic agents, and antianxiety agents.

6-6. ANALGESIC AGENTS

Analgesic agents relieve pain. Although a general anesthetic agent will produce unconsciousness, the patient might still be able to feel some pain. In these cases, a preanesthetic medication might be administered to the patient in order to relieve the pain. A variety of analgesic agents are available to achieve this purpose. Following are some commonly used agents:

a.   Meperidine (Demerol®).

b.   Morphine.

c.   Nubain®.

d.   Stadol®.

6-7. DRYING AGENTS

It is sometimes advantageous during an operation to have the patient's mucous membranes (that is, nose, throat) dry. Drying agents are administered for just this reason. You are probably familiar with the use of drying agents in certain over-the-counter cold medications. Following are two commonly used drying medications:

    a.   Atropine sulfate.

    b.   Glycopyrrolate (Robinul®).

6-8. NEUROMUSCULAR BLOCKING AGENTS

In some types of surgery (for example, abdominal surgery) it is highly advantageous to have the patient's skeletal muscles (for example, abdominal surgery) in a state of relaxation. Most general anesthetic agents do not produce a sufficient level of skeletal muscle relaxation. Therefore, neuromuscular blocking agents are administered to achieve the desired muscle relaxation effects. Two commonly used neuromuscular blocking agents:

    a.   Vecuronium (Norcuron®).

    b.   Succinylcholine (Anectine®).

6-9. SEDATIVE AND HYPNOTIC AGENTS

To ensure a good night's sleep prior to a surgical procedure, patients are sometimes administered either a sedative or a hypnotic agent. Agents commonly used for this purpose are:

    a.   Pentobarbital (Nembutal®).

    b.   Secobarbital (Seconal®).

6-10. ANTIANXIETY AGENTS

As one might expect, some patients are highly anxious about upcoming surgical procedures. Such increased anxiety interferes with the functioning of the patient (interferes with rest and decreases appetite). Anti-anxiety agents help to control this anxiety. Diazepam (Valium®) is sometimes used to control anxiety.

Continue with Exercises

EXERCISES, LESSON 6

INSTRUCTIONS: Answer the following exercises by marking the lettered response that best answers the exercise, by completing the incomplete statement, or by writing the answer in the space provided at the end of the exercise.

After you have completed all of these exercises, turn to "Solutions to Exercises" at the end of the lesson and check your answers. For each exercise answered incorrectly, reread the material referenced with the solution.

1.   From the definitions below, select the definition of the term general anesthetic.

     a.   An agent that depresses the central nervous system irreversibly to produce a loss of consciousness, analgesia) and muscle relaxation.

     b.   An agent that stimulates the central nervous system, thus making it possible for a physician to perform various types of surgeries.

     c.   An agent used to produce localized analgesia in a patient.

     d.   An agent that depresses the central nervous system reversibly to produce a loss of consciousness, analgesia, and muscle relaxation.

2.   From the list below, select the type(s) of general anesthetic.

     a.   Local.

     b.   Intravenous.

     c.   Induction.

     d.   Clinical.

3.   From the list below, select the agent that is classified as an inhalation anesthetic agent.

     a.   Thiopental sodium (Pentothal®).

     b.   Enflurane (Ethrane®).

     c.   Glycopyrrolate (Robinal®).

     d.   Succinylcholine (Anectine®).

4. From the list below, select the agent classified as an intravenous anesthetic agent.

    a. Fentanyl (Sublimaze®) and droperidol (Innovar®).

    b. Glycopyrrolate (Robinal®).

    c. Meperidine hydrochloride (Demerol®).

    d. Succinylcholine (Anectine®).

5. From the list of uses below, select the use of glycopyolate (Robinal®)

    a. Intravenous anesthetic agent.

    b. Skeletal muscle relaxant.

    c. Drying agent.

    d. Inhalation anesthetic agent.

6. From the list of uses below, select the use of succinylcholine (Anectine®).

    a. An antianxiety agent used the night before surgery.

    b. A sedative used the day before surgery.

    c. An analgesic agent used after surgery.

    d. A neuromuscular blocking agent used during surgery.

7. From the list of uses below, select the use of meperidine hydrochloride (Demerol®).

    a. An agent often used as a preanesthetic analgesic.

    b. An analgesic used to produce unconsciousness.

    c. An analgesic agent used for its ability to dry the patient's mouth.

    d. An analgesic agent used to stimulate a patient's breathing during surgery.

8. From the list below, select the use of ketamine (Ketalar®).

    a. An inhalation anesthetic used to induce anesthesia for diagnostic purposes.

    b. An intravenous anesthetic used to perform major surgery in adults over the age of 60.

    c. An intravenous anesthetic used to perform minor surgical procedures in children.

    d. An inhalation anesthetic agent used because of its ability to produce analgesia.

9. From the group below, select the use of the agent fentanyl (Sublimaze®) and droperidol (Innovar®).

    a. An agent that is used because it produces a dissociative type of anesthesia.

    b. An agent used because the patient easily inhales it.

    c. An agent used when the surgeon needs the cooperation of the patient because it produces a semiconscious state in the patient.

    d. An agent used during surgery because it produces a drying effect in the patient's mucous membranes.

10. From the group below, select the use of the agent diazepam (Valium®).

    a. A drying agent used to reduce saliva product in comatose patients.

    b. An analgesic agent administered after surgery.

    c. An antianxiety agent used to reduce a patient's apprehension before surgery.

    d. A nonbarbiturate anesthetic used before surgery.

Check Your Answers on Next Page

SOLUTIONS TO EXERCISES, LESSON 6

1. d An agent that depresses the central nervous system reversibly to produce a loss of consciousness, analgesia, and muscle relaxation. (para 6-2)

2. b Intravenous. (para 6-4b)

3. b Enflurane (Ethrane®). (para 6-4a(3))

4. a Fentanyl (Sublimaze®) and droperidol (Innovar®). (para 6-4b(2))

5. c Drying agent. (para 6-7)

6. d A neuromuscular blocking agent used during surgery. (para 6-8)

7. a An agent used as a preanesthetic analgesic. (para 6-6)

8. c An intravenous agent used to perform minor surgical procedures in children. (para 6-4b(3))

9. c An agent used when the surgeon needs the cooperation of the patient because it produces a semiconscious state in the patient. (para 6-4b(2))

10. c Antianxiety agent used to reduce a patient's apprehension before surgery. (para 6-10)

End of Lesson 6

LESSON ASSIGNMENT

LESSON 7   Sedative and Hypnotic Agents.

TEXT ASSIGNMENT   Paragraphs 7-1--7-9.

LESSON OBJECTIVES After completing this lesson, you should be able to:

7-1. Given a group of statements, select the best definition of a sedative-hypnotic.

7-2. From a group of statements, select the statement that best describes the mechanism of action of sedative-hypnotics.

7-3. Given a list of possible effects, select the effect(s) produced by sedative-hypnotics.

7-4. Given an effect produced by the sedative-hypnotics and a group of statements, select the statement that best describes that effect.

7-5. From a list of possible clinical uses, select the clinical use(s) of the sedative-hypnotics.

7-6. From a list of adverse reactions, select the adverse effect(s) associated with sedative-hypnotics.

7-7. From a list of cautions and warnings, select the caution(s) and warning(s) associated with the sedative-hypnotics.

7-8. Given a group of statements and two types of barbiturates (for example, ultra short-acting and short-acting), select the statement which best differentiates between the two types.

7-9. Given the trade name of a sedative-hypnotic agent and a list of generic names, match the trade name with its generic name.

7-10. Given the trade or generic name of a sedative-hypnotic agent and a group of possible clinical uses or side effects, select the use(s) or side effect(s) associated with that agent.

SUGGESTION

After studying the assignment, complete the exercises at the end of this lesson. These exercises will help you to achieve the lesson objectives.

LESSON 7

SEDATIVE AND HYPNOTIC AGENTS

Section I. BACKGROUND

7-1. INTRODUCTION

Sedative and hypnotic agents form an important class of drugs that are widely used in modern medical practice. The names of many of the agents should be fairly familiar to you since these drugs are so widely used in hospitals and dispensed to patients on an outpatient basis. You probably know that most sedative-hypnotic agents are controlled because of their abuse/misuse potential. The barbiturates have been regarded as the prototypes of this class of drugs because of their extensive use over the past 80 years. Because of their potential for addiction, physical dependence, and side effects, the barbiturates have been replaced by the benzodiazepines (for example, Valium®). The benzodiazepines are currently the most important sedative hypnotics because of their efficacy and safety.

7-2. DEFINITION OF SEDATIVE-HYPNOTIC

A sedative-hypnotic agent is a substance, which, if given in progressively larger doses, produces calm (sedation), sleep (hypnosis), general anesthesia, and ultimately death (because of medullary depression). Sedative-hypnotic agents are commonly used for symptomatic relief of anxiety and for the induction of sleep. Sedatives may be also referred to as anti-anxiety agents.

Section II. CLINICALLY IMPORTANT INFORMATION
CONCERNING SEDATIVE-HYPNOTICS

7-3. INTRODUCTION

Sedative-hypnotic agents are an important group of drugs, which are often prescribed to a variety of patients. You should be familiar with the effects and the clinical uses of these drugs.

7-4. THE PHARMACOLOGICAL ACTIONS OF SEDATIVE-HYPNOTIC AGENTS

a. **Mechanism of Action.** Sedatives and hypnotics selectively depress the reticular activating system (RAS), the mechanism responsible for keeping us awake.

b. **Effects Produced by Sedative-Hypnotic Agents.**

(1) Sedation. To sedate means to calm; therefore, sedation refers to the act of producing calm in a patient. You can also think of sedation as referring to a decreased responsiveness to a constant level of stimulation. Small doses (small amounts) of a sedative-hypnotic drug administered to a patient will produce sedation.

(2) Disinhibition. Disinhibition refers to actions a person may perform while under the effects of a drug that he would not perform if he were not taking the drug. This effect may be seen as euphoria, (feeling of well being or elation) in some patients and is a potential source of abuse of these agents. Disinhibition is presumed because of depression of a higher cortical (brain) center, which results in a resultant release of lower brain centers from constant inhibitory influence. Larger doses of a sedative-hypnotic agent will produce this effect.

(3) Relief of anxiety. This particular effect probably cannot be separated from the sedative and euphoriant effects produced by the sedative-hypnotic agents.

(4) Sleep. Sedative-hypnotic induced sleep differs in several ways from normal sleep. If a sufficiently large dose of any sedative-hypnotic agent is administered to a patient, sleep will result; however, the dose of a particular agent required to produce sleep will vary with the physiologic and psychologic state of the individual and the environmental situation in which the drug is given.

(5) Anesthesia. State III of general anesthesia (surgical anesthesia-- unconsciousness and paralysis of reflexes) can be induced in humans with large doses of sedative-hypnotic agents. Short- and ultra short-acting barbiturates are the only drugs used as anesthetic agents from this class.

(6) Analgesia. Patients who have been deeply anesthetized with barbiturates are totally unresponsive to pain.

(7) Anticonvulsant activity. All the barbiturates commonly used in clinical practice are capable of inhibiting convulsions. Phenobarbital and other long-acting drugs are selectively more effective at lower therapeutic doses in the treatment of epilepsy.

(8) Cardiovascular and respiratory effects. Sedative-hypnotic agents are respiratory depressants that depress the respiratory system. Sedative-hypnotic agents do not, when administered orally, produce significant cardiovascular effects.

(9) Dependence. Both psychic and physical dependence has been reported with both the barbiturate and nonbarbiturate sedative-hypnotic agents. Dependence usually occurs when sedative-hypnotics are given over a long period in large doses. Therefore, continued administration of these agents is usually necessary to prevent a withdrawal state in the patient.

7-5. CLINICAL USES OF SEDATIVE-HYPNOTIC AGENTS

Sedative-hypnotic agents are used to treat a variety of conditions. These include:

a. **Relief of Anxiety**. Sedative-hypnotics are effectively used to temporarily relieve anxiety associated with threatening or fearful situations (for example, anxiety that typically occurs before a surgical procedure).

b. **Treatment of Depression**. Depression is the most common manifestation of anxiety. Treatment of depression with sedative-hypnotic agents may be effective. It should be noted that major (psychotic) depressions might be intensified with sedative-hypnotics.

c. **Induction of Sleep (Hypnosis)**. Short-acting sedative-hypnotics are generally used because of less hangover or persistent effects. When used to produce sleep, sedative-hypnotics should not be administered continuously and should only be part of an overall plan of management and counseling.

d. **Anticonvulsant Therapy**. Some sedative-hypnotics (for example, phenobarbital) have been successfully used in the treatment of various types of convulsive disorders.

e. **Skeletal Muscle Relaxation**. Some sedative-hypnotics have been used to produce muscle relaxation in patients. However, the effectiveness of sedative-hypnotics for this use may be related more to their sedative properties than to their ability to produce true muscle relaxation.

f. **Anesthesia**. The ultra short-acting barbiturates (for example, thiopental) are used for surgical procedures of short duration.

7-6. ADVERSE EFFECTS OF SEDATIVE HYPNOTICS

Sedative-hypnotics, although safe when taken as directed, are not without their side effects. You should be familiar with the side effects produced by these agents:

a. **Drowsiness**. As you might anticipate, all of the sedative-hypnotic agents will cause drowsiness if a large enough dose is given to the patient. Furthermore, because of individual reactions to drugs, some patients will be made drowsy even by small doses of these agents. Patients who are prescribed sedative-hypnotics should be told not to drink alcoholic beverages while taking the drug since the alcohol could intensify the drowsiness effect.

b. **Impaired Performance and Judgment.** These agents interfere with a person 5 ability to think and to perform certain "hands-on" tasks. Sedative-hypnotic agents are equivalent to alcohol in their effects on distorting judgment and minor motor skills.

c. **Hangover Effect**. When a patient arises from a night's sleep after having taken a bedtime dose of a sedative-hypnotic, the patient may complain of feeling dizzy, lethargic, or exhausted. This is referred to as the "hangover effect." This effect is more prevalent with the long-acting sedative-hypnotics.

d. **Chronic Toxicity**.

(1) Drug abuse. The relief of anxiety and the euphoria provided by these drugs has led to the compulsive misuse of every member of this group. Because of their rapid onset of action and intense effect, the short-or intermediate-acting sedative-hypnotics are more apt to be misused than are the other types of sedative-hypnotics. These agents do not cause chronic organic toxicity.

(2) Withdrawal state. A patient who has been taking therapeutic doses of a sedative-hypnotic may find that he has a disturbed pattern of sleep with restlessness and nightmares when he suddenly stops taking the drug. Discontinuing larger doses of sedative-hypnotics may produce a hyperexcitable state in the patient characterized by weakness, tremor, anxiety, elevated blood pressure, and elevated pulse rate. The sudden withdrawal of even larger doses may produce convulsions or toxic psychosis with agitation, confusion, and hallucinations.

e. **Acute Toxicity**. The amount of a particular sedative-hypnotic required to produce death in a patient depends upon a variety of factors. An extremely large dose of a sedative-hypnotic will produce a state of prolonged, deep anesthesia. If the stage of severe medullary depression is reached, circulatory shock occurs. In case of acute toxicity, it is necessary for the patient to be immediately taken to the nearest medical treatment facility for emergency treatment.

7-7. CAUTIONS AND WARNINGS ASSOCIATED WITH THE USE OF SEDATIVE-HYPNOTICS

a. Ambulatory patients (those patients able to walk) should be warned to avoid activities that require mental alertness, judgment, and physical coordination while taking sedative-hypnotics.

b. Alcohol should not be consumed with sedative-hypnotic agents. This is because both the alcohol and the sedative-hypnotic would both act to depress the central nervous system.

c. Caution should be observed when these drugs are given to patients who have impaired liver function, since the sedative-hypnotics are broken down in the liver.

d. Sedative-hypnotic agents are probably best prescribed and taken only on an irregular basis when needed. Some physicians believe that a short (that is, week long) course of scheduled sedative-hypnotic therapy is the most desirable. The aim is not to offer the patient the opportunity to become physically or psychologically dependent upon the drugs.

Section III. CLASSIFICATION OF SEDATIVE-HYPNOTIC AGENTS

NOTE: The agents in this section are classified according to their duration of action and whether they are barbiturates or nonbarbiturates.

7-8. BARBITURATE SEDATIVES AND HYPNOTICS

a. **Ultra Short-Acting Barbiturates.**

(1) <u>Basic information</u>. Ultra short-acting barbiturates usually have a duration of action of 15 to 30 minutes. They are administered intravenously in order to induce anesthesia because of their high degree in lipid (fatty) materials. Ultra short-acting barbiturates are used to counteract the convulsions associated with some chemical substances (for example, tetanus toxin) or by the overdosage of certain drugs.

(2) <u>Examples of ultra short-acting barbiturates</u>.

(a) Methohexital (Brevital®).

(b) Thiopental (Pentothal®).

b. **Short-Acting Barbiturates.**

(1) <u>Basic information</u>. Short-acting barbiturates usually have a duration of action that lasts from 2 hours to 4 hours. Short-acting barbiturates are effective treatment--when taken by mouth--for the initial and short-term treatment of insomnia. These agents are widely used intramuscularly (IM) for preanesthetic sedation in order to calm the patient and to reduce anxiety often found in patients about to undergo surgery. Pentobarbital and secobarbital (see below) may be used for short-term daytime sedation in patients who suffer from anxiety.

(2) <u>Examples of short-acting barbiturates</u>.

(a) Pentobarbital (Nembutal®).

(b) Secobarbital (Seconal®).

c. **Intermediate-Acting Barbiturates**.

(1) Basic information. Intermediate-acting barbiturates have a duration of action that lasts from 4 hours to 6 hours. These agents are mainly use for the initial and short-term treatment of insomnia.

(2) Example of intermediate-acting barbiturate. Amobarbital (Amytal®).

d. **Long-Acting Barbiturates.**

(1) Basic information. Long-acting barbiturates have a duration of action that lasts from 6 hours to 8 hours. These agents are used orally to maintain daylong sedation in anxiety-tension states. Furthermore, long-acting barbiturates are useful in the treatment of various convulsive disorders.

(2) Examples of long-acting barbiturates.

(a) Phenobarbital.

(b) Mephobarbital (Mebaral®).

7-9. NONBARBITURATE SEDATIVES AND HYPNOTICS

a. **Short-Acting Agents.**

(1) Background information. Short-acting nonbarbiturate sedative-hypnotics are generally used orally in the initial and short-term treatment of insomnia.

(2) Examples of short-acting nonbarbiturate sedative-hypnotics.

(a) Chloral hydrate (Noctec®). Drug interactions may occur between chloral hydrate and anticoagulants, furosemide, alcohol, or other drugs that are CNS depressants.
(b) Triazolam (Halcion®). Triazolam is rapidly absorbed through the oral route and is as effective as the barbiturates in inducing sleep. It is excreted in breast milk and should not be administered to nursing mothers.

b. **Intermediate-Acting Agents**.

(1) Background information. Intermediate-acting nonbarbiturate agents are administered orally to effectively control moderate to severe daytime anxiety and tension in patients who have neuroses and mild depressive states.

(2) Examples of intermediate-acting nonbarbiturates.

(a) Diazepam (Valium®). Diazepam may be useful in the treatment of alcohol withdrawal symptoms (for example, delirium tremens, agitation, and so forth.) This agent produces skeletal muscle relaxant effects in humans and has been used with limited success in various neurologic and musculoskeletal disorders. Diazepam may be administered parenterally as a preanesthetic medication to reduce anxiety and to calm the patient. Diazepam is also administered intravenously in the treatment of status epilepticus. It is available in tablet form (2, 5, and 10 milligrams) and in injection form (5 milligrams per milliliter in 2 and 10 milliliter containers). Diazepam is a Note Q controlled substance in the military.

(b) Meprobamate (Equanil®, Miltown®). Meprobamate can produce skeletal muscle relaxant effects in humans; therefore, it has been used with some success in the treatment of various neurologic and musculoskeletal disorders. It appears to be less effective than diazepam in the treatment of anxiety and tension. The most common side effect associated with the agent is drowsiness. It is supplied in tablet and suspension forms. Meprobamate is a Note Q controlled item in the military.

(c) Other examples of nonbarbiturates used in the treatment of anxiety disorders include Lorazepam (Ativan®), Alprazolam (Xanax®), and Buspirone (Buspar®). Lorazepam is used primarily as an antianxiety agent, but is useful for treating insomnia due to stress and anxiety. Lorazepam is also used as a preanesthetic medication to produce sedation and decrease the patient's ability to recall events related to the day of surgery.

(d) Temazepam (Restoril®). Temazepam is administered in a nightly dose of 15 to 30 mg. It is an effective inducer of sleep with a good safety profile. Animal studies indicate a potential for Temazepam to cause teratogenic effects. Therefore, it should not be administered during pregnancy.

c. **Long-Acting Nonbarbiturate Agents.**

(1) Background information. These agents depress the central nervous system. Patients taking these drugs should be cautioned against performing hazardous activities while under their effects.

(2) Examples of long-acting nonbarbiturate agents.

(a) Chlordiazepoxide hydrochloride (Librium®). Chlordiazepoxide is orally administered as an antianxiety agent. It is also effective when administered parenterally in the treatment of alcohol withdrawal. Side effects associated with the agent include drowsiness, ataxia, and lethargy.

(b) Oxazepam (Serax®). Oxazepam is generally less effective than either diazepam or chlordiazepoxide in the treatment of tension and anxiety. Drowsiness is the most common side effect associated with this agent.

Continue with Exercises

EXERCISES, LESSON 7

INSTRUCTIONS: Answer the following exercises by marking the lettered response that best answers the exercise, by completing the incomplete statement, or by writing the answer in the space provided at the end of the exercise.

After you have completed all of the exercises, turn to "Solutions to Exercises" at the end of the lesson and check your answers. For each exercise answered incorrectly, reread the material referenced with the solution.

1.   Which statement best describes the mechanism of action of sedative-hypnotics?

      a. They inhibit the flow of potassium and sodium ions across the semipermeable membranes of the nerves.

      b. They inhibit the depolarization of the nerve fibers and thus produce calm or sleep.

      c. They depress the reticular activating system (RAS).

      d. They inhibit the transmission of electrical impulses from the brain by interfering with the passage of certain ions through the nerve fibers.

2.   Select the effect(s) produced by the sedative-hypnotics.

      a.   Relief of anxiety.

      b.   Disinhibition.

      c.   Analgesia.

      d.   All the above.

3. Which of the following statements best describes the analgesia produced by sedative-hypnotics?

    a. Patients who have been given extremely large doses of barbiturates are unresponsive to pain.

    b. Patients who are administered intravenous doses of sedative-hypnotics are unable to feel any painful stimuli.

    c. Patients who are given sedative-hypnotics seem to be more tolerant of pain than those patients who are not given these drugs.

    d. Patients who are given any amount of sedative-hypnotics are unable to feel pain, but they are also unable to maintain consciousness for long periods.

4. Select the clinical use(s) associated with the sedative-hypnotics.

    a. To induce sleep.

    b. To treat minimal brain dysfunction (MBD).

    c. To treat pain.

    d. All the above.

5. Select the adverse effect(s) associated with the use of sedative-hypnotic agents.

    a. Drowsiness.

    b. Hangover.

    c. Impaired judgment.

    d. All the above.

6. Select the caution(s) and warning(s) associated with the use of sedative-hypnotics.

    a. Caution should be observed when giving these drugs to patients who have impaired liver function.

    b. These agents should not be prescribed to those persons who are likely to become dependent upon them.

    c. Sedative-hypnotics should be taken on a continuous and regular basis to ensure desired therapeutic effects.

    d. All the above.

INSTRUCTIONS: Match the generic name of the drug with its corresponding trade name. (Exercise items 7 through 10.)

7. Pentobarbital _____   a. Librium®

8. Oxazepam _____   b. Nembutal®

9. Chlordiazepoxide _____   c. Serax®

10. Triazolam _____   d. Halcion®

11. Select the clinical use(s) of diazepam (Valium®).

    a. A treatment for minimal brain dysfunction (MBD).

    b. An anoretic for the suppression of appetite.

    c. A preanesthetic medication used to calm the patient.

    d. A drug used for induction of sleep.

12. Select the clinical use(s) of chlordiazepoxide.

   a. Antianxiety agent.

   b. Sleep inducer.

   c. Skeletal muscle constrictor.

   d. All the above.

13. What is the most common side effect associated with oxazepam (Serax®)?

   a. Ataxia.

   b. Lethargy.

   c. Drowsiness.

   d. Blurred vision.

14. What is the duration of action for ultra-short acting barbiturates?

   a. 6 to 8 hours.

   b. 4 to 6 hours.

   c. 2 to 4 hours.

   d. 15 to 30 minutes.

Check Your Answers on Next Page

SOLUTIONS TO EXERCISES, LESSON 7

1. c   They depress the reticular activating system (RAS).
        (para 7-4a)

2. d   All the above. (para 7-4b(2), (3), and (4))

3. a   Patients who have been given extremely large doses of barbiturates are
        unresponsive to pain. (para 7-4b(6))

4. a   To induce sleep. (para 7-5a)

5. d   All the above. (para 7-6)

6. a   Caution should be observed when prescribing these drugs to patients who
        have impaired liver function. (para 7-7c)

7. b   Nembutal®. (para 7-8b(2))

8. c   Serax®. (para 7-9c(2)(b))

9. a   Librium®. (para 7-9c(2)(a))

10. d   Halcion®. (para 7-9a(2)(b))

11. c   A preanesthetic medication used to calm the patient.
        (para 7-9b(2)(a))

12. a   Antianxiety agent. (para 7-9c(2)(a))

13. c   Drowsiness. (para 7-9c(2)(b))

14. d   15 to 30 minutes. (para 7-8a(1))

End of Lesson 7

LESSON ASSIGNMENT

LESSON 8   Anticonvulsant Agents.

TEXT ASSIGNMENT   Paragraphs 8-1--8-5.

LESSON OBJECTIVES   After completing this lesson, you should be able to:

8-1.   Given one of the following terms: epilepsy or convulsions, and a group of statements, select the meaning of that term.

8-2.   Given a group of statements, select the statement that best differentiates between clonic and tonic convulsions.

8-3.   Give the name of a type of epilepsy and a group of descriptions, select the best description of that type of epilepsy.

8-4.   From a group of potential causes, select the cause(s) of epilepsy in either a child or an adult.

8-5.   Given a group of statements, select the statement that best describes the mechanism of action for anticonvulsants.

8-6.   Given the trade name of an anticonvulsant agent and a group of generic names, match the trade name with its generic name.

8-7.   Given a trade or generic name of an anticonvulsant agent and a group of statements, select the statement that best describes the clinical use(s) or adverse reaction(s) associated with that agent.

8-8.   Given a trade or generic name of an anticonvulsant agent, a description of a situation involving the dispensing of that agent, and a group of statements describing cautions and/or warnings to the patient, select the statement that should be made to the patient receiving that medication.

SUGGESTION   After completing the assignment, complete the
                        exercises at the end of this lesson. These exercises
                        will help you to achieve the lesson objectives.

LESSON 8

ANTICONVULSANT AGENTS

Section I. REVIEW OF EPILEPSY

8-1. BASIC DEFINITIONS

Before studying about anticonvulsants, you should review/study the definitions that relate to the topic:

a. **Epilepsy**. Epilepsy is a chronic convulsive disorder of cerebral function. Epilepsy is characterized by recurrent attacks of motor, sensory, psychic, or autonomic nature. The attacks may involve changes in the state of patient consciousness and are usually sudden in onset and brief.

b. **Convulsion**. A convulsion is a violent involuntary contraction or series of contractions of the voluntary muscles. There are two types of convulsions.

   (1) Clonic convulsions. A clonic convulsion has alternating periods of contraction and relaxation of the voluntary muscles.

   (2) Tonic convulsions. A tonic convulsion is a state of sustained contraction of voluntary muscles.

8-2. TYPES OF EPILEPSY

There are four types of epilepsy. Certain signs and symptoms characterize each type.

a. **Grand Mal.** Grand Mal is the most common type of epilepsy. In this type of epilepsy, the person often experiences an aura (this can consist of certain sounds, fear discomfort) immediately before a seizure. Then the patient loss consciousness and has tonic-clonic convulsions. The seizures generally last from 2 to 5 minutes.

b. **Petit Mal**. This type of epilepsy is most frequently found in children. Brief periods of blank spells or loss of speech characterizes petit mal. During the seizures, which usually last from 1 to 30 seconds, the person stops what he is doing and after the seizure resumes what he was doing before the seizure. Many persons are not aware that they have had a seizure.

c. **Jacksonian (Focal).** This type of epilepsy is rare. It is usually associated with an organic lesion of a certain part of the brain (cerebral cortex). Jacksonian epilepsy is characterized by focal or local clonic type convulsions of localized muscle groups (for example, thumb, big toe, and so forth). The seizures normally last from 1-2 minutes.

d. **Psychomotor.** Psychomotor epilepsy is rare. Psychomotor epilepsy is characterized by periods of abnormal types of behavior (for example, extensive chewing or swallowing). The localized seizures may advance to generalized convulsions with resultant loss of consciousness.

8-3. CAUSES OF EPILEPSY

a. **In Children.** Epilepsy that occurs in infancy usually results from developmental defects, metabolic diseases, or injuries sustained during birth.

b. **In Adults.** Epilepsy that begins in adulthood usually is caused by trauma (an accident), cerebrovascular accident (a "stroke"), tumors, or diseases associated with the brain.

Section II. ANTICONVULSANT THERAPY

8-4. MECHANISM OF ACTION OF ANTICONVULSANTS

The mode and the site of action anticonvulsants are not known for sure. However, it is believed that the anticonvulsants suppress seizures by depressing the cerebral (motor) cortex of the brain, thereby raising the threshold of the central nervous system (CNS) to convulsive stimuli. Therefore, the person is less likely to undergo seizures.

8-5. SPECIFIC ANTICONVULSANT DRUGS

a. **Phenobarbital.**

(1) Clinical uses. Phenobarbital is orally administered in the treatment of grand mal epilepsy. It is less effective in the treatment of petit mal and psychomotor epilepsy. The injectable from of the drug is used to treat other types of convulsions.

(2) Adverse effects. The most common adverse effects associated with phenobarbital are related to sedation and disinhibition (see lesson 7 of this subcourse). These include dizziness, drowsiness, ataxia (lack of muscular coordination), and nystagmus (a rapid involuntary movement of the eyeball). Furthermore, as discussed in lesson 7 of this subcourse, persons taking phenobarital can experience withdrawal symptoms when they suddenly stop taking the drug. Epileptic patients are unusually susceptible to the hyperexcitable state induced by too rapid reduction of dosage or too rapid withdrawal of phenobarbital.

(3) <u>Cautions and warnings</u>. Patients who take phenobarbital should be warned about drowsiness. Patients who take phenobarbital should not drink alcohol while taking phenobarbital. Dosage of the drug should be reduced by small amounts in order to avoid hastening convulsions. Lastly, phenobarbital may stimulate the activity of a number of enzyme systems and affect the metabolism of various drugs (for example, anticoagulants, phenytoin).

b. **Phenytoin (Dilantin®).**

(1) <u>Clinical uses.</u> Phenytoin is used alone or in combination with phenobarbital in the treatment of grand mal and psychomotor epilepsy. It is also used in the treatment of other types of convulsions.

(2) <u>Adverse effects.</u> Adverse effects associated with phenytoin include ataxia (lack of muscular coordination, staggering walk), nystagmus (a rapid, involuntary movement of the eyeball), and slurred speech. Drowsiness and fatigue may accompany these adverse effects in some patients by tremors and nervousness and in others.

(3) <u>Caution and warning</u>. Drug interactions can occur between phenytoin and alcohol, barbiturates, folic acid, coumarin-type anticoagulants, disulfirams, the sulfonamides, and sympathomimetic agents. Phenytoin should be used cautiously with patients who are alcoholics or who have blood dyscrasias.

c. **Ethosuximide (Zarontin®).**

(1) <u>Clinic use</u>. Ethosuxamide is the drug of first choice for the treatment of petit mal epilepsy.

(2) <u>Adverse effects</u>. Drowsiness, ataxia, and gastrointestinal irritation are adverse effects associated with the use of ethosuxamide.

(3) <u>Caution and warning</u>. Ethosuxamide should be used cautiously with patients who have blood dyscrasias or liver or kidney impairment.

d. **Clonazepam (Klonopin®).**

(1) <u>Clinical uses</u>. Clonazepam is used in the treatment of grand mal epilepsy. It is the alternate drug for the treatment of petit mal in patients who fail to respond to ethosuxamide (Zarontin®) therapy.

(2) <u>Adverse effects</u>. The primary side effect associated with clonazepam is central nervous system depression. Drowsiness is frequently seen in patients who take this medication.

e. **Diazepam (Valium®), lorazepam (Ativan®).**

(1) <u>Clinical uses</u>. Diazepam or lorazepam are drugs of first choice for the treatment of status epilepticus (a particular type of convulsive disorder) when it is given intravenously.

(2) <u>Adverse effects.</u> Drowsiness, fatigue, and ataxia are the most common adverse effects seen with diazepam.

NOTE: Midazolam (Versed®) may be used as a continuous infusion for the treatment of status epilepticus in patients that fail diazepam or lorazepam.

Continue with Exercises

EXERCISES, LESSON 8

INSTRUCTIONS: Answer the following exercises by marking the lettered response that best answers the exercise, by completing the incomplete statement, or by writing the answer in the space provided at the end of the exercise.

After you have completed all of these exercises, turn to "Solutions to Exercises" at the end of the lesson and check your answers. For each exercise answered incorrectly, reread the material referenced with the solution.

1. Which of the following statements best describes epilepsy?

    a.   A mental condition that can be transmitted from one person to another.

    b.   A chronic convulsive disorder of brain function.

    c.   A chronic mental condition that is always characterized by violent contractions of the involuntary muscles.

    d.   A condition that harms the brain in such a way that the person cannot live a normal life.

2. Which of the following statements best describes grand mal epilepsy?

    a.   A type of epilepsy characterized by brief periods of blank spells or loss speech.

    b.   A type of epilepsy characterized by focal or local clonic type convulsions of localized muscle groups (for example, thumb, big toe, and so forth).

    c.   A type of epilepsy characterized by seizures which generally last from 2 to 5 minutes.

    d.   A rare type of epilepsy characterized by periods of abnormal behavior (for example, extensive chewing).

3. Which of the following cause epilepsy in adults?

    a.   Tumors.

    b.   Trauma.

    c.   Cerebrovascular accident.

    d.   All the above.

4. The anticonvulsants act by _____.

      a.   Depressing the cerebral cortex of the brain, thereby lowering the threshold of the CNS to convulsive stimuli.

      b.   Stimulating the cerebral cortex of the brain, thereby raising the threshold of the CNS to convulsive stimuli.

      c.   Depressing the cerebral cortex of the brain, thereby raising the threshold of the CNS to convulsive stimuli.

      d.   Depressing the cerebral cortex of the brain, thereby deadening the part of the brain that is responsible for the seizures.

INSTRUCTIONS: For exercises 5 through 8, match the generic name with its corresponding trade name.

5. Clonazepam _____   a. Zarontin®

6. Diazepam _____   b. Klonopin®

7. Phenytoin _____   c. Valium®

8. Ethosuximide _____   d. Dilantin®

9. Phenobarbital is orally administered in the treatment of _____.

      a.   Grand mal epilepsy.

      b.   Petit mal epilepsy.

      c.   Jackson epilepsy.

      d.   Psychomotor epilepsy.

10. Patients who take phenobarbital should be cautioned not to_____.

    a. Take aspirin with the drug.

    b. Take the drug with meals.

    c. Take the medication immediately after a seizure.

    d. Take the medication with alcohol.

11. Which adverse effect(s) is/are associated with the use of ethosuximide?

    a. Dizziness.

    b. Ataxia.

    c. Nystagmus.

    d. All the above.

12. Which adverse effect(s) is/are associated with the use of phenytoin.

    a. Nystagmus.

    b. Ataxia.

    c. Slurred speech.

    d. All the above.

Check Your Answers on Next Page

SOLUTIONS TO EXERCISES, LESSON 8

1. b A chronic convulsive disorder of brain function. (para 8-1a)

2. c A type of epilepsy characterized by seizures, which generally last from 2 to 5, minutes. (para 8-2a)

3. d All the above. (para 8-3b)

4. c Depressing the cerebral cortex of the brain, thereby raising the threshold of the CNS to convulsive stimuli. (para 8-4)

5. b Klonopin®. (para 8-5d)

6. c Valium®. (para 8-5e)

7. d Dilantin®. (para 8-5b)

8. a Zarontin®. (para 8-5c)

9. a Grand mal epilepsy. (para 8-5a)

10. d Take the medication with alcohol. (para 8-5a(3))

11. b Ataxia. (para 8-5c(2))

12. d All the above. (para 8-5b(2))

End of Lesson 8

LESSON 9	Psychotherapeutic Agents.
TEXT ASSIGNMENT	Paragraphs 9-1--9-20.
LESSON OBJECTIVES	After completing this lesson, you should be able to:

9-1. Given a group of statements and one of the four classes of functional mental disorders, select the best description of that class of mental disorders.

9-2. From a group of statements, select the statement that best differentiates between fear and anxiety.

9-3. Given one of the following terms: fear, anxiety, antianxiety agent, depression, antidepressant, antipsychotic agent, or tranquilizer and a group of definitions, select the correct definition of that term.

9-4. Given one of the following categories of drugs: antianxiety agents, antidepressant agents, and antipsychotic agents and a group of statements that describe uses, advantages, disadvantages, adverse effects, or precautions and warnings select the statement that best describes the use(s) advantage(s), disadvantage(s), adverse effect(s), or caution(s) and warning(s) associated with that category of drug.

9-5. Given a group of statements, select the statement that best describes the advantages of antianxiety agents over drugs that were previously used to calm or sedate patients.

9-6. Given the generic and/or trade name of a psychotherapeutic agent and a group of uses, adverse effects, or cautions and warnings, select the use(s), adverse effects, or cautions and warnings associated with that agent.

SUGGESTION   After completing the assignment, complete the
                        exercises at the end of this lesson. These exercises
                        will help you to achieve the lesson objectives.

LESSON 9

PSYCHOTHERAPEUTIC AGENTS

Section I. OVERVIEW

9-1. INTRODUCTION

Stress, anxiety, and depression are frequently used words in today's world. Every living person has problems of one type or another. Some people seem to cope quite well with stress most of the time, while other persons need assistance to make adjustments to life. The wise use of psychotherapeutic agents has become an integral part of assisting others to adjust to certain situations. Of course, psychologists and psychiatrists combine other treatment means with the wise use of drugs in their efforts to help others.

9-2. THE FOUR MAJOR CLASSES OF FUNCTIONAL MENTAL DISORDERS

Later in this lesson, certain drugs and their uses will be discussed. In order for you to understand the use of some of the drugs, you must be aware of the four major classes of functional mental disorders.

NOTE: Reality testing is an ego function that consists of an individual's ability to recognize and interpret the surrounding world (that is, what's going on?). The ability to recognize and interpret the surrounding world allows an individual to meet the demands of life and make survival judgments.

a. Neuroses (Neurotic Disorders). Neuroses are a group of conditions characterized by the development of anxiety because of unresolved unconscious conflicts. The neurotic person is anxious, but he does not know the cause of his anxiety. These conditions tend to become chronic. Reality testing is maintained. That Is, the neurotic remains in touch with reality.

b. **Psychoses (Psychotic Disorders).** Psychoses are a group of disorders with more or less severe disturbances of thought, mood, and/or behavior. Psychoses are usually chronic, but short episodes of psychosis do sometimes occur. Reality testing is always lost in one or more important respects. That is, a psychotic is not entirely in touch with his environment.

c. **Personality Disorders.** Personality disorders are types of mental disorders characterized by lifelong maladaptive patterns of adjustment to life. These types of disorders tend to be chronic. Personality disorders are usually recognized by adolescence. Reality testing is usually preserved.

d.   **Transient Situational Disturbances (Adjustment Disorders).** Transient situational disturbances (TSD) are temporary emotional disorders of any severity, which occur as reactions to overwhelming environmental stress. Reality testing may or may not be impaired during the acute phase of these disorders.

9-3. TERMINOLOGY ASSOCIATED WITH PSYCHOTHERAPEUTIC AGENTS

Before discussing the various psychotherapeutic agents, some terms and their definitions will be presented. These terms will be used later in the discussion of the psychotherapeutic agents.

a.   **Fear**. Fear is a feeling of apprehension caused by a real object in the environment. For example, a person who is unexpectedly confronted with a rattlesnake would probably display fear of the snake. If you closely observed such a surprised person, you would see such signs as increased blood pressure, increased respiratory rate, and increased heart rate. These physiological responses are mediated by the sympathetic nervous system.

b.   **Anxiety**. Anxiety is a feeling of apprehension that has no specific object. Most people have experienced the feeling of anxiety that occurs during test-taking time. Anxiety has both positive and negative components. On the positive side, anxiety motivates you to study for the exam rather than to go to the movies. On the negative side, anxiety can interfere with performance on the examination (that is, "black outs" during a pencil and paper test). Interestingly enough, a person who is frightened (that is, with a snake) or is anxious (as with a test) will display the same body signs such as increased blood pressure, increased heart rate, and increased respiratory rate.

c.   **Antianxiety Agent**. An antianxiety agent is a drug that is used to calm a patient. Although the drug reduces the subjective feeling of anxiety, it will have no effect on the cause of the anxiety.

d.   **Depression**. Depression is a disturbance of mood manifested by decreased self-esteem, decreased vitality, and increased sadness.

e.   **Antidepressant**. An antidepressant is a drug that will, after a period, cause an improvement in a depressed patient's mood.

f.   **Antipsychotic Agent**. An antipsychotic agent is a drug that will reduce specific symptoms (that is, hallucinations, delusions) in patients experiencing a psychosis.

g.   **Tranquilizer**. The term tranquilizer refers to a wide-variety of drugs that produce a calming change in patient attitude and behavior. At one time, these drugs were categorized into two major categories: the major tranquilizers and the minor tranquilizers. The major tranquilizers are now generally referred to as antipsychotic agents and the minor tranquilizers are referred to as antianxiety agents.

Section II. ANTIANXIETY AGENTS

9-4. INTRODUCTION TO ANTIANXIETY AGENTS

It is not unusual for a person to experience stress and anxiety. Most people can deal with the minor stresses of life without using antianxiety agents. However, when the degree of anxiety increases to the point of causing social and/or economic impairment, the attending physician may decide to prescribe an antianxiety agent. It should be remembered that the antianxiety agent will calm the patient, but the drug cannot remove the cause of anxiety. Often the antianxiety therapy is combined with counseling or therapy to help the patient deal with the stress and anxiety.

9-5. INDICATIONS FOR ANTIANXIETY AGENTS

Antianxiety agents are indicated in patients to control moderate to severe degrees of anxiety. Antianxiety agents are also extremely useful in treating patients when periods of overwhelming stress occur.

9-6. USES OF ANTIANXIETY AGENTS

Antianxiety agents are used in a variety of situations. Listed below are some of those situations.

a. **Control Moderate to Severe Stress and Anxiety in Neurotic and Depressed Patients**. Some neurotic and depressed patients are prescribed antianxiety agents to reduce the amount of subjective anxiety; thus enabling them to more productively participate in counseling or therapy.

b. **Control Stress and Anxiety in Previously Normal Persons in Periods of Overwhelming Stress**. In most cases, normal individuals are able to cope with the stress and anxiety of life. However, when unusual circumstances of extreme stress arise, physicians sometimes prescribe antianxiety agents to assist people during these periods. Antianxiety agents should not be prescribed for dealing with the stresses of everyday life (Food and Drug Administration ruling).

c. **Treat Withdrawal Symptoms in Alcoholism.** These agents are very effective in the treatment of delirium tremens associated with the withdrawal of alcohol from alcoholics.

d. **Treat Psychotic Patients in Periods of Acute Agitation.** Sometimes patients who have certain psychotic conditions undergo periods of acute agitation. Antianxiety agents are used to calm these types of patients during these periods. Thus, the patients become much more manageable. Generally speaking, antipsychotic drugs are more effective when used for this particular purpose.

e. **Decrease Preoperative and Postoperative Apprehension**. Patients who will undergo or have undergone surgery frequently have periods of apprehension. Antianxiety agents have been used to reduce this type of stress and tension.

9-7. ADVANTAGES OF THE USE OF ANTIANXIETY AGENTS

Anti-anxiety agents have two main advantages over drugs that were previously used to calm or sedate patients:

a. **Antianxiety Agents Do Not Cause Excessive Loss of Alertness**. Barbiturates were frequently used to calm patients. Unfortunately, the barbiturates sometimes calmed the patients to an undesirable degree. Although the antianxiety agents produce some degree of sedation during the initial days of therapy, this sedation is usually short-lived.

b. **Overdosage of Antianxiety Agents Rarely Results in Death to the Patient**. As previously stated, the barbiturates were previously used to calm patients. Unfortunately, overdose of barbiturates can frequently result in coma, respiratory depression, and death. Antianxiety agents, on the other hand, are somewhat safe in terms of the amount of drug required to produce coma, respiratory depression, and death. This factor makes the wise use of antianxiety agents in special circumstances useful in the treatment of extremely anxious patients who are entertaining thoughts about suicide.

9-8. DISADVANTAGES OF THE USE OF ANTIANXIETY AGENTS

Although the antianxiety agents do have many advantages over previously used drugs, they are not free from potentially harmful effects. The discussion below focuses on two major disadvantages of the group of drugs classified as antianxiety agents.

a. **Drowsiness.** Antianxiety agents, especially during the first few days of therapy, produce drowsiness in many patients. Further, many patients who take antianxiety drugs experience loss of judgment and a loss of mental powers. Consequently, patients who are on antianxiety therapy should be cautioned not to operate machinery.

b. **Drug Interaction Effects**. The antianxiety agents can interact with central nervous system depressants to produce a further degree of depression to the central nervous system. Thus, patients who are on antianxiety therapy should be cautioned against drinking alcohol or taking other central nervous system depressants.

9-9. EXAMPLES OF ANTIANXIETY AGENTS

This area of the subcourse is designed to provide you with a brief overview of some commonly prescribed antianxiety agents. If you desire further information about the agents discussed below, you should consult a reference (for example, <u>AMA Drug Evaluations</u>) which is well written and easy to understand.

a.   **Chlordiazepoxide Hydrochloride (Librium®).**

(1)   <u>Uses.</u> Chlordiazepoxide hydrochloride is widely used as an antianxiety agent to help people deal with stress. Further, it is used preoperatively to reduce patient apprehension. As an antianxiety agent, it has less anticonvulsant activity, and it produces less drowsiness than diazepam, another antianxiety drug.

(2)   <u>Adverse effects.</u> Chlordiazepoxide is likely to produce such adverse effects as drowsiness and lethargy. These adverse effects are more likely to occur in older patients.

(3)   <u>Cautions and warnings.</u> Patients taking chlordiazepoxide should be cautioned not to take a central nervous system depressant like alcohol since the additive effect might produce depression of the central nervous system. Furthermore, patients taking chlordiazepoxide should be cautioned against operating machinery (for example, driving an automobile).

b.   **Diazepam (Valium®).**

(1)   <u>Uses.</u> Diazepam is widely used for the treatment of anxiety and tension. Further, it is used in the treatment of muscle spasms.

(2)   <u>Adverse effects</u>. Diazepam produces such adverse effects as drowsiness,   fatigue, and ataxia (lack of coordination). Physical dependence can develop over a period with resultant withdrawal symptoms to include seizures.

(3)   <u>Cautions and warnings</u>. An individual taking diazepam should be cautioned against taking central nervous system depressants (that is, alcohol) and operating machinery.

c.   **Lorazepam (Ativan®).**

(1)   <u>Uses.</u> Lorazepam is primarily used in the treatment of anxiety.

(2)   <u>Adverse effects.</u> Lorazepam produces such adverse effects as drowsiness, fatigue, and ataxia (lack of coordination). Physical dependence can develop over a period of time with resultant withdrawal symptoms to include seizures.

(3)   <u>Cautions and warnings.</u> An individual taking lorazepam should be cautioned against taking central nervous system depressants (that is, alcohol) and operating machinery.

d. **Alprazolam (Xanax®).**

(1) <u>Uses.</u> Alprazolam is primarily used in the treatment of anxiety and has been useful in the management of panic attacks.

(2) <u>Adverse effects</u>. Alprazoam produces such adverse effects as drowsiness, fatigue, and ataxia (lack of coordination). Physical dependence can develop over a period with resultant withdrawal symptoms to include seizures.

(3) <u>Cautions and warnings</u>. An individual taking alprazolam should be cautioned against taking central nervous system depressants (that is, alcohol) and operating machinery.

e. **Hydroxyzine Hydrochloride (Atarax®) or Hydroxyzine Pamoate (Vistaril®).**

(1) <u>Uses</u>. Hydroxyzine has the following three primary uses:

(a) Antianxiety agent. The drug is used to treat anxiety, tension, and agitation.

(b) Antiemetic agent. Because hydroxyzine does have some antiemetic (antinausea and vomiting) properties, it is used in its injectable form (hydroxyzine pamoate) to manage postoperative nausea and vomiting.

(c) Antipruritic agent. Hydroxyzine has been used because of its antipruritic (anti-itch) properties.

NOTE: Atarax® is sometimes used as a sedative.

(2) <u>Adverse effects</u>. There is an extremely low incidence of adverse reactions with this drug. Some drowsiness may occur during the initial days of therapy; however, this drowsiness is short-lived.

(3) <u>Cautions and warnings</u>. An individual taking hydroxyzine should be cautioned against drinking alcohol and taking other central nervous system depressants because of the additive effect that may be produced. Furthermore, persons taking this drug should be cautioned against operating machinery (for example, driving an automobile).

f. **Buspirone (Buspar®).**

(1) <u>Uses</u>. Buspirone is used in the management of anxiety or the short term relief of symptoms of anxiety. It is unrelated to the benzodiazepines and therefore lacks the sedative and addictive properties of these agents.

(2) Adverse effects. The most common adverse effects include dizziness, nausea, and headache.

(3) Cautions and warnings. Although buspirone does not produce significant drowsiness, patients should be cautioned about driving or operating machinery until they are certain that this drug does not affect them adversely.

NOTE: Antidepressants, which are discussed in the next section, are becoming the agents of choice for anxiety disorders.

Section III. ANTIDEPRESSANT AGENTS

9-10. INTRODUCTION TO ANTIDEPRESSANT AGENTS

Depression is a frequently occurring psychiatric disorder. Patients with medical and surgical conditions frequently have signs and symptoms associated with depression. People who are depressed usually have low moods, decreased physical activity and mental alertness, decreased appetite, abnormal sleep patterns, and morbid preoccupations. Depression can be of rapid or slow onset. For example, a soldier who has been denied leave might display several signs of depression. This type of depression could be of rapid onset.

9-11. INDICATIONS FOR ANTIDEPRESSANT AGENTS

a. Most people undergo changes in mood. You can probably remember when you have been "up" (that is, right before a three-day weekend) and when you have been "down" (that is, right after a three-day weekend). Physicians have found antidepressant agents to be useful in the treatment of depression, which is not time limited and causes the patient social and economic difficulties.

b. Depression can be caused by chemical imbalances in the body, by stress, and by situations in the environment. It has been found that psychotherapy, reduction of stress, and improvement in the environment can be successful in treating some types of depression. However, in depression that results from chemical imbalances in the body, these types of treatment have not proven to be very effective.

9-12. EFFECTS OF ANTIDEPRESSANT AGENTS

Antidepressant agents elevate mood, increase physical activity and mental alertness, improve appetite and sleep patterns, and reduce morbid preoccupations. These effects are not seen immediately upon beginning antidepressant therapy. Instead, one to four weeks may pass before the patient shows any signs of improvement in the depression. This period is called the therapeutic lag period.

9-13. PRECAUTIONS ASSOCIATED WITH THE USE OF ANTIDEPRESSANT AGENTS

Although the antidepressant agents are safe for patient use, there are some precautions associated with their use:

a. Antidepressants should be used cautiously with patients who are hyperactive or agitated.

b. Antidepressants should be used cautiously with the elderly, with patients who have glaucoma, and with patients who have hypertension (high blood pressure).

c. Antidepressants may interact with other types of drugs. For example, references should be consulted to determine if any interaction could occur between a particular antidepressant and a drug a patient is taking to control high blood pressure, since some antidepressants partially block the action of some antihypertensive drugs. In addition, the action of some drugs (that is, the barbiturates) is increased in duration when they are administered to patients who are taking certain antidepressant agents.

9-14. SPECIFIC ANTIDEPRESSANT AGENTS

Immediately following is a discussion of several antidepressant agents. By no means is the listing below complete in terms of the number of agents available to the physician. Further, no attempt has been made to provide an in-depth discussion of each individual agent. If you desire additional information about any of the agents discussed below, you should consult a pharmacology reference (for example, AMA Drug Evaluations).

a. **Fluoxetine (Prozac®).**

(1) Uses. Fluoxetine belongs to a class of antidepressants called Selective Serotonin Reuptake Inhibitors (SSRIs). SSRIs are usually regarded as the treatment of choice for depression due to fewer side effects and a better safety profile than older agents. Fluoxetine is used to treat depression and anxiety disorders. The Serafem® product is approved for premenstrual dysphoric disorder (PMDD).

(2) Adverse effects. Fluoxetine may produce the following adverse effects:

(a) Miscellaneous effects (that is, sexual dysfunction).

(b) Central nervous system effects (for example, agitation and insomnia).

(c) Gastrointestinal effects (that is, nausea and diarrhea).

(3) Cautions and warnings.

      (a) Do not overlap with other antidepressants or monoamine oxidase inhibitors.

      (b) The drug may produce drowsiness.

      (c) The patient should not consume any alcohol while taking the drug.

NOTE: Other SSRIs include sertraline (Zoloft®), paroxetine (Paxil®), citalopram (Celexa®), and fluvoxamine (Luvox®).

b. **Imipramine Hydrochloride (Tofranil®).**

(1) Uses. Imipramine is used to treat depression; however, it can paradoxically aggravate the anxiety sometimes associated with depression. Imipramine also produces an anticholinergic effect and is therefore approved by the Food and Drug Administration (FDA) for the treatment of enuresis (bedwetting) in children.

(2) Adverse effects. Imipramine may produce the following adverse effects:

      (a) Cardiovascular effects (that is, orthostatic hypotension).

      (b) Central nervous system effects (for example, confusion and anxiety).

      (c) Gastrointestinal effects (that is, nausea and vomiting).

      (d) Anticholinergic effects (for example, dry mouth and constipation).

(3) Cautions and warnings.

      (a) Abruptly taking the drug away from the patient after long-term therapy may produce withdrawal symptoms.

      (b) The drug may produce drowsiness.

      (c) The patient should not consume any alcohol while taking the drug.

      (d) The drug should be used with caution in patients with glaucoma or urinary retention because of its anticholinergic effects.

c. **Desipramine (Norpramin®).**

(1) Uses. Desipramine is used to treat depression. It has also been used in facilitating withdrawal from cocaine.

(2) Adverse effects. Desipramine is closely related to imipramine but has only minimal cardiovascular, CNS, GI, and anticholinergic effects.

(3) Cautions and warnings.

(a) Abruptly taking the drug away from the patient after long-term therapy may produce withdrawal symptoms.

(b) The drug may produce drowsiness.

(c) The patient should not consume any alcohol while taking the drug.

(d) The drug should be used with caution in patients with glaucoma or urinary retention because of its anticholinergic effects.

d. **Amitriptyline Hydrochloride (Elavil®).**

(1) Uses. Amitriptyline is used in the treatment of depression and neuropathic pain syndromes.

(2) Adverse effects. Amitriptyline tends to cause confusion in elderly patients. In addition, it has other adverse effects that are similar to those produced by imipramine hydrochloride.

(3) Cautions and warnings.

(a) Abruptly taking the drug away from the patient after long-term therapy may produce withdrawal symptoms.

(b) The drug may produce drowsiness.

(c) The patient should not consume any alcohol while taking the drug.

(d) The drug should be used with caution in patients who have glaucoma or urinary retention due to its anticholinergic effects.

(4) Precautions. Amitriptyline can be cardiotoxic to some individuals.

d. **Nortriptyline Hydrochloride (Aventyl®).**

(1) Uses. Nortriptyline is used in the treatment of depression and neuropathic pain disorders.

(2) Adverse effects. The adverse effects produced by nortriptyline are the same as those produced by imipramine hydrochloride (see para 9-14b).

(3) Cautions and warnings. The adverse effects produced by nortriptyline are the same as those produced by imipramine hydrochloride (see para 9-14b).

e. **Trazodone (Desyrel®).**

(1) Uses. Trazodone is used in the treatment of depression. It is unrelated to any of the antidepressants discussed thus far.

(2) Adverse effects. The adverse effects produced by trazodone include skin rash, chest pain, drowsiness, tachycardia, vivid dreams/nightmares, and muscle aches.

(3) Cautions and warnings. Trazodone may produce drowsiness and may cause irregular heartbeat. The patient should observe caution when driving or performing other tasks requiring alertness. Alcohol and other depressant drugs should be avoided while taking trazodone.

f. **Nefazodone Hydrochloride (Serzone®).**

(1) Uses. Nefazodone hydrochloride is an oral antidepressant that is totally unrelated to the other available antidepressants.

(2) Adverse effects. The adverse effects of nefazodone hydrochloride are similar to selective serotonin reuptake inhibitors.

(3) Contraindications.

(a) The drug is contraindicated in patients who are taking other monoamine oxidase (MAO) inhibitors, and those having hypersensitivity to nefazodone or other phenylpiperazine antidepressants.

(b) The drug is contraindicated on patients who are taking nonsedating antihistimines (that is, Terfenadine and Astemizole).

(4) Cautions and warnings. Patients taking nefazodone hydrocloride should be cautioned against the following:

(a) The drug may produce drowsiness.

(b)   The patient should not consume any alcohol while taking the drug.

(c)   Patients with cardiovascular or cerebrovascular disease that could be exacerbated by hypotension should use with caution.

(d)   The potential for a fatal outcome is significantly increased by the concurrent use of alprazolam and triazolam.

Section IV. ANTIPSYCHOTIC AGENTS

9-15. INTRODUCTION TO ANTIPSYCHOTIC AGENTS

The general term psychoses encompass a wide variety of conditions. Each specific condition has particular signs and/or symptoms that assist the psychiatrist in making a diagnosis. Some psychotic conditions require long-term hospitalization, while others can be managed on an outpatient basis. Many psychotic patients show marked disorganization of thought patterns and behavior with either increased or decreased psychomotor activity. Antipsychotic agents help psychotic patients better organize their thoughts and coordinate their motor activities. In some cases, the use of antipsychotic agents can mean the difference between hospitalization and home-care.

9-16. INDICATIONS FOR USE OF ANTIPSYCHOTIC AGENTS

In order for an antipsychotic agent to be wisely used to treat a psychotic patient, the attending psychiatrist must carefully examine the patient and diagnose the specific condition. Proper diagnosis is the key word for beginning drug therapy for the psychotic patient.

9-17. USES OF ANTIPSYCHOTIC AGENTS

a.   The antipsychotic agents are used to treat various conditions of psychosis. When used in this manner, they help reduce the patient's fear, panic, and hostility. With this help, the patient is better able to organize life and more realistically respond to the environment.

b.   Some antipsychotic agents are used as adjuncts in anesthesia to control nausea and vomiting.

c.   The state of psychotic hyperarousal is the first group of symptoms to respond to antipsychotic medication. Delusions and hallucinations resolve more gradually over a period.

9-18. ADVERSE EFFECTS ASSOCIATED WITH ANTIPSYCHOTIC AGENTS

As with most drugs, the antipsychotic agents produce some adverse effects. Discussed below are some of those reactions:

a. **Extrapyramidal Reactions**. Extrapyramidal reactions are manifested by a parkinson-like syndrome. That is, the patient has tremors, muscular rigidity, postural abnormalities, pill-rolling movements with the fingers, and hypersalivation. Fortunately, these symptoms may be relieved or lessened, or the reactions may be prevented before they occur by the administration of diphenhydramine (Benadryl).

b. **Drowsiness, Dizziness, and Fatigue**. Although a sedative-effect is produced by many of the antipsychotic agents, this effect is short-lived because tolerance develops after one to three days.

c. **Orthostatic Hypotension.** Orthostatic hypotension (low blood pressure) is an adverse reaction produced by some of the antipsychotic agents. Patients experiencing this problem are at risk of fainting and injuring themselves.

d. **Anticholinergic Effects.**

9-19. DOSAGE PRINCIPLE ASSOCIATED WITH THE ANTIPSYCHOTIC AGENTS

You should be familiar with a dosage principle associated with the antipsychotic agents. This principle is: "High dosage-low potency/low dosage-high potency."

a. **High Dosage/Low Potency.** Initially when treating a psychotic patient, a psychiatrist might choose to select a drug that can be given in a high dosage (large amount of drug) because of its low potency. This allows the psychiatrist some freedom in dosage-especially if the patient is uncontrollable--without potential harm to the patient. High dosage/low potency drugs usually have a high incidence of anticholinergic side effects, but low incidence of extrapyramidal side effects.

b. **Low Dosage/High Potency.** After a patient has been on one antipsychotic agent and has been stabilized, the psychiatrist may choose to use another agent that can be given in smaller amounts (low dosage) because of its high potency. Usually, more potent drugs are easier to administer (that is, in tablet form). Low dosage/high potency drugs usually have a low incidence of anticholinergic side effects, but high incidence of extrapyramidal side effects

9-20. SPECIFIC ANTIPSYCHOTIC AGENTS

a. **Chlorpromazine (Thorazine®).**

(1) <u>Uses</u>. Chlorpromazine is a phenothiazine drug (a particular class of drugs) used in the treatment of acute and chronic psychoses. It is also used as a pre- or postoperative agent in the prevention of nausea and vomiting.

(2) <u>Adverse effects</u>. Chlorpromazine produces three major adverse effects:

(a) Extrapyramidal reactions. These reactions are frequently seen in both young and elderly patients who are taking large doses of the drug.

(b) Drowsiness.

(c) Orthostatic hypotension. Orthostatic hypotension is most likely to occur when the patient has been administered the drug intravenously. This can be prevented by having the patient remain reclined for at least one hour after the administration of the drug.

(d) Dryness of the mouth.

(3) <u>Cautions and warnings</u>. Chlorpromazine should not be prescribed to patients who have liver disease or glaucoma. Furthermore, patients taking the drug should be cautioned not to drink alcoholic beverages.

b. **Fluphenazine Hydrochloride (Prolixin®, Permitil®).**

(1) <u>Use</u>. Fluphenazine hydrochloride is used in the treatment of psychotic disorders.

(2) <u>Adverse effects</u>.

(a) Extrapyramidal reactions.

(b) Drowsiness or lethargy.

(c) Hypertension (increased blood pressure).

(3) <u>Cautions and warnings</u>. Abrupt withdrawal of the drug may result in nausea and vomiting, gastritis, and dizziness.

c. **Thioridazine Hydrochloride (Mellaril®).**

(1) <u>Use</u>. This is a phenothiazine used to treat acute and chronic types of psychosis. Thioridazine is safe in treating psychotic patients who also have liver disease.

(2) <u>Adverse effects</u>. Thioridazine produces the following adverse effects:

(a) Sedation and lethargy.

(b) Gastric irritation.

d. **Perphenazine (Trilafon®).**

(1) <u>Uses</u>. Perphenazine is used in the management of psychotic disorders.

(2) <u>Adverse effects</u>. Perphenazine, like chlorpromazine, can produce extrapyramidal reactions, orthostatic hypotension, drowsiness, and dry mouth (drowsiness and orthostatic hypotension are less than that seen with chlorpromazine).

(3) <u>Cautions and warnings</u>. Perphenazine may cause drowsiness. Patients should avoid alcohol and other CNS depressants while taking this drug.

e. **Trifluoperazine Hydrochloride (Stelazine®).**

(1) <u>Use</u>. This phenothiazine is used in the treatment of various types of acute and chronic psychoses. This drug is used primarily in the maintenance treatment of psychotic patients.

(2) <u>Adverse effects</u>. Two adverse effects are produced by this drug:

(a) Drowsiness may occur with the use of this drug.

(b) Extrapyramidal reactions may occur with the use of this drug.

(3) <u>Cautions and warnings</u>. The following cautions and warnings are associated with trifluoperazine:

(a) The use of alcohol with this agent should be avoided because of the possible interaction between the two substances.

(b) Since the drug can produce sedation, the patient should be cautioned against operating vehicles while under the effects of this drug.

f. **Haloperidol (Haldol®).**

(1) Use. This drug is used in the treatment of acute and chronic psychosis. In its parenteral (injectable) form (10 milligrams per milliliter of solution), haloperidol is a potent antipsychotic medication which is well suited for emergency room use. Haloperidol can be safely prescribed to patients who have liver disease.

NOTE: Haloperidol is considered the gold standard for antipsychotics.

(2) Adverse effects. Two adverse effects are seen with this drug:

(a) Extrapyramidal reactions.

(b) Depression, anxiety, and/or dizziness.

g. **Lithium Carbonate (Eskalith®, Lithane®).**

(1) Use. Lithium carbonate is used in the treatment of manic-depressive psychosis. After initial administration, approximately 7 to 10 days are required before the effects of the drug can be observed in the patient.

(2) Adverse effects. The following are some of the adverse effects associated with lithium carbonate:

IMPORTANT NOTE: The level of lithium carbonate in the bloodstream of the patient is very significant. The severity of the toxic symptoms tends to increase as the level of the drug in the patient's blood increases.

(a) Nausea, vomiting, cramps diarrhea.

(b) Drowsiness and muscular weakness.

(c) Tremors.

(d) Height loss or weight gain.

(3) Cautions and warnings. Cautions and warnings associated with the use of this agent are:

(a) Patients who are administered lithium carbonate should be kept under close medical supervision at all times. This is necessary because the amount of drug required to produce the desired effects is very close to the amount of drug that will produce toxic effects.

(b)   Blood levels of lithium carbonate should always be performed at regular intervals to ensure that the appropriate therapeutic levels of the drug are maintained.

(c)   Lithium carbonate should not be administered to patients who are taking diuretics (that is, some antihypertensive medications), because diuretics tend to cause an accumulation of the drug, and toxic levels of the drug could rapidly occur.

(d)   The efficacy (clinical effectiveness) of lithium carbonate in the treatment of the depressive phase of manic depressive illness remains controversial. The drug is the most effective treatment for true bipolar illness, particularly in the control of manic episodes. The drug is not effective in established depressed episodes. It may prevent reoccurrence of both manic and depressive episodes.

(e)   Drowsiness. Patients taking the drug should be cautioned against operating heavy machinery (for example, driving an automobile).

h.   **Risperidone (Risperdal®).**

(1)   Use. This drug belongs to the class of antipsychotics called "atypical". They are used for treatment resistance in older agents and reduce the likelihood of extrapyramidal side effects. They may be used as first line agents.

(2)   Adverse effects. Adverse effects seen with this drug are:

(a)   Extrapyramidal reactions.

(b)   Orthostatic hypotension.

NOTE: Other atypical antipsychotics include Olazapine (Zyprexa®), Clozapine (Clozaril®), and Quetiapine (Seroquel®).

Continue with Exercises

EXERCISES, LESSON 9

INSTRUCTIONS: Answer the following exercises by marking the lettered response that best answers the exercise, by completing the incomplete statement, or by writing the answer in the space provided at the end of the exercise.

After you have completed all of these exercises, turn to "Solutions to Exercises" at the end of the lesson and check your answers. For each exercise answered incorrectly, reread the material referenced with the solution.

1. Select the best description of personality disorders.

    a. Types of conditions characterized by the development of anxiety because of unresolved unconscious conflicts.

    b. Temporary emotional disorders that occur as reactions to overwhelming environmental stress.

    c. Types of mental disorders characterized by lifelong maladaptive patterns of adjustment to life.

    d. A group of disorders with more or less severe disturbances of thought, mood, and/or behavior.

2. From the statements below, select the statement that best differentiates between fear and anxiety.

    a. Fear is a feeling of apprehension caused by a real object in the environment, while anxiety is a feeling of apprehension that has no specific object in the environment.

    b. Fear and anxiety produce entirely different physiological reactions.

    c. Fear cannot be controlled, while anxiety can be controlled without the use of drugs.

    d. Fear is a feeling of apprehension that has no specific object in the environment, while anxiety is a feeling of apprehension caused by a real object in the environment.

3. Select the correct definition of the term antianxiety agent.

    a. A drug used to improve the depressed mood of a patient.

    b. A drug used to calm a patient.

    c. A drug which will reduce certain symptoms such as hallucinations and delusions.

    d. A drug which will remove a patient's fear.

4. Select the statement that best describes the use(s) of antidepressant agents.

    a. The treatment of depression that results because of chemical imbalances in the body.

    b. The treatment of depression that is not a result of chemical imbalances in the body.

    c. The treatment of patients who are experiencing periods of overwhelming stress.

    d. The treatment of acute and chronic psychoses.

5. Select the statement that best describes the adverse effects associated with antipsychotic agents.

    a. Antipsychotic agents are noted for the lack of adverse effects they produce.

    b. Antipsychotic agents can cause severe stimulation in many patients.

    c. Antipsychotic agents produce orthostatic hypertension.

    d. Antipsychotic agents can produce reactions that consist of tremors, muscular rigidity, and hypersalivation.

6. Select the statement that best describes the disadvantage(s) of antianxiety agents.

    a. Antianxiety agents can produce drowsiness in patients and can interact with central nervous system (CNS) depressants to produce a greater degree of CNS depression.

    b. Antianxiety agents produce an excessive loss of alertness.

    c. Because of their side effects, overdosage of antianxiety agents frequently results in death.

    d. Antianxiety agents produce tremors, muscular rigidity, and hypersalivation in many patients.

7. From the statements below, select the statement which best describes the advantage(s) of antianxiety agents over drugs which were previously used to calm or sedate patients.

    a. Antianxiety agents do not cause excessive loss of alertness.

    b. Antianxiety agents can be safely taken while driving or operating machinery.

    c. Overdosage of antianxiety agents rarely results in death to the patient.

    d. Both a and c.

    e. Both b and c.

8. Select the use of hydroxyzine hydrochloride (Atarax®).

    a. Antidiarrheal agent.

    b. Antianxiety agent.

    c. Antipsychotic agent.

    d. Antipyretic agent.

9.   Select the statement that best describes an adverse reaction associated with haloperidol (Haldol®).

   a. This drug may cause extrapyramidal reactions.

   b. This drug may produce hypotension.

   c. This drug may produce overstimulation.

   d. This drug may produce withdrawal.

10. Select the statement which best describes the use(s) associated with chlorpromazine (Thorazine®):

   a. The drug is used to treat acute and chronic types of psychosis.

   b. The drug is used as an antiemetic to prevent pre- or postoperative nausea and vomiting.

   c. The drug is used as an antianxiety agent.

   d. a and b.

   e. b and c.

Check Your Answers on Next Page

SOLUTIONS TO EXERCISES, LESSON 9

1. c Types of mental disorders characterized by lifelong maladaptive patterns of adjustment to life. (para 9-2c)

2. a Fear is a feeling of apprehension caused by a real object in the environment, while anxiety is a feeling of apprehension which has no specific object in the environment. (para 9-3a, b)

3. b A drug used to calm a patient. (para 9-3c)

4. b The treatment of depression that is not a result of chemical imbalances in the body. (para 9-11b)

5. d Antipsychotic agents can produce reactions that consist of tremors, muscular rigidity, and hypersalivation. (para 9-18a)

6. a Anxiety agents can produce drowsiness in patients and can interact with central nervous system (CNS) depressants to produce a greater degree of CNS depression. (para 9-8a, b)

7. e Both b and c. (para 9-7a, b)

8. b Antianxiety agent. (para 9-9e)

9. a This drug may cause extrapyramidal reactions. (para 9-20f)

10. d Both a and b. (para 9-20a)

End of Lesson 9

LESSON 10	Central Nervous System Stimulants.
TEXT ASSIGNMENT	Paragraphs 10-1--10-9.
LESSON OBJECTIVES	After completing this lesson, you should be able to:

10-1.　Given several categories, select the category(ies) of central nervous system (CNS) stimulants.

10-2.　Given a group of possible effects, select the pharmacological effect associated with xanthine derivatives.

10-3.　Given the trade name of a CNS stimulant and a group of generic names, match the trade name with its generic name.

10-4.　Given the trade or generic name of a CNS stimulant and a group of possible clinical uses, side effects, or cautions and warnings, select the clinical use, side effect, or caution and warning associated with that agent.

SUGGESTION	After completing the assignment, complete the exercises at the end of this lesson. These exercises will help you to achieve the lesson objectives.

LESSON 10

CENTRAL NERVOUS SYSTEM STIMULANTS

Section I. BACKGROUND

10-1. INTRODUCTION TO THE CENTRAL NERVOUS SYSTEM

a. Many people are familiar with the class of drugs known as CNS stimulants. Unfortunately, most people are aware of these agents because of the abuse/misuse associated with these drugs. The central nervous system stimulants do have a variety of medically approved uses. This subcourse lesson will focus on those uses.

b. This lesson will introduce you to the topic of CNS stimulants, how they act, their approved uses, and drugs representative of the drug class. Much has been written on CNS stimulants. If you wish to learn more about these agents, you should obtain an appropriate reference (see the lesson on reference selection, lesson 1 of this subcourse).

10-2. OTHER DRUGS WHICH ACT UPON THE CENTRAL NERVOUS SYSTEM

This lesson will focus on drugs that <u>stimulate</u> the central nervous system. There are, as you know, many classes of drugs that have other effects on the central nervous system. These drug classes include sedative and hypnotic agents (lesson 7), antianxiety agents (lesson 9), and anti-psychotic agents (lesson 9), centrally acting skeletal muscle relaxants (SC MD0805), and anticonvulsants (lesson 8). You should be familiar with the types of responses produced by these agents because, as you know, patients take a variety of medications. Some combinations of medications may not be desirable.

10-3. CLASSIFICATION OF CENTRAL NERVOUS SYSTEM (STIMULANTS)

a. Central nervous system stimulants excite the nerve cells of the central nervous system. These agents are classified according to their main site of action and their primary pharmacological effects. Following are the three categories of agents:

      (1) Cerebral of psychomotor agents.

      (2) Analeptics (brain stem stimulants).

      (3) Convulsants (spinal cord stimulants).

b.   As you might anticipate, when increasingly larger doses of a drug are administered to the patient, the effects produced by the drug cause stimulation of more than one area.

c.   Some central nervous system stimulants produce high levels of stimulation at other sites in the body (for example, the heart). In some cases, the usefulness of several CNS agents is limited because of the stimulation they produce in body organs.

Section II. CEREBRAL OR PSYCHOMOTOR AGENTS

10-4. INTRODUCTION

A variety of agents are classified as cerebral or psychomotor central nervous system agents. These drugs have one characteristic in common: they primarily stimulate the cerebral cortex of the brain.

10-5. CLASSES OF CEREBRAL OR PSYCHOMOTOR CENTRAL NERVOUS SYSTEM STIMULANTS

a.   **The Xanthine Derivatives**. The xanthine derivatives have several pharmacological effects. One, they directly relax the smooth muscle of the bronchi and pulmonary blood vessels. By such dilation of the bronchi, more oxygen can be drawn into the lungs. Two, they stimulate the central nervous system and produce diuresis (they increase the production of urine) by direct action on the kidney. There are several examples of xanthine derivatives:

(1)   Caffeine. Caffeine is found in coffee, tea, and in kola nuts (used to make some soft drinks). Caffeine is a stimulant that has been long used as a morning "picker-upper" for workers and students. Caffeine is found in some headache remedies products promoted to prevent drowsiness, and in some products designed to suppress appetite (in these preparations caffeine acts to stimulate the person). Although caffeine does have some desirable qualities (that is, small doses of the drug can promote better performance on tasks like typing and thinking), it is possible for a person to develop a psychological dependence on the drug. Withdrawal of the drug results in some persons' having mild withdrawal symptoms (for example, headaches).

(2)   Aminophylline (Theophylline ethylenediamine). This drug is used in the treatment of bronchial asthma. It is given intravenously to provide rapid relief of pulmonary edema and dyspnea seen in the acute congestive heart failure patient because it increases cardiac output, slightly increases venous pressure, and relaxes the bronchial muscle. Side effects associated with the oral administration of this agent include nausea, vomiting, and nervousness. The patient should be informed to take this medication with food. The medication is supplied in 100 and 200-milligram tablets, 250

and 500-milligram suppositories, and in injectable form (25 milligrams per milliliter in a 10-milliliter ampule).

(3)   Theophylline (Theo-dur®, Elixophyllin®). This xanthine derivative is used for the symptomatic relief of asthma because of its bronchial dilation effect. Theolair is but only one of many anhydrous theophylline products in use today. The side effects usually associated with the use of the drug are nausea, vomiting, and nervousness. The patient should be told to take theophylline with food. The drug is usually administered in a dosage of 3 to 5 milligrams per kilogram of body weight. It is supplied in various dosage forms (elixir, tablets, capsules, and sprinkles).

b.   **The Amphetamines.** Many health care professionals are concerned about the abuse/misuse of the amphetamines. These Schedule II medications certainly have been abused in the past. Today, physicians and pharmacists cooperate to ensure these drugs are wisely used for medically acceptable purposes. Amphetamines act pharmacologically to produce two primary effects. One, they increase an individual's state of alertness. Two, they elevate a person's mood. Now, several agents will be discussed. The particular use(s) for each agent will be presented.

(1)   Methylphenidate (Ritalin®). Methylphenidate (Ritalin®) is used to treat attention deficit hyperactivity disorder (ADHD), formerly known as minimal brain dysfunction, and narcolepsy. Observed abnormalities in ADHD include impulsiveness, short attention span, purposeless hyperactivity, emotional overreactivity, coordination and learning deficits, distractibility, and deficits in the perception of space, form, movement, and time. Since the first clinical sign seen with ADHD is purposeless hyperactivity, the terms hyperkinetic and hyperkinesia are sometimes used in place of attention deficit hyperactivity disorder (ADHD). Narcolepsy can be defined as an inability to stay awake. The most common side effect associated with this agent is nervousness. Methylphenidate is a Schedule II drug (Note R). The usual dosage of methylphenidate is 20 to 30 milligrams daily in divided doses. It is supplied in the form of 5 milligram, 10 milligram, and 20-milligram tablets.

(2)   Dextroamphetamine sulfate (Dexedrine®). Dextroamphetamine was once prescribed as an anoretic (an appetite depressant) for many years. Recently, it has been found that dextroamphetamine's inhibitory effect on the appetite lasts only for four or five weeks. This finding, coupled with its increased abuse, has drastically reduced the quantity of the prescriptions for this drug. This agent is not used in the military for the inhibition of appetite. It is used only for the treatment of attention deficity hyperactivity disorder (ADHD) and narcolepsy. Most military and civilian physicians believe that exercise and the restriction of food (caloric) intake is the method of choice for weight reduction. The most common side effects associated with dextroamphetamine are nervousness and headaches. This drug has a very high abuse potential. It is controlled as a Schedule II (Note R) item. Dextroamphetamine is supplied in 5-milligram tablets, 10- and 15-milligram capsules.

(3) Methamphetamine hydrochloride (Desoxyn®). This drug is similar to dextroamphetamine in terms of its ability to suppress the appetite. However, its abuse potential is such that it is rarely used any longer for this purpose.

c. **Other Agents**. Many other drugs produce pharmacological effects similar to those produced by the amphetamines. These are most often used for their ability to suppress the patient's appetite. Sometimes you will find these medications combined with other drugs (for example, a sedative or an antianxiety agent) in order to counteract the stimulation they produce.

(1) Pemoline (Cylert®). This drug is used in the treatment of ADHD. It is usually prescribed in a graduated dose - beginning with a 37.5-milligram daily dose. It is then gradually increased at 1-week intervals of 18.75 milligrams until a desired clinical response is observed. The most common side effect seen with this agent is insomnia. Pemoline appears to have a lower abuse potential than methylphenidate; pemoline is classified as a Note Q drug. The drug is supplied in the form of 18.75, 37.5, and 75 milligram tablets.

(2) Diethylpropion hydrochloride (Tenuate®). Diethylpropion hydrochloride is used as an appetite suppressant. It is less effective in this use than the amphetamines. It produces such side effects as dryness of the mouth, nausea, and headaches. It is available in both 25-milligram tablets and 75-milligram (timed-release) tablets. Diethylpropion is a Note Q drug.

(3) Phendimetrazine tartrate (Prelu-2®). This drug is used as an appetite suppressant. Long-term use of the drug, especially in large doses, may produce psychic dependence. It produces such side effects as nervousness, excitement, euphoria, and dryness of the mouth. It is supplied in 35-mllligram tablets and capsules and 105-milligram (timed-release) capsules. Phendimetrazine is a Note Q drug.

Section III. ANALEPTIC AGENTS (BRAIN STEM STIMULANTS)

10-6. INTRODUCTION

a. Analeptic agents are drugs that produce two primary effects. One, they stimulate the nerve cells of the body's respiratory center when it has been depressed by some condition (for example, illness or drugs). Two, they stimulate nerve cell centers responsible for keeping a person conscious.

b. Analeptic agents are not commonly used today because of the stimulation they produce in doses sufficient to produce their analeptic effect. These agents can produce such undesirable effects as convulsions, respiratory problems, or vomiting.

10-7. EXAMPLE OF AN ANALEPTIC AGENT

Doxapram (Dopram®) is an analeptic agent used for postanesthetic arousal and drug-induced central nervous system depression. It has the ability to arouse the patient after surgery without reducing the analgesia produced by opiates (for example, morphine). Thus, it is used to hasten recovery time. The faster the patient becomes aware of his or her surroundings, the faster nursing personnel are relieved of intensive care responsibilities. Doxapram is also used to stimulate respiration and hasten arousal in patients who have mild to moderate respiratory and central nervous system depression because of overdose. The most common side effects associated with this drug are headaches, nausea, and vomiting. The usual dose of the drug is 0.5 to 2.0 milligrams per kilogram of body weight. It is supplied as an injectable containing 20 milligrams per milliliter of solution.

Section IV. CONVULSANTS (SPINAL CORD STIMULANTS)

10-8. INTRODUCTION

Some chemical substances can so stimulate the motor areas of the central nervous system that a person's muscles begin to powerfully convulse (begin uncontrollable violent contractions). Some natural and manmade chemicals are capable of producing such reactions. For example, tetanospasmin, a chemical produced by the bacteria Clostridium tetani, is such a natural agent. Strychnine, a poison, once was used as a respiratory stimulant; however, its medicinal use has been stopped because of its toxicity.

10-9. THERAPEUTIC USE OF CONVULSANTS

Drugs in this classification have little clinical usefulness. Some drugs in this class have been used in the treatment of some types of psychotic agents.

Continue with Exercises

EXERCISES, LESSON 10

INSTRUCTIONS: Answer the following exercises by marking the lettered response that best answers the exercise, by completing the incomplete statement, or by writing the answer in the space provided at the end of the exercise. After you have completed all of the exercises, turn to "Solutions to Exercises" at the end of the lesson and check your answers. For each exercise answered incorrectly, reread the material referenced with the solution.

1.   Select the category(ies) of central nervous system stimulants.

    a.   Cerebral agents.

    b.   Convulsants.

    c.   Analeptics.

    d.   All the above.

2.   Select the pharmacological effect(s) associated with xanthine derivatives.

    a.   Bronchoconstriction.

    b.   Smooth muscle relaxation.

    c.   Enuresis.

    d.   All the above.

Match the generic names below with their corresponding trade names.

3.   Diethylpropion hydrochloride_____   a. Dopram®

4.   Methyl phenidate_____   b. Aminophylline®

5.   Theophylline ethylenediamine_____   c. Ritalin®

6.   Theophylline_____   d. Desoxyn®

7.   Methamphetamine hydrochloride_____   e. Elixophylline®

8.   Doxapram_____   f. Cylert®

9.   Pemoline_____   g. Tenuate®

10. What is the clinical use of diethylpropion hydrochloride?

    a. Used in the treatment of attention deficit hyperactivity disorder (ADHD).

    b. Used to suppress a patient's appetite.

    c. Used to treat a patient's anxiety.

    d. Used to stimulate a patient's respiratory system.

11. Long-term use of phendimetrazine tartrate (Prelu-2®) may produce
_____.

    a. Nausea or vomiting.

    b. Decreased metabolic rate.

    c. Psychic dependence.

    d. Insomnia.

12. What is the clinical use of dextroamphetamine sulfate (Dexedrine®)?

    a. To suppress a patient's appetite.

    b. To increase a patient's ability to concentrate.

    c. To treat narcolepsy.

    d. To stimulate respiration.

13. When taking Aminophylline orally, the patient should be cautioned
_____.

    a. Not to take the medication with alcohol.

    b. Take the medication with food.

    c. Discontinue the medication immediately if any slight nervousness is
detected.

    d. Not to drive while taking the medication.

Check Your Answers on Next Page

SOLUTIONS TO EXERCISES, LESSON 10

1. d   All the above. (para 10-3a)

2. b   Smooth muscle relaxation. (para 10-5a)

3. g   Tenuate®. (para 10-5c(2))

4. c   Ritalin®. (para 10-5b(1))

5. b   Aminophylline. (para 10-5a(2))

6. e   Elixophylline®. (para 10-5a(3))

7. d   Desoxyn®. (para 10-5b(3))

8. a   Dopram®. (para 10-7)

9. f   Cylert®. (para 10-5c(1))

10. b   Used to suppress a patient's appetite. (para 10-5c(2))

11. c   Psychic dependence. (para 10-5c(3))

12. c   To treat narcolepsy. (para 10-5b(2))

13. b   Take the medication with food. (para 10-5a(2))

End of Lesson 10

LESSON 11	Narcotic Agents.
LESSON ASSIGNMENT	Paragraphs 11-1--11-7
LESSON OBJECTIVES	After completing this lesson, you should be able to:

11-1. Given a group of definitions, select the definition of analgesia.

11-2. Given a group of pharmacological effects, select those that are produced by narcotic agents.

11-3. Given a group of definitions, select the meaning of the following terms: dysphoria, euphoria, tolerance, and miosis.

11-4. Given a general pharmacological effect produced by the narcotics and a group of statements, select the term that best describes that effect.

11-5. Given several statements, select the statement that best contrasts psychological and physiological dependence.

11-6. Given a group of side effects, select those side effects associated with the narcotic agents.

11-7. Given the trade and/or generic name of a specific narcotic agent, and a list of uses, side effects, or cautions and warnings, select the use, side effect, or caution and warning associated with that agent.

11-8. Given a group of cautions, select the caution associated with the use of narcotic agents.

11-9. Given the name naloxone (Narcan®) and a group of uses/indications, select the use/indication associated with the drug.

SUGGESTION   After studying the assignment, complete the exercises at the end of this lesson. These exercises will help you to achieve the lesson objectives.

LESSON 11

NARCOTIC AGENTS

Section I. BACKGROUND

11-1. GENERAL COMMENTS

Most people have legally used narcotic agents. Conditions characterized by a degree of discomfort (that is, pain, diarrhea, or cough), often are treated with medications that have narcotics as the active ingredient. It is very important for all medical personnel to be familiar with narcotic agents.

11-2. HISTORY OF NARCOTIC AGENTS

a. There is evidence that the opium poppy was used in Sumeria as early as 4000 B.C., and it is mentioned in the medical records of ancient Greece and Rome. During the Dark Ages, it passed to the Arabs, who took it to China about 900 A.D. It was either smoked or taken orally.

b. Opium was first used injectably around 1800; the U.S. Civil War saw the first widespread use in this manner. Because of a lack of knowledge and caution, a condition called "Soldier's Disease" was described--addiction. This coupled with the large influx of Chinese laborers who smoked, and the ready availability of opium caused a great deal of concern. There were no packaging or distribution laws; indeed, a children's formulation was marketed called "Mrs. Winslow's Soothing Syrup." This concern was an important factor in motivation for the Pure Food and Drug Act of 1906.

c. In 1805, a German Pharmacist's assistant isolated a pure alkaloid (a basic substance found usually in plant parts) from opium that he called morphine. It was subsequently found that opium contains two general categories of alkaloids; narcotics (phenanthrene) such as morphine and codeine, and nonnarcotics (benzylisoquinoline)

11-3. PHARMACOLOGICAL EFFECTS OF THE NARCOTICS

Narcotics produce pharmacological effects when administered to a patient. Some of these effects are desirable, while others are undesirable. Always remember that the legitimate use of these agents is implied in our discussion.

a. **Analgesic Effect.** Analgesia means relief of pain without the loss of consciousness. Analgesia is the most common use of narcotics. Although the exact mechanism of action by which narcotics act is unknown, it is thought that analgesia is obtained by the action of these agents on the cerebral cortex. The relief of pain is enhanced because narcotics raise a patient's pain threshold and thus produce a calming and soothing effect. Narcotic agents have particular application in the relief of continuous, dull pain. Consequently, these drugs are widely used in patients who are terminally ill.

b. **Antitussive Effect.** An antitussive agent acts to control or prevent cough. Some narcotics will depress the cough center of the brain and produce this antitussive effect. In general, the antitussive dose of a narcotic is lower than the analgesic dose of that same drug. Before progressing, it should be noted that a narcotic is not indicated for all types of coughs. Indeed, sometimes it is useful for a patient to cough in order to remove substances from the lungs.

c. **Mood Alteration Effect**. Some narcotics will produce a mood alteration in patients. The types of mood changes can be classified in two categories.

(1) Dysphoria. Dysphoria is a mood alteration characterized by feelings of anxiety, fidgetiness, or being ill at ease.

(2) Euphoria. Euphoria is characterized by an exaggerated feeling of well-being.

d. **Gastrointestinal Effect**. Narcotics produce some significant effects upon the gastrointestinal system (that is, stomach and intestines). Some narcotics are used specifically for their effect upon this system of the body.

(1) Decrease gastrointestinal motility. Narcotics decrease the peristaltic (wavelike) movements of the gastrointestinal tract. Consequently, they may cause constipation. This effect of narcotics is the basis of their being used to treat diarrhea. When used to treat diarrhea, the agents are referred to as antidiarrheals.

(2) Stimulate the chemoreceptor trigger zone. The chemoreceptor trigger zone (CTZ) is located at the base of the brain. When stimulated, the CTZ produces nausea and vomiting. Like many other categories of drugs, narcotics can stimulate the chemoreceptor trigger zone and cause nausea and vomiting.

e. **Respiratory System Effect**. Narcotics cause respiratory system depression because they reduce the sensitivity of the medullary centers to carbon dioxide in the blood. This depression of the respiratory system usually occurs at higher narcotic doses.

11-4. SIDE EFFECTS OF NARCOTICS

Side effects are frequently seen with the use of narcotics. Some of these side effects are characteristics of the narcotic agents.

a. **Dependence.** Dependence is a side effect of narcotics, which has caused much concern among many health-care professionals. There are two types of dependence.

(1) Psychological. Psychological dependence is produced when the drug causes an emotional or mental desire to repeat the use of the drug. Consequently, the individual taking the drug has a craving for the pleasurable mental effects produced by the drug (that is, euphoria, and so forth).

(2) Physiological (physical). Physical dependence is produced by prolonged use of a drug whose pharmacological action causes the body to adapt to its presence. When the drug is withdrawn after the person has become physically dependent, the body of the individual reacts in a hyperexcited way. You have probably read about or seen heroin (narcotic) addicts who are undergoing withdrawal. These episodes of withdrawal are characterized by stimulation of the central nervous system.

b. **Tolerance.** Tolerance is the body's ability to adapt to the presence of a foreign chemical substance (drug). This results in the requirement for progressively larger doses of the drug in order to obtain the same effect in the patient. It should be noted that tolerance is frequently seen in patients who abuse narcotics. Tolerance is not of great concern in narcotic therapy of short duration. However, for those chronically ill patients who are on long-term narcotic therapy, increased doses of the narcotic agents might be indicated to maintain the desired level of analgesia.

c. **Drowsiness.** Drowsiness is another side effect of narcotics. For this reason, individuals who are receiving narcotics should seriously examine their activities that is, driving) for safety purposes.

d. **Miosis.** Miosis (constricted pupils) is an effect commonly known as "pinpoint" pupils. Miosis is commonly seen in patients who are taking narcotic agents.

Section II. NARCOTIC AGENTS AND NARCOTIC ANTAGONISTS

11-5. SPECIFIC NARCOTIC AGENTS

a. **Morphine.** Morphine is the basis of the narcotic effect of opium and is the standard by which other analgesics are judged. It is used in moderate to severe pain, is the analgesic of choice for myocardial infarction, and is used to treat acute pulmonary edema. Morphine is most frequently given IM or SC, 10-15 mg every 4 hours, or IV, where 4-10 mg are diluted and given slowly over 4-5 minutes. It is used less frequently by the oral route (1/15--1/6 the effectiveness of parenteral administration) in a dose of 8-20 mg every 4 hours. The most common side effects associated with morphine are drowsiness, nausea, and vomiting. Morphine is supplied as an injection containing 8, 10, and 15 milligrams per milliliter; in tablets of 10, 15, and 30 milligrams; and as an oral solution containing 10-milligrams per 5-milliliters. Morphine in all forms is a Note R substance.

b. **Codeine**. Codeine is the second naturally occurring narcotic. Its use is very widespread; in some states it can be sold without prescription in combination products if its concentration is weak enough (ETH & codeine, Robitussin AC®). For our purposes, however, when codeine is dispensed as a single agent, it is Note R, when in combination, it is Note Q. Codeine is used as an antitussive, 5-15 mg every 4-6 hours, and as an analgesic in mild to moderate pain, 30-60mg every 4-6 hours. Its most common side effects include drowsiness, nausea/vomiting, and constipation; patients must be cautioned about the drowsiness and the additive effect seen with concurrent use of alcohol. Codeine is available as an injection of 15, 30, and 60 mg/ml, and in 15 and 30 mg tablets. A powder form for compounding is also available.

c. **Hydromorphone (Dilaudid®)**. Hydromorphone (Dilaudid®) is a drug that was obtained by chemical modification of morphine, used as an analgesic in moderate to severe pain. It is frequently used in pain associated with cancer. Its usual dose is 2 mg every 4 to 6 hours. Its major side effects are nausea and vomiting, dizziness, and constipation. Although the manufacturer states that drowsiness occurs infrequently, patients should be made aware of this possibility; also alcohol may intensify its effects. Dilaudid® is a Note R drug and is supplied in tablet or injectable form, both in 1, 2, 3, and 4 mg strengths.

d. **Meperidine (Demerol®)**. Meperidine was the first synthetically produced narcotic. It is one of the first widely used agents for moderate to severe pain. Usual doses of this agent (50-150 mg every 3-4 hours) produce some drowsiness, nausea, and vomiting. Patients who are prescribed meperidine should be cautioned that drowsiness might occur. Further, they should be advised that alcohol might intensify this drowsiness. Meperidine is a Note R drug, which is available as an injection (25, 50, 75, and 100 mg/ml), a tablet (50 or 100 mg tablets), and in a syrup (50 mg/5ml).

e. **Fentanyl (Sublimaze®, Duragesic®, Oralet®, Actiq®)**. Fentanyl is a synthetic agent with actions similar to morphine, but on a weight basis, Sublimaze® is 80-100 times more potent. It is used as an analgesic component in general anesthesia or conscious sedation and given intramuscularly (IM) or intravenously (IV). The dosage is dependent upon its intended role during anesthesia, and ranges from 0.025 to 0.1 mg. Respiratory depression is the side effect of concern for this agent. Fentanyl is unique in that it is available as an injection (Sublimaze®), in a topical patch formulation (Duragesic®), a lozenge (Fentanyl Oralet®) and a lozenge on a stick ("lollipop") (Actiq®) formulation. The latter three formulations are prescribed primarily for severe pain conditions. Fentanyl is handled as a Note R product.

f. **Methadone (Dolophine®)**. Methadone (Dolophine®) is a synthetic agent that has been used as an analgesic for moderate to severe pain, and to treat withdrawal symptoms of narcotics in a dose-tapering fashion. The usual dose for analgesia is 2.5-10 mg every 4 hours, and common side effects include drowsiness and nausea/vomiting. The effects of methadone may be intensified by alcohol, and the patient also should be cautioned about drowsiness. The injection, 10 mg/ml, and the tablets, 5 and 10 mg, are all Note R.

g. **Percodan®**. Percodan® is a popular semisynthetic narcotic intended for the relief of moderate pain that contains two salts of oxycodone, combined with aspirin. It is, of course, a fixed combination and is given in a usual dose of one tablet every 6 hours. In addition to the side effects of drowsiness and nausea/vomiting, pruritis is also a fairly frequent complaint. Patient cautionary statements regarding drowsiness and alcohol apply to this agent. It is a Note R product even though it is a combination. Percodan® is available in tablet form, and a half-strength product called Percodan-Demi® is also produced.

NOTE: Combination products of acetaminophen with oxycodone are Tylox® and Percocet®.

h. **Combination Products**. Codeine is combined with aspirin or acetaminophen (Tylenol®) to produce products that are used to treat mild to moderate pain. Common side effects of these combination products include nausea, vomiting, and drowsiness. Patients who are taking these products should be cautioned about the drowsiness. Further, patients should be warned against taking these with alcohol. These combination products are handled as Note Q items.

(1) Empirin® with codeine. Empirin® with codeine is a combination of aspirin and codeine. The usual dosage of these products is from one to two tablets every four hours. The various products are numbered based upon the amount of codeine contained in each product as noted below:

(a) Empirin® with Codeine #2 - 15 mg of codeine per tablet.

(b) Empirin® with Codeine #3 - 30 mg of codeine per tablet (most widely used of these products).

(c) Empirin® with Codeine #4 - 60 mg of codeine per tablet.

(2) Tylenol® with codeine. Tylenol® with codeine is a combination acetaminophen with codeine. The usual dosage of these products is from one to two tablets every four hours. As with Empirin® with codeine, the products are numbered based upon the amount of codeine contained in each tablet as noted below:

(a) Tylenol® with Codeine #1 - 7.5 mg of codeine per tablet.

(b) Tylenol® with Codeine #2 - 15 mg of codeine per tablet.

(c) Tylenol® with Codeine #3 - 30 mg of codeine per tablet (most widely used of these products).

(d) Tylenol® with Codeine #4 - 60 mg of codeine per tablet.

11-6. CAUTIONS OF NARCOTIC USE

a. Narcotics should not be used in patients experiencing any form of respiratory depression (that is, asthma).

b. Narcotics cause an increase in intracranial pressure (pressure within the skull). Therefore, they should not be used in the presence of head injuries.

c. Narcotics should be used cautiously in combination with other drugs that depress the central nervous system.

11-7. NARCOTIC ANTAGONISM

a. **Explanation**. As previously mentioned, narcotics depress the respiratory system. Sometimes it is necessary to reverse this respiratory depression (that is, overdose of narcotics) in order to save a patient's life.

b. **Naloxone (Narcan®)**. Naloxone (Narcan®) is the only true narcotic antagonist in that it does not possess agonist or morphine-like properties and, most importantly, it has no respiratory depressant action in therapeutic doses. Because it does not depress respiration, naloxone is the drug of choice in the treatment of respiratory depression of unknown causes, but which is suspected of being produced by a narcotic. Narcan® is given in a usual dose of 0.4 mg IM, SC, or IV, and may produce some nausea and vomiting. It is not a controlled substance, and is available as an injection, 0.4 mg/ml or 0.2 mg/ml for pediatric use.

c. **Indications/Uses**. Naloxone (Narcan®) is indicated/used to reverse respiratory depression caused by natural and synthetic narcotics, pentazocine (Talwin®), and propoxyphene (Darvon®). It is not effective against the respiratory depression caused by the barbiturates or benzodiazepines. Naloxone is a competitive antagonist.

Continue with Exercises

EXERCISES, LESSON 11

INSTRUCTIONS: Answer the following exercises by marking the lettered response that best answers the exercise, by completing the incomplete statement, or by writing the answer in the space provided at the end of the exercise.

After you have completed all of the exercises, turn to "Solutions to Exercises" at the end of the lesson and check your answers. For each exercise answered incorrectly, reread the material referenced with the solution.

1. From the group of definitions below, select the meaning of the term analgesia.

    a. The decrease in a patient's pain threshold.

    b. The relief of pain with loss of consciousness.

    c. The relief of pain without the loss of consciousness.

    d. The loss of consciousness with no effect on pain level.

2. From the group of pharmacological effects below, select the response that contains those produced by narcotic agents.

(1) Relief of pain.	(6) Depress respiratory rate.
(2) Antitussive.	(7) Increase blood pressure.
(3) Antipyretic.	(8) Increase respiratory rate.
(4) Decrease gastrointestinal motility.	(9) Decrease clotting time.
(5) Produce diarrhea.	(10) Produce loss of consciousness.

    a. (1), (2), (3), (6) and (10).

    b. (1), (2), (4) and (6).

    c. (1), (2) and (5).

    d. (1), (2), (4), (5), (6), (7) and (10).

3. From the group of definitions below, select the meaning of the term euphoria.

    a. A mood alteration characterized by feelings of anxiety.

    b. A mood alteration characterized by feelings of being ill at ease.

    c. A mood alteration effect characterized by analgesia.

    d. A mood alteration characterized by exaggerated feelings of well-being.

4. Narcotic agents produce an effect on a patient's respiratory system. From the list of descriptions below, select the best description of the specific effect produced by the narcotic agents.

    a. Narcotic agents stimulate a patient's respiratory system.

    b. Narcotic agents depress a patient's respiratory system.

    c. Narcotic agents decrease the levels of carbon dioxide in the blood.

    d. Narcotic agents depress the respiratory rate only in small doses.

5. Narcotic agents produce an effect on a patient's gastrointestinal system. From the list of descriptions below, select the best description of that specific effect.

    a. Narcotic agents stimulate the patient's CTZ to produce nausea and vomiting.

    b. Narcotic agents stimulate the patient's CTZ to produce diarrhea.

    c. Narcotic agents stimulate the patient's CTZ to produce constipation.

    d. Narcotic agents stimulate the patient's CTZ to produce peristalsis.

6. From the group of side effects below, select the response that contains the side effects associated with the narcotic agents.

(1) Independence.

(4) Miosis.

(2) Mitosis.

(5) Dependence.

(3) Tolerance.

(6) Drowsiness.

a. (1), (2), (3), (6).

b. (1), (3), (5), (6).

c. (3), (4), (5), (6).

d. (1), (2), (5), (6).

7. From the definitions below, select the best definition of the term tolerance.

a. The ability of the body to adapt to the presence of foreign substances that result in the requirement for progressively larger doses of the drug to obtain the same effect.

b. The ability of the body to adapt to the presence of foreign substances that result in the requirement for progressively smaller doses of the drug to obtain the same effect.

c. The ability of the body to adapt to the presence of foreign substances that result in the requirement for changing the route of administration of the drug.

d. The ability of the body to adapt to the presence of foreign substances that result in the requirement for changing the dosage form of the drug.

8. From the list of uses below, select the use of codeine.

a. Antitussive.

b. Antiemetic.

c. Antipyretic.

d. Sedative.

9. From the list of uses below, select the use of hydromorphone (Dilaudid®).

   a. Analgesic for moderate to severe pain.

   b. Analgesic for mild to moderate pain.

   c. Antidiarrheal in severe diarrhea.

   d. Emetic in poisoning.

10. From the list of cautions and warnings, select the caution and warning associated with the use of meperidine hydrochloride (Demerol®).

   a. The patient should be cautioned against taking aspirin with meperidine.

   b. The patient should be warned that alcohol can intensify the drowsiness caused by meperidine.

   c. The patient should be warned against not taking the drug on a regular basis.

   d. The patient should be cautioned against exercise when taking the drug.

11. From the list of uses below, select the use associated with Methadone (Dolophine®).

   a. An agent used to treat withdrawal symptoms associated with narcotic antagonists.

   b. An agent used in the treatment of mild to moderate pain.

   c. An agent used in the treatment of alcohol withdrawal symptoms.

   d. An agent used in the treatment of the withdrawal symptoms associated with narcotic agents.

12. From the group of cautions below, select the caution associated with the use of narcotic agents.

     a.   Narcotics should not be administered to patients over the age of 65.

     b.   Narcotics should not be administered intravenously.

     c.   Narcotics should be used cautiously with drugs that depress the central nervous system.

     d.   Narcotics should not be used by cardiac patients.

13. Select the use of Naloxone (Narcan®) from the list of uses below.

     a.   Narcotic.

     b.   Narcotic analgesic.

     c.   Narcotic suppressant.

     d.   Narcotic antagonist

Check Your Answers on Next Page

SOLUTIONS TO EXERCISES, LESSON 11

1. c   The relief of pain without the loss of consciousness. (para 11-3a)

2. b   (1), (2), (4), and (6). (para 11-3a, b, d(1), and e)

3. d   A mood alteration characterized by exaggerated feelings of well being. (para 11-3c(2))

4. b   Narcotic agents depress a patient's respiratory system. (para 11-3e)

5. a   Narcotic agents stimulate the patient's CTZ to produce nausea and vomiting. (para 11-3d(2))

6. c   (3), (4), (5), and (6). (para 11-4a, b, c, and d)

7. a   The ability of the body to adapt to the presence of foreign substances which results in the requirement for progressively larger doses of the drug to obtain the same effect. (para 11-4b)

8. a   Antitussive. (para 11-5b)

9. a   Analgesic for moderate to severe pain. (para 11-5c)

10. b   The patient should be warned that alcohol can intensify the drowsiness caused by meperidine. (para 11-5d)

11. d   An agent used in the treatment of the withdrawal symptoms associated with narcotic agents. (para 11-5f)

12. c   Narcotics should be used cautiously with drugs which depress the central nervous system. (para 11-6c)

13. d   Narcotic antagonist. (para 11-7b)

End of Lesson 11

ANNEX

DRUG PRONUNCIATION GUIDE

This Drug Pronunciation Guide was developed to help you to learn how the trade and generic names of commonly prescribed medications are frequently pronounced. Not all the drugs in the guide are discussed in this subcourse. Remember, it is not enough to be able to know the uses, indications, cautions and warnings, and contraindications for a drug--you must also know how to pronounce that drug's name.

Trade Name	*Generic Name*
Actifed (Ak'-ti-fed)	Triprolidine (Tri-pro'-li-deen) and Pseudoephedrine (Soo-do-e-fed'-rin)
Adapin (Ad'-a-pin)	Doxepin (Dok'-se-pin)
Sinequan (Sin'-a-kwan)	" "
Afrin (Af'-rin)	Oxymetazoline (Ok-see-met-az'-o-leen)
Aldactazide (Al-dak'-ta-zide)	Spironolactone (Spi-ro-no-lak'-tone) and Hydrochlorothiazide (Hy-dro-klor-thi'-a-zide)
Aldactone (Al-dak'-tone)	Spironolactone (Spi-ro-no-lak'-tone)
Aldomet (Al'-do-met)	Methyldopa (Meth-il-do'-pah)
Alupent (Al'-u-pent)	Metaproterenol (Met-a-pro-ter'-eh-nol)
Amoxil (Am-ok'-sil)	Amoxicillin (Ah-moks'-i-sil-in)
Amphojel (Am'-fo-jel)	Aluminum (Al-loo'-mi-num) Hydroxide (Hy-drok'-side)
Ampicillin (Amp'-I-sil-in)	Same
Antepar (Ab'-te-par)	Piperazine (Pi-per'-ah-zeen)
Anturane (An'-tu-rain)	Sulfinpyrazone (Sul-fin-pie'-ra-zone)
Anusol (An'-u-sol)	Pramoxine (Pram-ok'-seen)
Apresoline (A-press'-o-leen)	Hydralazine (Hy-dral'-ah-zeen)
Aralen (Ar'-a-len)	Chloroquine (Klor'-o-kwin)
Aristocort (A-ris'-to-cort)	Triamcinolone (Tri-am-sin'-o-lone)
Artane (Ar'-tane)	Trihexyphenidyl(Tri-hek-see-fen'-i-dil)
A.S.A.	Aspirin (As'-per-in)
Atromid S (A'-tro-mid)	Clofibrate (Klo-fi'-brate)
Avlosulfon (Av-lo-sul'-fon)	Dapsone (Dap'-sone)
Azolid (Az'-o-lid)	Phenylbutazone (Fen-il-bute'-a-zone)
Bactrim (Bak'-trim)	Sulfamethoxazole (Sul-fah-meth-oks'-ah-zole) and Trimethoprim (Tri-meth'-o-prim)
Bellergal (Bel'-er-gal)	Ergotamine (Er-got'-a-meen), Phenobarbital (Feen-o-bar'-bi-tal) and Belladonna (Bel-la-don'-na) Alkaloids
Benadryl (Ben'-a-dril)	Diphenhydramine (Di-fen-hy'-dra-meen)

Trade Name	Generic Name
Bendectin (Ben-dek'-tin)	Doxylamine (Dok-sil'-a-meen)
Benemid (Ben'-eh-mid)	Probenecid (Pro-ben'-eh-sid)
Bonine (Bo'-neen)	Meclizine (Mek'-li-zeen)
Cafergot (Kaf'-er-got)	Ergotamine (Er-got'-a-meen) and Caffeine (Kaf'-feen)
Calamine (Kal'-a-mine)	Same
Catapres (Kat'-a-press)	Clonidine (Klo'-ni-deen)
CeeNu (See'-new)	Lomustine (Lo-mus'-teen)
Chlor-Trimeton (Klo-tri '-meh-ton)	Chlorpheniramine (Klor-fen-it'-a-meen)
Clomid (Klo'-mid)	Clomiphene (Klo'-mi-feen)
Clonopin (Klo-o-pin)	Clonazepam (Klo-na'-ze-pam)
Codeine (Ko'-deen)	Same
Cogentin (Ko-jen'-tin)	Benztropine (Benz'-tro-peen)
Colace (Ko'-lace)	Dioctyl(Di-ok'-til) Sodium (So'-dee-um) Sulfosuccinate (Sul-fo-suk'-si-nate)
Colchicine (Kol'-chi-seen)	Same
Compazine (Kom'-pa-zeen)	Prochiorperazine (Pro-klor-per'-a-zeen)
Cordran (Kor'-dran)	Flurandrenolide (Floor-an-dren'-o-lide)
Coumadin (Koo'-mah-din)	Warfarin (War'-fah-rin)
CP	Cloroquine (Klor'-o-kwin) and Primaquine (Prim'-a-kwin)
Cyclogyl (Si'-klo-jel)	Cyclopentolate (Si-klo-pen'-to-late)
Cytomel (Si'-to-mel)	Liothyronine (Li-o-thy-ro-neen)
Cytoxan (Si-tok'-san)	Cyclophosphamide (Si-klo-fos'-fa-mide)
Dalmane (Dal '-mane)	Flurazepam (Floor-az'-e-pam)
Darvocet (Dar'-vo-set)	Propoxyphene (Pro-pok'-se-feen) and Acetaminopen (As-et-am'-ino-fen)
Darvon (Dar'-von)	Propoxyphene (Pro-pok-se-feen)
Decadron (Dek'-a-dron)	Dexamethasone (Dek-sa-meth'-ah-sone)
Deltasone (Del '-ta-sone)	Prednisone (Pred'-ni-sone)
Demerol (Dem'-er-ol)	Meperidine (Meh-pair'-i-deen)
Dexedrine (Deks '-eh-dreen)	Dextroamphetamine (Deks-tro-am-fet'-a-meen)
Diabinese (Di-ab'-i-nees)	Chlorpropamide (Klor-prop'-a-mide)
Diethylstilbestrol (Di-eth-il-stil-bes'-trol)	Same
Dilantin (Di-lan'-tin)	Phenytoin (Fen'-i-toin)
Dilaudid (Di-law'-did)	Hydromorphone (Hy-dro-more' -fon)
Dimetane (Di'-meh-tane)	Brompheniramine (Brom-fen-ir'-a-meen)

Trade Name	Generic Name
Dimetapp (Di'-meh-tap)	Brompheniramine (Brom-fen-ir'-a-meen) Phenylephrine (Fen-il-ef'-rin) and Phenylpropanolamine (Fen-il-pro-pan-ol'-a-meen)
Disophrol (Dice'-o-frol)	Dexbrompheniramine (Deks-brom-fen-ir'-a-meen) and Pseudoephedrine (Soo-do-e-fed'-rin)
Dolophine (Dol'-o-feen)	Methadone (Meth'-a-done)
Domeboro (Dome-bor'-o)	Aluminum (Ah-loo'-mi-num) Acetate (As'-e-tate)
Donnatal (Don'-na-tal)	Belladonna (Bel-la-don'-na) Alkaloids (Al'-ka-loids) and Phenobarbital (Feen-o-barb'-i-tal)
Doxidan (Dok'-si-dan)	Danthron (Dan'-thron) and Dicctyl (Di-ok'-til) Calcium (Kal'-see-um) Sulfosuccinate (Sul-fo-suk'-si-nate)
Drixoral (Driks'-or-al)	Dexbrompheniramine (Deks-brom-fen-ir'-a-meen) and Pseudoephedrine (Soo-do-e-fed'-rin)
Dulcolax (Dul'-ko-laks)	Bisacodyl (Bis-a'-ko-dil)
Dyazine (Di'-a-zide)	Triamterene (Tri-am'-ter-een) and Hydrochlorothiazide (Hy-dro-klor-o-thi'-a-zide)
Dymelor (Die'-meh-lor)	Acetohexamide (As-e-to-heks'-a-mide)
Dyrenium (Die-ren'-i-um)	Triamterene (Tri-am'-ter-een)
Efudex (Ef'-u-deks)	Fluorouracil (Floo-ro-ur'-ah-sil)
Elavil (El'-ah-vil)	Amitriptyline (Am-i-trip'-til-een)
Elixir Terpin (Ter'-pin) Hydrate	Same
Empirin (Em'-per-in)	Codeine (Ko'-deen) and Aspirin (As'-per-in)
E-Mycin (E-mie'-sin)	Erythromycin (E-rith-ro-mie'-sin)
Equanil (Ek'-wa-nil)	Meprobamate (Me-pro-bam'-ate)
Ergomar (Er'-go-mar)	Ergotamine (Er-got'-a-meen)
Ergotrate (Er'-go-trate)	Ergonovine (Er-go-no'-veen)
Erythrocin (Er-eeth'-ro-sin)	Erythromycin (Er-eeth-ro-my'-sin) Stearate (Stare'-rate)
Esidrix (Es'-i-driks)	Hyrochlorothiazide (Hy-dro-klor-o-thi'-a-zide)
Feosol (Fe'-o-sol)	Ferrous (Fer'-rus) Sulfate (Sul'-fate)
Fergon (Fer'-gon)	Ferrous (Fer'-rus) Gluconate (Glu'-con-ate)

Trade Name	Generic Name
Fiorinal (Fee-or'-i-nal)	Butalbi tal (Bu-tal'-bi-tal), Apririn, Phenacetin (Fen-ass'-eh-tin), and Caffeine (Kaf'-feen)
Flagyl (Fla'-jil)	Metronidazole (Me-tro-ni'-dah-zole)
Flexeril (Flek'-sa-ril)	Cyclobenzaprine (Si-klo-benz'-a-preen)
Fulvicin (Ful'-vi-sin)	Griseofulvin (Griz-e-o-ful'-vin)
Guantanol (Gan'-ta-nol)	Suiphamethoxazole (Sul-fah-meth-oks'-ah-zole)
Gantrisin (Gan'-tri-sin)	Sulfisoxazole (Sul-fi-sok'-sah-zole)
Gelusil (Jel'-u-sil)	Aluminum (Ah-loo'-mi-num) Hydroxide (Hy-drok'-side) and Magnesium (Mag-nee'-zee-um) Hydroxide
Grifulvin (Gri-ful'-vin)	Griseofulvin (Griz-e-o-ful'-vin)
Gynergen (Jin'-er-jen)	Ergotamine (Er-got'-a-meen)
Haldol (Hal'-dol)	Haloperidol (Hal-o-pair'-i-dol)
Halotestin (Hal-o-tes'-tin)	Fluoxymesterone (Floo-ok-see-mes-teh-rone)
Hexadrol (Hek'-sa-drol)	Dexamethasone (Dek-sa-meth'-a-sone)
Hydrodiuril (Hy-dro-di'-ur-il)	Hydroclorothiazide (Hy-dro-kior-thi'-a-zide)
Hygroton (Hy-grow'-ton)	Chiorthalidone (Kior-thal'-i-done)
Ilosone (I'-low-sone)	Erythromycin (Er-ith-ro-mi'-sin) Estolate (Es'-to-late)
Inderal (In'-der-al)	Propranolol (Pro-pran'-o-lol)
Indocin (In'-do-sin)	Indomethacin (In-do-meth'-a-sin)
INH	Isoniazid (I-so-ni'-a-zid)
Insulin (In'-sul-in)	Same
Intal	Cromolyn (Kro'-mo-lin)
Ismelin (Is'-meh-lin)	Guanethidine (Gwan-eth'-i-dine)
Isopto-Atropine (I-sop-to-at'-ro-peen)	Atropine (At'-ro-peen)
Isopto-Carpine (I-sop-to-car'-peen)	Pilocarpine (Pile-o-car'-peen)
Isordil (I'-sor-dil)	Isosorbide (I-so-sor'-bide)
Keflex (Kef'-lex)	Cephalexin (Sef-ah-lek'-sin)
Lanoxin (Lan-ok'-sin)	Digoxin (Di-jok'-sin)
Larodopa (Lar-o-do'-pa)	Levodopa (Le-o-do'-pa)
Larotid (Lar'-o-tid)	Amoxicillin (Ah-moks'-i-sil-in)
Lasix (La'-siks)	Furosemide (Fu-ro'-se-mide)
Leukeran (Lu'-ker-an)	Chlorambucil (Klor-ram'-bu-sil)
Librium (Lib'-ree-um)	Chlordiazepoxide (Klor-die-az-eh-pok'-side)

Trade Name	Generic Name
Lidex (Lie'-deks)	Fluocinoide (Floo-o-sin'-o-nide)
Lomotil (Lo'-mo-til)	Diphenoxylate (Die-fen-ok'-si-late)
Lopressor (Lo'-pres-sor)	Metoprolol (Met-o-pro'-lol)
Lotrimin (Lo'-tri-min)	Chlotrimazole (Klo-trim'-ah-zole)
Maalox (May'-loks)	Aluminum (Ah-loo'-mi-num) and Magnesium (Mag-nee'-zee-um) Hydroxides
Macrodanton (Ma-kro-dan'-tin)	Nitrofurantoin (Ni-tro-fur-an'-toin)
Mandelamine (Man-del'-a-meen)	Methenamine (Meth-en'-a-meen) Mandelate (Man'-deh-late)
Medihaler-Iso (Med-i-hail-er-I'-so)	Isoproterenol (I-so-pro-ter'-en-ol)
Mellaril (Mel'-la-ril)	Thioridazine (Thi-o-rid'-a-zeen)
Metamucil (Met-a-mu'-sil)	Psyllium (Sil'-e-um)
Metaprel (Meh'-ta-prel)	Metaproterenol (Meh'-ta-pro-ter'-eh-nol)
Methotrexate (Meth-o-treks'-ate)	Amethopterin (Ah-meth-op'-ter-in)
Milk of Magnesia	Same
Minipress (Min'-i-press)	Prazosin (Pra'-zo-sin)
Minocin (Min'-o-sin)	Minocycline (Mi-no-si'-kleen)
Monistat (Mon'-i-stat)	Miconazole (Mi-kon'-ah-zole)
Motrin (Mo'-trin)	Ibuprofen (I-bu'-pro-fen)
Myambutol (My-am'-bu-tol)	Ethambutol (Eth-am'-bu-tol)
Mycostatin (My-co-stat'-in)	Nystatin (Ny-stat'-in)
Mylanta (My-lan'-ta)	Aluminum (Ah-loo'-mi-num) and Magnesium (Mag-nee'-zee-um) Hydroxides and Simethicone (Si-meth'-i-kone)
Myleran (My-ler-an)	Busulfan (Bu-sul'-fan)
Mylicon (My'-li-kon)	Simethicone (Si-meth'-i-kone)
Mysoline (My'-so-leen)	Primidone (Pri'-mi-done)
Nalfon (Nal'-fon)	Fenoprofen (Fen-o-pro'-fen)
Naprosyn (Na'-pro-sin)	Naproxen (Na-prok'-sen)
Nembutal (Nem'-bu-tal)	Pentobarbital (Pen-to-barb'-i-tal)
Neosynephrine (Nee-o-sin-eh'-frin)	Phenylephrine (Fen-il-eh'-frin)
Nitrobid (Ni'-tro-bid)	Nitroglycerin (Ni-tro-gli'-ser-in)
Nitrol (Ni'-trol)	" "
Nitrostat (Ni-tro-stat)	" "
Noctec (Nok'-tek)	Chloral Hydrate (Klor'-al- Hy'-drate)
Norfiex (Nor'-fleks)	Orphenadrine Citrate (Or-fen'-a-dreen)
Norpace (Nor'-pace)	Disopyramide (Di-so-peer'-a-mide)

Trade Name	Generic Name
Novahistine (No-va-his'-teen) Expectorant	Guaifenesin (Gwi-fen'-eh-sin), Phenylpropanolamine (Fen-il-pro-pan-ol'-a-meen), and Codeine (Ko'-deen)
NTG	Nitroclycerin (Ni-tro-gli'-ser-in)
Nupercainal (New-per-kain'-al)	Dibucaine (Die'-bu-kain)
Oretic (O-ret'-ik)	Hydrochiorothiazide (Hy-dro-kior-thi'-a-zide)
Orinase (Or'-in-ase)	Tolbutamide (Tol-bu'-tah-mide)
Ornade (Or'-nade)	Chlorpheniramine (Klor-fen-ir'-a-meen), Triprolidine (Tri-pro-li-deen) and Pseudoephedrine (Su-do-eh-fed'-rin)
Parafon Forte (Pair'-a-fon For'-tay)	Chlorzoxazone (Klor-zok'-sa-zone)
Percodan (Per'-ko-dan)	Oxycodone (Ok-si-ko'-done)
Periactin (Per-ee-ak'-tin)	Cyproheptadine (Si-pro-hep'-tah-deen)
Persantine (Per-san'-teen)	Dipyridamole (Di-pi-rid'-ah-mole)
Phenobarbital (Feen-o-barb'-it-al)	Same
Phenylpropanolamine (Fen-il-pro-pan-ol'-a-meen)	Same
Pitocin (Pi-tow'-sin)	Oxytocin (Ok-see-tow'-sin)
Pontocaine (Pon'-to-kain)	Tetracaine (Teh'-tra-kain)
Povan (Po'-van)	Pyrvinium (Pire-vin'-ee-um)
Premarin (Prem'-ar-in)	Conjugated (Kon'-joo-gay-ted) Estrogens (Es-tro-jens)
Presamine (Press'-a-meen)	Imipramine (Im-ip'-rah-meen)
Primaquine (Pri'-mah-kwin)	Same
Probanthine (Pro-ban'-theen)	Propantheline (Pro-pan'-the-leen)
Pronestyl (Pro-nes'-til)	Procainamide (Pro-kain'-a-mide)
Prophylthiouracil (Pro-pil-thi-o-u'-rah-sil)	Same
Prostaphlin (Pro-staff'-lin)	Oxacillin (Oks'-ah-sil-in)
Provera (Pro-ver'-ah)	Medroxyprogesterone (Med-rok-see-pro-jes'-ter-one)
Pyridium (Pie-rid'-ee-um)	Phenazopyridine (Fen-ahs-o-per'-i-deen)
Quinidine (Kwin'-i-deen)	Same
Quinine (Kwie'-nine)	Same
Reserpine (Ree-ser'-peen)	Same
Retin A (Reh'-tin A)	Tretinoin (Tret'-i-noin)
Rifadin (Rie-fad'-in)	Rifampin (Rie-fam'-pin)
Riopan (Rie'-o-pan)	Magaidrate (Mag'-al-drate)

Trade Name	Generic Name
Rimactane (Rim-act'-ane)	Rifampin (Rie-fam'-pin)
Ritalin (Rit'-a-lin)	Methylphenidate (Meth-il-fen'-i-date)
Robaxin (Ro-bak'-sin)	Methocarbamol (Meth-o-kar'-ba-mol)
Robitussin (Row-i-tus'-sin)	Guaifenesin (Gwie-fen'-eh-sin)
Robitussin DM	Guiafenesin and Dextromethorphan (Dek-tro-meh-or'-fan)
Sansert (San'-sert)	Methysergide (Meth-ee-ser'-jide)
Seconal (Sek'-o-nal)	Secobarbital (Sek-o-bar'-bi-tal)
Selsun (Sel'-sun)	Selenium (Se-leh'-nee-um)
Septra (Sep'-tra)	Sulfamethoxazole (Sul-fah-meth-oks'-a-zole) and Trimethroprim (Tri-meth'-o-prim)
Serax (See'-raks)	Oxazepam (Oks-az'-eh-pam)
Silvadene (Sil'-va-deen)	Silver Sulfadiazine (Sul-fa-die'-a-zeen)
Sinemet (Si'-ne-met)	Levodopa (Le-vo-do'-pa)
Sinequan (Sin'-a-kwan)	Doxepin (Dok'-seh-pin)
Sorbitrate (Sor'-bi-trate)	Isosorbide (I-so-sor'-bide)
Stelazine (Stel'-a-zeen)	Trifluoperazine(Tri-floo-o-per'-a-zeen)
Sudafed (Soo'-da-fed)	Pseudophedrine (Soo-do-eh-feh'-drin)
Sulamyd (Sul'-a-mid)	Sulfacetamide (Sul-fah-set'-a-mide)
Sulfamylon (Sul-fa-mie'-lon)	Mafenide (Maf'-eh-nide)
Sultrin (Sul'-trin)	Sulfathiazole (Sul-fah-thi'-ah-zole) Sulfacetamide (Sul-fah-set'-ah-mide) and Sulfabenzamide (Sul-fah-benz'-ah-mide)
Surfak (Sur'-fak)	Dioctyl (Di-ok'-til) Calcium (Kal'-see-um) Sulfosuccinate (Sul-fo-suk'-si-nate)
Synalar (Sine'-a-lar)	Fluocinolone (Floo-o-sin'-o-lone)
Synthroid (Sin'-throid)	Levothyroxine (Lee-vo-thi-rok'-sin)
Tace (Tace)	Chlorotrianisene (Klor-o-tri-an'-I-seen)
Tagamet (Tag'-a-met)	Cimetidine (Si-met'-i-deen)
Talwin (Tal'-win)	Pentazocine (Pen-taz'-o-seen)
Tandearil (Tan'-da-ril)	Oxyphenbutazone (Ok-see-fen-bute'-a-zone)
Tegretol (Teg'-reh-tol)	Carbamazepine (Kar-ba-maz'-eh-peen)
Tessalon (Tess'-a-lon)	Benzonatate (Benz-on'-a-tate)
Tetracycline (Tet-ra-si'-kleen)	
Thorazine (Thor'-a-zeen)	Chlorpromazine (Klor-pro'-ma-zeen)
Thyroid (Thy'-roid)	Same
Tigan (Tie'-gan)	Trimethobenzamide (Tri-meth-o-benz'-a-mide)
Timoptic (Tim-op'-tic)	Timilol (Tim'-o-lol)

Trade Name	Generic Name
Tinactin (Tin-act'-in)	Tolnaftate (Tol-naf'-tate)
Titralac (Ti'-tra-lak)	Calcium (Kal-see-um) Carbonate (Kar'-bon-ate) and Glycine (Gly'-seen)
Tofranil (Toe'-fra-nil)	Imipramine (I-mip'-rah-meen)
Tolectin (Tow-lek'-tin)	Tolmetin (Tol-met'-in)
Triavil (Tri'-a-vil)	Perphenazine (Per-fen'-a-zeen) and Amitriptlyline (Am-i-trip'-ti-leen)
Trilafon (Try'-la-fon)	Perphenazine (Per-fen-a-zeen)
Tylenol (Tie'-leh-nol)	Acetaminophen (As-et-am'-ino-fen)
Tylenol #3	Acetaminophen and Codeine (Ko'-deen)
Unipen (U'-ni-pen)	Nafcillin (Naf-sil-lin)
Urecholine (Ur-eh-ko'-leen)	Bethanecol (Beth-an'-eh-kol)
Valisone (Val'-i-sone)	Betamethasone (Beh-tah-meth'-a-sone)
Valium (Val'-ee-um)	Diazepam (Die-aze-eh-pam)
Vermox (Ver'-moks)	Mebendazole (Meh-ben'-dah-zole)
Vibramycin (Vie-bra-my'-sin)	Doxycycline (Doks-see-si'-kleen)
Xylocaine (Zie'-low-kain)	Lidocaine (Lie-do-kain)
Zarontin (Zar-on'-tin)	Ethosuximide (Eh-tho-suks'-a-mide)
Zyloprim (Zie'-low-prim)	Allopurinol (Al-lo-pure'-in-ol)

COMMENT SHEET

SUBCOURSE MD0804   Pharmacology I   **EDITION 100**

Your comments about this subcourse are valuable and aid the writers in refining the subcourse and making it more usable. Please enter your comments in the space provided. ENCLOSE THIS FORM (OR A COPY) WITH YOUR ANSWER SHEET **ONLY** IF YOU HAVE COMMENTS ABOUT THIS SUBCOURSE..

FOR A WRITTEN REPLY, WRITE A SEPARATE LETTER AND INCLUDE SOCIAL SECURITY NUMBER, RETURN ADDRESS (and e-mail address, if possible), SUBCOURSE NUMBER AND EDITION, AND PARAGRAPH/EXERCISE/EXAMINATION ITEM NUMBER.

PLEASE COMPLETE THE FOLLOWING ITEMS:
(Use the reverse side of this sheet, if necessary.)

1.   List any terms that were not defined properly.

_____
_____
_____
_____

2.   List any errors.

   paragraph   error   correction

_____
_____
_____
_____
_____
_____
_____
_____

3.   List any suggestions you have to improve this subcourse.

_____
_____
_____
_____

4.   Student Information (optional)

Name/Rank _____
SSN _____
Address _____
         _____
E-mail Address _____
Telephone number (DSN) _____
MOS/AOC _____

U.S. ARMY MEDICAL DEPARTMENT CENTER AND SCHOOL   Fort Sam Houston, Texas 78234-6130

Pharmacology II

Subcourse MD0805

This page intentionally left blank.

U.S. ARMY MEDICAL DEPARTMENT CENTER AND SCHOOL
FORT SAM HOUSTON, TEXAS 78234-6100

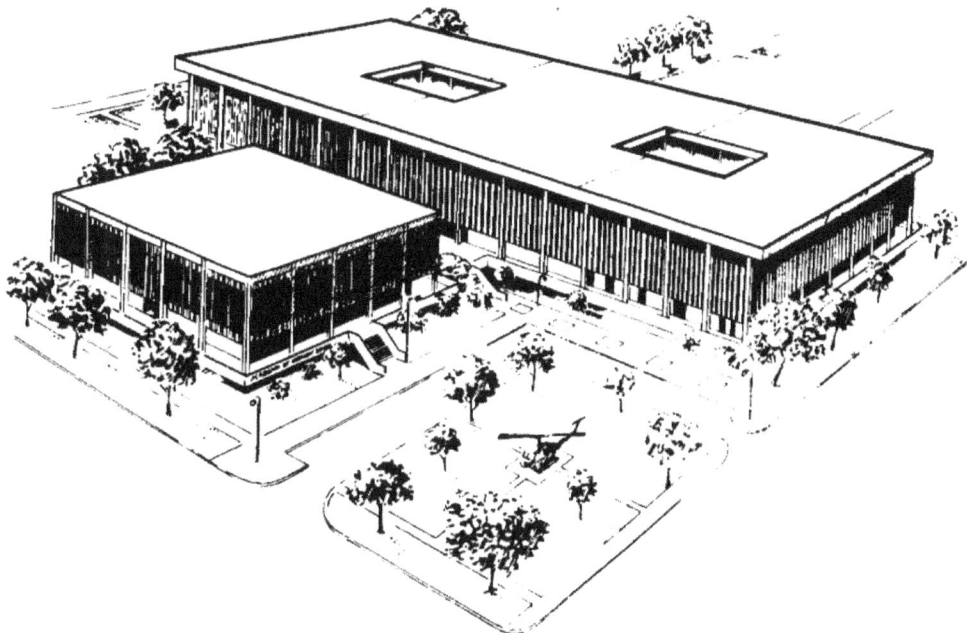

PHARMACOLOGY II

SUBCOURSE MD0805   **EDITION 100**

DEVELOPMENT

This subcourse is approved for resident and correspondence course instruction. It reflects the current thought of the Academy of Health Sciences and conforms to printed Department of the Army doctrine as closely as currently possible. Development and progress render such doctrine continuously subject to change.

ADMINISTRATION

For comments or questions regarding enrollment, student records, or shipments, contact the Nonresident Instruction Branch at DSN 471-5877, commercial (210) 221-5877, toll-free 1-800-344-2380; fax: 210-221-4012 or DSN 471-4012, e-mail accp@amedd.army.mil, or write to:

> COMMANDER
> AMEDDC&S
> ATTN MCCS HSN
> 2105 11TH STREET SUITE 4192
> FORT SAM HOUSTON TX 78234-5064

Approved students whose enrollments remain in good standing may apply to the Nonresident Instruction Branch for subsequent courses by telephone, letter, or e-mail.

Be sure your social security number is on all correspondence sent to the Academy of Health Sciences.

CLARIFICATION OF TRAINING LITERATURE TERMINOLOGY

When used in this publication, words such as "he," "him," "his," and "men" are intended to include both the masculine and feminine genders, unless specifically stated otherwise or when obvious in context.

TABLE OF CONTENTS

TABLE OF CONTENTS (cont'd)

LIST OF ILLUSTRATIONS

CORRESPONDENCE COURSE OF THE
U.S. ARMY MEDICAL DEPARTMENT CENTER AND SCHOOL

SUBCOURSE MD0805

PHARMACOLOGY II

INTRODUCTION

In Subcourse MD0804, Pharmacology I, the basics of pharmacology were reviewed. MD0804 stressed the identification and use of references pertaining to drug information. Furthermore, you were given specific information on eight specific categories of drugs.

Subcourse MD0805, Pharmacology II, is intended to give you a review of certain essential anatomical and physiological concepts important to pharmacology and to introduce six categories of drugs. The review of anatomy and physiology should help you gain a better understanding of how the drugs work in the body and how they produce the side effects that are commonly associated with their use.

Remember that this subcourse is not intended to be used as an authoritative source of drug information. New drugs are being discovered and new uses for existing drugs are being found through research. Therefore, you should rely on this subcourse to review concepts or to learn new information. You should then use other sources (see MD0804, Pharmacology I--Lesson 1) to gain additional information which will help you to do your job in a better way.

Subcourse Components:

This subcourse consists of 10 lessons. The lessons are:

Lesson 1. Dermatological Agents.

Lesson 2. The Human Muscular System.

Lesson 3. Skeletal Muscle Relaxants.

Lesson 4. Analgesic, Anti-inflammatory, and Anti-gout Agents.

Lesson 5. Review of Ocular and Auditory Anatomy and Physiology.

Lesson 6. Review of the Autonomic Nervous System.

Lesson 7. Adrenergic Agents.

Lesson 8. Adrenergic Blocking Agents.

Lesson 9. Cholinergic Agents.

Lesson 10. Cholinergic Blocking Agents (Anticholinergic Agents).

Credit Awarded:

To receive credit hours, you must be officially enrolled and complete an examination furnished by the Nonresident Instruction Branch at Fort Sam Houston, Texas. Upon successful completion of the examination for this subcourse, you will be awarded 14 credit hours.

You can enroll by going to the web site http://atrrs.army.mil and enrolling under "Self Development" (School Code 555).

A listing of correspondence courses and subcourses available through the Nonresident Instruction Section is found in Chapter 4 of DA Pamphlet 350-59, Army Correspondence Course Program Catalog. The DA PAM is available at the following website: http://www.usapa.army.mil/pdffiles/p350-59.pdf.

LESSON ASSIGNMENT

LESSON 1	Dermatological Agents.
TEXT ASSIGNMENT	Paragraphs 1-1--1-5.
LESSON OBJECTIVES	After completing this lesson, you should be able to:

1-1.   Given a group of definitions and one of the following terms: dermatological agent, antiseborrheic agent, astringent, keratolytic agent, or keratoplastic agent, select the definition of that term.

1-2.   Given a group of statements, select the statement that best describes a general consideration pertaining to dermatological agents.

1-3.   Given a group of statements and the name of a particular category of dermatological agents, select the statement which best describes a general consideration or indication of that particular category.

1-4.   Given the trade or generic name of a dermatological agent and a list of trade and/or generic names, select the agent's corresponding name.

1-5.   Given the generic and/or trade name of a dermatological agent and a group of statements, select the statement which best describes the indication, use, or side effect associated with that agent.

SUGGESTION   After studying the assignment, complete the exercises at the end of this lesson. These exercises will help you to achieve the lesson objectives.

LESSON 1

DERMATOLOGICAL AGENTS

Section I. BACKGROUND INFORMATION

1-1. DEFINITION OF DERMATOLOGICAL AGENTS

Dermatological agents are drugs that exert either a chemical or physical action on the skin to aid in the correction of a disorder of the skin.

1-2. GENERAL CONSIDERATIONS INVOLVING DERMATOLOGICAL AGENTS

a.   The vehicles (creams, lotions, ointments, and so forth.) in which therapeutic ingredients are incorporated and diluted have been found to have pharmacological properties of their own. This subcourse will not mention these pharmacological properties of the vehicles. Instead, it will focus strictly on the pharmacological actions and effects of the therapeutic ingredients.

b.   There is a great variation in the manner in which vehicles hold, release, or assist in the absorption of their therapeutic ingredients. Therefore, it is important that the vehicle selected to contain a therapeutic ingredient be suitable for use on the portion of skin on which it will be applied.

c.   The distribution of the therapeutic ingredient(s) throughout a vehicle is an important factor in the determination of a dermatological's effectiveness. You must be aware of this fact because you might one day be required to compound or manufacture some of the dermatological products discussed in this subcourse.

Section II. THERAPEUTIC CATEGORIES OF DERMATOLOGICAL AGENTS

1-3. ANTISEBORRHEICS

a.   **Definition.** Antiseborrheics are used in the management of seborrheic dermatitis. Seborrheic dermatitis is characterized by a yellowish and greasy scaling of the scalp and/or mid-parts of the face (around eyebrows and nose) and ears.

b.   **General Considerations.** The ideal antiseborrheic agent should be nontoxic, relieve pruritus (itching), modify excessive dryness, and demonstrate wide antifungal and antibacterial spectra.

c. **Specific Antiseborrheic Agents.**

(1) Chloroxine (Capitrol®). This agent is used in the treatment of dandruff and seborrheic dermatitis of the scalp. The patient should be instructed not to use this medication if blistered, raw, or oozing areas are present on the scalp and to keep the medication away from the eyes. This medication may slightly discolor light-colored hair.

(2) Selenium sulfide (Selsun®). This shampoo product is used to treat dandruff and seborrheic dermatitis of the scalp. The patient should be instructed not to use this medication if blistered, raw, or oozing areas are present on the scalp and to keep the medication away from the eyes. This medication should be thoroughly rinsed from the hair of persons with light-colored hair because it can cause discoloration.

(3) Sebulex® or Sebra® Shampoo. This product is made of salicylic acid (2%) and sulfur (2%). It is used as a shampoo to treat seborrheic dermatitis, dandruff, and psoriasis of the scalp. Present in these concentrations, salicylic acid and sulfur are used for their keratoplastic (mild keratolytic) actions. The patient using this product should be informed of two things. One, this product may discolor light-colored hair. Two, the patient should not use this product on the same area to which has been applied any topical mercury-containing product (such as ammoniated mercury ointment) because doing so might stain that area of skin and produce a foul odor (interaction between sulfur and mercury).

(4) Sebutone® or Sebra T® Shampoo. This product is made of salicylic acid (2%), coal tar (0.5%), and sulfur (2%). In these concentrations, the salicylic acid and sulfur are used for their keratoplastic (mild keratolytic) actions, and coal tar is used for its antipruritic (controls itching), antibacterial, and keratoplastic actions. The patient using this product should be informed of two things. One, this product may discolor light-colored hair. Two, the patient should not use this product on the same area to which has been applied any topical mercury-containing product (such as ammoniated mercury ointment) because doing so might stain that area and produce a foul odor.

1-4. ASTRINGENTS

a. **Definition.** An astringent is an agent that dries mucous secretions, shrinks skin, and causes blanching (whitening).

b. **Indications for the use of Astringents.** Astringents are used to reduce inflammation of mucous membranes, to promote healing, and to toughen skin.

c. **Specific Astringent Agents.**

(1) Aluminum acetate tablets (Domeboro®. Burow's solution). When these tablets are added to water, aluminum acetate solution is prepared. This product is used as an astringent for inflammatory skin conditions such as insect bites, poison ivy, and athlete's foot. The patient receiving these tablets should be warned that they are for

external use only. The patient should be told to see his physician if the inflammatory condition does not improve and to avoid getting the prepared solution in contact with his eyes. Usually one or two of the tablets are dissolved in a pint of water. The patient is then to soak the affected area two or three times daily in the freshly prepared solution for 15 minutes.

(2) Calamine lotion (calamine and zinc oxide lotion). This product is used as an astringent and as a protectant (used to cover and protect epithelial surfaces). Both these actions aid in reducing inflammation associated with insect bites, poison ivy, and sunburn. The patient receiving this product should be told that the preparation is for external use only and that he should shake the product well before using it.

(3) Phenolated and mentholated calamine lotion. Phenol and menthol have been added to the product above because they produce an antipruritic effect.

1-5. KERATOLYTICS

a. **Definition**. A keratolytic is an agent that induces sloughing of cornified epithelium (horny or hard layer of the skin).

b. **General Considerations**. Keratolytic drugs act to damage the cornified layer of skin that is then sloughed off to whatever depth the agent has acted. A keratoplastic (mild keratolytic) effect is seen when the drug does not produce a rapid destruction and sloughing, thereby softening the keratin and loosening the cornified epithelium.

c. **Indications for the Use of Keratolytic Agents**. Keratolytic agents are used to remove warts and corns. They are also used in the treatment of severe acne.

d. **Indications for the Use of Keratoplastic Agents**. Keratoplastic agents are used in the treatment of acne, eczema, psoriasis, and seborrheic dermatitis.

e. **Specific Keratolytic Agents**.

NOTE: You will see chemicals (1) through (4) present in several manufactured products. You might be called upon to compound or manufacture products containing one or more of these substances. If you handle these chemicals, remember that they are irritating to the skin. You should wash your hands immediately after working with them.

(1) Coal tar (chemical name). This agent is used as a keratoplastic in the treatment of eczema, psoriasis, and seborrheic dermatitis.

(2) Salicylic acid (chemical name). It is used as a keratolytic when present in concentrations of from 5% to 20%. It is used as a kerato- plastic when present in concentrations of from 1% to 2%.

(3) Sulfur (chemical name). Sulfur is used as a keratoplastic in the treatment of acne and seborrheic dermatitis.

(4) Tretinoin (topical) (Retin A®). This agent is used in the treatment of severe acne. The application of this agent to the skin will produce a horny layer of skin that is more easily removed. It is important that the patient use this preparation as directed by the physician and package directions. This medicine should not be applied to windburned or sunburned skin. It should not be applied to open wounds. Furthermore, the medication should not be applied inside the nose, around the eyes, or around the mouth. While the patient is using the medication, he should avoid exposing the area being treated to too much wind or sun (or sun lamp). When the patient begins using this product, he may find that he is more sensitive to cold temperatures and to wind than before; therefore, protection should be worn until the persons sees how he reacts. This product is available in cream, liquid, and gel.

(5) Salicylic acid 2% and sulfur 2% (Fostex®). This preparation is available in cream or soap. It is used to treat acne.

(6) Salicylic acid 2% and Sulfur 2% shampoo (Sebulex® or Sebra®). This shampoo is used to treat dandruff.

(7) Salicylic acid 2%, coal tar 0.5%, and sulfur 2% shampoo (Sebutone® or Sebra T®). This product is used to treat dandruff.

Continue with Exercises

End of Lesson 1

EXERCISES, LESSON 1

INSTRUCTIONS: Answer the following exercises by marking the lettered response which best answers the question.

After you have completed all the exercises, turn to "Solutions to Exercises" at the end of the lesson, and, check your answers. For each exercise answered incorrectly, reread the material referenced with the solution.

1. Select the definition of the term antiseborrheic agent.

    a. An agent that dries mucous secretions, shrinks skin, and causes blanching.

    b. An agent used to manage a skin condition characterized by a yellowish and greasy scaling of the scalp and/or mid-parts of the face and ears.

    c. An agent used in the treatment of severe acne and in the removal of warts or corns.

    d. An agent used in the treatment of acne, eczema, and psoriasis.

2. Which of the following statements best describes a general consideration associated with the use of keratolytic agents?

    a. These agents are not to be used on mucous membranes.

    b. These agents sometimes produce a yellowish and greasy scaling around the mid-parts of the face when they are applied as a treatment for acne.

    c. These agents usually make a person excessively sensitive to the effects of cold and wind.

    d. These agents are used to damage the cornified layer of skin so that it will be sloughed off.

3. Select the correct use of Burow's solution.

    a. An astringent for inflammatory skin conditions.

    b. An agent used in the treatment of seborrheic dermatitis.

    c. An agent used in the treatment of eczema.

    d. An astringent used in the treatment of warts and corns.

4. Match the generic name in Column A with its corresponding trade name in Column B.

Column A	Column B
A. Salicylic acid 2% and sulfur 2% soap	_____ Fostex®
B. Selenium sulfide	_____ Retin A®
C. Tretinoin	_____ Selsun®
D. Aluminum acetate tablets	_____ Capitrol®
E. Coal tar	_____ Burow's solution

5. Select the information you should give a patient who has been prescribed selenium sulfide shampoo for the first time.

   a. "You should wear some sort of protection because you might be more sensitive to cold temperatures and to wind."

   b. "You should not use this medication if you have applied any medicine containing mercury on your scalp."

   c. "You should not use this medication if your scalp is raw or blistered."

   d. "You should stop using this medication if your scalp condition has not improved within five days."

6. Select the information you should give to a person who has been prescribed aluminum acetate tablets for the first time.

   a. "These tablets are not to be taken by mouth. Instead, make a solution as prescribed on the container label and use the prepared solution as a soak."

   b. "Do not be alarmed if your hair turns slightly orange for a few days after you use this product."

   c. "Do not expose the portion of your body you are soaking in the prepared solution to sunlight or wind."

   d. "Do not use the solution you prepare from these tablets on any part of your body to which has been applied any medication containing mercury."

7. Select the correct use of coal tar.

   a. A keratoplastic agent used in the treatment of eczema, psoriasis, and seborrheic dermatitis.

   b. A keratolytic agent used in the treatment of severe acne.

   c. An astringent used in the treatment of acne and seborrheic dermatitis.

   d. A product used as a protectant and astringent in the treatment of inflammation associated with insect bites and sunburn.

Check Your Answers on Next Page

SOLUTIONS TO EXERCISES, LESSON 1

1.   b   An agent used to manage a skin condition characterized by a yellowish and greasy scaling of the scalp and/or mid-parts of the face and ears. (para 1-3a)

2.   d   These agents are used to damage the cornified layer of skin so that it will be sloughed off. (para 1-5b)

3.   a   An astringent for inflammatory skin conditions. (para 1-4c(1))

4.   <u>A</u>   Fostex® (para 1-5e(5))

        <u>C</u>   Retin A® (para 1-5e(4))

        <u>B</u>   Selsun® (para 1-3c(2))

        <u>E</u>   Capitrol® (para 1-3c(1))

        <u>D</u>   Burow's Solution (para 1-4c(1))

5.   c   "You should not use this medication if your scalp is raw or blistered." (para 1-3c(2))

6.   a   "These tablets are not to be taken by mouth. Instead, make a solution as prescribed on the container label and use the prepared solution as a soak." (para 1-4c(1))

7.   a   A keratoplastic agent used in the treatment of eczema, psoriasis, and seborrheic dermatitis. (para 1-5e(1))

End of Lesson 1

ANNEX

DRUG PRONUNCIATION GUIDE

This Drug Pronunciation Guide was developed to help you to learn how the trade and generic names of commonly prescribed medications are frequently pronounced. Not all the drugs in the guide are discussed in this subcourse. Remember, it is not enough to be able to know the uses, indications, cautions and warnings, and contraindications for a drug--you must also know how to pronounce that drug's name.

Trade Name	*Generic Name*
Actifed (Ak'-ti-fed)	Triprolidine (Tri-pro'-li-deen) and Pseudoephedrine (Soo-do-e-fed'-rin)
Adapin (Ad'-a-pin)	Doxepin (Dok'-se-pin)
Sinequan (Sin'-a-kwan)	" "
Afrin (Af'-rin)	Oxymetazoline (Ok-see-met-az'-o-leen)
Aldactazide (Al-dak'-ta-zide)	Spironolactone (Spi-ro-no-lak'-tone) and Hydrochlorothiazide (Hy-dro-klor-thi'-a-zide)
Aldactone (Al-dak'-tone)	Spironolactone (Spi-ro-no-lak'-tone)
Aldomet (Al'-do-met)	Methyldopa (Meth-il-do'-pah)
Alupent (Al'-u-pent)	Metaproterenol (Met-a-pro-ter'-eh-nol)
Amoxil (Am-ok'-sil)	Amoxicillin (Ah-moks'-i-sil-in)
Amphojel (Am'-fo-jel)	Aluminum (Al-loo'-mi-num) Hydroxide (Hy-drok'-side)
Ampicillin (Amp'-I-sil-in)	Same
Antepar (Ab'-te-par)	Piperazine (Pi-per'-ah-zeen)
Anturane (An'-tu-rain)	Sulfinpyrazone (Sul-fin-pie'-ra-zone)
Anusol (An'-u-sol)	Pramoxine (Pram-ok'-seen)
Apresoline (A-press'-o-leen)	Hydralazine (Hy-dral'-ah-zeen)
Aralen (Ar'-a-len)	Chloroquine (Klor'-o-kwin)
Aristocort (A-ris'-to-cort)	Triamcinolone (Tri-am-sin'-o-lone)
Artane (Ar'-tane)	Trihexyphenidyl(Tri-hek-see-fen'-i-dil)
A.S.A.	Aspirin (As'-per-in)
Atromid S (A'-tro-mid)	Clofibrate (Klo-fi'-brate)
Avlosulfon (Av-lo-sul'-fon)	Dapsone (Dap'-sone)
Azolid (Az'-o-lid)	Phenylbutazone (Fen-il-bute'-a-zone)
Bactrim (Bak'-trim)	Sulfamethoxazole (Sul-fah-meth-oks'-ah-zole) and Trimethoprim (Tri-meth'-o-prim)
Bellergal (Bel'-er-gal)	Ergotamine (Er-got'-a-meen), Phenobarbital (Feen-o-bar'-bi-tal) and Belladonna (Bel-la-don'-na) Alkaloids
Benadryl (Ben'-a-dril)	Diphenhydramine (Di-fen-hy'-dra-meen)

Trade Name	Generic Name
Bendectin (Ben-dek'-tin)	Doxylamine (Dok-sil'-a-meen)
Benemid (Ben'-eh-mid)	Probenecid (Pro-ben'-eh-sid)
Bonine (Bo'-neen)	Meclizine (Mek'-li-zeen)
Cafergot (Kaf'-er-got)	Ergotamine (Er-got'-a-meen) and Caffeine (Kaf'-feen)
Calamine (Kal'-a-mine)	Same
Catapres (Kat'-a-press)	Clonidine (Klo'-ni-deen)
CeeNu (See'-new)	Lomustine (Lo-mus'-teen)
Chlor-Trimeton (Klo-tri '-meh-ton)	Chlorpheniramine (Klor-fen-it'-a-meen)
Clomid (Klo'-mid)	Clomiphene (Klo'-mi-feen)
Clonopin (Klo-o-pin)	Clonazepam (Klo-na'-ze-pam)
Codeine (Ko'-deen)	Same
Cogentin (Ko-jen'-tin)	Benztropine (Benz'-tro-peen)
Colace (Ko'-lace)	Dioctyl(Di-ok'-til) Sodium (So'-dee-um) Sulfosuccinate (Sul-fo-suk'-si-nate)
Colchicine (Kol'-chi-seen)	Same
Compazine (Kom'-pa-zeen)	Prochiorperazine (Pro-klor-per'-a-zeen)
Cordran (Kor'-dran)	Flurandrenolide (Floor-an-dren'-o-lide)
Coumadin (Koo'-mah-din)	Warfarin (War'-fah-rin)
CP	Cloroquine (Klor'-o-kwin) and Primaquine (Prim'-a-kwin)
Cyclogyl (Si'-klo-jel)	Cyclopentolate (Si-klo-pen'-to-late)
Cytomel (Si'-to-mel)	Liothyronine (Li-o-thy-ro-neen)
Cytoxan (Si-tok'-san)	Cyclophosphamide (Si-klo-fos'-fa-mide)
Dalmane (Dal '-mane)	Flurazepam (Floor-az'-e-pam)
Darvocet (Dar'-vo-set)	Propoxyphene (Pro-pok'-se-feen) and Acetaminopen (As-et-am'-ino-fen)
Darvon (Dar'-von)	Propoxyphene (Pro-pok-se-feen)
Decadron (Dek'-a-dron)	Dexamethasone (Dek-sa-meth'-ah-sone)
Deltasone (Del '-ta-sone)	Prednisone (Pred'-ni-sone)
Demerol (Dem'-er-ol)	Meperidine (Meh-pair'-i-deen)
Dexedrine (Deks '-eh-dreen)	Dextroamphetamine (Deks-tro-am-fet'-a-meen)
Diabinese (Di-ab'-i-nees)	Chlorpropamide (Klor-prop'-a-mide)
Diethylstilbestrol (Di-eth-il-stil-bes'-trol)	Same
Dilantin (Di-lan'-tin)	Phenytoin (Fen'-i-toin)
Dilaudid (Di-law'-did)	Hydromorphone (Hy-dro-more' -fon)
Dimetane (Di'-meh-tane)	Brompheniramine (Brom-fen-ir'-a-meen)

Trade Name	Generic Name
Dimetapp (Di'-meh-tap)	Brompheniramine (Brom-fen-ir'-a-meen) Phenylephrine (Fen-il-ef'-rin) and Phenylpropanolamine (Fen-il-pro-pan-ol'-a-meen)
Disophrol (Dice'-o-frol)	Dexbrompheniramine (Deks-brom-fen-ir'-a-meen) and Pseudoephedrine (Soo-do-e-fed'-rin)
Dolophine (Dol'-o-feen)	Methadone (Meth'-a-done)
Domeboro (Dome-bor'-o)	Aluminum (Ah-loo'-mi-num) Acetate (As'-e-tate)
Donnatal (Don'-na-tal)	Belladonna (Bel-la-don'-na) Alkaloids (Al'-ka-loids) and Phenobarbital (Feen-o-barb'-i-tal)
Doxidan (Dok'-si-dan)	Danthron (Dan'-thron) and Dicctyl (Di-ok'-til) Calcium (Kal'-see-um) Sulfosuccinate (Sul-fo-suk'-si-nate)
Drixoral (Driks'-or-al)	Dexbrompheniramine (Deks-brom-fen-ir'-a-meen) and Pseudoephedrine (Soo-do-e-fed'-rin)
Dulcolax (Dul'-ko-laks)	Bisacodyl (Bis-a'-ko-dil)
Dyazine (Di'-a-zide)	Triamterene (Tri-am'-ter-een) and Hydrochlorothiazide (Hy-dro-klor-o-thi'-a-zide)
Dymelor (Die'-meh-lor)	Acetohexamide (As-e-to-heks'-a-mide)
Dyrenium (Die-ren'-i-um)	Triamterene (Tri-am'-ter-een)
Efudex (Ef'-u-deks)	Fluorouracil (Floo-ro-ur'-ah-sil)
Elavil (El'-ah-vil)	Amitriptyline (Am-i-trip'-til-een)
Elixir Terpin (Ter'-pin) Hydrate	Same
Empirin (Em'-per-in)	Codeine (Ko'-deen) and Aspirin (As'-per-in)
E-Mycin (E-mie'-sin)	Erythromycin (E-rith-ro-mie'-sin)
Equanil (Ek'-wa-nil)	Meprobamate (Me-pro-bam'-ate)
Ergomar (Er'-go-mar)	Ergotamine (Er-got'-a-meen)
Ergotrate (Er'-go-trate)	Ergonovine (Er-go-no'-veen)
Erythrocin (Er-eeth'-ro-sin)	Erythromycin (Er-eeth-ro-my'-sin) Stearate (Stare'-rate)
Esidrix (Es'-i-driks)	Hyrochlorothiazide (Hy-dro-klor-o-thi'-a-zide)
Feosol (Fe'-o-sol)	Ferrous (Fer'-rus) Sulfate (Sul'-fate)
Fergon (Fer'-gon)	Ferrous (Fer'-rus) Gluconate (Glu'-con-ate)

Trade Name	Generic Name
Fiorinal (Fee-or'-i-nal)	Butalbi tal (Bu-tal'-bi-tal), Apririn, Phenacetin (Fen-ass'-eh-tin), and Caffeine (Kaf'-feen)
Flagyl (Fla'-jil)	Metronidazole (Me-tro-ni'-dah-zole)
Flexeril (Flek'-sa-ril)	Cyclobenzaprine (Si-klo-benz'-a-preen)
Fulvicin (Ful'-vi-sin)	Griseofulvin (Griz-e-o-ful'-vin)
Guantanol (Gan'-ta-nol)	Suiphamethoxazole (Sul-fah-meth-oks'-ah-zole)
Gantrisin (Gan'-tri-sin)	Sulfisoxazole (Sul-fi-sok'-sah-zole)
Gelusil (Jel'-u-sil)	Aluminum (Ah-loo'-mi-num) Hydroxide (Hy-drok'-side) and Magnesium (Mag-nee'-zee-um) Hydroxide
Grifulvin (Gri-ful'-vin)	Griseofulvin (Griz-e-o-ful'-vin)
Gynergen (Jin'-er-jen)	Ergotamine (Er-got'-a-meen)
Haldol (Hal'-dol)	Haloperidol (Hal-o-pair'-i-dol)
Halotestin (Hal-o-tes'-tin)	Fluoxymesterone (Floo-ok-see-mes-teh-rone)
Hexadrol (Hek'-sa-drol)	Dexamethasone (Dek-sa-meth'-a-sone)
Hydrodiuril (Hy-dro-di'-ur-il)	Hydroclorothiazide (Hy-dro-kior-thi'-a-zide)
Hygroton (Hy-grow'-ton)	Chiorthalidone (Kior-thal'-i-done)
Ilosone (I'-low-sone)	Erythromycin (Er-ith-ro-mi'-sin) Estolate (Es'-to-late)
Inderal (In'-der-al)	Propranolol (Pro-pran'-o-lol)
Indocin (In'-do-sin)	Indomethacin (In-do-meth'-a-sin)
INH	Isoniazid (I-so-ni'-a-zid)
Insulin (In'-sul-in)	Same
Intal	Cromolyn (Kro'-mo-lin)
Ismelin (Is'-meh-lin)	Guanethidine (Gwan-eth'-i-dine)
Isopto-Atropine (I-sop-to-at'-ro-peen)	Atropine (At'-ro-peen)
Isopto-Carpine (I-sop-to-car'-peen)	Pilocarpine (Pile-o-car'-peen)
Isordil (I'-sor-dil)	Isosorbide (I-so-sor'-bide)
Keflex (Kef'-lex)	Cephalexin (Sef-ah-lek'-sin)
Lanoxin (Lan-ok'-sin)	Digoxin (Di-jok'-sin)
Larodopa (Lar-o-do'-pa)	Levodopa (Le-o-do'-pa)
Larotid (Lar'-o-tid)	Amoxicillin (Ah-moks'-i-sil-in)
Lasix (La'-siks)	Furosemide (Fu-ro'-se-mide)
Leukeran (Lu'-ker-an)	Chlorambucil (Klor-ram'-bu-sil)
Librium (Lib'-ree-um)	Chlordiazepoxide (Klor-die-az-eh-pok'-side)

Trade Name	Generic Name
Lidex (Lie'-deks)	Fluocinoide (Floo-o-sin'-o-nide)
Lomotil (Lo'-mo-til)	Diphenoxylate (Die-fen-ok'-si-late)
Lopressor (Lo'-pres-sor)	Metoprolol (Met-o-pro'-lol)
Lotrimin (Lo'-tri-min)	Chlotrimazole (Klo-trim'-ah-zole)
Maalox (May'-loks)	Aluminum (Ah-loo'-mi-num) and Magnesium (Mag-nee'-zee-um) Hydroxides
Macrodanton (Ma-kro-dan'-tin)	Nitrofurantoin (Ni-tro-fur-an'-toin)
Mandelamine (Man-del'-a-meen)	Methenamine (Meth-en'-a-meen) Mandelate (Man'-deh-late)
Medihaler-Iso (Med-i-hail-er-I'-so)	Isoproterenol (I-so-pro-ter'-en-ol)
Mellaril (Mel'-la-ril)	Thioridazine (Thi-o-rid'-a-zeen)
Metamucil (Met-a-mu'-sil)	Psyllium (Sil'-e-um)
Metaprel (Meh'-ta-prel)	Metaproterenol (Meh'-ta-pro-ter'-eh-nol)
Methotrexate (Meth-o-treks'-ate)	Amethopterin (Ah-meth-op'-ter-in)
Milk of Magnesia	Same
Minipress (Min'-i-press)	Prazosin (Pra'-zo-sin)
Minocin (Min'-o-sin)	Minocycline (Mi-no-si'-kleen)
Monistat (Mon'-i-stat)	Miconazole (Mi-kon'-ah-zole)
Motrin (Mo'-trin)	Ibuprofen (I-bu'-pro-fen)
Myambutol (My-am'-bu-tol)	Ethambutol (Eth-am'-bu-tol)
Mycostatin (My-co-stat'-in)	Nystatin (Ny-stat'-in)
Mylanta (My-lan'-ta)	Aluminum (Ah-loo'-mi-num) and Magnesium (Mag-nee'-zee-um) Hydroxides and Simethicone (Si-meth'-i-kone)
Myleran (My-ler-an)	Busulfan (Bu-sul'-fan)
Mylicon (My'-li-kon)	Simethicone (Si-meth'-i-kone)
Mysoline (My'-so-leen)	Primidone (Pri'-mi-done)
Nalfon (Nal'-fon)	Fenoprofen (Fen-o-pro'-fen)
Naprosyn (Na'-pro-sin)	Naproxen (Na-prok'-sen)
Nembutal (Nem'-bu-tal)	Pentobarbital (Pen-to-barb'-i-tal)
Neosynephrine (Nee-o-sin-eh'-frin)	Phenylephrine (Fen-il-eh'-frin)
Nitrobid (Ni'-tro-bid)	Nitroglycerin (Ni-tro-gli'-ser-in)
Nitrol (Ni'-trol)	" "
Nitrostat (Ni-tro-stat)	" "
Noctec (Nok'-tek)	Chloral Hydrate (Klor'-al- Hy'-drate)
Norfiex (Nor'-fleks)	Orphenadrine Citrate (Or-fen'-a-dreen)
Norpace (Nor'-pace)	Disopyramide (Di-so-peer'-a-mide)

Trade Name	Generic Name
Novahistine (No-va-his'-teen) Expectorant	Guaifenesin (Gwi-fen'-eh-sin), Phenylpropanolamine (Fen-il-pro-pan-ol'-a-meen), and Codeine (Ko'-deen)
NTG	Nitroclycerin (Ni-tro-gli'-ser-in)
Nupercainal (New-per-kain'-al)	Dibucaine (Die'-bu-kain)
Oretic (O-ret'-ik)	Hydrochiorothiazide (Hy-dro-kior-thi'-a-zide)
Orinase (Or'-in-ase)	Tolbutamide (Tol-bu'-tah-mide)
Ornade (Or'-nade)	Chlorpheniramine (Klor-fen-ir'-a-meen), Triprolidine (Tri-pro-li-deen) and Pseudoephedrine (Su-do-eh-fed'-rin)
Parafon Forte (Pair'-a-fon For'-tay)	Chlorzoxazone (Klor-zok'-sa-zone)
Percodan (Per'-ko-dan)	Oxycodone (Ok-si-ko'-done)
Periactin (Per-ee-ak'-tin)	Cyproheptadine (Si-pro-hep'-tah-deen)
Persantine (Per-san'-teen)	Dipyridamole (Di-pi-rid'-ah-mole)
Phenobarbital (Feen-o-barb'-it-al)	Same
Phenylpropanolamine (Fen-il-pro-pan-ol'-a-meen)	Same
Pitocin (Pi-tow'-sin)	Oxytocin (Ok-see-tow'-sin)
Pontocaine (Pon'-to-kain)	Tetracaine (Teh'-tra-kain)
Povan (Po'-van)	Pyrvinium (Pire-vin'-ee-um)
Premarin (Prem'-ar-in)	Conjugated (Kon'-joo-gay-ted) Estrogens (Es-tro-jens)
Presamine (Press'-a-meen)	Imipramine (Im-ip'-rah-meen)
Primaquine (Pri'-mah-kwin)	Same
Probanthine (Pro-ban'-theen)	Propantheline (Pro-pan'-the-leen)
Pronestyl (Pro-nes'-til)	Procainamide (Pro-kain'-a-mide)
Prophylthiouracil (Pro-pil-thi-o-u'-rah-sil)	Same
Prostaphlin (Pro-staff'-lin)	Oxacillin (Oks'-ah-sil-in)
Provera (Pro-ver'-ah)	Medroxyprogesterone (Med-rok-see-pro-jes'-ter-one)
Pyridium (Pie-rid'-ee-um)	Phenazopyridine (Fen-ahs-o-per'-i-deen)
Quinidine (Kwin'-i-deen)	Same
Quinine (Kwie'-nine)	Same
Reserpine (Ree-ser'-peen)	Same
Retin A (Reh'-tin A)	Tretinoin (Tret'-i-noin)
Rifadin (Rie-fad'-in)	Rifampin (Rie-fam'-pin)
Riopan (Rie'-o-pan)	Magaidrate (Mag'-al-drate)

Trade Name	Generic Name
Rimactane (Rim-act'-ane)	Rifampin (Rie-fam'-pin)
Ritalin (Rit'-a-lin)	Methylphenidate (Meth-il-fen'-i-date)
Robaxin (Ro-bak'-sin)	Methocarbamol (Meth-o-kar'-ba-mol)
Robitussin (Row-i-tus'-sin)	Guaifenesin (Gwie-fen'-eh-sin)
Robitussin DM	Guiafenesin and Dextromethorphan (Dek-tro-meh-or'-fan)
Sansert (San'-sert)	Methysergide (Meth-ee-ser'-jide)
Seconal (Sek'-o-nal)	Secobarbital (Sek-o-bar'-bi-tal)
Selsun (Sel'-sun)	Selenium (Se-leh'-nee-um)
Septra (Sep'-tra)	Sulfamethoxazole (Sul-fah-meth-oks'-a-zole) and Trimethroprim (Tri-meth'-o-prim)
Serax (See'-raks)	Oxazepam (Oks-az'-eh-pam)
Silvadene (Sil'-va-deen)	Silver Sulfadiazine (Sul-fa-die'-a-zeen)
Sinemet (Si'-ne-met)	Levodopa (Le-vo-do'-pa)
Sinequan (Sin'-a-kwan)	Doxepin (Dok'-seh-pin)
Sorbitrate (Sor'-bi-trate)	Isosorbide (I-so-sor'-bide)
Stelazine (Stel'-a-zeen)	Trifluoperazine(Tri-floo-o-per'-a-zeen)
Sudafed (Soo'-da-fed)	Pseudophedrine (Soo-do-eh-feh'-drin)
Sulamyd (Sul'-a-mid)	Sulfacetamide (Sul-fah-set'-a-mide)
Sulfamylon (Sul-fa-mie'-lon)	Mafenide (Maf'-eh-nide)
Sultrin (Sul'-trin)	Sulfathiazole (Sul-fah-thi'-ah-zole) Sulfacetamide (Sul-fah-set'-ah-mide) and Sulfabenzamide (Sul-fah-benz'-ah-mide)
Surfak (Sur'-fak)	Dioctyl (Di-ok'-til) Calcium (Kal'-see-um) Sulfosuccinate (Sul-fo-suk'-si-nate)
Synalar (Sine'-a-lar)	Fluocinolone (Floo-o-sin'-o-lone)
Synthroid (Sin'-throid)	Levothyroxine (Lee-vo-thi-rok'-sin)
Tace (Tace)	Chlorotrianisene (Klor-o-tri-an'-I-seen)
Tagamet (Tag'-a-met)	Cimetidine (Si-met'-i-deen)
Talwin (Tal'-win)	Pentazocine (Pen-taz'-o-seen)
Tandearil (Tan'-da-ril)	Oxyphenbutazone (Ok-see-fen-bute'-a-zone)
Tegretol (Teg'-reh-tol)	Carbamazepine (Kar-ba-maz'-eh-peen)
Tessalon (Tess'-a-lon)	Benzonatate (Benz-on'-a-tate)
Tetracycline (Tet-ra-si'-kleen)	
Thorazine (Thor'-a-zeen)	Chlorpromazine (Klor-pro'-ma-zeen)
Thyroid (Thy'-roid)	Same
Tigan (Tie'-gan)	Trimethobenzamide (Tri-meth-o-benz'-a-mide)
Timoptic (Tim-op'-tic)	Timilol (Tim'-o-lol)

Trade Name	Generic Name
Tinactin (Tin-act'-in)	Tolnaftate (Tol-naf'-tate)
Titralac (Ti'-tra-lak)	Calcium (Kal-see-um) Carbonate (Kar'-bon-ate) and Glycine (Gly'-seen)
Tofranil (Toe'-fra-nil)	Imipramine (I-mip'-rah-meen)
Tolectin (Tow-lek'-tin)	Tolmetin (Tol-met'-in)
Triavil (Tri'-a-vil)	Perphenazine (Per-fen'-a-zeen) and Amitriptlyline (Am-i-trip'-ti-leen)
Trilafon (Try'-la-fon)	Perphenazine (Per-fen-a-zeen)
Tylenol (Tie'-leh-nol)	Acetaminophen (As-et-am'-ino-fen)
Tylenol #3	Acetaminophen and Codeine (Ko'-deen)
Unipen (U'-ni-pen)	Nafcillin (Naf-sil-lin)
Urecholine (Ur-eh-ko'-leen)	Bethanecol (Beth-an'-eh-kol)
Valisone (Val'-i-sone)	Betamethasone (Beh-tah-meth'-a-sone)
Valium (Val'-ee-um)	Diazepam (Die-aze-eh-pam)
Vermox (Ver'-moks)	Mebendazole (Meh-ben'-dah-zole)
Vibramycin (Vie-bra-my'-sin)	Doxycycline (Doks-see-si'-kleen)
Xylocaine (Zie'-low-kain)	Lidocaine (Lie-do-kain)
Zarontin (Zar-on'-tin)	Ethosuximide (Eh-tho-suks'-a-mide)
Zyloprim (Zie'-low-prim)	Allopurinol (Al-lo-pure'-in-ol)

End of Lesson 1 Annex

LESSON 2	The Human Muscular System.
TEXT ASSIGNMENT	Paragraphs 2-1--2-4.
LESSON OBJECTIVES	After completing this lesson, you should be able to:

2-1. Given one of the following terms: motor unit, tonus, or all or none law and a group of definitions, select the definition of that term.

2-2. Given a list of properties, select the properties of muscle tissue.

2-3. Given one of the properties of muscle tissue and a group of statements, select the statements that best describe that property.

2-4. From a list, select the types of muscle tissue found in the human body.

2-5. Given the name of a type of muscle tissue found in the body and a group of statements, select the statement that best describes that type of muscle tissue.

2-6. Given the name of a type of muscle tissue found in the body and a group of statements, select the statement that best describes the physiology of that type of tissue.

2-7. Given a statement relating to muscle physiology and a list of the types of muscle tissue, select the type of muscle tissue to which the statement applies.

SUGGESTION After studying the assignment, complete the exercises at the end of this lesson. These exercises will help you to achieve the lesson objectives.

LESSON 2

THE HUMAN MUSCULAR SYSTEM

2-1. BACKGROUND

Muscular tissue is useful to the body because it contracts and thereby produces movement. The contraction of striated muscle attached to bone results in movement of the skeleton. Cardiac muscle contracts rhythmically and acts as a pump to move blood through the cardiovascular system. The contraction of smooth or visceral muscle results in the movement of materials inside the body, such as the propulsion of food through the digestive tract.

2-2. TERMS ASSOCIATED WITH THE HUMAN MUSCULAR SYSTEM

a. **Motor Unit**. A motor unit is a single motor neuron and the number of striated muscle fibers activated by it (innervation). The importance of the motor unit is that its fibers work in unison.

b. **Tonus**. Tonus is defined as a slight continuous contraction of muscle tissue that aids in the maintenance of posture and in the return of blood to the heart.

c. **All or None Law.** Under the influence of nervous stimulation, a single muscle fiber will always contract to its maximum capacity.

2-3. PROPERTIES OF MUSCLE TISSUE

Muscles have certain key properties:

a. **Irritability.** Irritability refers to the ability of a muscle to respond to a stimulus.

b. **Contractability.** Contractability refers to the muscle's ability to shorten in length.

c. **Extensibility**. Extensibility refers to a muscle's ability to extend in length.

d. **Elasticity**. Elasticity refers to a muscle's ability to stretch and return to its normal position.

2-4. TYPES OF MUSCLE TISSUE

a. **Skeletal Muscle.** Each skeletal muscle is an individual organ of the human body. Each is composed of several types of tissues, mainly striated muscle fibers, and fibrous connective tissue (FCT). Each is attached to and moves bones. Bones are parts of the skeleton serving as levers. The large portion of a muscle is known as its belly or fleshy belly. The muscle is attached to bones by tendons or aponeuroses. Tendons and aponeuroses are similar to each other. However, tendons are cord-like, and aponeuroses are broad and flat. The fleshy portion may be directly connected to the bone. If it is attached to the bone, it is called a "fleshy attachment."

(1) Anatomy. The muscle cells of skeletal muscles are elongated and are called fibers. The fibers of the skeletal muscles are striated (a striped appearance) to give strength. Movement of the skeleton, such as lifting a leg, is voluntary, as are all of the movements characterized by the skeletal system.

(2) Physiology. The neuromuscular junction consists of a nerve fiber and a skeletal muscle fiber. The nerve fiber is branched at the end to form a structure called the end plate. This end plate invaginates into the muscle fiber, but it always stays outside the membrane of the muscle. The sole feet are located at the tips of the numerous branches of the end plate. The space between the fiber membrane and the sole foot are referred to as the synaptic cleft. A gelatinous substance fills the synaptic cleft. Mitochondria that supposedly synthesize the substance acetylcholine are located in the sole foot. Numerous small vesicles (bags) serve as storage locations for acetylcholine. The enzyme cholinesterase, which is used to destroy acetylcholine, is also found in the area of the synaptic cleft.

(a) Secretion of acetylcholine. The vesicles release acetylcholine when a nerve impulse reaches the neuromuscular junction. Shortly after the acetylcholine is released (around two milliseconds), it diffuses and no longer has any effect upon the muscle. During the short time, the acetylcholine produces its effects upon the muscle; the muscle becomes very permeable to sodium ions (Nat). Because of the influx of sodium ions into the muscle, the electrical potential of the membrane increases. Hence, the muscle fiber is stimulated. Figure 2-1 illustrates the contraction of skeletal muscle.

(b) Destruction of acetylcholine. Shortly after the acetylcholine is released, cholinesterase begins to destroy it. Such a rapid destruction of the acetylcholine prevents it from re-stimulating the muscle until another nerve impulse reaches the neuromuscular junction. Figure 2-2 illustrates the relaxation of the muscle tissue.

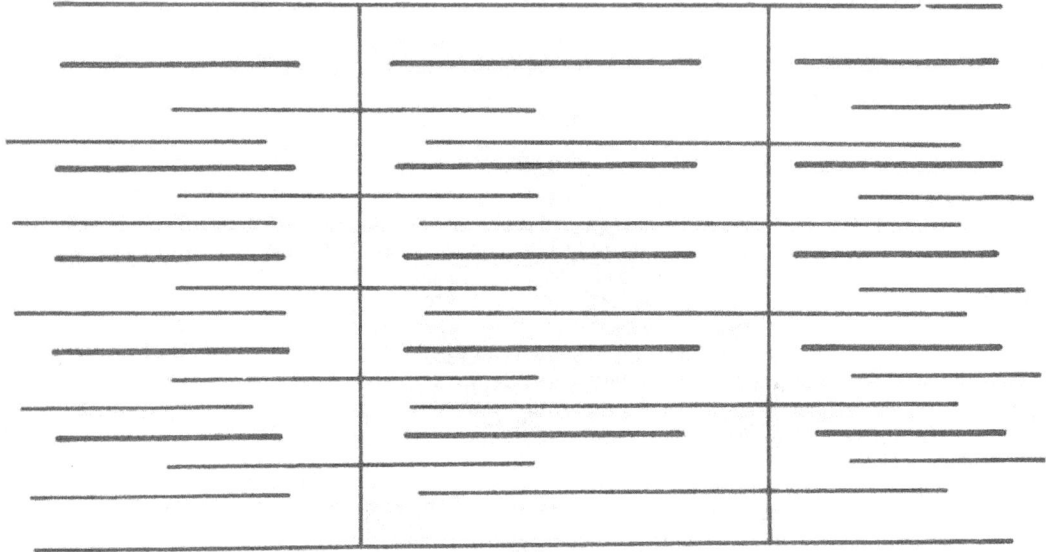

Figure 2-1. Contracted skeletal muscle.

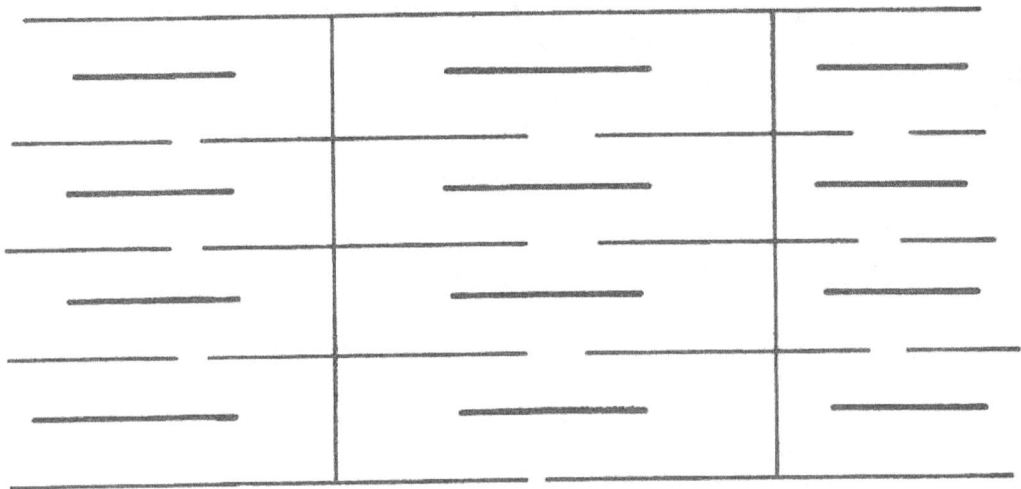

Figure 2-2. Relaxed skeletal muscle.

(3) <u>Disorders</u>.

(a) Muscle cramps. Muscle cramps are persistent involuntary contractions of the skeletal muscles. Muscle cramps can be caused by over-exercise, lack of blood flow, or severe cold.

(b) Myasthenia gravis. Myasthenia gravis is a major disorder of the skeletal muscle system. Muscle weakness and excessive fatigue characterize it. In myasthenia gravis, the muscular system is marked by progressive paralysis of the muscles, which is caused by an abnormal condition at the neuromuscular junction due to a lack of acetylcholine or an excess of cholinesterase. If there is either too little acetylcholine or an excess of cholinesterase, a contraction will not occur.

b. **Cardiac Muscle.** The muscles of the heart are called <u>cardiac muscles</u>.

(1) <u>Anatomy</u>. Cardiac muscle is made up of branched, striated fibers and responds to stimuli as if it were a single muscle fiber. Cardiac tissue is responsible for the propulsion of blood through the circulatory system. The contraction and relaxation of the heart move the blood.

(2) <u>Physiology</u>. In order for an individual to live (without the assistance of life-support equipment), his heart must never stop beating. Cardiac muscle must maintain a steady rhythm and not become fatigued. Cardiac muscle does not become fatigued because it can use both glucose and lactic acid, its waste product. The contraction of the cardiac muscle is involuntary and does not directly respond to any nervous stimulation. This property is referred to as <u>inherent rhythmicity</u>. The heart rate may be modified by the autonomic nervous system. Sympathetic or adrenergic stimulation will increase heart rate and parasympathetic or cholinergic stimulation will decrease heart rate. To ensure rhythmical contractibility, cardiac muscle must be supplied with appropriate ions in proper concentrations. These ions are supplied in the blood. Too little sodium leads to weak and rapid heart contractions. Too much potassium makes the cardiac muscle cells lose their excitability and complete heart blockage can occur. Excessive levels of calcium in the blood can lead to increased contractibility of the cardiac muscle. Extremely high levels of the calcium ion in the heart tissue can cause the heart to remain in a state of contraction.

(3) <u>Disorders</u>. An irregular heart beat pattern is called an arrhythmia. There are different types of cardiac arrhythmias (that is, flutter or fibrillation). Arrhythmias can sometimes be treated with drugs. More specific information on arrhythmias and the drugs used to treat them will be given to you in another subcourse (MD0806, Pharmacology III).

c. **Smooth Muscle.** All muscles that are not found in the heart or are not attached to the skeletal system are called smooth muscles.

(1) Anatomy. The fibers of smooth muscles are elongated and nonstriated. The size of the fiber varies with the location of the muscle. For example, the smallest smooth muscles are found in the blood vessels and the largest are found in the digestive tract. Smooth muscle is responsible for such important functions as peristalsis, blood pressure, and air volume. Peristalsis is the rhythmic wave-like motion of the alimentary canal and other tubular organs caused by waves of contraction passing along the smooth muscle in the tube. Smooth muscle is involved in blood pressure by altering the diameter of blood vessels. It is involved in the control of air volume by altering the diameter of the bronchial tubes. Smooth muscle contracts involuntarily-it is an unconscious act.

(2) Physiology. The same chemical substances are found in smooth muscle as are found in skeletal muscle. Contraction of smooth muscle tissue occurs by the activation by ions--just the same as with skeletal muscles: Contraction occurs during depolarization of the muscle membrane, and it stops after repolarization. Smooth muscle tissue does not contract as rapidly as skeletal muscle tissue. Furthermore, the relaxation of the smooth muscle following contraction is likewise slower than in skeletal muscle. Smooth muscle is capable of maintaining tonic contractions over a long period of time. Smooth muscle can undergo changes in length without significant change in tension. This is called stress-relaxation.

Continue with Exercises

EXERCISES, LESSON 2

INSTRUCTIONS: Answer the following exercises by marking the lettered response which best answers the question.

After you have completed all the exercises, turn to "Solutions to Exercises" at the end of the lesson, and check your answers. For each exercise answered incorrectly, reread the material referenced with the solution.

1. The term tonus is best defined as:

    a. The process by which all muscle fibers always contract to their maximum capacity.

    b. The ability of a muscle to stretch and return to its normal position.

    c. A slight continuous contraction of muscle tissue which aids in the maintenance of posture and in the return of blood to the heart.

    d. The ability of a muscle fiber to contract and expand in order to meet the requirements of extension.

2. Which of the following is a property of muscle tissue? (More than one response may be correct.)

    a. Irritability.

    b. Malleability.

    c. Extensibility.

3. Elasticity, one of the properties of muscle tissue, is best defined as:

    a. The ability of a muscle to stretch and return to its normal position.

    b. The ability of a muscle to shorten in length.

    c. The ability of a muscle to respond to a stimulus.

    d. The ability of a muscle to extend in length.

4. Which of the following is a type of muscle tissue found in the human body? (More than one response may be correct.)

    a. Skeletal muscle tissue.

    b. Adipose muscle tissue.

    c. Cardiac muscle tissue.

    d. Smooth muscle tissue.

5. Select the statement that best describes skeletal muscle.

    a. Muscle tissue that is made up of branched, striated fibers and responds to stimuli as if it were a single muscle fiber.

    b. Muscle fibers that are striated and elongated.

    c. Muscle fibers that are elongated and non-striated.

    d. Muscle tissue which is branched and striated and is found in the alimentary canal.

6. Which of the following statements best describes the physiology involved with cardiac muscle tissue?

    a. The contraction is involuntary and does not respond directly to any nervous stimulation.

    b. In this tissue, relaxation occurs during depolarization of the muscle membrane and stops after repolarization.

    c. In this tissue, the chemical acetylcholine is released by the vesicles in the neuromuscular junction with a resultant influx of potassium ions into the muscle.

    d. The secretion of acetylcholinesterase near the neuromuscular junction produces the contraction of this type of tissue.

Check Your Answers on Next Page

SOLUTIONS TO EXERCISES, LESSON 2

1. c   A slight continuous contraction of muscle tissue which aids in the maintenance of posture and in the return of blood to the heart. (para 2-2b)

2. a   Irritability   (para 2-3a)
    c   Extensibility   (para 2-3c)

3. a   The ability of a muscle to stretch and return to its normal position. (para 2-3d)

4. a   Skeletal muscle tissue. (para 2-4a)
    c   Cardiac muscle tissue. (para 2-4b)
    d   Smooth muscle tissue. (para 2-4c)

5. b   Muscle fibers which are striated and elongated. (para 2-4a(1))

6. a   The contraction is involuntary and does not respond directly to any nervous stimulation. (para 2-4b(2))

End of Lesson 2

ANNEX

DRUG PRONUNCIATION GUIDE

This Drug Pronunciation Guide was developed to help you to learn how the trade and generic names of commonly prescribed medications are frequently pronounced. Not all the drugs in the guide are discussed in this subcourse. Remember, it is not enough to be able to know the uses, indications, cautions and warnings, and contraindications for a drug--you must also know how to pronounce that drug's name.

Trade Name	*Generic Name*
Actifed (Ak'-ti-fed)	Triprolidine (Tri-pro'-li-deen) and Pseudoephedrine (Soo-do-e-fed'-rin)
Adapin (Ad'-a-pin)	Doxepin (Dok'-se-pin)
Sinequan (Sin'-a-kwan)	" "
Afrin (Af'-rin)	Oxymetazoline (Ok-see-met-az'-o-leen)
Aldactazide (Al-dak'-ta-zide)	Spironolactone (Spi-ro-no-lak'-tone) and Hydrochlorothiazide (Hy-dro-klor-thi'-a-zide)
Aldactone (Al-dak'-tone)	Spironolactone (Spi-ro-no-lak'-tone)
Aldomet (Al'-do-met)	Methyldopa (Meth-il-do'-pah)
Alupent (Al'-u-pent)	Metaproterenol (Met-a-pro-ter'-eh-nol)
Amoxil (Am-ok'-sil)	Amoxicillin (Ah-moks'-i-sil-in)
Amphojel (Am'-fo-jel)	Aluminum (Al-loo'-mi-num) Hydroxide (Hy-drok'-side)
Ampicillin (Amp'-I-sil-in)	Same
Antepar (Ab'-te-par)	Piperazine (Pi-per'-ah-zeen)
Anturane (An'-tu-rain)	Sulfinpyrazone (Sul-fin-pie'-ra-zone)
Anusol (An'-u-sol)	Pramoxine (Pram-ok'-seen)
Apresoline (A-press'-o-leen)	Hydralazine (Hy-dral'-ah-zeen)
Aralen (Ar'-a-len)	Chloroquine (Klor'-o-kwin)
Aristocort (A-ris'-to-cort)	Triamcinolone (Tri-am-sin'-o-lone)
Artane (Ar'-tane)	Trihexyphenidyl(Tri-hek-see-fen'-i-dil)
A.S.A.	Aspirin (As'-per-in)
Atromid S (A'-tro-mid)	Clofibrate (Klo-fi'-brate)
Avlosulfon (Av-lo-sul'-fon)	Dapsone (Dap'-sone)
Azolid (Az'-o-lid)	Phenylbutazone (Fen-il-bute'-a-zone)
Bactrim (Bak'-trim)	Sulfamethoxazole (Sul-fah-meth-oks'-ah-zole) and Trimethoprim (Tri-meth'-o-prim)
Bellergal (Bel'-er-gal)	Ergotamine (Er-got'-a-meen), Phenobarbital (Feen-o-bar'-bi-tal) and Belladonna (Bel-la-don'-na) Alkaloids
Benadryl (Ben'-a-dril)	Diphenhydramine (Di-fen-hy'-dra-meen)

Trade Name	Generic Name
Bendectin (Ben-dek'-tin)	Doxylamine (Dok-sil'-a-meen)
Benemid (Ben'-eh-mid)	Probenecid (Pro-ben'-eh-sid)
Bonine (Bo'-neen)	Meclizine (Mek'-li-zeen)
Cafergot (Kaf'-er-got)	Ergotamine (Er-got'-a-meen) and Caffeine (Kaf'-feen)
Calamine (Kal'-a-mine)	Same
Catapres (Kat'-a-press)	Clonidine (Klo'-ni-deen)
CeeNu (See'-new)	Lomustine (Lo-mus'-teen)
Chlor-Trimeton (Klo-tri '-meh-ton)	Chlorpheniramine (Klor-fen-it'-a-meen)
Clomid (Klo'-mid)	Clomiphene (Klo'-mi-feen)
Clonopin (Klo-o-pin)	Clonazepam (Klo-na'-ze-pam)
Codeine (Ko'-deen)	Same
Cogentin (Ko-jen'-tin)	Benztropine (Benz'-tro-peen)
Colace (Ko'-lace)	Dioctyl(Di-ok'-til) Sodium (So'-dee-um) Sulfosuccinate (Sul-fo-suk'-si-nate)
Colchicine (Kol'-chi-seen)	Same
Compazine (Kom'-pa-zeen)	Prochlorperazine (Pro-klor-per'-a-zeen)
Cordran (Kor'-dran)	Flurandrenolide (Floor-an-dren'-o-lide)
Coumadin (Koo'-mah-din)	Warfarin (War'-fah-rin)
CP	Cloroquine (Klor'-o-kwin) and Primaquine (Prim'-a-kwin)
Cyclogyl (Si'-klo-jel)	Cyclopentolate (Si-klo-pen'-to-late)
Cytomel (Si'-to-mel)	Liothyronine (Li-o-thy-ro-neen)
Cytoxan (Si-tok'-san)	Cyclophosphamide (Si-klo-fos'-fa-mide)
Dalmane (Dal '-mane)	Flurazepam (Floor-az'-e-pam)
Darvocet (Dar'-vo-set)	Propoxyphene (Pro-pok'-se-feen) and Acetaminopen (As-et-am'-ino-fen)
Darvon (Dar'-von)	Propoxyphene (Pro-pok-se-feen)
Decadron (Dek'-a-dron)	Dexamethasone (Dek-sa-meth'-ah-sone)
Deltasone (Del '-ta-sone)	Prednisone (Pred'-ni-sone)
Demerol (Dem'-er-ol)	Meperidine (Meh-pair'-i-deen)
Dexedrine (Deks '-eh-dreen)	Dextroamphetamine (Deks-tro-am-fet'-a-meen)
Diabinese (Di-ab'-i-nees)	Chlorpropamide (Klor-prop'-a-mide)
Diethylstilbestrol (Di-eth-il-stil-bes'-trol)	Same
Dilantin (Di-lan'-tin)	Phenytoin (Fen'-i-toin)
Dilaudid (Di-law'-did)	Hydromorphone (Hy-dro-more' -fon)
Dimetane (Di'-meh-tane)	Brompheniramine (Brom-fen-ir'-a-meen)

Trade Name	Generic Name
Dimetapp (Di'-meh-tap)	Brompheniramine (Brom-fen-ir'-a-meen) Phenylephrine (Fen-il-ef'-rin) and Phenylpropanolamine (Fen-il-pro-pan-ol'-a-meen)
Disophrol (Dice'-o-frol)	Dexbrompheniramine (Deks-brom-fen-ir'-a-meen) and Pseudoephedrine (Soo-do-e-fed'-rin)
Dolophine (Dol'-o-feen)	Methadone (Meth'-a-done)
Domeboro (Dome-bor'-o)	Aluminum (Ah-loo'-mi-num) Acetate (As'-e-tate)
Donnatal (Don'-na-tal)	Belladonna (Bel-la-don'-na) Alkaloids (Al'-ka-loids) and Phenobarbital (Feen-o-barb'-i-tal)
Doxidan (Dok'-si-dan)	Danthron (Dan'-thron) and Dicctyl (Di-ok'-til) Calcium (Kal'-see-um) Sulfosuccinate (Sul-fo-suk'-si-nate)
Drixoral (Driks'-or-al)	Dexbrompheniramine (Deks-brom-fen-ir'-a-meen) and Pseudoephedrine (Soo-do-e-fed'-rin)
Dulcolax (Dul'-ko-laks)	Bisacodyl (Bis-a'-ko-dil)
Dyazine (Di'-a-zide)	Triamterene (Tri-am'-ter-een) and Hydrochlorothiazide (Hy-dro-klor-o-thi'-a-zide)
Dymelor (Die'-meh-lor)	Acetohexamide (As-e-to-heks'-a-mide)
Dyrenium (Die-ren'-i-um)	Triamterene (Tri-am'-ter-een)
Efudex (Ef'-u-deks)	Fluorouracil (Floo-ro-ur'-ah-sil)
Elavil (El'-ah-vil)	Amitriptyline (Am-i-trip'-til-een)
Elixir Terpin (Ter'-pin) Hydrate	Same
Empirin (Em'-per-in)	Codeine (Ko'-deen) and Aspirin (As'-per-in)
E-Mycin (E-mie'-sin)	Erythromycin (E-rith-ro-mie'-sin)
Equanil (Ek'-wa-nil)	Meprobamate (Me-pro-bam'-ate)
Ergomar (Er'-go-mar)	Ergotamine (Er-got'-a-meen)
Ergotrate (Er'-go-trate)	Ergonovine (Er-go-no'-veen)
Erythrocin (Er-eeth'-ro-sin)	Erythromycin (Er-eeth-ro-my'-sin) Stearate (Stare'-rate)
Esidrix (Es'-i-driks)	Hyrochlorothiazide (Hy-dro-klor-o-thi'-a-zide)
Feosol (Fe'-o-sol)	Ferrous (Fer'-rus) Sulfate (Sul'-fate)
Fergon (Fer'-gon)	Ferrous (Fer'-rus) Gluconate (Glu'-con-ate)

Trade Name	Generic Name
Fiorinal (Fee-or'-i-nal)	Butalbi tal (Bu-tal'-bi-tal), Apririn, Phenacetin (Fen-ass'-eh-tin), and Caffeine (Kaf'-feen)
Flagyl (Fla'-jil)	Metronidazole (Me-tro-ni'-dah-zole)
Flexeril (Flek'-sa-ril)	Cyclobenzaprine (Si-klo-benz'-a-preen)
Fulvicin (Ful'-vi-sin)	Griseofulvin (Griz-e-o-ful'-vin)
Guantanol (Gan'-ta-nol)	Suiphamethoxazole (Sul-fah-meth-oks'-ah-zole)
Gantrisin (Gan'-tri-sin)	Sulfisoxazole (Sul-fi-sok'-sah-zole)
Gelusil (Jel'-u-sil)	Aluminum (Ah-loo'-mi-num) Hydroxide (Hy-drok'-side) and Magnesium (Mag-nee'-zee-um) Hydroxide
Grifulvin (Gri-ful'-vin)	Griseofulvin (Griz-e-o-ful'-vin)
Gynergen (Jin'-er-jen)	Ergotamine (Er-got'-a-meen)
Haldol (Hal'-dol)	Haloperidol (Hal-o-pair'-i-dol)
Halotestin (Hal-o-tes'-tin)	Fluoxymesterone (Floo-ok-see-mes-teh-rone)
Hexadrol (Hek'-sa-drol)	Dexamethasone (Dek-sa-meth'-a-sone)
Hydrodiuril (Hy-dro-di'-ur-il)	Hydroclorothiazide (Hy-dro-kior-thi'-a-zide)
Hygroton (Hy-grow'-ton)	Chiorthalidone (Kior-thal'-i-done)
Ilosone (I'-low-sone)	Erythromycin (Er-ith-ro-mi'-sin) Estolate (Es'-to-late)
Inderal (In'-der-al)	Propranolol (Pro-pran'-o-lol)
Indocin (In'-do-sin)	Indomethacin (In-do-meth'-a-sin)
INH	Isoniazid (I-so-ni'-a-zid)
Insulin (In'-sul-in)	Same
Intal	Cromolyn (Kro'-mo-lin)
Ismelin (Is'-meh-lin)	Guanethidine (Gwan-eth'-i-dine)
Isopto-Atropine (I-sop-to-at'-ro-peen)	Atropine (At'-ro-peen)
Isopto-Carpine (I-sop-to-car'-peen)	Pilocarpine (Pile-o-car'-peen)
Isordil (I'-sor-dil)	Isosorbide (I-so-sor'-bide)
Keflex (Kef'-lex)	Cephalexin (Sef-ah-lek'-sin)
Lanoxin (Lan-ok'-sin)	Digoxin (Di-jok'-sin)
Larodopa (Lar-o-do'-pa)	Levodopa (Le-o-do'-pa)
Larotid (Lar'-o-tid)	Amoxicillin (Ah-moks'-i-sil-in)
Lasix (La'-siks)	Furosemide (Fu-ro'-se-mide)
Leukeran (Lu'-ker-an)	Chlorambucil (Klor-ram'-bu-sil)
Librium (Lib'-ree-um)	Chlordiazepoxide (Klor-die-az-eh-pok'-side)

Trade Name	Generic Name
Lidex (Lie'-deks)	Fluocinoide (Floo-o-sin'-o-nide)
Lomotil (Lo'-mo-til)	Diphenoxylate (Die-fen-ok'-si-late)
Lopressor (Lo'-pres-sor)	Metoprolol (Met-o-pro'-lol)
Lotrimin (Lo'-tri-min)	Chlotrimazole (Klo-trim'-ah-zole)
Maalox (May'-loks)	Aluminum (Ah-loo'-mi-num) and Magnesium (Mag-nee'-zee-um) Hydroxides
Macrodanton (Ma-kro-dan'-tin)	Nitrofurantoin (Ni-tro-fur-an'-toin)
Mandelamine (Man-del'-a-meen)	Methenamine (Meth-en'-a-meen) Mandelate (Man'-deh-late)
Medihaler-Iso (Med-i-hail-er-I'-so)	Isoproterenol (I-so-pro-ter'-en-ol)
Mellaril (Mel'-la-ril)	Thioridazine (Thi-o-rid'-a-zeen)
Metamucil (Met-a-mu'-sil)	Psyllium (Sil'-e-um)
Metaprel (Meh'-ta-prel)	Metaproterenol (Meh'-ta-pro-ter'-eh-nol)
Methotrexate (Meth-o-treks'-ate)	Amethopterin (Ah-meth-op'-ter-in)
Milk of Magnesia	Same
Minipress (Min'-i-press)	Prazosin (Pra'-zo-sin)
Minocin (Min'-o-sin)	Minocycline (Mi-no-si'-kleen)
Monistat (Mon'-i-stat)	Miconazole (Mi-kon'-ah-zole)
Motrin (Mo'-trin)	Ibuprofen (I-bu'-pro-fen)
Myambutol (My-am'-bu-tol)	Ethambutol (Eth-am'-bu-tol)
Mycostatin (My-co-stat'-in)	Nystatin (Ny-stat'-in)
Mylanta (My-lan'-ta)	Aluminum (Ah-loo'-mi-num) and Magnesium (Mag-nee'-zee-um) Hydroxides and Simethicone (Si-meth'-i-kone)
Myleran (My-ler-an)	Busulfan (Bu-sul'-fan)
Mylicon (My'-li-kon)	Simethicone (Si-meth'-i-kone)
Mysoline (My'-so-leen)	Primidone (Pri'-mi-done)
Nalfon (Nal'-fon)	Fenoprofen (Fen-o-pro'-fen)
Naprosyn (Na'-pro-sin)	Naproxen (Na-prok'-sen)
Nembutal (Nem'-bu-tal)	Pentobarbital (Pen-to-barb'-i-tal)
Neosynephrine (Nee-o-sin-eh'-frin)	Phenylephrine (Fen-il-eh'-frin)
Nitrobid (Ni'-tro-bid)	Nitroglycerin (Ni-tro-gli'-ser-in)
Nitrol (Ni'-trol)	" "
Nitrostat (Ni-tro-stat)	" "
Noctec (Nok'-tek)	Chloral Hydrate (Klor'-al- Hy'-drate)
Norfiex (Nor'-fleks)	Orphenadrine Citrate (Or-fen'-a-dreen)
Norpace (Nor'-pace)	Disopyramide (Di-so-peer'-a-mide)

Trade Name	Generic Name
Novahistine (No-va-his'-teen) Expectorant	Guaifenesin (Gwi-fen'-eh-sin), Phenylpropanolamine (Fen-il-pro-pan-ol'-a-meen), and Codeine (Ko'-deen)
NTG	Nitroclycerin (Ni-tro-gli'-ser-in)
Nupercainal (New-per-kain'-al)	Dibucaine (Die'-bu-kain)
Oretic (O-ret'-ik)	Hydrochiorothiazide (Hy-dro-kior-thi'-a-zide)
Orinase (Or'-in-ase)	Tolbutamide (Tol-bu'-tah-mide)
Ornade (Or'-nade)	Chlorpheniramine (Klor-fen-ir'-a-meen), Triprolidine (Tri-pro-li-deen) and Pseudoephedrine (Su-do-eh-fed'-rin)
Parafon Forte (Pair'-a-fon For'-tay)	Chlorzoxazone (Klor-zok'-sa-zone)
Percodan (Per'-ko-dan)	Oxycodone (Ok-si-ko'-done)
Periactin (Per-ee-ak'-tin)	Cyproheptadine (Si-pro-hep'-tah-deen)
Persantine (Per-san'-teen)	Dipyridamole (Di-pi-rid'-ah-mole)
Phenobarbital (Feen-o-barb'-it-al)	Same
Phenylpropanolamine (Fen-il-pro-pan-ol'-a-meen)	Same
Pitocin (Pi-tow'-sin)	Oxytocin (Ok-see-tow'-sin)
Pontocaine (Pon'-to-kain)	Tetracaine (Teh'-tra-kain)
Povan (Po'-van)	Pyrvinium (Pire-vin'-ee-um)
Premarin (Prem'-ar-in)	Conjugated (Kon'-joo-gay-ted) Estrogens (Es-tro-jens)
Presamine (Press'-a-meen)	Imipramine (Im-ip'-rah-meen)
Primaquine (Pri'-mah-kwin)	Same
Probanthine (Pro-ban'-theen)	Propantheline (Pro-pan'-the-leen)
Pronestyl (Pro-nes'-til)	Procainamide (Pro-kain'-a-mide)
Prophylthiouracil (Pro-pil-thi-o-u'-rah-sil)	Same
Prostaphlin (Pro-staff'-lin)	Oxacillin (Oks'-ah-sil-in)
Provera (Pro-ver'-ah)	Medroxyprogesterone (Med-rok-see-pro-jes'-ter-one)
Pyridium (Pie-rid'-ee-um)	Phenazopyridine (Fen-ahs-o-per'-i-deen)
Quinidine (Kwin'-i-deen)	Same
Quinine (Kwie'-nine)	Same
Reserpine (Ree-ser'-peen)	Same
Retin A (Reh'-tin A)	Tretinoin (Tret'-i-noin)
Rifadin (Rie-fad'-in)	Rifampin (Rie-fam'-pin)
Riopan (Rie'-o-pan)	Magaidrate (Mag'-al-drate)

Trade Name	Generic Name
Rimactane (Rim-act'-ane)	Rifampin (Rie-fam'-pin)
Ritalin (Rit'-a-lin)	Methylphenidate (Meth-il-fen'-i-date)
Robaxin (Ro-bak'-sin)	Methocarbamol (Meth-o-kar'-ba-mol)
Robitussin (Row-i-tus'-sin)	Guaifenesin (Gwie-fen'-eh-sin)
Robitussin DM	Guiafenesin and Dextromethorphan (Dek-tro-meh-or'-fan)
Sansert (San'-sert)	Methysergide (Meth-ee-ser'-jide)
Seconal (Sek'-o-nal)	Secobarbital (Sek-o-bar'-bi-tal)
Selsun (Sel'-sun)	Selenium (Se-leh'-nee-um)
Septra (Sep'-tra)	Sulfamethoxazole (Sul-fah-meth-oks'-a-zole) and Trimethroprim (Tri-meth'-o-prim)
Serax (See'-raks)	Oxazepam (Oks-az'-eh-pam)
Silvadene (Sil'-va-deen)	Silver Sulfadiazine (Sul-fa-die'-a-zeen)
Sinemet (Si'-ne-met)	Levodopa (Le-vo-do'-pa)
Sinequan (Sin'-a-kwan)	Doxepin (Dok'-seh-pin)
Sorbitrate (Sor'-bi-trate)	Isosorbide (I-so-sor'-bide)
Stelazine (Stel'-a-zeen)	Trifluoperazine(Tri-floo-o-per'-a-zeen)
Sudafed (Soo'-da-fed)	Pseudophedrine (Soo-do-eh-feh'-drin)
Sulamyd (Sul'-a-mid)	Sulfacetamide (Sul-fah-set'-a-mide)
Sulfamylon (Sul-fa-mie'-lon)	Mafenide (Maf'-eh-nide)
Sultrin (Sul'-trin)	Sulfathiazole (Sul-fah-thi'-ah-zole) Sulfacetamide (Sul-fah-set'-ah-mide) and Sulfabenzamide (Sul-fah-benz'-ah-mide)
Surfak (Sur'-fak)	Dioctyl (Di-ok'-til) Calcium (Kal'-see-um) Sulfosuccinate (Sul-fo-suk'-si-nate)
Synalar (Sine'-a-lar)	Fluocinolone (Floo-o-sin'-o-lone)
Synthroid (Sin'-throid)	Levothyroxine (Lee-vo-thi-rok'-sin)
Tace (Tace)	Chlorotrianisene (Klor-o-tri-an'-I-seen)
Tagamet (Tag'-a-met)	Cimetidine (Si-met'-i-deen)
Talwin (Tal'-win)	Pentazocine (Pen-taz'-o-seen)
Tandearil (Tan'-da-ril)	Oxyphenbutazone (Ok-see-fen-bute'-a-zone)
Tegretol (Teg'-reh-tol)	Carbamazepine (Kar-ba-maz'-eh-peen)
Tessalon (Tess'-a-lon)	Benzonatate (Benz-on'-a-tate)
Tetracycline (Tet-ra-si'-kleen)	
Thorazine (Thor'-a-zeen)	Chlorpromazine (Klor-pro'-ma-zeen)
Thyroid (Thy'-roid)	Same
Tigan (Tie'-gan)	Trimethobenzamide (Tri-meth-o-benz'-a-mide)
Timoptic (Tim-op'-tic)	Timilol (Tim'-o-lol)

Trade Name	Generic Name
Tinactin (Tin-act'-in)	Tolnaftate (Tol-naf'-tate)
Titralac (Ti'-tra-lak)	Calcium (Kal-see-um) Carbonate (Kar'-bon-ate) and Glycine (Gly'-seen)
Tofranil (Toe'-fra-nil)	Imipramine (I-mip'-rah-meen)
Tolectin (Tow-lek'-tin)	Tolmetin (Tol-met'-in)
Triavil (Tri'-a-vil)	Perphenazine (Per-fen'-a-zeen) and Amitriptlyline (Am-i-trip'-ti-leen)
Trilafon (Try'-la-fon)	Perphenazine (Per-fen-a-zeen)
Tylenol (Tie'-leh-nol)	Acetaminophen (As-et-am'-ino-fen)
Tylenol #3	Acetaminophen and Codeine (Ko'-deen)
Unipen (U'-ni-pen)	Nafcillin (Naf-sil-lin)
Urecholine (Ur-eh-ko'-leen)	Bethanecol (Beth-an'-eh-kol)
Valisone (Val'-i-sone)	Betamethasone (Beh-tah-meth'-a-sone)
Valium (Val'-ee-um)	Diazepam (Die-aze-eh-pam)
Vermox (Ver'-moks)	Mebendazole (Meh-ben'-dah-zole)
Vibramycin (Vie-bra-my'-sin)	Doxycycline (Doks-see-si'-kleen)
Xylocaine (Zie'-low-kain)	Lidocaine (Lie-do-kain)
Zarontin (Zar-on'-tin)	Ethosuximide (Eh-tho-suks'-a-mide)
Zyloprim (Zie'-low-prim)	Allopurinol (Al-lo-pure'-in-ol)

End of Lesson 2 Annex

LESSON ASSIGNMENT

LESSON 3	Skeletal Muscle Relaxants.
TEXT ASSIGNMENT	Paragraphs 3-1--3-7.
LESSON OBJECTIVES	After completing this lesson, you should be able to:

3-1. Given a group of definitions, select the definition of the term muscle relaxant.

3-2. Given a group of statements, select the statement that best describes the mechanism of action of neuromuscular blocking agents.

3-3. Given a group of statements, select the statement that best describes the process of normal nerve transmission.

3-4. Given a list of uses, select the use of neuromuscular blocking agents.

3-5. Given one of the two classifications of neuromuscular blocking agents and a group of statements, select the statement that best describes that classification's mechanism of action.

3-6. Given a group of statements, select the statement that best describes the mechanism of action of centrally-acting skeletal muscle relaxants.

3-7. Given the trade or generic name of a skeletal muscle relaxant and a list of trade or generic names select the appropriate name of that particular drug.

3-8. Given the trade or generic name of a skeletal muscle relaxant and a group of uses or side effects, select the use or side effect of that agent.

SUGGESTION   After studying the assignment, complete the exercises at the end of this lesson. These exercises will help you to achieve the lesson objectives.

LESSON 3

SKELETAL MUSCLE RELAXANTS

Section I. GENERAL

3-1. BACKGROUND

Some Indian tribes in South America have used muscle relaxants for centuries. They have used curare, a potent muscle relaxant, to kill game and to protect themselves because of curare's ultimate pharmacological effect-death. Today, anesthesiologists use this agent to relax skeletal muscles in some surgical procedures. This lesson will focus on skeletal muscle relaxants and their use in modern medicine.

3-2. DEFINITION OF A MUSCLE RELAXANT

A skeletal muscle relaxant may be defined as an agent that reduces skeletal muscle tone. Even when muscles are at rest, there is a certain amount of tension or tautness that is present. This remaining degree of contraction of skeletal muscle is called skeletal muscle tone. It is believed that skeletal muscle tone results entirely from nerve impulses originating from the spinal cord. If these nerve impulses are blocked in some manner, the result is decreased skeletal muscle tone: skeletal muscle relaxation. The degree of skeletal muscle relaxation ranges from partial to complete depending upon the effectiveness of the skeletal muscle relaxant being used and its site of activity.

Section II. THE NEUROMUSCULAR BLOCKING AGENTS

3-3. MECHANISM OF ACTION

a.   The neuromuscular blocking agents act by blocking the action of acetylcholine (Ach) at the neuromuscular junction or at the muscle receptor site.

b.   What occurs at the neuromuscular junction during normal nerve transmission? The nerve impulse enters the terminal knob, and the neurotransmitter acetylcholine (Ach) is released and attaches to appropriate receptor sites on the muscle receptor site, much like a lock and key (Figure 3-1). When Ach attaches, there is a great influx of sodium into the muscle receptor site, and potassium flows out. This causes the receptor site to depolarize; therefore, muscle contraction results.

c.   The Ach does not remain in the receptor sites forever. When it releases, it is destroyed by acetylcholinesterase (Ache). The resultant release causes an influx of potassium back into the muscle receptor site, and sodium is pumped out. The nerve that stimulates the muscle receptor site repolarizes and returns to normal. Because of repolarization, the skeletal muscle relaxes.

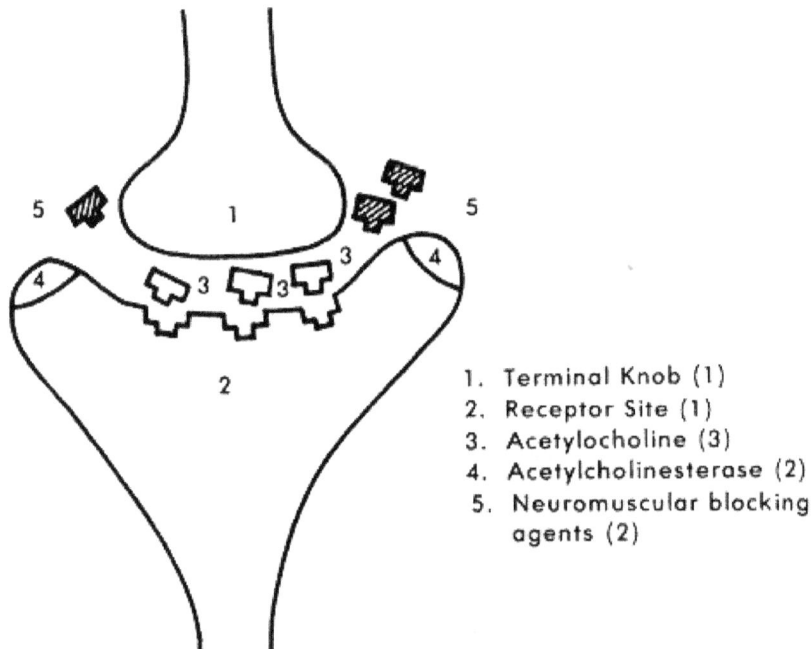

1. Terminal Knob (1)
2. Receptor Site (1)
3. Acetylocholine (3)
4. Acetylcholinesterase (2)
5. Neuromuscular blocking agents (2)

Figure 3-1. Muscle depolarization.

3-4. USE OF THE NEUROMUSCULAR BLOCKING AGENTS

The neuromuscular blocking agents are used with general anesthetics to provide sustained muscle relaxation. This sustained muscle relaxation reduces the tone of the skeletal muscles (that is makes them flaccid or flabby) during surgical procedures. Because of this skeletal muscle relaxation, the surgeon can easily cut through the muscle.

3-5. CLASSIFICATION OF THE NEUROMUSCULAR BLOCKING AGENTS

The neuromuscular blocking agents are classified as either non-depolarizing agents or depolarizing agents.

a. The non-depolarizing agents compete with the neurotransmitter, acetylcholine, for the muscle receptor site. Therefore, they prevent depolarization. This produces flaccid paralysis of the skeletal muscles for a period of about one hour-depending upon the concentration of the agent administered. The non-depolarizing blocking agents are often referred to as competitive neuromuscular blocking agents. Examples of non-depolarizing blocking agents are curare, vecuronium (Norcuron®), pancuronium (Pavulon®), and cisatricurium (Nimbex®).

(1) Curare. Curare is used to produce a complete skeletal muscle relaxation or flaccid paralysis of skeletal muscle during general anesthesia and other procedures. It is a potentially dangerous drug for obvious reasons: Too much of a drug administered too quickly can result in paralysis of the muscles that control respiration. The primary side effects associated with curare are bradycardia and hypotension. The individual responsible for administering the curare during anesthesia must monitor the vital signs of the patient to ensure that the patient does not experience toxic effects from the curare. That person will also have to ensure that the patient is able to breathe (sometimes mechanical assistance is required) when curare is administered since curare relaxes all the skeletal muscles of the body, and the patient sometimes finds difficulty in breathing. Curare is supplied in an injectable form.

(2) Pancuronium (Pavulon®). Pancuronium is five times more potent than curare and it produces complete skeletal muscle relaxation. It poses the same risk factors for the patient, as does curare. The primary side effects seen with pancuronium are cardiac arrhythmias of various types.

b. The depolarizing blocking agents act like an excess of acetylcholine to depolarize the muscle receptor site and prevent its repolarization. Thus, there is an initial depolarization at the neuromuscular junction producing muscle contraction; but since the muscle receptor site cannot depolarize, complete skeletal muscle relaxation follows. In general, the relaxation effects produced by the depolarizing agents are of shorter duration than the relaxation produced by the non-depolarizing agents.

(1) Succinylcholine (Anectine®). Succinylcholine is a depolarizing agent used to produce complete muscle relaxation for various surgical procedures. The primary side effects associated with succinylcholine are cardiac arrhythmias and post-operative apnea (temporary stoppage of breathing).

(2) Decamethonium bromide (Syncurine®). Decamethonium bromide is used as a muscle relaxant for relatively short surgical procedures. Side effects associated with this agent include muscle soreness, respiratory depression, and prolonged apnea.

Section III. CENTRALLY ACTING SKELETAL MUSCLE RELAXANTS

3-6. BACKGROUND

Centrally acting skeletal muscle relaxants are so called because they act on the central nervous system to decrease muscle tone. They decrease muscle tone by depressing the internuncial neurons at the spinal cord (Figures 3-2 and 3-3). When given in normal therapeutic doses, these agents are not potent enough to produce flaccid paralysis. However, large oral or injectable doses of these drugs may produce hypotension, flaccid paralysis, and respiratory depression. Many of these drugs are similar in chemical structure to antianxiety agents. These agents are used to relieve skeletal muscle spasms. Whether relief of pain achieved by patients taking these drugs is due to their muscle relaxant effect or to their sedative effect is unknown.

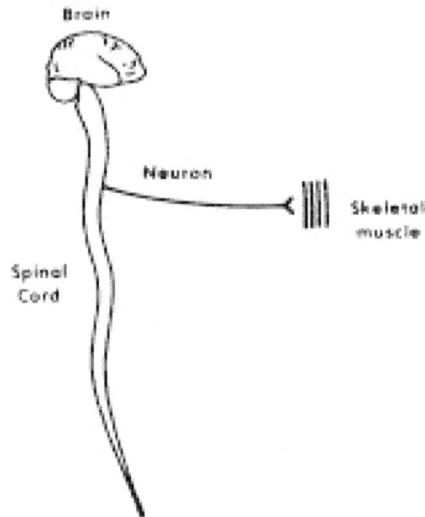

Figure 3-2. The somatic nervous system.

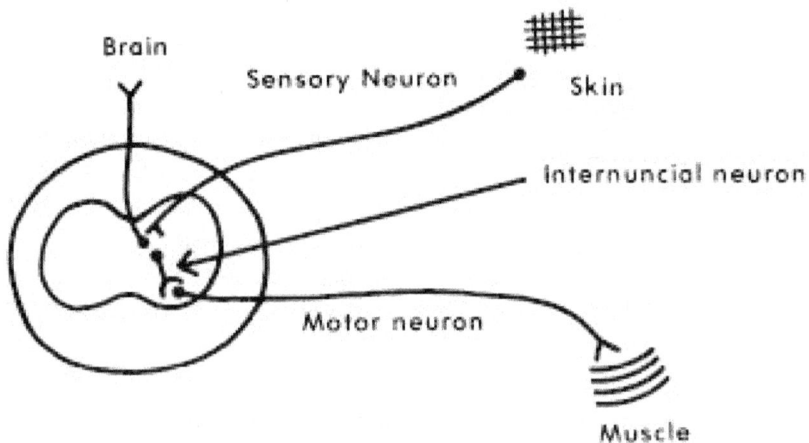

Figure 3-3. Cross section of spinal cord showing internuncial neuron.

3-7. EXAMPLES OF CENTRALLY ACTING SKELETAL MUSCLE RELAXANTS

a. **Diazepam (Valium®).** Diazepam is an antianxiety agent that is also used as a skeletal muscle relaxant in a dosage of from 2 to 10 milligrams three or four times daily. The main side effect of diazepam is central nervous system depression. The patient taking diazepam should be warned that the drug might cause drowsiness. Furthermore, the patient should be warned not to drink alcoholic beverages while taking diazepam. Diazepam is a controlled substance (Note Q).

b. **Cyclobenzaprine (Flexeril®).** This skeletal muscle relaxant is usually given in a dosage of between 20 to 40 milligrams in 2 to 4 divided doses on a daily basis. Central nervous system depression is the primary side effect of this drug. The patient taking cyclobenzaprine should be warned that he might experience drowsiness because of the drug. He should also be warned not to drink alcoholic beverages while taking the drug. This agent is supplied in tablet form.

c. **Orphenadrine Citrate (Norflex®).** This skeletal muscle relaxant is given in a dosage of 100 milligrams twice daily. The drug causes central nervous system depression. The patient should be warned that he might become drowsy while taking the drug. Furthermore, the patient should be warned not to drink alcoholic beverages while taking Norflex®. Norflex® is available in tablet form.

d. **Chlorzoxazone (Paraflex®, Parafon Forte DSC®).** This skeletal muscle relaxant is used as an adjunct to rest, physical therapy, and other measures to relieve the discomfort associated with acute, painful musculoskeletal conditions. It does not directly relax tense muscles. Chlorzoxazone has some antianxiety properties and causes some CNS depression. The patient taking this medication should be warned of the potential drowsiness and should not drink alcohol while taking this medication. The usual adult dosage is 250-mg three or four times a day. Initial dosage for painful musculoskeletal conditions is 500-mg three or four times daily and increased to 750 mg three or four times daily if needed. Chlorzoxazone is supplied as 250-mg tablets (Paraflex®) and 500-mg tablets (Parafon Forte DSC®).

e. **Methocarbamol (Robaxin®).** Methocarbamol is a skeletal muscle relaxant which is usually administered in a dosage of 1 gram four times daily for muscle spasms. Since it can produce central nervous system depression, the patient should be warned of the drowsiness that could accompany its use. When administered intravenously, methocarbamol is used to treat acute muscle spasms associated with trauma and inflammation. Methocarbamol is also used in producing skeletal muscle relaxation for orthopedic procedures when it is administered intravenously.

f. **Dantrolene (Dantrium®).** Dantrolene is a skeletal muscle relaxant that reduces skeletal muscle tone through a direct effect on muscle contraction. It is believed that dantrolene affects the uptake of calcium by muscle tissue. This drug is used to relieve the muscle spasticity associated with such diseases as multiple sclerosis or cerebral palsy. It is given in oral form initially in a dose of 25 milligrams once or twice daily; the dosage of the drug is then increased in increments until the desired therapeutic effect is attained. Although it does not produce its effects on the central nervous system like the other oral skeletal muscle relaxants, it may cause drowsiness. You should warn the patient about this potential drowsiness. Dantrolene may also cause nausea and vomiting. Dantrolene is used in the treatment of malignant hyperthermia.

Continue with Exercises

EXERCISES, LESSON 3

INSTRUCTIONS: Answer the following exercises by marking the lettered response which best answers the question.

After you have completed all the exercises, turn to "Solutions to Exercises" at the end of the lesson, and check your answers. For each exercise answered incorrectly, reread the material referenced with the solution.

1. Select the best definition of the term muscle relaxant.

    a. An agent that prevents the transmission of any nerve impulses.

    b. An agent that causes a patient to become less anxious.

    c. An agent that reduces skeletal muscle tone.

    d. An agent that causes muscles to be relaxed because it increases the amount of acetylcholine present at the neuromuscular junction.

2. Which of the following statements best describes the mechanism of action of neuromuscular blocking agents?

    a. They decrease muscle tone by depressing the internuncial neurons at the spinal cord.

    b. They block the action of acetylcholine at the neuromuscular junction or at the muscle receptor site.

    c. They act on the terminal knob to cause a release of acetylcholine at the neuromuscular junction to produce the depolarization of the receptor site.

    d. They cause a great influx of sodium into the muscle receptor site and a great influx of potassium out of the receptor site in order to make the muscle become relaxed.

3. Centrally acting skeletal muscle relaxants act by:

    a. Decreasing the muscle tone by depressing the internuncial neurons at the spinal cord.

    b. Blocking the action of acetylcholine at the neuromuscular junction or the muscle receptor site.

    c. Causing the sodium and potassium at the receptor site to flow into and out of the area.

    d. Destroying the acetylcholine at the neuromuscular junction.

4. Match the generic names in Column I with the appropriate trade name in Column II.

Column I	Column II
_____ Cyclobenzaprine	A. Flexeril®
_____ Pancuronium	B. Parafon Forte DSC®
_____ Orphenadrine citrate	C. Anectine®
_____ Succinylcholine	D. Pavulon®
_____ Chlorzoxazone	E. Norfiex®
	F. Syncurine®
	G. Dantrium®

5. Select the use of decamethonium bromide.

   a. Used to produce complete muscle relaxation during general anesthesia.

   b. Used to calm or relax a patient prior to surgery.

   c. Used to relieve muscle spasms.

   d. Used as a muscle relaxant for relatively short procedures.

6. The patient taking Parafon Forte DSC® should be warned:

   a. Not to drink alcoholic beverages while taking the drug.

   b. That the drug may produce muscle spasms if taken in excess.

   c. That the drug may produce hypertension and bradycardia.

   d. That the drug may produce cardiac arrhythmias.

7. The person who administers curare during general anesthesia must carefully observe the patient because curare might produce:

    a. Cardiac arrhythmias.

    b. Too deep a level of analgesia in a patient.

    c. Respiratory depression.

    d. Tachycardia.

8. The patient taking orphenadrine citrate should be warned that:

    a. He may become drowsy while taking the drug.

    b. The drug may produce skeletal muscle relaxation.

    c. He may experience cardiac arrhythmias.

    d. The drug may produce tachycardia.

9. Methocarbamol (Robaxin®) when administered intravenously is used to treat:

    a. Multiple sclerosis and cerebral palsy.

    b. Hypercalcemia.

    c. Trauma.

    d. Acute muscle spasms associated with trauma and inflammation.

Check Your Answers on Next Page

SOLUTIONS TO EXERCISES, LESSON 3

1.   c   An agent that reduces skeletal muscle tone. (para 3-2)

2.   b   They block the action of acetylcholine at the neuromuscular junction or at the muscle receptor site. (para 3-3a)

3.   a   Decreasing the muscle tone by depressing the internuncial neurons at the spinal cord. (para 3-6)

4.   <u>A</u>   Cyclobenzaprine (para 3-7b)

     <u>D</u>   Pancuronium (para 3-5a(2))

     <u>E</u>   Orphenadrine citrate (para 3-7c)

     <u>C</u>   Succinylcholine (para 3-5b(1))

     <u>B</u>   Chlorzoxazone (para 3-7d)

5.   d   Used as a muscle relaxant for relatively short procedures. (para 3-5b(2))

6.   a   Not to drink alcoholic beverages while taking the drug. (para 3-7d)

7.   c   Respiratory depression. (para 3-5a(1))

8.   a   He may become drowsy while taking the drug. (para 3-7c)

9.   d   Acute muscle spasms associated with trauma and inflammation. (para 3-7e)

End of Lesson 3

ANNEX

DRUG PRONUNCIATION GUIDE

This Drug Pronunciation Guide was developed to help you to learn how the trade and generic names of commonly prescribed medications are frequently pronounced. Not all the drugs in the guide are discussed in this subcourse. Remember, it is not enough to be able to know the uses, indications, cautions and warnings, and contraindications for a drug--you must also know how to pronounce that drug's name.

Trade Name	*Generic Name*
Actifed (Ak'-ti-fed)	Triprolidine (Tri-pro'-li-deen) and Pseudoephedrine (Soo-do-e-fed'-rin)
Adapin (Ad'-a-pin)	Doxepin (Dok'-se-pin)
Sinequan (Sin'-a-kwan)	" "
Afrin (Af'-rin)	Oxymetazoline (Ok-see-met-az'-o-leen)
Aldactazide (Al-dak'-ta-zide)	Spironolactone (Spi-ro-no-lak'-tone) and Hydrochlorothiazide (Hy-dro-klor-thi'-a-zide)
Aldactone (Al-dak'-tone)	Spironolactone (Spi-ro-no-lak'-tone)
Aldomet (Al'-do-met)	Methyldopa (Meth-il-do'-pah)
Alupent (Al'-u-pent)	Metaproterenol (Met-a-pro-ter'-eh-nol)
Amoxil (Am-ok'-sil)	Amoxicillin (Ah-moks'-i-sil-in)
Amphojel (Am'-fo-jel)	Aluminum (Al-loo'-mi-num) Hydroxide (Hy-drok'-side)
Ampicillin (Amp'-I-sil-in)	Same
Antepar (Ab'-te-par)	Piperazine (Pi-per'-ah-zeen)
Anturane (An'-tu-rain)	Sulfinpyrazone (Sul-fin-pie'-ra-zone)
Anusol (An'-u-sol)	Pramoxine (Pram-ok'-seen)
Apresoline (A-press'-o-leen)	Hydralazine (Hy-dral'-ah-zeen)
Aralen (Ar'-a-len)	Chloroquine (Klor'-o-kwin)
Aristocort (A-ris'-to-cort)	Triamcinolone (Tri-am-sin'-o-lone)
Artane (Ar'-tane)	Trihexyphenidyl(Tri-hek-see-fen'-i-dil)
A.S.A.	Aspirin (As'-per-in)
Atromid S (A'-tro-mid)	Clofibrate (Klo-fi'-brate)
Avlosulfon (Av-lo-sul'-fon)	Dapsone (Dap'-sone)
Azolid (Az'-o-lid)	Phenylbutazone (Fen-il-bute'-a-zone)
Bactrim (Bak'-trim)	Sulfamethoxazole (Sul-fah-meth-oks'-ah-zole) and Trimethoprim (Tri-meth'-o-prim)
Bellergal (Bel'-er-gal)	Ergotamine (Er-got'-a-meen), Phenobarbital (Feen-o-bar'-bi-tal) and Belladonna (Bel-la-don'-na) Alkaloids
Benadryl (Ben'-a-dril)	Diphenhydramine (Di-fen-hy'-dra-meen)

Trade Name	Generic Name
Bendectin (Ben-dek'-tin)	Doxylamine (Dok-sil'-a-meen)
Benemid (Ben'-eh-mid)	Probenecid (Pro-ben'-eh-sid)
Bonine (Bo'-neen)	Meclizine (Mek'-li-zeen)
Cafergot (Kaf'-er-got)	Ergotamine (Er-got'-a-meen) and Caffeine (Kaf'-feen)
Calamine (Kal'-a-mine)	Same
Catapres (Kat'-a-press)	Clonidine (Klo'-ni-deen)
CeeNu (See'-new)	Lomustine (Lo-mus'-teen)
Chlor-Trimeton (Klo-tri '-meh-ton)	Chlorpheniramine (Klor-fen-it'-a-meen)
Clomid (Klo'-mid)	Clomiphene (Klo'-mi-feen)
Clonopin (Klo-o-pin)	Clonazepam (Klo-na'-ze-pam)
Codeine (Ko'-deen)	Same
Cogentin (Ko-jen'-tin)	Benztropine (Benz'-tro-peen)
Colace (Ko'-lace)	Dioctyl(Di-ok'-til) Sodium (So'-dee-um) Sulfosuccinate (Sul-fo-suk'-si-nate)
Colchicine (Kol'-chi-seen)	Same
Compazine (Kom'-pa-zeen)	Prochlorperazine (Pro-klor-per'-a-zeen)
Cordran (Kor'-dran)	Flurandrenolide (Floor-an-dren'-o-lide)
Coumadin (Koo'-mah-din)	Warfarin (War'-fah-rin)
CP	Cloroquine (Klor'-o-kwin) and Primaquine (Prim'-a-kwin)
Cyclogyl (Si'-klo-jel)	Cyclopentolate (Si-klo-pen'-to-late)
Cytomel (Si'-to-mel)	Liothyronine (Li-o-thy-ro-neen)
Cytoxan (Si-tok'-san)	Cyclophosphamide (Si-klo-fos'-fa-mide)
Dalmane (Dal '-mane)	Flurazepam (Floor-az'-e-pam)
Darvocet (Dar'-vo-set)	Propoxyphene (Pro-pok'-se-feen) and Acetaminopen (As-et-am'-ino-fen)
Darvon (Dar'-von)	Propoxyphene (Pro-pok-se-feen)
Decadron (Dek'-a-dron)	Dexamethasone (Dek-sa-meth'-ah-sone)
Deltasone (Del '-ta-sone)	Prednisone (Pred'-ni-sone)
Demerol (Dem'-er-ol)	Meperidine (Meh-pair'-i-deen)
Dexedrine (Deks '-eh-dreen)	Dextroamphetamine (Deks-tro-am-fet'-a-meen)
Diabinese (Di-ab'-i-nees)	Chlorpropamide (Klor-prop'-a-mide)
Diethylstilbestrol (Di-eth-il-stil-bes'-trol)	Same
Dilantin (Di-lan'-tin)	Phenytoin (Fen'-i-toin)
Dilaudid (Di-law'-did)	Hydromorphone (Hy-dro-more' -fon)
Dimetane (Di'-meh-tane)	Brompheniramine (Brom-fen-ir'-a-meen)

Trade Name	Generic Name
Dimetapp (Di'-meh-tap)	Brompheniramine (Brom-fen-ir'-a-meen) Phenylephrine (Fen-il-ef'-rin) and Phenylpropanolamine (Fen-il-pro-pan-ol'-a-meen)
Disophrol (Dice'-o-frol)	Dexbrompheniramine (Deks-brom-fen-ir'-a-meen) and Pseudoephedrine (Soo-do-e-fed'-rin)
Dolophine (Dol'-o-feen)	Methadone (Meth'-a-done)
Domeboro (Dome-bor'-o)	Aluminum (Ah-loo'-mi-num) Acetate (As'-e-tate)
Donnatal (Don'-na-tal)	Belladonna (Bel-la-don'-na) Alkaloids (Al'-ka-loids) and Phenobarbital (Feen-o-barb'-i-tal)
Doxidan (Dok'-si-dan)	Danthron (Dan'-thron) and Dicctyl (Di-ok'-til) Calcium (Kal'-see-um) Sulfosuccinate (Sul-fo-suk'-si-nate)
Drixoral (Driks'-or-al)	Dexbrompheniramine (Deks-brom-fen-ir'-a-meen) and Pseudoephedrine (Soo-do-e-fed'-rin)
Dulcolax (Dul'-ko-laks)	Bisacodyl (Bis-a'-ko-dil)
Dyazine (Di'-a-zide)	Triamterene (Tri-am'-ter-een) and Hydrochlorothiazide (Hy-dro-klor-o-thi'-a-zide)
Dymelor (Die'-meh-lor)	Acetohexamide (As-e-to-heks'-a-mide)
Dyrenium (Die-ren'-i-um)	Triamterene (Tri-am'-ter-een)
Efudex (Ef'-u-deks)	Fluorouracil (Floo-ro-ur'-ah-sil)
Elavil (El'-ah-vil)	Amitriptyline (Am-i-trip'-til-een)
Elixir Terpin (Ter'-pin) Hydrate	Same
Empirin (Em'-per-in)	Codeine (Ko'-deen) and Aspirin (As'-per-in)
E-Mycin (E-mie'-sin)	Erythromycin (E-rith-ro-mie'-sin)
Equanil (Ek'-wa-nil)	Meprobamate (Me-pro-bam'-ate)
Ergomar (Er'-go-mar)	Ergotamine (Er-got'-a-meen)
Ergotrate (Er'-go-trate)	Ergonovine (Er-go-no'-veen)
Erythrocin (Er-eeth'-ro-sin)	Erythromycin (Er-eeth-ro-my'-sin) Stearate (Stare'-rate)
Esidrix (Es'-i-driks)	Hyrochlorothiazide (Hy-dro-klor-o-thi'-a-zide)
Feosol (Fe'-o-sol)	Ferrous (Fer'-rus) Sulfate (Sul'-fate)
Fergon (Fer'-gon)	Ferrous (Fer'-rus) Gluconate (Glu'-con-ate)

Trade Name	Generic Name
Fiorinal (Fee-or'-i-nal)	Butalbi tal (Bu-tal'-bi-tal), Apririn, Phenacetin (Fen-ass'-eh-tin), and Caffeine (Kaf'-feen)
Flagyl (Fla'-jil)	Metronidazole (Me-tro-ni'-dah-zole)
Flexeril (Flek'-sa-ril)	Cyclobenzaprine (Si-klo-benz'-a-preen)
Fulvicin (Ful'-vi-sin)	Griseofulvin (Griz-e-o-ful'-vin)
Guantanol (Gan'-ta-nol)	Suiphamethoxazole (Sul-fah-meth-oks'-ah-zole)
Gantrisin (Gan'-tri-sin)	Sulfisoxazole (Sul-fi-sok'-sah-zole)
Gelusil (Jel'-u-sil)	Aluminum (Ah-loo'-mi-num) Hydroxide (Hy-drok'-side) and Magnesium (Mag-nee'-zee-um) Hydroxide
Grifulvin (Gri-ful'-vin)	Griseofulvin (Griz-e-o-ful'-vin)
Gynergen (Jin'-er-jen)	Ergotamine (Er-got'-a-meen)
Haldol (Hal'-dol)	Haloperidol (Hal-o-pair'-i-dol)
Halotestin (Hal-o-tes'-tin)	Fluoxymesterone (Floo-ok-see-mes-teh-rone)
Hexadrol (Hek'-sa-drol)	Dexamethasone (Dek-sa-meth'-a-sone)
Hydrodiuril (Hy-dro-di'-ur-il)	Hydroclorothiazide (Hy-dro-kior-thi'-a-zide)
Hygroton (Hy-grow'-ton)	Chiorthalidone (Kior-thal'-i-done)
Ilosone (I'-low-sone)	Erythromycin (Er-ith-ro-mi'-sin) Estolate (Es'-to-late)
Inderal (In'-der-al)	Propranolol (Pro-pran'-o-lol)
Indocin (In'-do-sin)	Indomethacin (In-do-meth'-a-sin)
INH	Isoniazid (I-so-ni'-a-zid)
Insulin (In'-sul-in)	Same
Intal	Cromolyn (Kro'-mo-lin)
Ismelin (Is'-meh-lin)	Guanethidine (Gwan-eth'-i-dine)
Isopto-Atropine (I-sop-to-at'-ro-peen)	Atropine (At'-ro-peen)
Isopto-Carpine (I-sop-to-car'-peen)	Pilocarpine (Pile-o-car'-peen)
Isordil (I'-sor-dil)	Isosorbide (I-so-sor'-bide)
Keflex (Kef'-lex)	Cephalexin (Sef-ah-lek'-sin)
Lanoxin (Lan-ok'-sin)	Digoxin (Di-jok'-sin)
Larodopa (Lar-o-do'-pa)	Levodopa (Le-o-do'-pa)
Larotid (Lar'-o-tid)	Amoxicillin (Ah-moks'-i-sil-in)
Lasix (La'-siks)	Furosemide (Fu-ro'-se-mide)
Leukeran (Lu'-ker-an)	Chlorambucil (Klor-ram'-bu-sil)
Librium (Lib'-ree-um)	Chlordiazepoxide (Klor-die-az-eh-pok'-side)

Trade Name	Generic Name
Lidex (Lie'-deks)	Fluocinoide (Floo-o-sin'-o-nide)
Lomotil (Lo'-mo-til)	Diphenoxylate (Die-fen-ok'-si-late)
Lopressor (Lo'-pres-sor)	Metoprolol (Met-o-pro'-lol)
Lotrimin (Lo'-tri-min)	Chlotrimazole (Klo-trim'-ah-zole)
Maalox (May'-loks)	Aluminum (Ah-loo'-mi-num) and Magnesium (Mag-nee'-zee-um) Hydroxides
Macrodanton (Ma-kro-dan'-tin)	Nitrofurantoin (Ni-tro-fur-an'-toin)
Mandelamine (Man-del'-a-meen)	Methenamine (Meth-en'-a-meen) Mandelate (Man'-deh-late)
Medihaler-Iso (Med-i-hail-er-I'-so)	Isoproterenol (I-so-pro-ter'-en-ol)
Mellaril (Mel'-la-ril)	Thioridazine (Thi-o-rid'-a-zeen)
Metamucil (Met-a-mu'-sil)	Psyllium (Sil'-e-um)
Metaprel (Meh'-ta-prel)	Metaproterenol (Meh'-ta-pro-ter'-eh-nol)
Methotrexate (Meth-o-treks'-ate)	Amethopterin (Ah-meth-op'-ter-in)
Milk of Magnesia	Same
Minipress (Min'-i-press)	Prazosin (Pra'-zo-sin)
Minocin (Min'-o-sin)	Minocycline (Mi-no-si'-kleen)
Monistat (Mon'-i-stat)	Miconazole (Mi-kon'-ah-zole)
Motrin (Mo'-trin)	Ibuprofen (I-bu'-pro-fen)
Myambutol (My-am'-bu-tol)	Ethambutol (Eth-am'-bu-tol)
Mycostatin (My-co-stat'-in)	Nystatin (Ny-stat'-in)
Mylanta (My-lan'-ta)	Aluminum (Ah-loo'-mi-num) and Magnesium (Mag-nee'-zee-um) Hydroxides and Simethicone (Si-meth'-i-kone)
Myleran (My-ler-an)	Busulfan (Bu-sul'-fan)
Mylicon (My'-li-kon)	Simethicone (Si-meth'-i-kone)
Mysoline (My'-so-leen)	Primidone (Pri'-mi-done)
Nalfon (Nal'-fon)	Fenoprofen (Fen-o-pro'-fen)
Naprosyn (Na'-pro-sin)	Naproxen (Na-prok'-sen)
Nembutal (Nem'-bu-tal)	Pentobarbital (Pen-to-barb'-i-tal)
Neosynephrine (Nee-o-sin-eh'-frin)	Phenylephrine (Fen-il-eh'-frin)
Nitrobid (Ni'-tro-bid)	Nitroglycerin (Ni-tro-gli'-ser-in)
Nitrol (Ni'-trol)	" "
Nitrostat (Ni-tro-stat)	" "
Noctec (Nok'-tek)	Chloral Hydrate (Klor'-al- Hy'-drate)
Norfiex (Nor'-fleks)	Orphenadrine Citrate (Or-fen'-a-dreen)
Norpace (Nor'-pace)	Disopyramide (Di-so-peer'-a-mide)

Trade Name	Generic Name
Novahistine (No-va-his'-teen) Expectorant	Guaifenesin (Gwi-fen'-eh-sin), Phenylpropanolamine (Fen-il-pro-pan-ol'-a-meen), and Codeine (Ko'-deen)
NTG	Nitroclycerin (Ni-tro-gli'-ser-in)
Nupercainal (New-per-kain'-al)	Dibucaine (Die'-bu-kain)
Oretic (O-ret'-ik)	Hydrochlorothiazide (Hy-dro-kior-thi'-a-zide)
Orinase (Or'-in-ase)	Tolbutamide (Tol-bu'-tah-mide)
Ornade (Or'-nade)	Chlorpheniramine (Klor-fen-ir'-a-meen), Triprolidine (Tri-pro-li-deen) and Pseudoephedrine (Su-do-eh-fed'-rin)
Parafon Forte (Pair'-a-fon For'-tay)	Chlorzoxazone (Klor-zok'-sa-zone)
Percodan (Per'-ko-dan)	Oxycodone (Ok-si-ko'-done)
Periactin (Per-ee-ak'-tin)	Cyproheptadine (Si-pro-hep'-tah-deen)
Persantine (Per-san'-teen)	Dipyridamole (Di-pi-rid'-ah-mole)
Phenobarbital (Feen-o-barb'-it-al)	Same
Phenylpropanolamine (Fen-il-pro-pan-ol'-a-meen)	Same
Pitocin (Pi-tow'-sin)	Oxytocin (Ok-see-tow'-sin)
Pontocaine (Pon'-to-kain)	Tetracaine (Teh'-tra-kain)
Povan (Po'-van)	Pyrvinium (Pire-vin'-ee-um)
Premarin (Prem'-ar-in)	Conjugated (Kon'-joo-gay-ted) Estrogens (Es-tro-jens)
Presamine (Press'-a-meen)	Imipramine (Im-ip'-rah-meen)
Primaquine (Pri'-mah-kwin)	Same
Probanthine (Pro-ban'-theen)	Propantheline (Pro-pan'-the-leen)
Pronestyl (Pro-nes'-til)	Procainamide (Pro-kain'-a-mide)
Prophylthiouracil (Pro-pil-thi-o-u'-rah-sil)	Same
Prostaphlin (Pro-staff'-lin)	Oxacillin (Oks'-ah-sil-in)
Provera (Pro-ver'-ah)	Medroxyprogesterone (Med-rok-see-pro-jes'-ter-one)
Pyridium (Pie-rid'-ee-um)	Phenazopyridine (Fen-ahs-o-per'-i-deen)
Quinidine (Kwin'-i-deen)	Same
Quinine (Kwie'-nine)	Same
Reserpine (Ree-ser'-peen)	Same
Retin A (Reh'-tin A)	Tretinoin (Tret'-i-noin)
Rifadin (Rie-fad'-in)	Rifampin (Rie-fam'-pin)
Riopan (Rie'-o-pan)	Magaidrate (Mag'-al-drate)

Trade Name	Generic Name
Rimactane (Rim-act'-ane)	Rifampin (Rie-fam'-pin)
Ritalin (Rit'-a-lin)	Methylphenidate (Meth-il-fen'-i-date)
Robaxin (Ro-bak'-sin)	Methocarbamol (Meth-o-kar'-ba-mol)
Robitussin (Row-i-tus'-sin)	Guaifenesin (Gwie-fen'-eh-sin)
Robitussin DM	Guiafenesin and Dextromethorphan (Dek-tro-meh-or'-fan)
Sansert (San'-sert)	Methysergide (Meth-ee-ser'-jide)
Seconal (Sek'-o-nal)	Secobarbital (Sek-o-bar'-bi-tal)
Selsun (Sel'-sun)	Selenium (Se-leh'-nee-um)
Septra (Sep'-tra)	Sulfamethoxazole (Sul-fah-meth-oks'-a-zole) and Trimethroprim (Tri-meth'-o-prim)
Serax (See'-raks)	Oxazepam (Oks-az'-eh-pam)
Silvadene (Sil'-va-deen)	Silver Sulfadiazine (Sul-fa-die'-a-zeen)
Sinemet (Si'-ne-met)	Levodopa (Le-vo-do'-pa)
Sinequan (Sin'-a-kwan)	Doxepin (Dok'-seh-pin)
Sorbitrate (Sor'-bi-trate)	Isosorbide (I-so-sor'-bide)
Stelazine (Stel'-a-zeen)	Trifluoperazine(Tri-floo-o-per'-a-zeen)
Sudafed (Soo'-da-fed)	Pseudophedrine (Soo-do-eh-feh'-drin)
Sulamyd (Sul'-a-mid)	Sulfacetamide (Sul-fah-set'-a-mide)
Sulfamylon (Sul-fa-mie'-lon)	Mafenide (Maf'-eh-nide)
Sultrin (Sul'-trin)	Sulfathiazole (Sul-fah-thi'-ah-zole) Sulfacetamide (Sul-fah-set'-ah-mide) and Sulfabenzamide (Sul-fah-benz'-ah-mide)
Surfak (Sur'-fak)	Dioctyl (Di-ok'-til) Calcium (Kal'-see-um) Sulfosuccinate (Sul-fo-suk'-si-nate)
Synalar (Sine'-a-lar)	Fluocinolone (Floo-o-sin'-o-lone)
Synthroid (Sin'-throid)	Levothyroxine (Lee-vo-thi-rok'-sin)
Tace (Tace)	Chlorotrianisene (Klor-o-tri-an'-I-seen)
Tagamet (Tag'-a-met)	Cimetidine (Si-met'-i-deen)
Talwin (Tal'-win)	Pentazocine (Pen-taz'-o-seen)
Tandearil (Tan'-da-ril)	Oxyphenbutazone (Ok-see-fen-bute'-a-zone)
Tegretol (Teg'-reh-tol)	Carbamazepine (Kar-ba-maz'-eh-peen)
Tessalon (Tess'-a-lon)	Benzonatate (Benz-on'-a-tate)
Tetracycline (Tet-ra-si'-kleen)	
Thorazine (Thor'-a-zeen)	Chlorpromazine (Klor-pro'-ma-zeen)
Thyroid (Thy'-roid)	Same
Tigan (Tie'-gan)	Trimethobenzamide (Tri-meth-o-benz'-a-mide)
Timoptic (Tim-op'-tic)	Timilol (Tim'-o-lol)

Trade Name	Generic Name
Tinactin (Tin-act'-in)	Tolnaftate (Tol-naf'-tate)
Titralac (Ti'-tra-lak)	Calcium (Kal-see-um) Carbonate (Kar'-bon-ate) and Glycine (Gly'-seen)
Tofranil (Toe'-fra-nil)	Imipramine (I-mip'-rah-meen)
Tolectin (Tow-lek'-tin)	Tolmetin (Tol-met'-in)
Triavil (Tri'-a-vil)	Perphenazine (Per-fen'-a-zeen) and Amitriptlyline (Am-i-trip'-ti-leen)
Trilafon (Try'-la-fon)	Perphenazine (Per-fen-a-zeen)
Tylenol (Tie'-leh-nol)	Acetaminophen (As-et-am'-ino-fen)
Tylenol #3	Acetaminophen and Codeine (Ko'-deen)
Unipen (U'-ni-pen)	Nafcillin (Naf-sil-lin)
Urecholine (Ur-eh-ko'-leen)	Bethanecol (Beth-an'-eh-kol)
Valisone (Val'-i-sone)	Betamethasone (Beh-tah-meth'-a-sone)
Valium (Val'-ee-um)	Diazepam (Die-aze-eh-pam)
Vermox (Ver'-moks)	Mebendazole (Meh-ben'-dah-zole)
Vibramycin (Vie-bra-my'-sin)	Doxycycline (Doks-see-si'-kleen)
Xylocaine (Zie'-low-kain)	Lidocaine (Lie-do-kain)
Zarontin (Zar-on'-tin)	Ethosuximide (Eh-tho-suks'-a-mide)
Zyloprim (Zie'-low-prim)	Allopurinol (Al-lo-pure'-in-ol)

End of Lesson 3 Annex

LESSON ASSIGNMENT

LESSON 4	Analgesic, Anti-inflammatory, and Anti-gout Agents.
TEXT ASSIGNMENT	Paragraphs 4-1--4-8.
LESSON OBJECTIVES	After completing this lesson, you should be able to:

4-1. Given one of the following terms: analgesic, anti-pyretic, anti-inflammatory agent, rheumatism, arthritis, or gout, and a list of definitions select the definition of the given term.

4-2. Given the trade or generic name of an analgesic, anti-inflammatory, or anti-gout agent and a list of trade and/or generic names, select the appropriate name for that agent.

4-3. Given the trade and/or generic name of an analgesic, anti-inflammatory, or anti-gout agent and a group of statements pertaining to indications, use, side effects, or cautions and warnings, select the statement that best applies to that drug.

4-4. Given a group of statements, select the statement that best describes the cause of gout.

SUGGESTION   After studying the assignment, complete the exercises at the end of this lesson. These exercises will help you to achieve the lesson objectives.

LESSON 4

ANALGESIC, ANTI-INFLAMMATORY, AND ANTIGOUT AGENTS

Section I. BACKGROUND

4-1. INTRODUCTION TO ANALGESIC, ANTI-INFLAMMATORY, AND ANTI-GOUT AGENTS

Since the beginning of time, every civilization has sought a perfect medicinal agent that would relieve pain. As far back as the third century, B.C., physicians were administering the juice of the opium poppy to patients for the relief of pain. Opium derivatives are still widely used in the treatment of severe pain. Fortunately, agents with less abuse potential have been discovered for the relief of pain. This lesson will focus on analgesics, anti-inflammatory, and anti-gout agents.

4-2. DEFINITIONS

a. **Analgesic**. An analgesic is an agent that relieves pain.

b. **Antipyretic**. An antipyretic is an agent that lowers elevated body temperature.

c. **Anti-Inflammatory Agent**. An anti-inflammatory agent is a drug that decreases inflammation.

d. **Rheumatism**. Rheumatism is a condition characterized by inflammation of connective tissue.

e. **Arthritis**. Arthritis is a form of rheumatism in which the inflammation is confined to body joints.

f. **Gout**. Gout is a form of arthritis that is caused by an excess of uric acid in the blood that periodically precipitates in the peripheral joints as monosodium urate.

Section II. ANALGESIC AGENTS

4-3. BACKGROUND

Analgesic agents relieve pain. Some agents (like morphine or meperidine) are used to relieve severe pain, while others (like acetaminophen) are administered to relieve less severe pain. The material in this section of the lesson will consider agents used to relieve less severe pain.

4-4. SPECIFIC ANALGESIC AGENTS

a. **Acetaminophen (Tylenol®).** Acetaminophen is used as an analgesic and as an antipyretic. It is not an anti-inflammatory agent: Acetaminophen will <u>not</u> relieve the swelling or redness found in arthritis or rheumatism. Side effects associated with this agent are itching or skin rash (most likely caused by hypersensitivity reactions), hemolytic anemia (persons with G-6-PD deficiency are especially susceptible), and kidney damage. This drug may cause liver damage with chronic use. Acetaminophen is available in capsule, elixir, suspension, syrup, tablet, chewable tablet, and suppository forms.

b. **Aspirin (A.S.A.).** Aspirin is used as an analgesic, anti-pyretic, and anti-inflammatory agent. Aspirin produces gastric irritation. Taking aspirin with a full glass of water or milk (8 fluid ounces) can help minimize stomach irritation. Tinnitus (ringing of the ears) is a symptom of aspirin overdose. Aspirin interacts with a variety of medications. One, the effects of oral hypoglycemic or insulin is increased when aspirin is administered concurrently with them. Two, since aspirin has some anti-coagulant effects, concurrent administration of aspirin, and some anti-coagulants can result in increased risk of patient bleeding. Patients should be cautioned against taking any oral aspirin preparation that has a strong vinegar-like odor. Aspirin is available in a variety of dosage forms (tablets, enteric coated tablets--dissolve in the intestines, and suppositories).

c. **Aspirin, Magnesium Hydroxide, and Aluminum Hydroxide Tablets (Cama®).** This aspirin-containing product is an analgesic, anti-inflammatory, and antipyretic agent. The magnesium hydroxide and aluminum hydroxide is in the formulation to reduce the stomach irritation associated with the aspirin. Patients taking this medication should be told not to take this medication with tetracyclines because the tetracycline's therapeutic effect might be decreased: This medication and tectracyclines should not be taken within one hour of each other. This product should be taken with at least 8 fluid ounces of water. Patients should be cautioned against taking this product if it has a strong vinegar-like odor.

d. **Propoxyphene Hydrochloride (Darvon®).** Propoxyphene is a centrally acting opioid analgesic. The drug may produce side effects such as dizziness, drowsiness, or blurred vision. Patients taking propoxyphene should be cautioned against taking alcohol or other central nervous system depressants while they are taking propoxyphene. Propoxyphene is a Note Q controlled substance.

e. **Propoxyphene Napsylate (Darvon N®).** Propoxyphene napsylate is used as an analgesic. It may produce such side effects as drowsiness and dizziness. Patients should be warned against taking alcohol or other central nervous system depressants when they are taking this drug. Darvon N® is a Note Q controlled substance.

f. **Pentazocine (Talwin®).** Pentazocine is a centrally acting opioid analgesic. Side effects associated with this agent are gastrointestinal upset, sedation, blurred vision, hallucinations, mental confusion, and shortness of breath. This medication should be used with caution in-patients who have a history of drug abuse or dependence. The oral dosage form (Talwin NX®) is combined with naloxone, a narcotic antagonist, to discourage the abuse of this substance. When the tablet is dissolved and then injected, the naloxone negates the euphoric effects of the pentazocine. Patients taking pentazocine should not take alcohol or any other central nervous system depressant at the same time, since this agent is a central nervous system depressant.

g. **Butalbital with Aspirin and Caffeine (Fiorinal®).** This product contains butalbital (a short-to-intermediate-acting barbiturate--50 mg), aspirin (325 mg), and caffeine (40 mg). The product is used as an analgesic. Side effects associated with this agent are gastrointestinal upset and sedation. This product may cause drug dependence. Patients taking this drug should not take any alcohol or any other central nervous system depressant. Fiorinal® is a Note Q controlled substance. (**NOTE:** Fiorinal® with Codeine is another formulation of this product. It is used to raise the threshold of pain.)

Section III. ANTI-INFLAMMATORY AGENTS

4-5. BACKGROUND

In certain conditions (that is, arthritis) or injuries, affected tissues become inflamed. The net effect of such inflammation is to surround the affected area and "wall it off" so that the movement of toxic products or bacteria from the affected part is delayed. Blood flow to the area is increased and certain changes happen in the capillaries to increase the fluid level of the tissues. Hence, the area becomes swollen. Redness of the area follows. Although this is a protective mechanism for the body, it is desirable at times to use drugs to decrease this effect.

4-6. SPECIFIC ANTI-INFLAMMATORY AGENTS

a. **Indomethacin (Indocin®).** Indomethacin is used in the treatment of various medical problems, including certain types of arthritis. Indomethacin is used to relieve swelling, inflammation, joint pain, stiffness, and fever. Patients hypersensitive to aspirin may also be hypersensitive to indomethacin. Side effects associated with the agent are gastrointestinal upset, headache, dizziness, and ringing or buzzing in the ears. Patients should be instructed to take this medication with food or milk or right after meals in order to lessen the possibility of gastrointestinal upset. Furthermore, in order to lessen gastrointestinal upset, patients should be instructed not to regularly drink alcoholic beverages or take aspirin unless their physician has told them otherwise. Since the drug does have the side effect of dizziness, the patient should be told not to drive or operate hazardous machinery until he or she has been taking the drug and has determined its effects on alertness.

b. **Ibuprofen (Motrin®).** Ibuprofen is used to treat the symptoms of arthritis. Ibuprofen relieves swelling, joint pain, stiffness, and inflammation. Some patients may have to take the drug for one to two weeks before they begin to feel its full effects. Side effects associated with the use of this agent include skin rashes, itching of skin, ringing or buzzing in the ears, dizziness, or a bloated feeling. Since the drug can cause some stomach irritation, the patient should not take alcohol or aspirin regularly while taking this drug unless the patient's physician has directed otherwise. Furthermore, since the drug does cause dizziness in some patients, the patient should be instructed not to drive or operate hazardous machinery until he or she has been taking the drug and has determined it affects on alertness.

c. **Fenoprofen (Nalfon®).** Fenoprofen is used to treat the symptoms of arthritis. Fenoprofen relieves swelling, joint pain, stiffness, and inflammation. Side effects associated with the use of this drug include ringing or buzzing in the ears, skin rash, black tarry stools, constipation, and drowsiness. Since the drug can cause some stomach irritation, the patient should not take alcohol or aspirin regularly while taking this drug unless the patient's physician directs otherwise. Furthermore, since the drug does cause drowsiness in some patients, the patient should be instructed not to drive or operate hazardous machinery until he or she has been taking the drug and has determined its effects on alertness.

d. **Tolmetin (Tolectin®).** Tolmetin is used to treat the symptoms of arthritis. The information for this drug is the same as for fenoprofen (Nalfon®)--see 4-6d above.

e. **Naproxen (Naprosyn®).** Naproxen is used to treat the symptoms of arthritis. Naproxen relieves swelling, joint pain, stiffness, and inflammation. Side effects associated with this agent include black tarry stools, blurred vision, skin rash, ringing or buzzing in the ears, and dizziness. Since this drug can cause some stomach irritation, the patient should not take alcohol or aspirin regularly while taking this drug unless the patient's physician directs otherwise. The drug may be taken with food, antacids, or milk to reduce stomach irritation.

f. **Sulindac (Clinoril®).** This drug is used to treat arthritis. This drug should be given with food twice daily; otherwise, the information for this drug is the same as is listed under naproxen (Naprosyn®).

g. **Piroxicam (Feldene®).** This drug is a unique agent because it has a 45-hour half-life. This long half-life permits once daily dosing. Piroxicam is used in the treatment of rheumatoid arthritis, ankylosing spondylitis, and osteoarthritis. The average daily dose is 20 mg. Gastrointestinal side effects are encountered in approximately 20 percent of patients.

h. **Celecoxib (Celebrex®).** This drug is unique because it may cause less risk of gastrointestinal side effects than other anti-inflammatory agents. Celecoxib is used in the treatment of rheumatoid and osteo arthritis.

Section IV. ANTIGOUT AGENTS

4-7. BACKGROUND

a. Gout is a metabolic disease characterized by attacks of acute pain, tenderness, and swelling of such joints as the instep, ankle, great toe, and elbow. Gout is caused by the deposition of sodium urate micro crystals. This condition is seen primarily in males. It is thought that heredity plays a major factor in gout, because gout occurs more often in relatives of those who have gout than in the population in general.

b. Gout is caused by defective purine metabolism. Humans lack the enzyme uricase, an enzyme that converts uric acid to allantoin. Uric acid is a major end product of the metabolism of purine (indirectly of amino acid metabolism). The level of uric acid in the plasma and urine is normally high (saturated). Sometimes a moderate increase in uric acid production can lead to the deposition of sodium urate microcrystals as described above.

c. The treatment of gout is usually designed to (1) relieve pain and (2) increase the elimination of uric acid from the body. Drugs administered to increase the elimination of uric acid from the body are referred to as uricosuric agents.

4-8. DRUGS USED TO TREAT GOUT

a. **Colchicine.** While the exact mechanism of action of colchicine is unknown, the administration of the drug causes a decrease in the amount of urate crystals deposited in the various parts of the body--the result is a decrease in the inflammatory process. This drug is the oldest and most effective agent used in the treatment of acute attacks of gout. The usual dose of an acute gout attack is 1.2 milligrams immediately, then 0.6 milligram every 30 minutes to one hour until nausea and vomiting or diarrhea starts or pain is relieved. Each patient must initially titrate his own dosage. If seven tablets caused adverse effects the first administration, the patient should reduce the dosage to six tablets on the next acute attack. The usual side effect associated with the administration of colchicine is gastrointestinal irritation. Occasionally antidiarreheals are prescribed to offset this adverse effect. The patient should be informed to allow an interval of at least three days between treatments--otherwise, toxic effects may occur from accumulation.

b. **Sulfinpyrazone (Anturane®).** Sulfinpyrazone potentiates the urinary excretion of uric acid. This anti-gout agent has the primary side effect of gastrointestinal upset. The patient taking this medication should be told to take this medication with food or milk. This medication should not be taken with salicylates.

c. **Allopurinol (Zyloprim®).** Allopurinol acts by decreasing the production of uric acid. This drug is not effective in the treatment of acute gout attacks, because it has no anti-inflammatory action. In fact, allopurinol may actually intensify the inflammation seen during an acute gout attack. Although the drug cannot be used to treat acute gout attacks, the patient should be instructed to continue taking allopurinol if he has such an attack. Allopurinol may produce such side effects as skin rash and gastrointestinal upset. If the drug causes too much gastrointestinal upset, the patient can take it after meals. The patient taking allopurinol should be instructed to drink at least 10 to 12 full glasses (8 fluid ounces per glass) of fluids each day--unless informed otherwise by his physician. This is done to prevent the formation of kidney stones while taking the drug.

    d. **Probenecid (Benemid®).** Probenecid increases the urinary excretion of uric acid. This anti-gout agent has the following side effects associated with its use: bloody urine, lower back pain, and painful urination. The patient should be instructed not to drink too much alcohol while taking this drug since doing so could lessen the therapeutic effect of probenecid. Furthermore, the patient should be told not to take aspirin with this agent because salicylates antagonize the uricosuric action of probenecid.

Continue with Exercises

EXERCISES, LESSON 4

INSTRUCTIONS: Answer the following exercises by marking the lettered response that best answers the question.

After you have completed all the exercises, turn to "Solutions to Exercises" at the end of the lesson, and check your answers. For each exercise answered incorrectly, reread the material referenced with the solution.

1. Rheumatism is best described as:

    a. A form of arthritis that is caused by an excess of uric acid in the blood.

    b. A painful inflammation of body joints.

    c. A condition characterized by inflammation of connective tissue.

    d. A painful form of arthritis that causes gradual destruction of body joints.

2. Arthritis is best described as:

    a. A form of rheumatism in which the inflammation is limited to body joints.

    b. A destructive condition that attacks body joints by the accumulation of uric acid.

    c. A chronic condition characterized by the inability of the body's joints to become lubricated.

    d. An acute inflammation of the body joints and related connective tissue caused by infection or excess amounts of certain chemical substances in the body.

3. A patient complains that some aspirin she has at home is beginning to smell like vinegar. What should you tell her?

    a. Take the medication as usual -- nothing is wrong with it.

    b. Take the aspirin with at least 8 fluid ounces of water or milk.

    c. Never take more than two of those aspirin tablets at one time since the vinegar-like smell indicates the aspirin has increased in potency.

    d. Discard the aspirin and obtain a fresh supply.

4. A patient has been prescribed propoxyphene napsylate (Darvon N®). What should the patient be told?

   a. Take the medication with at least eight fluid ounces of water or milk.

   b. This medication should be taken at least one hour after taking tetracyclines.

   c. This medication should not be taken with alcohol or other CNS depressants.

   d. This medication should not be taken if it has a strong vinegar-like odor.

5. An elderly patient complains that he has been taking Motrin® for three days without experiencing much relief from his arthritis. What should the patient be told?

   a. Continue taking the drug since some patients have to take it for one or two weeks before they begin to feel its full effects.

   b. See the physician because the dosage probably needs to be increased.

   c. Stop taking the drug until pharmacy personnel ensure that the medication is not expired.

   d. Double the dose of the medication so the effects can be felt faster.

6. Gout is caused by:

   a. The defective metabolism of allantoin.

   b. The inflammation of connective tissue surrounding the body joints.

   c. Defective purine metabolism that causes sodium urate micro-crystals to be deposited in certain body joints.

   d. The incomplete elimination of uric acid from the body.

7. Sulfinpyrazone (Anturane®) is used in the treatment of:

   a. Rheumatism.

   b. Arthritis.

   c. Gout.

8. What should a patient who is taking Benemid® be told?

    a. This medication should not be taken with aspirin.

    b. This medication should not be taken with alcohol or other CNS depressants since Benemid® is a CNS depressant.

    c. This medication should not be taken on an empty stomach since it causes severe tissue irritation.

    d. This medication should be taken with antidiarrheals to lessen gastrointestinal irritation.

9. Select the use of pentazocine (Talwin®).

    a. Anti-gout agent.

    b. Anti-inflammatory agent.

    c. Antipyretic.

    d. Analgesic.

10. Match the drug name in Column A with its corresponding name in Column B.

COLUMN A		COLUMN B
_____ Anturane®	a.	Ibuprofen
_____ Benemid®	b.	Butazolidin®
_____ Motrin®	c.	Aspirin, magnesium hydroxide, and aluminum hydroxide tablets
_____ Cama®	d.	Probenecid
_____ Allopurinol	e.	Zyloprim®
	f.	Colchicine
	g.	Sulfinpyrazone

Check Your Answers on Next Page

SOLUTIONS TO EXERCISES, LESSON 4

1. c   A condition characterized by inflammation of connective tissue. (para 4-2d)

2. a   A form of rheumatism in which the inflammation is limited to body joints. (para 4-2e)

3. d   Discard the aspirin and obtain a fresh supply. (para 4-4b)

4. c   This medication should not be taken with alcohol or other CNS depressants. (para 4-4d)

5. a   Continue taking the drug since some patients have to take it for one to two weeks before they begin to feel its full effects. (para 4-6b)

6. c   Defective purine metabolism that causes sodium urate microcrystals to be deposited in certain body joints. (para 4-7a,b)

7. c   Gout. (para 4-8b)

8. a   This medication should not be taken with aspirin because aspirin will decrease its effectiveness. (para 4-8d)

9. d   Analgesic. (para 4-4f)

10. g   Anturane®. (para 4-8b)

    d   Benemid®. (para 4-8d)

    a   Motrin®. (para 4-6b)

    c   Cama®. (para 4-4c)

    e   Allopurinol. (para 4-8c)

End of Lesson 4

ANNEX

DRUG PRONUNCIATION GUIDE

This Drug Pronunciation Guide was developed to help you to learn how the trade and generic names of commonly prescribed medications are frequently pronounced. Not all the drugs in the guide are discussed in this subcourse. Remember, it is not enough to be able to know the uses, indications, cautions and warnings, and contraindications for a drug--you must also know how to pronounce that drug's name.

Trade Name	*Generic Name*
Actifed (Ak'-ti-fed)	Triprolidine (Tri-pro'-li-deen) and Pseudoephedrine (Soo-do-e-fed'-rin)
Adapin (Ad'-a-pin)	Doxepin (Dok'-se-pin)
Sinequan (Sin'-a-kwan)	" "
Afrin (Af'-rin)	Oxymetazoline (Ok-see-met-az'-o-leen)
Aldactazide (Al-dak'-ta-zide)	Spironolactone (Spi-ro-no-lak'-tone) and Hydrochlorothiazide (Hy-dro-klor-thi'-a-zide)
Aldactone (Al-dak'-tone)	Spironolactone (Spi-ro-no-lak'-tone)
Aldomet (Al'-do-met)	Methyldopa (Meth-il-do'-pah)
Alupent (Al'-u-pent)	Metaproterenol (Met-a-pro-ter'-eh-nol)
Amoxil (Am-ok'-sil)	Amoxicillin (Ah-moks'-i-sil-in)
Amphojel (Am'-fo-jel)	Aluminum (Al-loo'-mi-num) Hydroxide (Hy-drok'-side)
Ampicillin (Amp'-I-sil-in)	Same
Antepar (Ab'-te-par)	Piperazine (Pi-per'-ah-zeen)
Anturane (An'-tu-rain)	Sulfinpyrazone (Sul-fin-pie'-ra-zone)
Anusol (An'-u-sol)	Pramoxine (Pram-ok'-seen)
Apresoline (A-press'-o-leen)	Hydralazine (Hy-dral'-ah-zeen)
Aralen (Ar'-a-len)	Chloroquine (Klor'-o-kwin)
Aristocort (A-ris'-to-cort)	Triamcinolone (Tri-am-sin'-o-lone)
Artane (Ar'-tane)	Trihexyphenidyl(Tri-hek-see-fen'-i-dil)
A.S.A.	Aspirin (As'-per-in)
Atromid S (A'-tro-mid)	Clofibrate (Klo-fi'-brate)
Avlosulfon (Av-lo-sul'-fon)	Dapsone (Dap'-sone)
Azolid (Az'-o-lid)	Phenylbutazone (Fen-il-bute'-a-zone)
Bactrim (Bak'-trim)	Sulfamethoxazole (Sul-fah-meth-oks'-ah-zole) and Trimethoprim (Tri-meth'-o-prim)
Bellergal (Bel'-er-gal)	Ergotamine (Er-got'-a-meen), Phenobarbital (Feen-o-bar'-bi-tal) and Belladonna (Bel-la-don'-na) Alkaloids
Benadryl (Ben'-a-dril)	Diphenhydramine (Di-fen-hy'-dra-meen)

Trade Name	Generic Name
Bendectin (Ben-dek'-tin)	Doxylamine (Dok-sil'-a-meen)
Benemid (Ben'-eh-mid)	Probenecid (Pro-ben'-eh-sid)
Bonine (Bo'-neen)	Meclizine (Mek'-li-zeen)
Cafergot (Kaf'-er-got)	Ergotamine (Er-got'-a-meen) and Caffeine (Kaf'-feen)
Calamine (Kal'-a-mine)	Same
Catapres (Kat'-a-press)	Clonidine (Klo'-ni-deen)
CeeNu (See'-new)	Lomustine (Lo-mus'-teen)
Chlor-Trimeton (Klo-tri '-meh-ton)	Chlorpheniramine (Klor-fen-it'-a-meen)
Clomid (Klo'-mid)	Clomiphene (Klo'-mi-feen)
Clonopin (Klo-o-pin)	Clonazepam (Klo-na'-ze-pam)
Codeine (Ko'-deen)	Same
Cogentin (Ko-jen'-tin)	Benztropine (Benz'-tro-peen)
Colace (Ko'-lace)	Dioctyl(Di-ok'-til) Sodium (So'-dee-um) Sulfosuccinate (Sul-fo-suk'-si-nate)
Colchicine (Kol'-chi-seen)	Same
Compazine (Kom'-pa-zeen)	Prochlorperazine (Pro-klor-per'-a-zeen)
Cordran (Kor'-dran)	Flurandrenolide (Floor-an-dren'-o-lide)
Coumadin (Koo'-mah-din)	Warfarin (War'-fah-rin)
CP	Cloroquine (Klor'-o-kwin) and Primaquine (Prim'-a-kwin)
Cyclogyl (Si'-klo-jel)	Cyclopentolate (Si-klo-pen'-to-late)
Cytomel (Si'-to-mel)	Liothyronine (Li-o-thy-ro-neen)
Cytoxan (Si-tok'-san)	Cyclophosphamide (Si-klo-fos'-fa-mide)
Dalmane (Dal '-mane)	Flurazepam (Floor-az'-e-pam)
Darvocet (Dar'-vo-set)	Propoxyphene (Pro-pok'-se-feen) and Acetaminopen (As-et-am'-ino-fen)
Darvon (Dar'-von)	Propoxyphene (Pro-pok-se-feen)
Decadron (Dek'-a-dron)	Dexamethasone (Dek-sa-meth'-ah-sone)
Deltasone (Del '-ta-sone)	Prednisone (Pred'-ni-sone)
Demerol (Dem'-er-ol)	Meperidine (Meh-pair'-i-deen)
Dexedrine (Deks '-eh-dreen)	Dextroamphetamine (Deks-tro-am-fet'-a-meen)
Diabinese (Di-ab'-i-nees)	Chlorpropamide (Klor-prop'-a-mide)
Diethylstilbestrol (Di-eth-il-stil-bes'-trol)	Same
Dilantin (Di-lan'-tin)	Phenytoin (Fen'-i-toin)
Dilaudid (Di-law'-did)	Hydromorphone (Hy-dro-more' -fon)
Dimetane (Di'-meh-tane)	Brompheniramine (Brom-fen-ir'-a-meen)

Trade Name	Generic Name
Dimetapp (Di'-meh-tap)	Brompheniramine (Brom-fen-ir'-a-meen) Phenylephrine (Fen-il-ef'-rin) and Phenylpropanolamine (Fen-il-pro-pan-ol'-a-meen)
Disophrol (Dice'-o-frol)	Dexbrompheniramine (Deks-brom-fen-ir'-a-meen) and Pseudoephedrine (Soo-do-e-fed'-rin)
Dolophine (Dol'-o-feen)	Methadone (Meth'-a-done)
Domeboro (Dome-bor'-o)	Aluminum (Ah-loo'-mi-num) Acetate (As'-e-tate)
Donnatal (Don'-na-tal)	Belladonna (Bel-la-don'-na) Alkaloids (Al'-ka-loids) and Phenobarbital (Feen-o-barb'-i-tal)
Doxidan (Dok'-si-dan)	Danthron (Dan'-thron) and Dicctyl (Di-ok'-til) Calcium (Kal'-see-um) Sulfosuccinate (Sul-fo-suk'-si-nate)
Drixoral (Driks'-or-al)	Dexbrompheniramine (Deks-brom-fen-ir'-a-meen) and Pseudoephedrine (Soo-do-e-fed'-rin)
Dulcolax (Dul'-ko-laks)	Bisacodyl (Bis-a'-ko-dil)
Dyazine (Di'-a-zide)	Triamterene (Tri-am'-ter-een) and Hydrochlorothiazide (Hy-dro-klor-o-thi'-a-zide)
Dymelor (Die'-meh-lor)	Acetohexamide (As-e-to-heks'-a-mide)
Dyrenium (Die-ren'-i-um)	Triamterene (Tri-am'-ter-een)
Efudex (Ef'-u-deks)	Fluorouracil (Floo-ro-ur'-ah-sil)
Elavil (El'-ah-vil)	Amitriptyline (Am-i-trip'-til-een)
Elixir Terpin (Ter'-pin) Hydrate	Same
Empirin (Em'-per-in)	Codeine (Ko'-deen) and Aspirin (As'-per-in)
E-Mycin (E-mie'-sin)	Erythromycin (E-rith-ro-mie'-sin)
Equanil (Ek'-wa-nil)	Meprobamate (Me-pro-bam'-ate)
Ergomar (Er'-go-mar)	Ergotamine (Er-got'-a-meen)
Ergotrate (Er'-go-trate)	Ergonovine (Er-go-no'-veen)
Erythrocin (Er-eeth'-ro-sin)	Erythromycin (Er-eeth-ro-my'-sin) Stearate (Stare'-rate)
Esidrix (Es'-i-driks)	Hyrochlorothiazide (Hy-dro-klor-o-thi'-a-zide)
Feosol (Fe'-o-sol)	Ferrous (Fer'-rus) Sulfate (Sul'-fate)
Fergon (Fer'-gon)	Ferrous (Fer'-rus) Gluconate (Glu'-con-ate)

Trade Name	Generic Name
Fiorinal (Fee-or'-i-nal)	Butalbi tal (Bu-tal'-bi-tal), Apririn, Phenacetin (Fen-ass'-eh-tin), and Caffeine (Kaf'-feen)
Flagyl (Fla'-jil)	Metronidazole (Me-tro-ni'-dah-zole)
Flexeril (Flek'-sa-ril)	Cyclobenzaprine (Si-klo-benz'-a-preen)
Fulvicin (Ful'-vi-sin)	Griseofulvin (Griz-e-o-ful'-vin)
Guantanol (Gan'-ta-nol)	Suiphamethoxazole (Sul-fah-meth-oks'-ah-zole)
Gantrisin (Gan'-tri-sin)	Sulfisoxazole (Sul-fi-sok'-sah-zole)
Gelusil (Jel'-u-sil)	Aluminum (Ah-loo'-mi-num) Hydroxide (Hy-drok'-side) and Magnesium (Mag-nee'-zee-um) Hydroxide
Grifulvin (Gri-ful'-vin)	Griseofulvin (Griz-e-o-ful'-vin)
Gynergen (Jin'-er-jen)	Ergotamine (Er-got'-a-meen)
Haldol (Hal'-dol)	Haloperidol (Hal-o-pair'-i-dol)
Halotestin (Hal-o-tes'-tin)	Fluoxymesterone (Floo-ok-see-mes-teh-rone)
Hexadrol (Hek'-sa-drol)	Dexamethasone (Dek-sa-meth'-a-sone)
Hydrodiuril (Hy-dro-di'-ur-il)	Hydroclorothiazide (Hy-dro-kior-thi'-a-zide)
Hygroton (Hy-grow'-ton)	Chiorthalidone (Kior-thal'-i-done)
Ilosone (I'-low-sone)	Erythromycin (Er-ith-ro-mi'-sin) Estolate (Es'-to-late)
Inderal (In'-der-al)	Propranolol (Pro-pran'-o-lol)
Indocin (In'-do-sin)	Indomethacin (In-do-meth'-a-sin)
INH	Isoniazid (I-so-ni'-a-zid)
Insulin (In'-sul-in)	Same
Intal	Cromolyn (Kro'-mo-lin)
Ismelin (Is'-meh-lin)	Guanethidine (Gwan-eth'-i-dine)
Isopto-Atropine (I-sop-to-at'-ro-peen)	Atropine (At'-ro-peen)
Isopto-Carpine (I-sop-to-car'-peen)	Pilocarpine (Pile-o-car'-peen)
Isordil (I'-sor-dil)	Isosorbide (I-so-sor'-bide)
Keflex (Kef'-lex)	Cephalexin (Sef-ah-lek'-sin)
Lanoxin (Lan-ok'-sin)	Digoxin (Di-jok'-sin)
Larodopa (Lar-o-do'-pa)	Levodopa (Le-o-do'-pa)
Larotid (Lar'-o-tid)	Amoxicillin (Ah-moks'-i-sil-in)
Lasix (La'-siks)	Furosemide (Fu-ro'-se-mide)
Leukeran (Lu'-ker-an)	Chlorambucil (Klor-ram'-bu-sil)
Librium (Lib'-ree-um)	Chlordiazepoxide (Klor-die-az-eh-pok'-side)

Trade Name	Generic Name
Lidex (Lie'-deks)	Fluocinoide (Floo-o-sin'-o-nide)
Lomotil (Lo'-mo-til)	Diphenoxylate (Die-fen-ok'-si-late)
Lopressor (Lo'-pres-sor)	Metoprolol (Met-o-pro'-lol)
Lotrimin (Lo'-tri-min)	Chlotrimazole (Klo-trim'-ah-zole)
Maalox (May'-loks)	Aluminum (Ah-loo'-mi-num) and Magnesium (Mag-nee'-zee-um) Hydroxides
Macrodanton (Ma-kro-dan'-tin)	Nitrofurantoin (Ni-tro-fur-an'-toin)
Mandelamine (Man-del'-a-meen)	Methenamine (Meth-en'-a-meen) Mandelate (Man'-deh-late)
Medihaler-Iso (Med-i-hail-er-I'-so)	Isoproterenol (I-so-pro-ter'-en-ol)
Mellaril (Mel'-la-ril)	Thioridazine (Thi-o-rid'-a-zeen)
Metamucil (Met-a-mu'-sil)	Psyllium (Sil'-e-um)
Metaprel (Meh'-ta-prel)	Metaproterenol (Meh'-ta-pro-ter'-eh-nol)
Methotrexate (Meth-o-treks'-ate)	Amethopterin (Ah-meth-op'-ter-in)
Milk of Magnesia	Same
Minipress (Min'-i-press)	Prazosin (Pra'-zo-sin)
Minocin (Min'-o-sin)	Minocycline (Mi-no-si'-kleen)
Monistat (Mon'-i-stat)	Miconazole (Mi-kon'-ah-zole)
Motrin (Mo'-trin)	Ibuprofen (I-bu'-pro-fen)
Myambutol (My-am'-bu-tol)	Ethambutol (Eth-am'-bu-tol)
Mycostatin (My-co-stat'-in)	Nystatin (Ny-stat'-in)
Mylanta (My-lan'-ta)	Aluminum (Ah-loo'-mi-num) and Magnesium (Mag-nee'-zee-um) Hydroxides and Simethicone (Si-meth'-i-kone)
Myleran (My-ler-an)	Busulfan (Bu-sul'-fan)
Mylicon (My'-li-kon)	Simethicone (Si-meth'-i-kone)
Mysoline (My'-so-leen)	Primidone (Pri'-mi-done)
Nalfon (Nal'-fon)	Fenoprofen (Fen-o-pro'-fen)
Naprosyn (Na'-pro-sin)	Naproxen (Na-prok'-sen)
Nembutal (Nem'-bu-tal)	Pentobarbital (Pen-to-barb'-i-tal)
Neosynephrine (Nee-o-sin-eh'-frin)	Phenylephrine (Fen-il-eh'-frin)
Nitrobid (Ni'-tro-bid)	Nitroglycerin (Ni-tro-gli'-ser-in)
Nitrol (Ni'-trol)	" "
Nitrostat (Ni-tro-stat)	" "
Noctec (Nok'-tek)	Chloral Hydrate (Klor'-al- Hy'-drate)
Norfiex (Nor'-fleks)	Orphenadrine Citrate (Or-fen'-a-dreen)
Norpace (Nor'-pace)	Disopyramide (Di-so-peer'-a-mide)

Trade Name	Generic Name
Novahistine (No-va-his'-teen) Expectorant	Guaifenesin (Gwi-fen'-eh-sin), Phenylpropanolamine (Fen-il-pro-pan-ol'-a-meen), and Codeine (Ko'-deen)
NTG	Nitroclycerin (Ni-tro-gli'-ser-in)
Nupercainal (New-per-kain'-al)	Dibucaine (Die'-bu-kain)
Oretic (O-ret'-ik)	Hydrochiorothiazide (Hy-dro-kior-thi'-a-zide)
Orinase (Or'-in-ase)	Tolbutamide (Tol-bu'-tah-mide)
Ornade (Or'-nade)	Chlorpheniramine (Klor-fen-ir'-a-meen), Triprolidine (Tri-pro-li-deen) and Pseudoephedrine (Su-do-eh-fed'-rin)
Parafon Forte (Pair'-a-fon For'-tay)	Chlorzoxazone (Klor-zok'-sa-zone)
Percodan (Per'-ko-dan)	Oxycodone (Ok-si-ko'-done)
Periactin (Per-ee-ak'-tin)	Cyproheptadine (Si-pro-hep'-tah-deen)
Persantine (Per-san'-teen)	Dipyridamole (Di-pi-rid'-ah-mole)
Phenobarbital (Feen-o-barb'-it-al)	Same
Phenylpropanolamine (Fen-il-pro-pan-ol'-a-meen)	Same
Pitocin (Pi-tow'-sin)	Oxytocin (Ok-see-tow'-sin)
Pontocaine (Pon'-to-kain)	Tetracaine (Teh'-tra-kain)
Povan (Po'-van)	Pyrvinium (Pire-vin'-ee-um)
Premarin (Prem'-ar-in)	Conjugated (Kon'-joo-gay-ted) Estrogens (Es-tro-jens)
Presamine (Press'-a-meen)	Imipramine (Im-ip'-rah-meen)
Primaquine (Pri'-mah-kwin)	Same
Probanthine (Pro-ban'-theen)	Propantheline (Pro-pan'-the-leen)
Pronestyl (Pro-nes'-til)	Procainamide (Pro-kain'-a-mide)
Prophylthiouracil (Pro-pil-thi-o-u'-rah-sil)	Same
Prostaphlin (Pro-staff'-lin)	Oxacillin (Oks'-ah-sil-in)
Provera (Pro-ver'-ah)	Medroxyprogesterone (Med-rok-see-pro-jes'-ter-one)
Pyridium (Pie-rid'-ee-um)	Phenazopyridine (Fen-ahs-o-per'-i-deen)
Quinidine (Kwin'-i-deen)	Same
Quinine (Kwie'-nine)	Same
Reserpine (Ree-ser'-peen)	Same
Retin A (Reh'-tin A)	Tretinoin (Tret'-i-noin)
Rifadin (Rie-fad'-in)	Rifampin (Rie-fam'-pin)
Riopan (Rie'-o-pan)	Magaidrate (Mag'-al-drate)

Trade Name	Generic Name
Rimactane (Rim-act'-ane)	Rifampin (Rie-fam'-pin)
Ritalin (Rit'-a-lin)	Methylphenidate (Meth-il-fen'-i-date)
Robaxin (Ro-bak'-sin)	Methocarbamol (Meth-o-kar'-ba-mol)
Robitussin (Row-i-tus'-sin)	Guaifenesin (Gwie-fen'-eh-sin)
Robitussin DM	Guiafenesin and Dextromethorphan (Dek-tro-meh-or'-fan)
Sansert (San'-sert)	Methysergide (Meth-ee-ser'-jide)
Seconal (Sek'-o-nal)	Secobarbital (Sek-o-bar'-bi-tal)
Selsun (Sel'-sun)	Selenium (Se-leh'-nee-um)
Septra (Sep'-tra)	Sulfamethoxazole (Sul-fah-meth-oks'-a-zole) and Trimethroprim (Tri-meth'-o-prim)
Serax (See'-raks)	Oxazepam (Oks-az'-eh-pam)
Silvadene (Sil'-va-deen)	Silver Sulfadiazine (Sul-fa-die'-a-zeen)
Sinemet (Si'-ne-met)	Levodopa (Le-vo-do'-pa)
Sinequan (Sin'-a-kwan)	Doxepin (Dok'-seh-pin)
Sorbitrate (Sor'-bi-trate)	Isosorbide (I-so-sor'-bide)
Stelazine (Stel'-a-zeen)	Trifluoperazine(Tri-floo-o-per'-a-zeen)
Sudafed (Soo'-da-fed)	Pseudophedrine (Soo-do-eh-feh'-drin)
Sulamyd (Sul'-a-mid)	Sulfacetamide (Sul-fah-set'-a-mide)
Sulfamylon (Sul-fa-mie'-lon)	Mafenide (Maf'-eh-nide)
Sultrin (Sul'-trin)	Sulfathiazole (Sul-fah-thi'-ah-zole) Sulfacetamide (Sul-fah-set'-ah-mide) and Sulfabenzamide (Sul-fah-benz'-ah-mide)
Surfak (Sur'-fak)	Dioctyl (Di-ok'-til) Calcium (Kal'-see-um) Sulfosuccinate (Sul-fo-suk'-si-nate)
Synalar (Sine'-a-lar)	Fluocinolone (Floo-o-sin'-o-lone)
Synthroid (Sin'-throid)	Levothyroxine (Lee-vo-thi-rok'-sin)
Tace (Tace)	Chlorotrianisene (Klor-o-tri-an'-I-seen)
Tagamet (Tag'-a-met)	Cimetidine (Si-met'-i-deen)
Talwin (Tal'-win)	Pentazocine (Pen-taz'-o-seen)
Tandearil (Tan'-da-ril)	Oxyphenbutazone (Ok-see-fen-bute'-a-zone)
Tegretol (Teg'-reh-tol)	Carbamazepine (Kar-ba-maz'-eh-peen)
Tessalon (Tess'-a-lon)	Benzonatate (Benz-on'-a-tate)
Tetracycline (Tet-ra-si'-kleen)	
Thorazine (Thor'-a-zeen)	Chlorpromazine (Klor-pro'-ma-zeen)
Thyroid (Thy'-roid)	Same
Tigan (Tie'-gan)	Trimethobenzamide (Tri-meth-o-benz'-a-mide)
Timoptic (Tim-op'-tic)	Timilol (Tim'-o-lol)

Trade Name	Generic Name
Tinactin (Tin-act'-in)	Tolnaftate (Tol-naf'-tate)
Titralac (Ti'-tra-lak)	Calcium (Kal-see-um) Carbonate (Kar'-bon-ate) and Glycine (Gly'-seen)
Tofranil (Toe'-fra-nil)	Imipramine (I-mip'-rah-meen)
Tolectin (Tow-lek'-tin)	Tolmetin (Tol-met'-in)
Triavil (Tri'-a-vil)	Perphenazine (Per-fen'-a-zeen) and Amitriptlyline (Am-i-trip'-ti-leen)
Trilafon (Try'-la-fon)	Perphenazine (Per-fen-a-zeen)
Tylenol (Tie'-leh-nol)	Acetaminophen (As-et-am'-ino-fen)
Tylenol #3	Acetaminophen and Codeine (Ko'-deen)
Unipen (U'-ni-pen)	Nafcillin (Naf-sil-lin)
Urecholine (Ur-eh-ko'-leen)	Bethanecol (Beth-an'-eh-kol)
Valisone (Val'-i-sone)	Betamethasone (Beh-tah-meth'-a-sone)
Valium (Val'-ee-um)	Diazepam (Die-aze-eh-pam)
Vermox (Ver'-moks)	Mebendazole (Meh-ben'-dah-zole)
Vibramycin (Vie-bra-my'-sin)	Doxycycline (Doks-see-si'-kleen)
Xylocaine (Zie'-low-kain)	Lidocaine (Lie-do-kain)
Zarontin (Zar-on'-tin)	Ethosuximide (Eh-tho-suks'-a-mide)
Zyloprim (Zie'-low-prim)	Allopurinol (Al-lo-pure'-in-ol)

End of Lesson 4 Annex

LESSON ASSIGNMENT

LESSON 5

Review of Ocular and Auditory Anatomy and Physiology.

TEXT ASSIGNMENT

Paragraphs 5-1 through 5-13.

LESSON OBJECTIVES

After completing this lesson, you should be able to:

5-1. Given the name of a part of the bulbus oculi and a group of statements, select the statement that best describes that part or its function.

5-2. Given the name of one of the structures associated with the bulbus oculi (the adnexa) and a group of statements, select the statement which best describes that part or its function.

5-3. Given the name of a disease/condition that affects the eye and a group of statements, select the statement that best describes that disease/condition.

5-4. From a list of possible methods, select the method(s) by which sound may be transmitted.

5-5. Given the name of one of the parts of the human ear and a group of statements, select the statement which best describes that part of the ear or its function.

5-6. Given a disorder/malfunction of the ear and a group of statements, select the statement that best describes that disorder/ malfunction.

5-7. Given a group of statements, select the statement that best describes how the body maintains equilibrium (balance).

SUGGESTION

After studying the assignment, complete the exercises at the end of this lesson. These exercises will help you to achieve the lesson objectives.

LESSON 5

REVIEW OF OCULAR AND AUDITORY ANATOMY AND PHYSIOLOGY

Section I. OCCULAR ANATOMY AND PHYSIOLOGY

5-1. BACKGROUND

a. **Stimulus.** Rays of light stimulate the receptor tissues of the eyeballs (bulbus oculi) to produce the special sense of vision. This includes both the sensation of vision or seeing and a variety of reactions known as the light reflexes. The actual reception of the light energy is a chemical reaction that in turn stimulates the neuron endings.

b. **Sense Organ.** The eyeball (bulbus oculi) is the special sense organ that contains the receptor tissues. The bulbus oculi is suspended in the orbit. The orbit is a skeletal socket of the skull that helps protect the bulbus oculi. Various structures associated with the functioning of the bulbus oculi are called the adnexa. The adnexa include the eyelids, the lacrimal system, and so forth.

5-2. THE BULBUS OCULI (Figure 5-1)

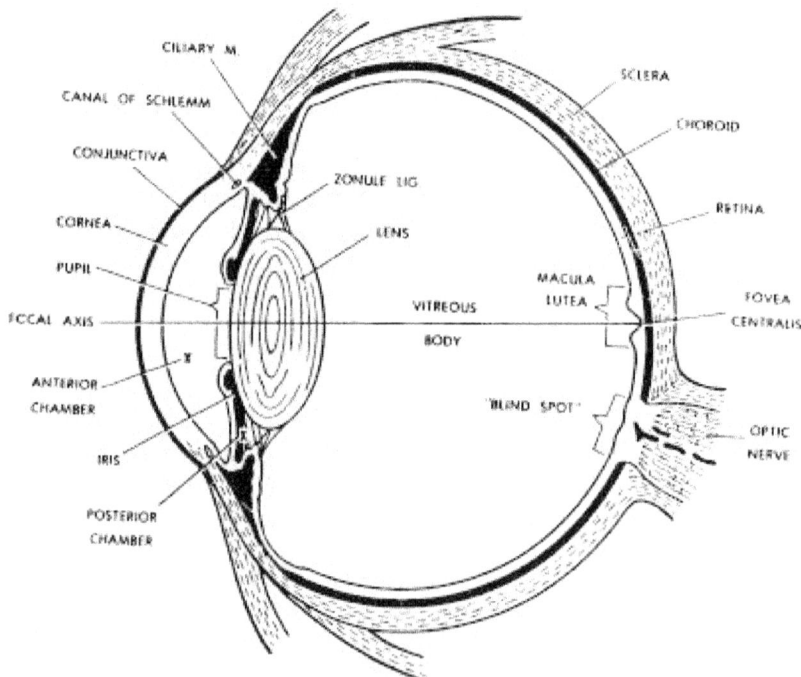

Figure 5-1. A focal-axis section of the bulbus oculi.

a. **Shape**. Normally the bulbus oculi is a spherical bulb-like structure. Its anterior surface, transparent and more curved, is known as the cornea of the bulbus oculi.

b. **Wall of the Bulbus Oculi**. The bulbus oculi is a hollow structure. Its wall is made up of three layers known as coats or tunics.

(1) Sclera. The outermost layer is white and very dense fibrous connective tissue (FCT). It is known as the sclera, scleral coat, or fibrous tunic. Its anterior portion is called the cornea. As already mentioned, the cornea is transparent and more curved than the rest of the sclera. The fixed curvature of the cornea enables it to serve as the major focusing device for the bulbus oculi.

(2) Choroid. The middle layer of the wall of the bulbus oculi is known as the choroid, the choroid coat, or the vascular tunic. This layer is richly supplied with blood vessels. It is also pigmented with a black material. The black color absorbs the light rays and prevents them from reflecting at random.

(3) Retina. The inner layer of the wall of the bulbus oculi is known as the retina, retinal coat, or internal tunic. The actual photoreceptor elements are located in the retina at the back and sides of the bulbus oculi. These elements are the rods and cones. They constitute the nervous portion of the retina. In the anterior part of the bulbus oculi, the retina continues as a non-nervous portion.

c. **Internal Structures of the Bulbus Oculi.**

(1) The nervous retina.

(a) The photoreceptors of the nervous portion of the retina (Figure 5-2) contain chemicals known as visual pigments (rhodopsin). The cones are more concentrated in the center at the back of the bulbus oculi. The cones can perceive colors and are used for acute vision. However, cones require more intense light than do rods. The rods are distributed more toward the sides of the nervous retina. Although the rods are capable of perceiving less intense light, rods perceive only black and white.

(b) If you look directly at an object, light from the object will fall in the small depression of the retina called the fovea centralis. The fovea centralis is at the posterior end of the bulbus oculi, exactly opposite the centers of the cornea, pupil, and lens. The fovea centralis is found in a small yellow area of the retina called the macula lutea. The macula lutea is the area of the retina where vision is the sharpest.

FOVEA	=	small depression
CENTRALIS	=	center
MACULA	=	spot
LUTEA	=	yellow

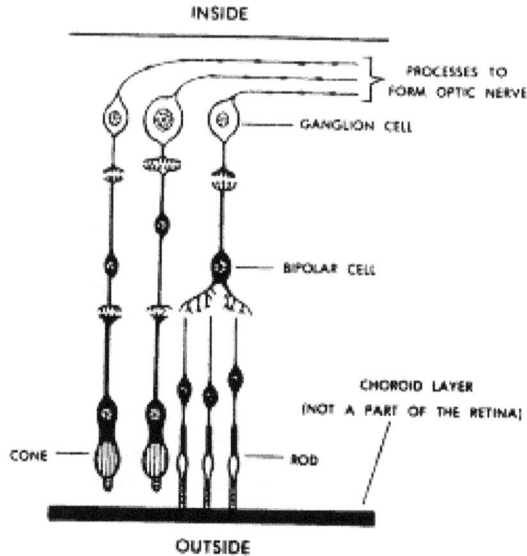

INSIDE

PROCESSES TO FORM OPTIC NERVE

GANGLION CELL

BIPOLAR CELL

CHOROID LAYER (NOT A PART OF THE RETINA)

CONE

ROD

OUTSIDE

Figure 5-2. Cellular detail of retina.

(c) Associated with the rods and cones are the beginnings of neurons of the optic nerve. These neurons pass out of the bulbus oculi at the posterior end (in a point medial and superior to the fovea centralis). At the point of exit, there are not rods or cones. Therefore, it is called the blind spot (optic papilla/optic disk).

(2) Ciliary body. The anterior end of the choroid layer thickens to form a circular "picture frame" around the lens of the bulbus oculi. This is also near the margin of the base of the cornea. The frame-like structure is called the ciliary body. It includes mostly radial muscle fibers, which form the ciliary muscle.

(3) Ligaments. The lens is suspended in place by ligaments. These ligaments connect the margin (equator) of the lens with the ciliary body.

(4) Crystalline lens. The crystalline lens is located in the center of the anterior of the bulbus oculi, just behind the cornea.

(a) The lens is biconvex. This means that it has two outwardly curved surfaces. The anterior surface is flatter (less curved) than the posterior surface.

(b) The lens is transparent and elastic. As one grows older, the lens becomes less and less elastic. The ligaments maintain a tension upon the lens. This tension keeps the lens flatter and allows the lens to focus on distant objects. When the ciliary muscle contracts, the tension on the lens is decreased. The decreased tension allows the lens to thicken. The greater thickness increases the anterior curvature and allows close objects to be seen clearly.

(c)   The process of focusing the crystalline lens for viewing close objects clearly is called accommodation. The process of accommodation is accompanied by a reduction in the pupil size as well as a convergence of the two central lines of sight (axes on bulbi oculi).

(5)   Iris. Another structure formed from the anterior portion of the choroid layer is the iris. The iris is located between the lens and the cornea.

(a)   The pupil is the hole in the middle of the iris. Radial and circular muscles in the iris control the size of the pupil. The radial muscles are dilators. The circular muscles are the constrictors. By changing the size of the pupil, the iris controls the amount of light entering the bulbus oculi.

(b)   The iris may have many different colors. Multiple genes determine the actual color.

(6)   Chambers. The space between the cornea and the lens is called the anterior cavity. The space between the cornea and the iris is referred to as the anterior chamber. The space between the iris and the lens is called the posterior chamber (see Figure 5-1). Both chambers of the anterior cavity are filled with a fluid called the aqueous humor. The aqueous humor is secreted into the chambers by the ciliary body. It drains into the encircling canal of Schlemm, located in the angle between the cornea and the iris. This angle is called the irioiocornealis angle.

(7)   Vitreous body. Behind the lens is a jelly-like material called the vitreous body. It fills the posterior cavity of the bulbus oculi.

5-3. THE ADNEXA

The adnexa are the various structures associated with the bulbus oculi.

a.   **Extrinsic Ocular Muscles**. Among the adnexa are the extrinsic ocular muscles that move the bulbus oculi within the orbit (the cavity in the upper facial skull that contains the bulbus oculi).

b.   **Eyelids.** Attached to the margins of the orbit, in front of the bulbus oculi, are the upper and lower eyelids. These have muscles for opening and closing the eyelids. The eyelashes (cilia) are special hairs of the eyelids that help protect these bulbus oculi. The margins of the eyelids have special oil to prevent the loss of fluids from the area. The inner lining of the eyelids is continuous with the conjunctiva, a membrane over the anterior surface of the bulbus oculi.

c.   **Lacrimal Apparatus**. The conjunctiva must be kept moist and clean at all times. To do this, a lacrimal apparatus is associated with the eyelids. In the upper outer corner of the orbit is a lacrimal gland, which secretes a lacrimal fluid (tears) into the junction between the upper eyelid and the conjunctiva. The motion of the bulbus oculi and the eyelids (blinking) moves this fluid moved across the surface of the conjunctiva to the medialinferior aspect. Here, the lacrimal fluid is collected and delivered into the nasal chamber by the nasal lacrimal duct.

d. **Eyebrow.** The eyebrow is a special group of hairs above the orbit. The eyebrow serves to keep rain and perspiration away from the bulbus oculi.

e. **Optic Nerve.** Neurons carry information from the photoreceptors of the nervous retina. They leave the bulbus oculi at the blind spot. At the optic nerve, or second cranial nerve, the neurons pass to the rear of the orbit. There, the optic nerve exits through the optic canal into the cranial cavity. Beneath the brain, the optic nerves from both sides join to form the optic chiasma, in which half of the neurons from each optic nerve cross to the opposite side. Rom the optic chiasma, the right and left optic tracts proceed to the brain proper.

5-4. DISEASES/CONDITIONS AFFECTING THE EYE

a. **Myopia ("Near-Sightedness").** In myopia the image from distant objects are focused in front of the retina. Myopia is caused by a lens that is too strong. Although the ciliary muscle is completely relaxed, the light rays entering the eye are not properly bent to be focused on the retina. This type of lens condition can be corrected by the use of a concave lens. Figure 5-3a illustrates this condition and correction with a concave lens.

b. **Hypermetropia (Hyperopia)("Far-Sightedness").** In hypermetropia, the parallel light rays entering the eye are not bent sufficiently by the lens and the image is focused behind the retina. In hypermetropia, the bulbus oculi is too short or the lens system is too weak when the ciliary muscle is relaxed. A convex lens is used to correct this condition. Figure 5-3b illustrates this condition and its correction with a convex lens.

c. **Astigmatism.** Astigmatism occurs when the light rays passing through an astigmatic lens are not all focused at the same point. A malformed lens or cornea causes astigmatism. A specially designed lens can be used to help correct this condition.

d. **Glaucoma.** Glaucoma is a common cause of blindness. In glaucoma, the intraocular pressure becomes too great and causes damage to the retina and optic nerve. The intraocular pressure of a normal person is approximately 15 to 20 mm Hg (millimeters of mercury), while the intraocular pressure of a person with glaucoma can reach from 80 to 90 mm Hg. As the intraocular pressure increases, damage is done to the delicate tissues of the eye. The retinal artery, which enters the bulbus oculi at the optic disk, becomes increasingly compressed. Hence, nutrition to the retina is reduced--damage to the retina and optic nerve follow. Glaucoma can be either of a sudden onset or of a slow onset. Glaucoma results from the high pressure caused by reduced drainage of a fluid (aqueous humor). Because of the decreased drainage and continued fluid output, the high pressure develops. A variety of medications can be used to treat glaucoma. Pilocarpine, acetazolamide (Diamox®) and timolol (Timoptic®) are just three examples of such medications. These medications will be presented in later lessons.

　　　e.　**Cataracts.** A cataract is an irreversible and progressive clouding of the lens leading to blindness. Cataracts are surgically removed.

　　　f.　**Conjunctivitis.** Conjunctivitis is an inflammation of the conjunctiva.

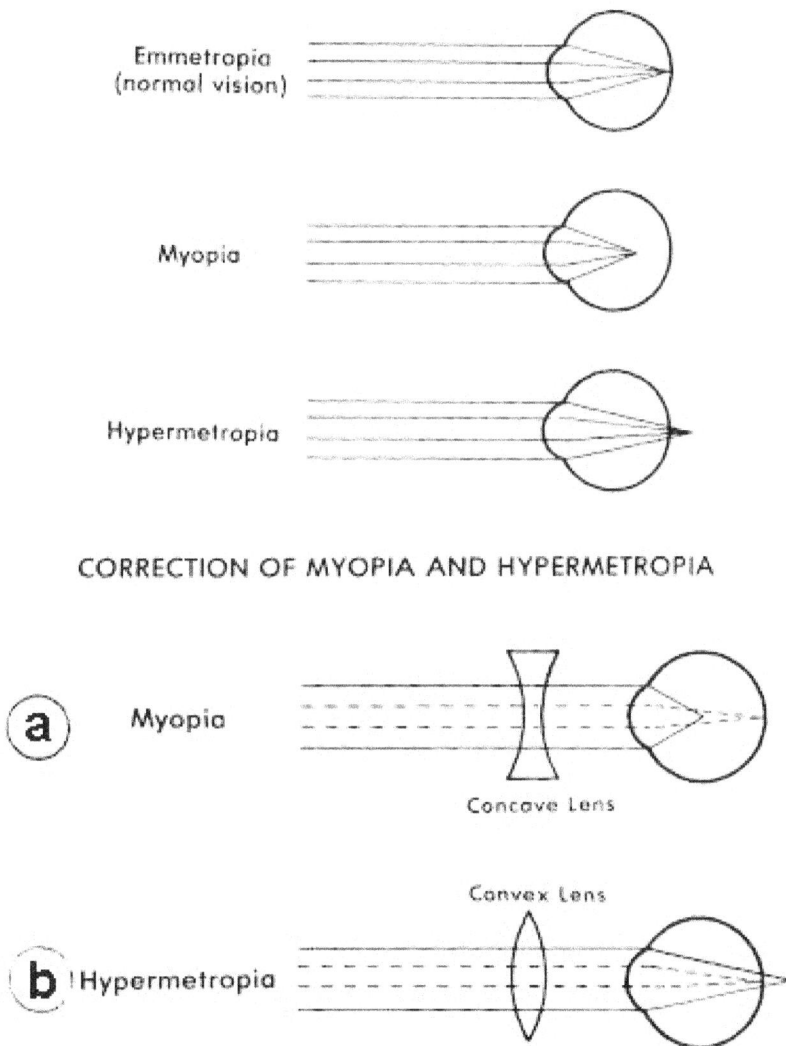

CORRECTION OF MYOPIA AND HYPERMETROPIA

Figure 5-3. Myopia and Hypermetropia contrasted with normal vision.

Section II. AUDITORY ANATOMY AND PHYSIOLOGY

5-5. BACKGROUND

The human ear serves two major special sensory functions: hearing (auditory) and equilibrium (balance). The stimulus for hearing is sound waves. The stimulus for equilibrium is gravity.

a. **Methods of Sound Transmission.** The sound stimulus is transmitted in a variety of ways. Regardless of the actual transmission method, the sound stimulus is unchanged. Sound may be transmitted by:

(1) Airborne waves, which have frequency (pitch) and amplitude (loudness or intensity).

(2) Mechanical oscillations (vibrations) of structures.

(3) Fluid-born pressure pulses.

(4) Electrical impulses along the neurons to and in the brain.

b. **Sections of the Human Ear (Figure 5-4).** The human ear has three major parts. Each part serves a specific function in the transmission and reception of the sound stimulus. The three parts are known as the external (outer) ear, the middle ear, and the internal (inner) ear.

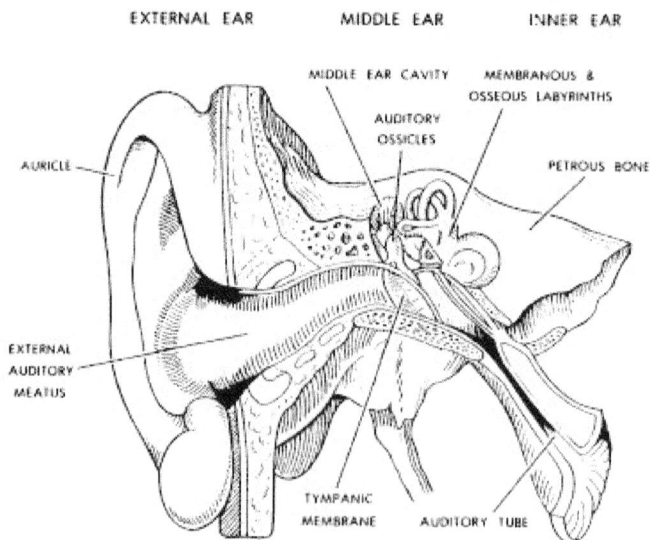

Figure 5-4. A frontal section of the human ear.

5-6. THE EXTERNAL EAR

The external ear begins on the outside of the head in the form of a funnel-shaped auricle (pinna). Actually serving as a funnel, the auricle directs airborne sound waves into the external auditory meatus. The external auditory meatus is a tubular canal extending into the temporal portion of the skull

5-7. THE MIDDLE EAR

a. **Tympanic Membrane.** At the inner end of the external auditory meatus is a tympanic membrane. The tympanic membrane (eardrum) is a circular membrane separating the external auditory meatus from the middle ear cavity. The tympanic membrane vibrates (mechanically oscillates) in response to airborne sound waves.

b. **Middle Ear Cavity.** On the medial side of the tympanic membrane is the middle ear cavity. The middle ear cavity is a space within the temporal bone.

c. **Auditory Ossicles.** The auditory ossicles (OSSICLE = small bone) are three very small bones which form a chain across the middle ear cavity. They join the tympanic membrane with the medial wall of the middle ear cavity. In order, the ossicles are named as follows: malleus, incus, and stapes. The malleus is attached to the tympanic membrane. A sound stimulus is transmitted from the tympanic membrane to the medial wall of the middle ear cavity by way of the ossicles. The ossicles vibrate (mechanically oscillate) in response to the sound stimulus.

d. **Auditory (Eustachian) Tube**. The auditory tube is a passage connecting the middle ear cavity with the nasopharynx. The auditory tube maintains equal air pressure on the two sides of the tympanic membrane.

e. **Association With Other Spaces**. The middle ear cavity is associated with other spaces in the skull. The thin roof of the middle ear cavity is the floor of part of the cranial cavity. The middle ear cavity is continuous posteriorly with the mastoid air cells via the antrum (an upper posterior recess of the middle ear cavity.

5-8. THE INTERNAL EAR

a. **Labyrinths (Figure 5-4).**

(1) <u>Bony labyrinth</u>. The bony labyrinth (LABYRINTH = a maze) is a complex cavity within the temporal bone. It has three semi-circular canals, a vestibule (hallway), and a snail-shaped cochlear portion.

(2) <u>Membranous labyrinth.</u> The membranous labyrinth is a hollow tubular structure suspended within the bony labyrinth.

b. **Fluids of the Internal Ear**. The endolymph is a fluid filling the space within the membranous labyrinth. The perilymph is a fluid filling the space between the membranous labyrinth and the bony labyrinth.

ENDO = within

PERI = around

These fluids are continuously formed and drained away.

c. **The Cochlea**. The cochlea is a spiral structure associated with hearing. It has 2 1/2 turns. The snail- shaped portion of the bony labyrinth forms its outer boundaries.

(1) The central column or axis of the cochlea is called the modiolus. Extending from this central column is a spiral shelf of bone called the spiral lamina. A fibrous membrane called the basilar membrane (or basilar lamina) connects the spiral lamina with the outer bony wall of the cochlea. The basilar membrane forms the floor of the cochlear duct, the spiral portion of the mebranous labyrinth. Within the cochlear duct, there is a structure on the basilar membrane called the organ of Corti. The organ of Corti has hairs that are the sensory receptors for the special sense of hearing.

LAMINA = thin plate

(2) Within the bony cochlea, the space above the cochlear duct is known as the scala vestibuli and the space below is known as the scala tympani. Since the scala are joined at their apex, they form a continuous channel and the connection between them is called the helicotrema.

d. **Transmission.**

(1) The sound stimulus is transferred from the stapes to the perilymph of the scala vestibuli. Here the stimulus is transmitted as a pressure pulse in the fluid.

(2) In response, the basilar membrane of the cochlea vibrates (mechanically oscillates). Only selected portions of the basilar membrane vibrate at any one time, depending on the frequency of the sound stimulus.

(3) The hair cells of the organ of Corti at that particular location are mechanically stimulated. This stimulation is transferred to the neurons of the acoustic nerve. The acoustic nerve passes out of the modiolus into the cranial cavity and goes to the brain.

5-9. DISORDERS OR MALFUNCTIONS OF THE EAR

a. **Deafness.** Deafness can be divided into two types. One type is caused by the inability of the middle ear mechanisms to transmit sounds into the cochlea. This is sometimes called conduction deafness. Another type, usually referred to as nerve deafness, is caused by the impairment of the auditory nerve or cochlea. As one might expect, if either the cochlea or auditory nerve is destroyed, the patient is permanently deaf. However, if the cochlea and auditory nerve are still capable of functioning and only the ossicular system has been destroyed, the patient can still hear because sound waves can be conducted into the cochlea by bone conduction.

b. **Tinnitus.** Tinnitus is ringing in the ears or the sensation of noise in the ears or head. Persons who take large doses of certain drugs (like aspirin) complain of tinnitus.

c. **Meniere's Syndrome**. Meniere's Syndrome is a disorder characterized by intermittent attacks of vertigo (dizziness), nausea, vomiting, and profuse sweating. It is a disorder of the membranous labyrinth of the inner ear.

d. **Swimmer's Ear.** Swimmer's ear is a fungal infection of the outer ear.

e. **Otitis Media**. Otitis media is the inflammation of the middle ear or eardrum.

f. **Otitis Externa**. Otitis externa is the inflammation of the outer ear.

Section III. ANATOMY AND PHYSIOLOGY OF EQUILIBRIUM (BALANCE)

5-10. BACKGROUND

a. **Posture**. Posture is the specific alignment of the body parts at any given time. Humans can assume an infinite variety of postures. However, the truly erect posture is unique to humans.

b. **Equilibrium**. Equilibrium is the state of balance of the body. An erect standing human has a highly unstable equilibrium. Therefore, the human can easily fall. Through a variety of sensory inputs (visual, and so forth) and postural reflexes, the body is maintained in its erect posture.

c. **Stimulus-Gravitational Forces.** A primary sensory input for equilibrium consists of gravitational forces. This input is received by the membranous labyrinth within the internal ear. The gravitational forces are of two types: static, when the body is standing still, and kinetic, when the body is moving in either linear (straight) or angular directions.

d. **Membranous Labyrinth**. The specific portions of the membranous labyrinth involved are the two sac-like structures--the sacculus and the utriculus. Each of these two structures has an area of special hair cells called the macula. In addition, there are three semi-circular ducts located within the osseous semi-circular canals of the temporal bone of the skull. Each semi-circular duct has a crista, a little ridge of hair cells across the axis of the duct.

e. **"Body Sense."** All of the various sensory inputs related to the maintenance of equilibrium and posture are integrated within the brain as "body sense." Correct information is sent to the muscles of the body by means of specific postural reflexes in order to maintain the proper posture.

5-11. SACCULUS AND UTRICULUS

a. The sacculus and the utriculus are two sac-like portions of the membranous labyrinth. They are filled with endolymph.

b. On the wall of each sac is a collection of special hair cells known as the macula, which serves as a receptor organ for static and linear kinetic gravitational forces. The saccular macula and the utricular macula are oriented at more or less right angles to each other. For the pair of maculae in the membranous labyrinth of the right side, there is a corresponding pair in the labyrinth of the left side. Information from all of these maculae is sent into the brain for continuous sensing of the position of the head in space.

5-12. SEMICIRCULAR DUCTS

Extending from and opening into the utriculus are three hollow structures called the semicircular ducts. Since the utriculus completes the circle for each duct, the ducts act as if they were complete (Figure 5-5).

a. **Orientation**. Two of the ducts are vertically oriented (one anterior and one posterior). The third duct is essentially horizontal. The three ducts are all oriented at right angles to each other. In addition, the three ducts of one membranous labyrinth are matched or paired by the three ducts of the opposite membranous labyrinth.

b. **Ampullae and Cristae**. Each semi-circular duct ends with an enlargement where it opens into the utriculus. This enlargement or swelling is called an ampulla. The crista is at a right angle to the axis of the duct. Movement of the endolymph within the duct--caused by movement of the head in space--deforms (bends) the hairs of the crista in specific directions. These are responses to linear and/or angular kinetic gravitational forces.

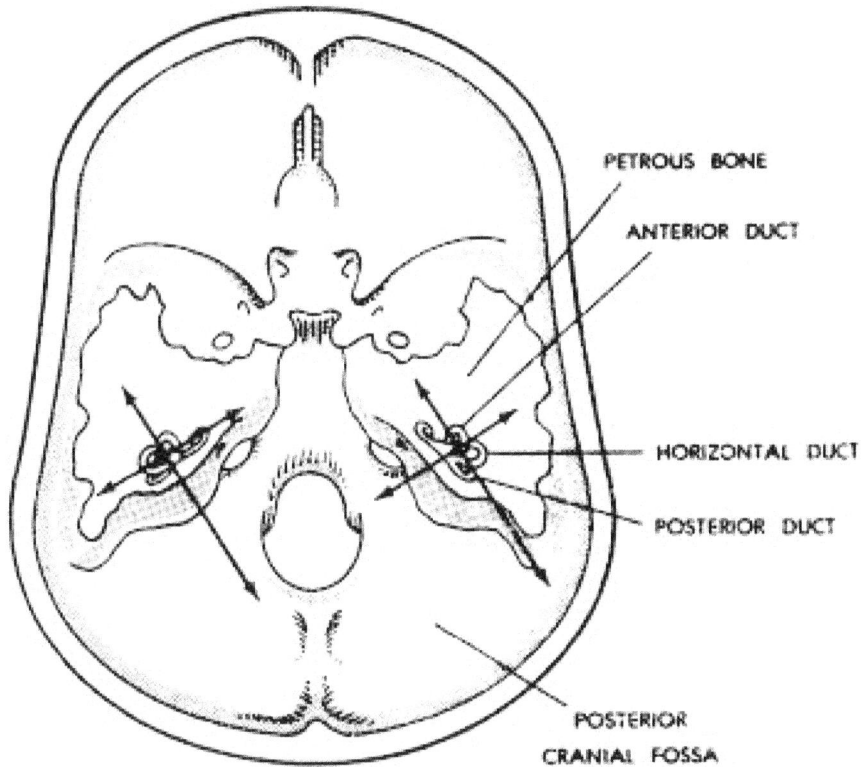

Figure 5-5. Diagram of semicircular duct orientation.

5-13. THE VESTIBULAR NERVE

The vestibular nerve carries all this information from the maculae and cristae to the brain. The vestibular nerve is part of the auditory nerve. The auditory nerve (acoustic nerve) is a combination of the vestibular nerve (balance) and the otic nerve (hearing).

Continue with Exercises

EXERCISES, LESSON 5

INSTRUCTIONS: Answer the following exercises by marking the lettered response which best answers the question.

After you have completed all the exercises, turn to "Solutions to Exercises" at the end of the lesson and check your answers. For each exercise answered incorrectly, reread the material referenced with the solution.

1. The sclera is best described as:

   a. The inner layer of the wall of the bulbus oculi where the rods and cones of the eye are located.

   b. The white and very dense fibrous connective tissue that is the outermost layer of the bulbus oculi.

   c. The middle layer of the wall of the bulbus oculi.

   d. The transparent layer that forms the outermost portion of the bulbus oculi.

2. The retina is:

   a. The middle layer of the bulbus oculi that is pigmented black to absorb light rays so they will not be reflected at random within the eye.

   b. The transparent portion of the bulbus oculi that serves as the major focusing device for the eye.

   c. The inner layer of the wall of the bulbus oculi where the photo-receptor elements of the eye are located.

   d. The non-nervous portion of the inner layer of the bulbus oculi.

3. The cones of the bulbus oculi function to:

   a. Perceive black and white.

   b. Perceive colors.

   c. Prevent random reflection of light rays within the eye.

   d. Provide vision in conditions of little or no light.

4. What is the blind spot?

    a. The blind spot is a place in the cornea where there are no cones.

    b. The blind spot is a place in the retina where the optic nerve enters the bulbus oculi.

    c. The blind spot is an area located in the center of the anterior of the bulbus oculi.

    d. The blind spot is the origin of the optic nerve where there are no rods or cones.

5. The vitreous body is best described as:

    a. The space between the cornea and the lens.

    b. The jelly-like material that fills the posterior cavity of the bulbus oculi.

    c. The group of muscles responsible for controlling the size of the pupil.

    d. The colored portion of the anterior part of the choroid layer that is between the lens and the cornea.

6. The function of the lacrimal apparatus of the eye is to:

    a. Produce oil to prevent the loss of fluids from the bulbus oculi.

    b. Keep rain and perspiration away from the bulbus oculi.

    c. Open and close the eyelids.

    d. Keep the eye clean and moist at all times.

7. Myopia is best defined as:

    a. A condition in which the image from a distant object is focused in front of the retina.

    b. A condition in which the light rays entering the eye are focused behind the retina.

    c. A condition characterized by increased intraocular pressure which can result in blindness.

    d. A condition characterized by an irreversible and progressive clouding of the lens.

8. What is the function of the auditory (Eustachian) tube?

    a. This tube transmits from the tympanic membrane to the middle ear cavity.

    b. This tube carries sound waves from the external ear to the auditory ossicles.

    c. This tube maintains equal air pressure on the two sides of the tympanic membrane.

    d. This tube carries the sound waves from the external ear to the tympanic membrane.

9. The cochlea of the internal ear is best described as:

    a. A complex cavity within the temporal bone.

    b. A spiral structure associated with hearing.

    c. A hollow tubular structure suspended within the bony labyrinth.

    d. A structure containing fluid which is located between the membranous labyrinth and the bony labyrinth.

10. Meniere's Syndrome is best described as:

   a. An inflammation of the outer ear.

   b. An acute fungal infection of the outer ear.

   c. A disorder characterized by intermittent attacks of dizziness, nausea, vomiting, and profuse sweating.

   d. An inflammation of the middle ear or eardrum.

11. Conduction deafness is best described as:

   a. The type of deafness caused by the inability of the middle ear mechanisms to transmit sounds into the cochlea.

   b. The type of deafness caused by the impairment of the auditory nerve or cochlea.

   c. The type of deafness caused by the ossification of the tympanic membrane.

12. Which of the following statements best describes how the body maintains equilibrium?

   a. Information from the membranous labyrinth is sent to the brain.

   b. The semicircular ducts input energy to the brain.

   c. Movement of the endolymph within the semicircular duct provides all the equilibrium information to the brain.

   d. The brain receives sensory inputs from many sources and integrates this knowledge as "body sense."

Check Your Answers on Next Page

SOLUTIONS TO EXERCISES, LESSON 5

1. b   The white and very dense fibrous connective tissue which is the outermost layer of the bulbus oculi. (para 5-2b(1))

2. c   The inner layer of the wall of the bulbus oculi where the photoreceptor elements of the eye are located. (para 5-2b)(3))

3. b   Perceive colors. (para 5-2c(1)(a))

4. d   The blind spot is the origin of the optic nerve where there are no rods or cones. (para 5-2c(1)(c))

5. b   The jelly-like material which fills the posterior cavity of the bulbus oculi. (para 5-2c(7))

6. d   Keep the eye clean and moist at all times. (para 5-3c)

7. a   A condition in which the image from a distant object is focused in front of the retina. (para 5-4a)

8. c   This tube maintains equal air pressure on the two sides of the tympanic membrane. (para 5-7d)

9. b   A spiral structure associated with hearing. (para 5-8c)

10. c   A disorder characterized by intermittent attacks of dizziness, nausea, vomiting, and profuse sweating. (para 5-9c)

11. a   The type of deafness caused by the inability of the middle ear mechanisms to transmit sounds into the cochlea. (para 5-9a)

12. d   The brain receives sensory inputs from many sources and integrates this knowledge into "body sense." (para 5-10e)

End of Lesson 5

ANNEX

DRUG PRONUNCIATION GUIDE

This Drug Pronunciation Guide was developed to help you to learn how the trade and generic names of commonly prescribed medications are frequently pronounced. Not all the drugs in the guide are discussed in this subcourse. Remember, it is not enough to be able to know the uses, indications, cautions and warnings, and contraindications for a drug--you must also know how to pronounce that drug's name.

Trade Name	*Generic Name*
Actifed (Ak'-ti-fed)	Triprolidine (Tri-pro'-li-deen) and Pseudoephedrine (Soo-do-e-fed'-rin)
Adapin (Ad'-a-pin)	Doxepin (Dok'-se-pin)
Sinequan (Sin'-a-kwan)	" "
Afrin (Af'-rin)	Oxymetazoline (Ok-see-met-az'-o-leen)
Aldactazide (Al-dak'-ta-zide)	Spironolactone (Spi-ro-no-lak'-tone) and Hydrochlorothiazide (Hy-dro-klor-thi'-a-zide)
Aldactone (Al-dak'-tone)	Spironolactone (Spi-ro-no-lak'-tone)
Aldomet (Al'-do-met)	Methyldopa (Meth-il-do'-pah)
Alupent (Al'-u-pent)	Metaproterenol (Met-a-pro-ter'-eh-nol)
Amoxil (Am-ok'-sil)	Amoxicillin (Ah-moks'-i-sil-in)
Amphojel (Am'-fo-jel)	Aluminum (Al-loo'-mi-num) Hydroxide (Hy-drok'-side)
Ampicillin (Amp'-I-sil-in)	Same
Antepar (Ab'-te-par)	Piperazine (Pi-per'-ah-zeen)
Anturane (An'-tu-rain)	Sulfinpyrazone (Sul-fin-pie'-ra-zone)
Anusol (An'-u-sol)	Pramoxine (Pram-ok'-seen)
Apresoline (A-press'-o-leen)	Hydralazine (Hy-dral'-ah-zeen)
Aralen (Ar'-a-len)	Chloroquine (Klor'-o-kwin)
Aristocort (A-ris'-to-cort)	Triamcinolone (Tri-am-sin'-o-lone)
Artane (Ar'-tane)	Trihexyphenidyl(Tri-hek-see-fen'-i-dil)
A.S.A.	Aspirin (As'-per-in)
Atromid S (A'-tro-mid)	Clofibrate (Klo-fi'-brate)
Avlosulfon (Av-lo-sul'-fon)	Dapsone (Dap'-sone)
Azolid (Az'-o-lid)	Phenylbutazone (Fen-il-bute'-a-zone)
Bactrim (Bak'-trim)	Sulfamethoxazole (Sul-fah-meth-oks'-ah-zole) and Trimethoprim (Tri-meth'-o-prim)
Bellergal (Bel'-er-gal)	Ergotamine (Er-got'-a-meen), Phenobarbital (Feen-o-bar'-bi-tal) and Belladonna (Bel-la-don'-na) Alkaloids
Benadryl (Ben'-a-dril)	Diphenhydramine (Di-fen-hy'-dra-meen)

Trade Name	Generic Name
Bendectin (Ben-dek'-tin)	Doxylamine (Dok-sil'-a-meen)
Benemid (Ben'-eh-mid)	Probenecid (Pro-ben'-eh-sid)
Bonine (Bo'-neen)	Meclizine (Mek'-li-zeen)
Cafergot (Kaf'-er-got)	Ergotamine (Er-got'-a-meen) and Caffeine (Kaf'-feen)
Calamine (Kal'-a-mine)	Same
Catapres (Kat'-a-press)	Clonidine (Klo'-ni-deen)
CeeNu (See'-new)	Lomustine (Lo-mus'-teen)
Chlor-Trimeton (Klo-tri '-meh-ton)	Chlorpheniramine (Klor-fen-it'-a-meen)
Clomid (Klo'-mid)	Clomiphene (Klo'-mi-feen)
Clonopin (Klo-o-pin)	Clonazepam (Klo-na'-ze-pam)
Codeine (Ko'-deen)	Same
Cogentin (Ko-jen'-tin)	Benztropine (Benz'-tro-peen)
Colace (Ko'-lace)	Dioctyl(Di-ok'-til) Sodium (So'-dee-um) Sulfosuccinate (Sul-fo-suk'-si-nate)
Colchicine (Kol'-chi-seen)	Same
Compazine (Kom'-pa-zeen)	Prochiorperazine (Pro-klor-per'-a-zeen)
Cordran (Kor'-dran)	Flurandrenolide (Floor-an-dren'-o-lide)
Coumadin (Koo'-mah-din)	Warfarin (War'-fah-rin)
CP	Cloroquine (Klor'-o-kwin) and Primaquine (Prim'-a-kwin)
Cyclogyl (Si'-klo-jel)	Cyclopentolate (Si-klo-pen'-to-late)
Cytomel (Si'-to-mel)	Liothyronine (Li-o-thy-ro-neen)
Cytoxan (Si-tok'-san)	Cyclophosphamide (Si-klo-fos'-fa-mide)
Dalmane (Dal '-mane)	Flurazepam (Floor-az'-e-pam)
Darvocet (Dar'-vo-set)	Propoxyphene (Pro-pok'-se-feen) and Acetaminopen (As-et-am'-ino-fen)
Darvon (Dar'-von)	Propoxyphene (Pro-pok-se-feen)
Decadron (Dek'-a-dron)	Dexamethasone (Dek-sa-meth'-ah-sone)
Deltasone (Del '-ta-sone)	Prednisone (Pred'-ni-sone)
Demerol (Dem'-er-ol)	Meperidine (Meh-pair'-i-deen)
Dexedrine (Deks '-eh-dreen)	Dextroamphetamine (Deks-tro-am-fet'-a-meen)
Diabinese (Di-ab'-i-nees)	Chlorpropamide (Klor-prop'-a-mide)
Diethylstilbestrol (Di-eth-il-stil-bes'-trol)	Same
Dilantin (Di-lan'-tin)	Phenytoin (Fen'-i-toin)
Dilaudid (Di-law'-did)	Hydromorphone (Hy-dro-more' -fon)
Dimetane (Di'-meh-tane)	Brompheniramine (Brom-fen-ir'-a-meen)

Trade Name	Generic Name
Dimetapp (Di'-meh-tap)	Brompheniramine (Brom-fen-ir'-a-meen) Phenylephrine (Fen-il-ef'-rin) and Phenylpropanolamine (Fen-il-pro-pan-ol'-a-meen)
Disophrol (Dice'-o-frol)	Dexbrompheniramine (Deks-brom-fen-ir'-a-meen) and Pseudoephedrine (Soo-do-e-fed'-rin)
Dolophine (Dol'-o-feen)	Methadone (Meth'-a-done)
Domeboro (Dome-bor'-o)	Aluminum (Ah-loo'-mi-num) Acetate (As'-e-tate)
Donnatal (Don'-na-tal)	Belladonna (Bel-la-don'-na) Alkaloids (Al'-ka-loids) and Phenobarbital (Feen-o-barb'-i-tal)
Doxidan (Dok'-si-dan)	Danthron (Dan'-thron) and Dicctyl (Di-ok'-til) Calcium (Kal'-see-um) Sulfosuccinate (Sul-fo-suk'-si-nate)
Drixoral (Driks'-or-al)	Dexbrompheniramine (Deks-brom-fen-ir'-a-meen) and Pseudoephedrine (Soo-do-e-fed'-rin)
Dulcolax (Dul'-ko-laks)	Bisacodyl (Bis-a'-ko-dil)
Dyazine (Di'-a-zide)	Triamterene (Tri-am'-ter-een) and Hydrochlorothiazide (Hy-dro-klor-o-thi'-a-zide)
Dymelor (Die'-meh-lor)	Acetohexamide (As-e-to-heks'-a-mide)
Dyrenium (Die-ren'-i-um)	Triamterene (Tri-am'-ter-een)
Efudex (Ef'-u-deks)	Fluorouracil (Floo-ro-ur'-ah-sil)
Elavil (El'-ah-vil)	Amitriptyline (Am-i-trip'-til-een)
Elixir Terpin (Ter'-pin) Hydrate	Same
Empirin (Em'-per-in)	Codeine (Ko'-deen) and Aspirin (As'-per-in)
E-Mycin (E-mie'-sin)	Erythromycin (E-rith-ro-mie'-sin)
Equanil (Ek'-wa-nil)	Meprobamate (Me-pro-bam'-ate)
Ergomar (Er'-go-mar)	Ergotamine (Er-got'-a-meen)
Ergotrate (Er'-go-trate)	Ergonovine (Er-go-no'-veen)
Erythrocin (Er-eeth'-ro-sin)	Erythromycin (Er-eeth-ro-my'-sin) Stearate (Stare'-rate)
Esidrix (Es'-i-driks)	Hyrochlorothiazide (Hy-dro-klor-o-thi'-a-zide)
Feosol (Fe'-o-sol)	Ferrous (Fer'-rus) Sulfate (Sul'-fate)
Fergon (Fer'-gon)	Ferrous (Fer'-rus) Gluconate (Glu'-con-ate)

Trade Name	Generic Name
Fiorinal (Fee-or'-i-nal)	Butalbi tal (Bu-tal'-bi-tal), Apririn, Phenacetin (Fen-ass'-eh-tin), and Caffeine (Kaf'-feen)
Flagyl (Fla'-jil)	Metronidazole (Me-tro-ni'-dah-zole)
Flexeril (Flek'-sa-ril)	Cyclobenzaprine (Si-klo-benz'-a-preen)
Fulvicin (Ful'-vi-sin)	Griseofulvin (Griz-e-o-ful'-vin)
Guantanol (Gan'-ta-nol)	Suiphamethoxazole (Sul-fah-meth-oks'-ah-zole)
Gantrisin (Gan'-tri-sin)	Sulfisoxazole (Sul-fi-sok'-sah-zole)
Gelusil (Jel'-u-sil)	Aluminum (Ah-loo'-mi-num) Hydroxide (Hy-drok'-side) and Magnesium (Mag-nee'-zee-um) Hydroxide
Grifulvin (Gri-ful'-vin)	Griseofulvin (Griz-e-o-ful'-vin)
Gynergen (Jin'-er-jen)	Ergotamine (Er-got'-a-meen)
Haldol (Hal'-dol)	Haloperidol (Hal-o-pair'-i-dol)
Halotestin (Hal-o-tes'-tin)	Fluoxymesterone (Floo-ok-see-mes-teh-rone)
Hexadrol (Hek'-sa-drol)	Dexamethasone (Dek-sa-meth'-a-sone)
Hydrodiuril (Hy-dro-di'-ur-il)	Hydroclorothiazide (Hy-dro-kior-thi'-a-zide)
Hygroton (Hy-grow'-ton)	Chiorthalidone (Kior-thal'-i-done)
Ilosone (I'-low-sone)	Erythromycin (Er-ith-ro-mi'-sin) Estolate (Es'-to-late)
Inderal (In'-der-al)	Propranolol (Pro-pran'-o-lol)
Indocin (In'-do-sin)	Indomethacin (In-do-meth'-a-sin)
INH	Isoniazid (I-so-ni'-a-zid)
Insulin (In'-sul-in)	Same
Intal	Cromolyn (Kro'-mo-lin)
Ismelin (Is'-meh-lin)	Guanethidine (Gwan-eth'-i-dine)
Isopto-Atropine (I-sop-to-at'-ro-peen)	Atropine (At'-ro-peen)
Isopto-Carpine (I-sop-to-car'-peen)	Pilocarpine (Pile-o-car'-peen)
Isordil (I'-sor-dil)	Isosorbide (I-so-sor'-bide)
Keflex (Kef'-lex)	Cephalexin (Sef-ah-lek'-sin)
Lanoxin (Lan-ok'-sin)	Digoxin (Di-jok'-sin)
Larodopa (Lar-o-do'-pa)	Levodopa (Le-o-do'-pa)
Larotid (Lar'-o-tid)	Amoxicillin (Ah-moks'-i-sil-in)
Lasix (La'-siks)	Furosemide (Fu-ro'-se-mide)
Leukeran (Lu'-ker-an)	Chlorambucil (Klor-ram'-bu-sil)
Librium (Lib'-ree-um)	Chlordiazepoxide (Klor-die-az-eh-pok'-side)

Trade Name	Generic Name
Lidex (Lie'-deks)	Fluocinoide (Floo-o-sin'-o-nide)
Lomotil (Lo'-mo-til)	Diphenoxylate (Die-fen-ok'-si-late)
Lopressor (Lo'-pres-sor)	Metoprolol (Met-o-pro'-lol)
Lotrimin (Lo'-tri-min)	Chlotrimazole (Klo-trim'-ah-zole)
Maalox (May'-loks)	Aluminum (Ah-loo'-mi-num) and Magnesium (Mag-nee'-zee-um) Hydroxides
Macrodanton (Ma-kro-dan'-tin)	Nitrofurantoin (Ni-tro-fur-an'-toin)
Mandelamine (Man-del'-a-meen)	Methenamine (Meth-en'-a-meen) Mandelate (Man'-deh-late)
Medihaler-Iso (Med-i-hail-er-I'-so)	Isoproterenol (I-so-pro-ter'-en-ol)
Mellaril (Mel'-la-ril)	Thioridazine (Thi-o-rid'-a-zeen)
Metamucil (Met-a-mu'-sil)	Psyllium (Sil'-e-um)
Metaprel (Meh'-ta-prel)	Metaproterenol (Meh'-ta-pro-ter'-eh-nol)
Methotrexate (Meth-o-treks'-ate)	Amethopterin (Ah-meth-op'-ter-in)
Milk of Magnesia	Same
Minipress (Min'-i-press)	Prazosin (Pra'-zo-sin)
Minocin (Min'-o-sin)	Minocycline (Mi-no-si'-kleen)
Monistat (Mon'-i-stat)	Miconazole (Mi-kon'-ah-zole)
Motrin (Mo'-trin)	Ibuprofen (I-bu'-pro-fen)
Myambutol (My-am'-bu-tol)	Ethambutol (Eth-am'-bu-tol)
Mycostatin (My-co-stat'-in)	Nystatin (Ny-stat'-in)
Mylanta (My-lan'-ta)	Aluminum (Ah-loo'-mi-num) and Magnesium (Mag-nee'-zee-um) Hydroxides and Simethicone (Si-meth'-i-kone)
Myleran (My-ler-an)	Busulfan (Bu-sul'-fan)
Mylicon (My'-li-kon)	Simethicone (Si-meth'-i-kone)
Mysoline (My'-so-leen)	Primidone (Pri'-mi-done)
Nalfon (Nal'-fon)	Fenoprofen (Fen-o-pro'-fen)
Naprosyn (Na'-pro-sin)	Naproxen (Na-prok'-sen)
Nembutal (Nem'-bu-tal)	Pentobarbital (Pen-to-barb'-i-tal)
Neosynephrine (Nee-o-sin-eh'-frin)	Phenylephrine (Fen-il-eh'-frin)
Nitrobid (Ni'-tro-bid)	Nitroglycerin (Ni-tro-gli'-ser-in)
Nitrol (Ni'-trol)	" "
Nitrostat (Ni-tro-stat)	" "
Noctec (Nok'-tek)	Chloral Hydrate (Klor'-al- Hy'-drate)
Norfiex (Nor'-fleks)	Orphenadrine Citrate (Or-fen'-a-dreen)
Norpace (Nor'-pace)	Disopyramide (Di-so-peer'-a-mide)

Trade Name	Generic Name
Novahistine (No-va-his'-teen) Expectorant	Guaifenesin (Gwi-fen'-eh-sin), Phenylpropanolamine (Fen-il-pro-pan-ol'-a-meen), and Codeine (Ko'-deen)
NTG	Nitroclycerin (Ni-tro-gli'-ser-in)
Nupercainal (New-per-kain'-al)	Dibucaine (Die'-bu-kain)
Oretic (O-ret'-ik)	Hydrochiorothiazide (Hy-dro-kior-thi'-a-zide)
Orinase (Or'-in-ase)	Tolbutamide (Tol-bu'-tah-mide)
Ornade (Or'-nade)	Chlorpheniramine (Klor-fen-ir'-a-meen), Triprolidine (Tri-pro-li-deen) and Pseudoephedrine (Su-do-eh-fed'-rin)
Parafon Forte (Pair'-a-fon For'-tay)	Chlorzoxazone (Klor-zok'-sa-zone)
Percodan (Per'-ko-dan)	Oxycodone (Ok-si-ko'-done)
Periactin (Per-ee-ak'-tin)	Cyproheptadine (Si-pro-hep'-tah-deen)
Persantine (Per-san'-teen)	Dipyridamole (Di-pi-rid'-ah-mole)
Phenobarbital (Feen-o-barb'-it-al)	Same
Phenylpropanolamine (Fen-il-pro-pan-ol'-a-meen)	Same
Pitocin (Pi-tow'-sin)	Oxytocin (Ok-see-tow'-sin)
Pontocaine (Pon'-to-kain)	Tetracaine (Teh'-tra-kain)
Povan (Po'-van)	Pyrvinium (Pire-vin'-ee-um)
Premarin (Prem'-ar-in)	Conjugated (Kon'-joo-gay-ted) Estrogens (Es-tro-jens)
Presamine (Press'-a-meen)	Imipramine (Im-ip'-rah-meen)
Primaquine (Pri'-mah-kwin)	Same
Probanthine (Pro-ban'-theen)	Propantheline (Pro-pan'-the-leen)
Pronestyl (Pro-nes'-til)	Procainamide (Pro-kain'-a-mide)
Prophylthiouracil (Pro-pil-thi-o-u'-rah-sil)	Same
Prostaphlin (Pro-staff'-lin)	Oxacillin (Oks'-ah-sil-in)
Provera (Pro-ver'-ah)	Medroxyprogesterone (Med-rok-see-pro-jes'-ter-one)
Pyridium (Pie-rid'-ee-um)	Phenazopyridine (Fen-ahs-o-per'-i-deen)
Quinidine (Kwin'-i-deen)	Same
Quinine (Kwie'-nine)	Same
Reserpine (Ree-ser'-peen)	Same
Retin A (Reh'-tin A)	Tretinoin (Tret'-i-noin)
Rifadin (Rie-fad'-in)	Rifampin (Rie-fam'-pin)
Riopan (Rie'-o-pan)	Magaidrate (Mag'-al-drate)

Trade Name	Generic Name
Rimactane (Rim-act'-ane)	Rifampin (Rie-fam'-pin)
Ritalin (Rit'-a-lin)	Methylphenidate (Meth-il-fen'-i-date)
Robaxin (Ro-bak'-sin)	Methocarbamol (Meth-o-kar'-ba-mol)
Robitussin (Row-i-tus'-sin)	Guaifenesin (Gwie-fen'-eh-sin)
Robitussin DM	Guiafenesin and Dextromethorphan (Dek-tro-meh-or'-fan)
Sansert (San'-sert)	Methysergide (Meth-ee-ser'-jide)
Seconal (Sek'-o-nal)	Secobarbital (Sek-o-bar'-bi-tal)
Selsun (Sel'-sun)	Selenium (Se-leh'-nee-um)
Septra (Sep'-tra)	Sulfamethoxazole (Sul-fah-meth-oks'-a-zole) and Trimethroprim (Tri-meth'-o-prim)
Serax (See'-raks)	Oxazepam (Oks-az'-eh-pam)
Silvadene (Sil'-va-deen)	Silver Sulfadiazine (Sul-fa-die'-a-zeen)
Sinemet (Si'-ne-met)	Levodopa (Le-vo-do'-pa)
Sinequan (Sin'-a-kwan)	Doxepin (Dok'-seh-pin)
Sorbitrate (Sor'-bi-trate)	Isosorbide (I-so-sor'-bide)
Stelazine (Stel'-a-zeen)	Trifluoperazine(Tri-floo-o-per'-a-zeen)
Sudafed (Soo'-da-fed)	Pseudophedrine (Soo-do-eh-feh'-drin)
Sulamyd (Sul'-a-mid)	Sulfacetamide (Sul-fah-set'-a-mide)
Sulfamylon (Sul-fa-mie'-lon)	Mafenide (Maf'-eh-nide)
Sultrin (Sul'-trin)	Sulfathiazole (Sul-fah-thi'-ah-zole) Sulfacetamide (Sul-fah-set'-ah-mide) and Sulfabenzamide (Sul-fah-benz'-ah-mide)
Surfak (Sur'-fak)	Dioctyl (Di-ok'-til) Calcium (Kal'-see-um) Sulfosuccinate (Sul-fo-suk'-si-nate)
Synalar (Sine'-a-lar)	Fluocinolone (Floo-o-sin'-o-lone)
Synthroid (Sin'-throid)	Levothyroxine (Lee-vo-thi-rok'-sin)
Tace (Tace)	Chlorotrianisene (Klor-o-tri-an'-I-seen)
Tagamet (Tag'-a-met)	Cimetidine (Si-met'-i-deen)
Talwin (Tal'-win)	Pentazocine (Pen-taz'-o-seen)
Tandearil (Tan'-da-ril)	Oxyphenbutazone (Ok-see-fen-bute'-a-zone)
Tegretol (Teg'-reh-tol)	Carbamazepine (Kar-ba-maz'-eh-peen)
Tessalon (Tess'-a-lon)	Benzonatate (Benz-on'-a-tate)
Tetracycline (Tet-ra-si'-kleen)	
Thorazine (Thor'-a-zeen)	Chlorpromazine (Klor-pro'-ma-zeen)
Thyroid (Thy'-roid)	Same
Tigan (Tie'-gan)	Trimethobenzamide (Tri-meth-o-benz'-a-mide)
Timoptic (Tim-op'-tic)	Timilol (Tim'-o-lol)

Trade Name	Generic Name
Tinactin (Tin-act'-in)	Tolnaftate (Tol-naf'-tate)
Titralac (Ti'-tra-lak)	Calcium (Kal-see-um) Carbonate (Kar'-bon-ate) and Glycine (Gly'-seen)
Tofranil (Toe'-fra-nil)	Imipramine (I-mip'-rah-meen)
Tolectin (Tow-lek'-tin)	Tolmetin (Tol-met'-in)
Triavil (Tri'-a-vil)	Perphenazine (Per-fen'-a-zeen) and Amitriptlyline (Am-i-trip'-ti-leen)
Trilafon (Try'-la-fon)	Perphenazine (Per-fen-a-zeen)
Tylenol (Tie'-leh-nol)	Acetaminophen (As-et-am'-ino-fen)
Tylenol #3	Acetaminophen and Codeine (Ko'-deen)
Unipen (U'-ni-pen)	Nafcillin (Naf-sil-lin)
Urecholine (Ur-eh-ko'-leen)	Bethanecol (Beth-an'-eh-kol)
Valisone (Val'-i-sone)	Betamethasone (Beh-tah-meth'-a-sone)
Valium (Val'-ee-um)	Diazepam (Die-aze-eh-pam)
Vermox (Ver'-moks)	Mebendazole (Meh-ben'-dah-zole)
Vibramycin (Vie-bra-my'-sin)	Doxycycline (Doks-see-si'-kleen)
Xylocaine (Zie'-low-kain)	Lidocaine (Lie-do-kain)
Zarontin (Zar-on'-tin)	Ethosuximide (Eh-tho-suks'-a-mide)
Zyloprim (Zie'-low-prim)	Allopurinol (Al-lo-pure'-in-ol)

End of Lesson 5 Annex

LESSON 6

Review of the Autonomic Nervous System.

TEXT ASSIGNMENT

Paragraphs 6-1 through 6-12.

LESSON OBJECTIVES

After completing this lesson, you should be able to:

6-1. From a list, select the names of the two major divisions of the human nervous system.

6-2. From a list, select the names of the two divisions of the peripheral nervous system.

6-3. Given a group of statements, select the statement that best describes the autonomic nervous system.

6-4. Given a list, select the names of the two divisions of the autonomic nervous system.

6-5. Given a group of statements, select the statement that best describes the sympathetic nervous system.

6-6. Given a group of that best describes the statements, select the statement parasympathetic nervous system.

6-7. Given a group of statements, select the statement that best describes the physiology of the sympathetic nervous system.

6-8. Given a list of chemical substances, select the neurotransmitters of the sympathetic nervous system.

6-9. Given a group of statements and the name of one of the types of receptor sites of the sympathetic nervous system (alpha or beta), select the physiological effect produced by the stimulation of that receptor.

6-10. Given the name of a part of the body and a group of effects, select the effect produced on that part of the body by the sympathetic nervous system.

6-11. Given a group of statements, select the statement that best describes the physiology of the parasympathetic nervous system.

6-12. Given a list of chemical substances, select the chemical transmitter of the parasympathetic nervous system.

6-13. Given the name of a part of the body and a group of effects, select the effect produced on that part by the parasympathetic nervous system.

SUGGESTION

After studying the assignment, complete the exercises at the end of this lesson. These exercises will help you to achieve the lesson objectives.

LESSON 6

REVIEW OF THE AUTONOMIC NERVOUS SYSTEM

Section I. INTRODUCTION

6-1. BACKGROUND

a. At some time in your life, you have faced a situation in which you have undergone a real scare. For example, have you ever been walking down a dark street at night and heard someone running toward you from behind? At that time, certain physiological changes took place in your body. Many of these changes directly involved the autonomic nervous system.

b. The autonomic nervous system (ANS) with its ability to make rapid internal adjustments is one of the most important systems present in the body in terms of the maintenance of body balance. The autonomic nervous system is very complex. Almost every organ of the body receives some type of effect produced by the autonomic nervous system.

c. Because of the wide distribution of the autonomic nervous system, many drugs produce definite effects upon it. This can occur as a blockade of natural activity or a direct effect mimicking natural stimulation. Many so-called side effects of drugs can also be traced to interference with normal autonomic function. Therefore, you must have an understanding of how the autonomic nervous system works and how various drugs can affect its operation. Many drugs used routinely and in emergencies are classified as autonomic nervous system drugs.

6-2. REVIEW OF THE HUMAN NERVOUS SYSTEM

a. The nervous system is divided into two major divisions--the central nervous system and the peripheral nervous system. As you will recall, the central nervous system is composed of the brain and spinal cord. The peripheral nervous system includes the parts of the nervous system other than the brain and spinal cord. Figure 6-1 illustrates the division of the human nervous system.

b. The peripheral nervous system has two divisions: the somatic nervous system and the autonomic nervous system. Figure 6-2 illustrates this division.

(1) Somatic nervous system. The somatic nervous system innervates skeletal muscle. It is under voluntary control and contains no ganglia. Acetylcholine is the chemical transmitter in the somatic nervous system (see lesson 2 of this subcourse).

(2) <u>Autonomic nervous system</u>. The autonomic nervous system is involuntary. It innervates smooth muscles, cardiac muscles, and gland cells. The autonomic nervous system aids the body in the fight or flight response.

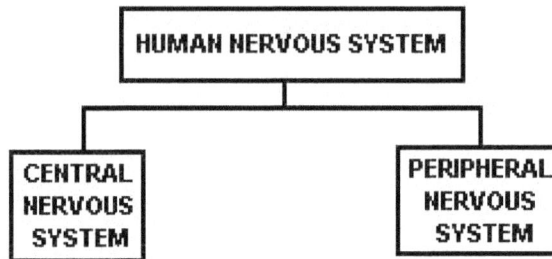

Figure 6-1. Divisions of the peripheral nervous system.

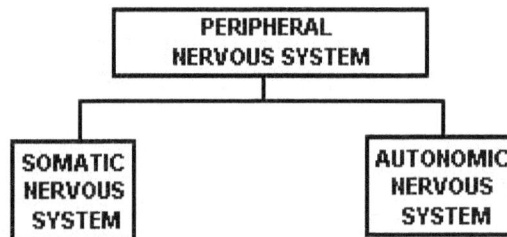

Figure 6-2. Divisions of the peripheral nervous system.

Section II. THE AUTONOMIC NERVOUS SYSTEM

6-3. INTRODUCTION

As was previously mentioned, the autonomic nervous system is one part of the peripheral nervous system. The autonomic nervous system is involuntary. It innervates smooth muscles, cardiac muscles, and gland cells. It aids the body in the fight or flight response. The autonomic nervous system helps to control urinary output, sweating, body temperature, arterial pressure, and gastrointestinal motility and secretion.

6-4. CONTROL OF THE AUTONOMIC NERVOUS SYSTEM

Centers located in the brain stem, hypothalamus, and spinal cord activate the autonomic nervous system.

6-5. ORGANIZATION OF THE AUTONOMIC NERVOUS SYSTEM

The autonomic nervous system is divided into two divisions: the <u>sympathetic</u> and the <u>parasympathetic</u>. Figure 6-3 illustrates this division.

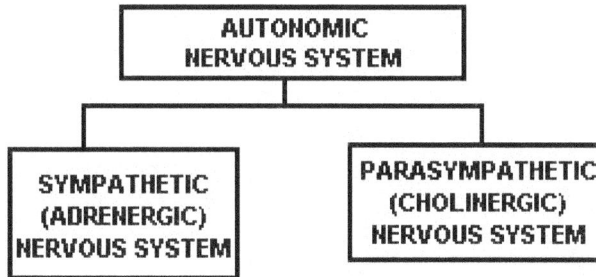

Figure 6-3. Divisions of the autonomic nervous system.

a. **Sympathetic Nervous System.** The sympathetic nervous system is frequently referred to as the <u>adrenergic nervous system</u>. Because of its transmitter epinephrine, which is more commonly known by its trade name "Adrenalin," it prepares the body for stress situations. Stimulation of the adrenergic nervous system has the general effect of expending energy. When a person is scared, this system prepares the body for the fight or flight response. In other words, it prepares the body to either fight or run. More information on this important system will be provided later in this lesson.

b. **Parasympathetic Nervous System.** The parasympathetic nervous system is usually referred to as the cholinergic nervous system. The cholinergic nervous system is responsible for bringing the body back to normal after the fight or flight response. The effects of the cholinergic nervous system are generally the opposite of those produced by the adrenergic nervous system. More information on the cholinergic nervous system will be provided later in this lesson.

Section III. THE SYMPATHETIC NERVOUS SYSTEM

6-6. INTRODUCTION TO THE SYMPATHETIC NERVOUS SYSTEM

You have already been told that the sympathetic nervous system is one component of the autonomic nervous system. Although this system is essential for a person in normal living, it is not crucial for a person to have this system if that individual is in a controlled environment (no stress, excitement, change in temperature, and so forth). Without the presence of this system, one's temperature would not adjust to the environmental temperature, one's level of blood glucose would not increase during times of stress, and one's resistance to fatigue would decrease.

6-7. PHYSIOLOGY OF THE SYMPATHETIC NERVOUS SYSTEM

a.   The sympathetic nervous system is stimulated by the hypothalamus. The nerves of the sympathetic nervous system arise from the thoracolumbar section of the spinal cord. These nerves have short postganglionic fibers. These fibers synapse in the sympathetic chain ganglia that lie near the spinal cord. A ganglion is a joining of nerve fibers. Following synapse, the impulses travel down long postganglionic fibers and synapse at the effector organ.

b.   The neurotransmitter at the preganglionic synapse is <u>acetylcholine</u>, while the neurotransmitters at the effector organ are <u>norepinephrine</u> and <u>epinephrine</u>. Norepinephrine and epinephrine are released by the adrenal medulla and circulate in the blood. Norepinephrine is also released by the postganglionic adrenergic neuron. The enzymes, catechol-o-methyltransferase (COMT) and monoamine oxidase (MAO) terminate transmission.

c.   Circulating epinephrine and norepinephrine are destroyed by COMT. The norepinephrine, which is released by the neuron, is either reabsorbed by the neuron or destroyed in the synapse by MAO.

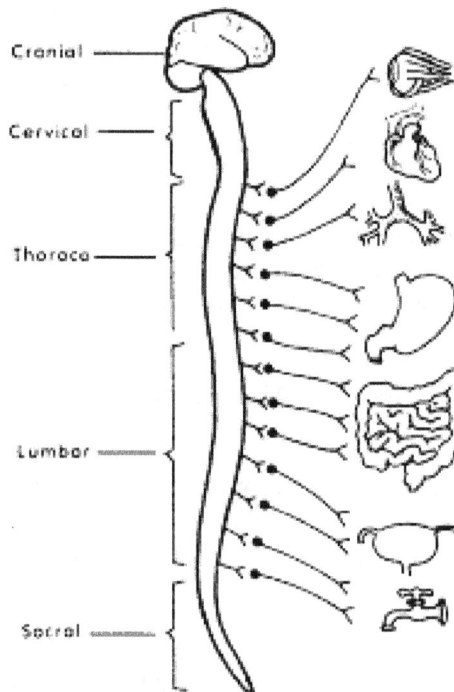

Figure 6-4. Sympathetic nervous system.

6-8. ALPHA AND BETA RECEPTOR SITES

It has been found that different effector organs have either alpha or beta predominant receptor sites.

a. **Alpha Receptors**. Alpha-receptors are associated mainly with increased contractibility of vascular smooth muscle and intestinal relaxation. Alpha-receptors have been classified into two types.

(1) Alpha$_1$. Alpha$_1$ receptors are located at the postsynaptic effector sites to stimulate transmitter release in smooth muscle (that is, contracts smooth muscle of peripheral blood vessels.

(2) Alpha$_2$. Alpha$_2$ receptors are located presynaptic on axon terminals to inhibit release of transmitter (norepinephrine). These predominate in the intestinal tract to cause relaxation.

b. **Beta Receptors**. Beta-receptors are associated with vasodilation and relaxation of nonintestinal smooth muscle and cardiac stimulation. Beta-receptors are divided into two types (example: bronchial dilation).

(1) Beta$_1$. Beta$_1$ receptors cause cardiac stimulation and lipolysis.

(2) Beta$_2$. Beta$_2$ receptors cause bronchodilatation, relaxation of blood vessels (usually skeletal muscles), and muscle glycogenolysis.

6-9. EFFECTS PRODUCED BY THE SYMPATHETIC NERVOUS SYSTEM

The sympathetic nervous system produces a variety of physiological effects upon the body. Listed below are some of these effects/responses:

a. **Eye (Pupil).** Mydriasis (dilation) of the pupil is produced by alpha stimulation.

b. **Heart.** Both an increase in heart rate and an increase in the contraction strength of the heart are produced by beta stimulation.

c. **Bronchi.** Relaxation of the bronchial muscle is produced by beta$_2$ stimulation.

d. **Blood Vessels.**

(1) Blood vessels in skeletal muscle. Constriction or dilation is produced-- over the usual concentration range of physiologically released and circulating epinephrine, the beta-receptor response (vasodilation) predominates in blood vessels of skeletal muscle and liver. The alpha-receptor response (vasoconstriction) is obtained in blood vessels of other abdominal organs.

(2) Blood vessels in the skin and mucous membranes. Constriction is produced by alpha stimulation.

e. **Salivary Glands**. Thick and viscous secretions are produced by alpha stimulation.

f. **Stomach.** The motility and tone of the stomach muscle is usually decreased (alpha$_2$ and beta? stimulation) and the stomach sphincters are contracted (alpha stimulation).

g. **Intestines**. The motility and tone of the intestinal muscles are decreased (alpha$_2$ and beta$_2$ stimulation) and secretions are inhibited.

h. **Urinary Bladder**. The wall of the bladder is usually relaxed (beta stimulation) and the sphincter of the bladder is contracted (alpha stimulation) by stimulation from the sympathetic nervous system.

Section IV. THE PARASYMPATHETIC NERVOUS SYSTEM

6-10. INTRODUCTION TO THE PARASYMPATHETIC NERVOUS SYSTEM

You have already been told that the parasympathetic nervous system is one component of the autonomic nervous system. The parasympathetic nervous system (also referred to as the cholinergic nervous system) is responsible for bringing the body back to normal after the fight or flight response. The effects of the cholinergic nervous system are generally the opposite of those produced by the sympathetic (adrenergic) nervous system. The parasympathetic nervous system is responsible for maintaining the daily functions performed within the body. This division of the autonomic nervous system serves to conserve energy--it is necessary for life. Without the presence of this nervous system, the absorption of necessary nutrients would be hindered, gastrointestinal motility would be decreased, gastrointestinal secretions would be increased, and the urinary bladder and rectum would fail to empty.

6-11. PHYSIOLOGY OF THE PARASYMPATHETIC NERVOUS SYSTEM

a. The parasympathetic nervous system is stimulated by the hypothalamus. It has long preganglionic fibers and short postganglionic fibers (Figure 6-5). The short postganglionic fibers are usually located within the effector organ.

b. The chemical transmitter at both the preganglionic synapse and at the effector organ is acetylcholine. As mentioned previously, acetycholine is also the transmitter at skeletal muscle for the somatic nervous system; however, the receptors for the two nervous systems are different. Transmission of impulses is terminated by the destruction of acetylcholine by the enzyme acetylcholinesterase.

Acetyicholinesterase is frequently referred to as cholinesterase. The general effects of parasympathetic stimulation are conservation and restoration of energy.

       c.   The parasympathetic nervous system does <u>not</u> have alpha and beta receptor sites.

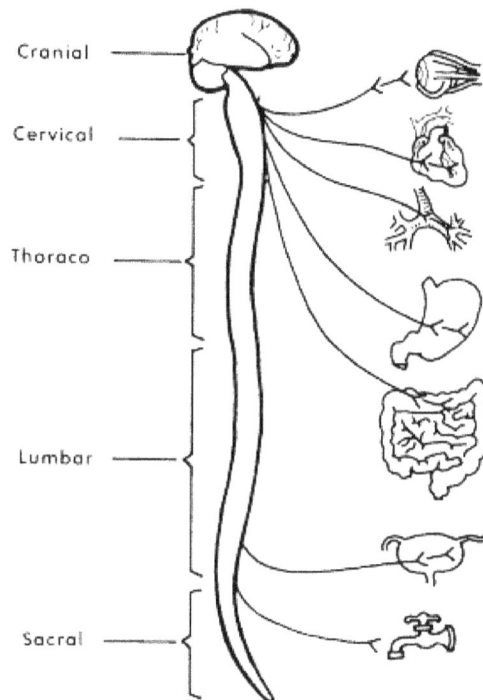

Figure 6-5. The parasympathetic nervous system.

6-12. EFFECTS PRODUCED BY THE PARASYMPATHETIC NERVOUS SYSTEM

       The parasympathetic physiological activity on the organs is generally the opposite of the sympathetic with a few exceptions. The effect of the parasympathetic nervous system effects on some areas of the body are listed below:

       a.   **Eye (Pupil).** Contraction of the pupil (miosis) is produced by parasympathetic stimulation.

       b.   **Heart.** The parasympathetic nervous system produces a decrease in heart rate and a slight decrease in the contraction strength of the heart.

       c.   **Bronch**i. The bronchi are contracted by parasympathetic stimulation.

d. **Salivary Glands**. Parasympathetic nervous system stimulation of the salivary glands leads to profuse, watery secretions.

e. **Stomach**. Parasympathetic stimulation of the stomach leads to increased motility and tone and relaxed (usually) sphincters.

f. **Intestines**. Increased intestinal motility and tone and stimulated secretion of intestinal fluids are products of parasympathetic stimulation.

g. **Urinary Bladder**. Parasympathetic stimulation causes contraction of the bladder wall and relaxation of the sphincter.

Continue with Exercises

EXERCISES, LESSON 6

INSTRUCTIONS: Answer the following exercises by marking the lettered response that best answers the question.

After you have completed all the exercises, turn to "Solutions to Exercises" at the end of the lesson and check your answers. For each exercise answered incorrectly, reread the material referenced with the solution.

1.   Select the names of the two major divisions of the human nervous system.

    a.   The central nervous system and the somatic nervous system.

    b.   The central nervous system and the peripheral nervous system.

    c.   The central nervous system and the autonomic nervous system.

    d.   The central nervous system and the parasympathetic nervous system.

2.   Select the names of the two divisions of the peripheral nervous system.

    a.   The central nervous system and the somatic nervous system.

    b.   The autonomic nervous system and the parasympathetic nervous system.

    c.   The somatic nervous system and the autonomic nervous system.

3.   The autonomic nervous system is best described as:

    a.   The part of the peripheral nervous system that is under voluntary control.

    b.   The part of the peripheral nervous system that innervates skeletal muscle and which has acetylcholine as the chemical transmitter.

    c.   The part of the peripheral nervous system that is involuntary and innervates smooth muscles, cardiac muscles, and gland cells.

    d.   The part of the peripheral nervous system that is involuntary and is frequently referred to as the adrenergic nervous system.

4. Which statement best describes the sympathetic nervous system?

   a. The component of the autonomic nervous system that has acetylcholine as its primary transmitter.

   b. The component of the autonomic nervous system that has epinephrine as its chemical transmitter.

   c. The component of the autonomic nervous system which is responsible for bringing the body back to normal after the fight or flight response.

   d. The component of the autonomic nervous system which is not crucial for a person to have if they live in a controlled environment (no stress).

5. The parasympathetic nervous system is best described as the component of the autonomic nervous system which:

   a. Has acetylcholinesterase as its chemical transmitter.

   b. Has epinephrine as its chemical transmitter.

   c. Is not crucial for a person to have if he/she lives in a controlled environment (no stress).

   d. Is responsible for bringing the body back to normal after the fight or flight response.

6. The neurotransmitter of the sympathetic nervous system at the preganglionic synapse is _____ while the neurotransmitters at the effector organ are _____ and _____.

   a. Epinephrine, norepinephrine, and acetylcholine.

   b. Acetylcholine, norepinephrine, and epinephrine.

   c. Epinephrine, acetylcholine, and acetylcholinesterase.

   d. Acetylcholine, Catechol-o-methyltransferase, and monoamine oxidase.

7. Stimulation of beta-receptor sites results in:

    a. Vasodilation and relaxation of nonintestinal smooth muscle and cardiac stimulation.

    b. Increased contractility of vascular smooth muscle and intestinal relaxation.

    c. Contraction of smooth muscle.

    d. Vasocontraction of vascular smooth muscle.

8. Select the effect produced on the eye by the sympathetic nervous system.

    a. Mydriasis (dilation) of the pupil.

    b. Miosis (contraction) of the pupil.

9. Select the effect produced on the eye by parasympathetic stimulation.

    a. Mydriasis (dilation) of the pupil.

    b. Miosis (contraction) of the pupil.

10. Parasympathetic stimulation of the salivary glands leads to:

    a. Profuse, watery secretions.

    b. Thick and viscous secretions.

    c. None of the above.

11. Sympathetic stimulation of the intestines results in:

    a. Decreased motility and tone of the muscles.

    b. Increased motility and tone of the muscles.

    c. None of the above.

12. The chemical transmitter of the parasympathetic nervous system is:

   a. Epinephrine.

   b. Norepinephrine.

   c. Acetylcholinesterase.

   d. Acetylcholine.

13. Parasympathetic stimulation of the heart results in: (more than one response can be correct)

   a. Increased heart rate.

   b. Decreased heart rate.

   c. Increased contraction strength.

   d. Decreased contraction strength.

Check Your Answers on Next Page

SOLUTIONS TO EXERCISES, LESSON 6

1. b   The central nervous system and the peripheral nervous system.
        (para 6-2a)

2. c   The somatic nervous system and the autonomic nervous system.
        (para 6-2b)

3. c   The part of the peripheral nervous system that is involuntary and
        innervates smooth muscles, cardiac muscles, and gland cells.
        (para 6-2b(2))

4. b   The component of the autonomic nervous system that has epinephrine
        as its chemical transmitter. (para 6-5a)

5. d   Is responsible for bringing the body back to normal after the fight
        or flight response. (para 6-5b)

6. b   Acetylcholine; norepinephrine and epinephrine. (para 6-7b)

7. a   Vasodilation and relaxation of nonintestinal smooth muscle and
        cardiac stimulation. (para 6-8b)

8. a   Hydriasis (dilation) of the pupil. (para 6-9a)

9. b   Miosis (contraction) of the pupil. (para 6-12a)

10. a   Profuse, water secretions. (para 6-12d)

11. a   Decreased motility and tone of the muscles. (para 6-9g)

12. d   Acetylcholine. (para 6-11b)

13. b   Decreased heart rate. (para 6-12b)
    d   Decreased contraction strength. (para 6-12b)

End of Lesson 6

ANNEX

DRUG PRONUNCIATION GUIDE

This Drug Pronunciation Guide was developed to help you to learn how the trade and generic names of commonly prescribed medications are frequently pronounced. Not all the drugs in the guide are discussed in this subcourse. Remember, it is not enough to be able to know the uses, indications, cautions and warnings, and contraindications for a drug--you must also know how to pronounce that drug's name.

Trade Name	Generic Name
Actifed (Ak'-ti-fed)	Triprolidine (Tri-pro'-li-deen) and Pseudoephedrine (Soo-do-e-fed'-rin)
Adapin (Ad'-a-pin)	Doxepin (Dok'-se-pin)
Sinequan (Sin'-a-kwan)	" "
Afrin (Af'-rin)	Oxymetazoline (Ok-see-met-az'-o-leen)
Aldactazide (Al-dak'-ta-zide)	Spironolactone (Spi-ro-no-lak'-tone) and Hydrochlorothiazide (Hy-dro-klor-thi'-a-zide)
Aldactone (Al-dak'-tone)	Spironolactone (Spi-ro-no-lak'-tone)
Aldomet (Al'-do-met)	Methyldopa (Meth-il-do'-pah)
Alupent (Al'-u-pent)	Metaproterenol (Met-a-pro-ter'-eh-nol)
Amoxil (Am-ok'-sil)	Amoxicillin (Ah-moks'-i-sil-in)
Amphojel (Am'-fo-jel)	Aluminum (Al-loo'-mi-num) Hydroxide (Hy-drok'-side)
Ampicillin (Amp'-I-sil-in)	Same
Antepar (Ab'-te-par)	Piperazine (Pi-per'-ah-zeen)
Anturane (An'-tu-rain)	Sulfinpyrazone (Sul-fin-pie'-ra-zone)
Anusol (An'-u-sol)	Pramoxine (Pram-ok'-seen)
Apresoline (A-press'-o-leen)	Hydralazine (Hy-dral'-ah-zeen)
Aralen (Ar'-a-len)	Chloroquine (Klor'-o-kwin)
Aristocort (A-ris'-to-cort)	Triamcinolone (Tri-am-sin'-o-lone)
Artane (Ar'-tane)	Trihexyphenidyl(Tri-hek-see-fen'-i-dil)
A.S.A.	Aspirin (As'-per-in)
Atromid S (A'-tro-mid)	Clofibrate (Klo-fi'-brate)
Avlosulfon (Av-lo-sul'-fon)	Dapsone (Dap'-sone)
Azolid (Az'-o-lid)	Phenylbutazone (Fen-il-bute'-a-zone)
Bactrim (Bak'-trim)	Sulfamethoxazole (Sul-fah-meth-oks'-ah-zole) and Trimethoprim (Tri-meth'-o-prim)
Bellergal (Bel'-er-gal)	Ergotamine (Er-got'-a-meen), Phenobarbital (Feen-o-bar'-bi-tal) and Belladonna (Bel-la-don'-na) Alkaloids
Benadryl (Ben'-a-dril)	Diphenhydramine (Di-fen-hy'-dra-meen)

Trade Name	Generic Name
Bendectin (Ben-dek'-tin)	Doxylamine (Dok-sil'-a-meen)
Benemid (Ben'-eh-mid)	Probenecid (Pro-ben'-eh-sid)
Bonine (Bo'-neen)	Meclizine (Mek'-li-zeen)
Cafergot (Kaf'-er-got)	Ergotamine (Er-got'-a-meen) and Caffeine (Kaf'-feen)
Calamine (Kal'-a-mine)	Same
Catapres (Kat'-a-press)	Clonidine (Klo'-ni-deen)
CeeNu (See'-new)	Lomustine (Lo-mus'-teen)
Chlor-Trimeton (Klo-tri '-meh-ton)	Chlorpheniramine (Klor-fen-it'-a-meen)
Clomid (Klo'-mid)	Clomiphene (Klo'-mi-feen)
Clonopin (Klo-o-pin)	Clonazepam (Klo-na'-ze-pam)
Codeine (Ko'-deen)	Same
Cogentin (Ko-jen'-tin)	Benztropine (Benz'-tro-peen)
Colace (Ko'-lace)	Dioctyl(Di-ok'-til) Sodium (So'-dee-um) Sulfosuccinate (Sul-fo-suk'-si-nate)
Colchicine (Kol'-chi-seen)	Same
Compazine (Kom'-pa-zeen)	Prochiorperazine (Pro-klor-per'-a-zeen)
Cordran (Kor'-dran)	Flurandrenolide (Floor-an-dren'-o-lide)
Coumadin (Koo'-mah-din)	Warfarin (War'-fah-rin)
CP	Cloroquine (Klor'-o-kwin) and Primaquine (Prim'-a-kwin)
Cyclogyl (Si'-klo-jel)	Cyclopentolate (Si-klo-pen'-to-late)
Cytomel (Si'-to-mel)	Liothyronine (Li-o-thy-ro-neen)
Cytoxan (Si-tok'-san)	Cyclophosphamide (Si-klo-fos'-fa-mide)
Dalmane (Dal '-mane)	Flurazepam (Floor-az'-e-pam)
Darvocet (Dar'-vo-set)	Propoxyphene (Pro-pok'-se-feen) and Acetaminopen (As-et-am'-ino-fen)
Darvon (Dar'-von)	Propoxyphene (Pro-pok-se-feen)
Decadron (Dek'-a-dron)	Dexamethasone (Dek-sa-meth'-ah-sone)
Deltasone (Del '-ta-sone)	Prednisone (Pred'-ni-sone)
Demerol (Dem'-er-ol)	Meperidine (Meh-pair'-i-deen)
Dexedrine (Deks '-eh-dreen)	Dextroamphetamine (Deks-tro-am-fet'-a-meen)
Diabinese (Di-ab'-i-nees)	Chlorpropamide (Klor-prop'-a-mide)
Diethylstilbestrol (Di-eth-il-stil-bes'-trol)	Same
Dilantin (Di-lan'-tin)	Phenytoin (Fen'-i-toin)
Dilaudid (Di-law'-did)	Hydromorphone (Hy-dro-more' -fon)
Dimetane (Di'-meh-tane)	Brompheniramine (Brom-fen-ir'-a-meen)

Trade Name	Generic Name
Dimetapp (Di'-meh-tap)	Brompheniramine (Brom-fen-ir'-a-meen) Phenylephrine (Fen-il-ef'-rin) and Phenylpropanolamine (Fen-il-pro-pan-ol'-a-meen)
Disophrol (Dice'-o-frol)	Dexbrompheniramine (Deks-brom-fen-ir'-a-meen) and Pseudoephedrine (Soo-do-e-fed'-rin)
Dolophine (Dol'-o-feen)	Methadone (Meth'-a-done)
Domeboro (Dome-bor'-o)	Aluminum (Ah-loo'-mi-num) Acetate (As'-e-tate)
Donnatal (Don'-na-tal)	Belladonna (Bel-la-don'-na) Alkaloids (Al'-ka-loids) and Phenobarbital (Feen-o-barb'-i-tal)
Doxidan (Dok'-si-dan)	Danthron (Dan'-thron) and Dicctyl (Di-ok'-til) Calcium (Kal'-see-um) Sulfosuccinate (Sul-fo-suk'-si-nate)
Drixoral (Driks'-or-al)	Dexbrompheniramine (Deks-brom-fen-ir'-a-meen) and Pseudoephedrine (Soo-do-e-fed'-rin)
Dulcolax (Dul'-ko-laks)	Bisacodyl (Bis-a'-ko-dil)
Dyazine (Di'-a-zide)	Triamterene (Tri-am'-ter-een) and Hydrochlorothiazide (Hy-dro-klor-o-thi'-a-zide)
Dymelor (Die'-meh-lor)	Acetohexamide (As-e-to-heks'-a-mide)
Dyrenium (Die-ren'-i-um)	Triamterene (Tri-am'-ter-een)
Efudex (Ef'-u-deks)	Fluorouracil (Floo-ro-ur'-ah-sil)
Elavil (El'-ah-vil)	Amitriptyline (Am-i-trip'-til-een)
Elixir Terpin (Ter'-pin) Hydrate	Same
Empirin (Em'-per-in)	Codeine (Ko'-deen) and Aspirin (As'-per-in)
E-Mycin (E-mie'-sin)	Erythromycin (E-rith-ro-mie'-sin)
Equanil (Ek'-wa-nil)	Meprobamate (Me-pro-bam'-ate)
Ergomar (Er'-go-mar)	Ergotamine (Er-got'-a-meen)
Ergotrate (Er'-go-trate)	Ergonovine (Er-go-no'-veen)
Erythrocin (Er-eeth'-ro-sin)	Erythromycin (Er-eeth-ro-my'-sin) Stearate (Stare'-rate)
Esidrix (Es'-i-driks)	Hyrochlorothiazide (Hy-dro-klor-o-thi'-a-zide)
Feosol (Fe'-o-sol)	Ferrous (Fer'-rus) Sulfate (Sul'-fate)
Fergon (Fer'-gon)	Ferrous (Fer'-rus) Gluconate (Glu'-con-ate)

Trade Name	Generic Name
Fiorinal (Fee-or'-i-nal)	Butalbi tal (Bu-tal'-bi-tal), Apririn, Phenacetin (Fen-ass'-eh-tin), and Caffeine (Kaf'-feen)
Flagyl (Fla'-jil)	Metronidazole (Me-tro-ni'-dah-zole)
Flexeril (Flek'-sa-ril)	Cyclobenzaprine (Si-klo-benz'-a-preen)
Fulvicin (Ful'-vi-sin)	Griseofulvin (Griz-e-o-ful'-vin)
Guantanol (Gan'-ta-nol)	Suiphamethoxazole (Sul-fah-meth-oks'-ah-zole)
Gantrisin (Gan'-tri-sin)	Sulfisoxazole (Sul-fi-sok'-sah-zole)
Gelusil (Jel'-u-sil)	Aluminum (Ah-loo'-mi-num) Hydroxide (Hy-drok'-side) and Magnesium (Mag-nee'-zee-um) Hydroxide
Grifulvin (Gri-ful'-vin)	Griseofulvin (Griz-e-o-ful'-vin)
Gynergen (Jin'-er-jen)	Ergotamine (Er-got'-a-meen)
Haldol (Hal'-dol)	Haloperidol (Hal-o-pair'-i-dol)
Halotestin (Hal-o-tes'-tin)	Fluoxymesterone (Floo-ok-see-mes-teh-rone)
Hexadrol (Hek'-sa-drol)	Dexamethasone (Dek-sa-meth'-a-sone)
Hydrodiuril (Hy-dro-di'-ur-il)	Hydroclorothiazide (Hy-dro-kior-thi'-a-zide)
Hygroton (Hy-grow'-ton)	Chiorthalidone (Kior-thal'-i-done)
Ilosone (I'-low-sone)	Erythromycin (Er-ith-ro-mi'-sin) Estolate (Es'-to-late)
Inderal (In'-der-al)	Propranolol (Pro-pran'-o-lol)
Indocin (In'-do-sin)	Indomethacin (In-do-meth'-a-sin)
INH	Isoniazid (I-so-ni'-a-zid)
Insulin (In'-sul-in)	Same
Intal	Cromolyn (Kro'-mo-lin)
Ismelin (Is'-meh-lin)	Guanethidine (Gwan-eth'-i-dine)
Isopto-Atropine (I-sop-to-at'-ro-peen)	Atropine (At'-ro-peen)
Isopto-Carpine (I-sop-to-car'-peen)	Pilocarpine (Pile-o-car'-peen)
Isordil (I'-sor-dil)	Isosorbide (I-so-sor'-bide)
Keflex (Kef'-lex)	Cephalexin (Sef-ah-lek'-sin)
Lanoxin (Lan-ok'-sin)	Digoxin (Di-jok'-sin)
Larodopa (Lar-o-do'-pa)	Levodopa (Le-o-do'-pa)
Larotid (Lar'-o-tid)	Amoxicillin (Ah-moks'-i-sil-in)
Lasix (La'-siks)	Furosemide (Fu-ro'-se-mide)
Leukeran (Lu'-ker-an)	Chlorambucil (Klor-ram'-bu-sil)
Librium (Lib'-ree-um)	Chlordiazepoxide (Klor-die-az-eh-pok'-side)

Trade Name	Generic Name
Lidex (Lie'-deks)	Fluocinoide (Floo-o-sin'-o-nide)
Lomotil (Lo'-mo-til)	Diphenoxylate (Die-fen-ok'-si-late)
Lopressor (Lo'-pres-sor)	Metoprolol (Met-o-pro'-lol)
Lotrimin (Lo'-tri-min)	Chlotrimazole (Klo-trim'-ah-zole)
Maalox (May'-loks)	Aluminum (Ah-loo'-mi-num) and Magnesium (Mag-nee'-zee-um) Hydroxides
Macrodanton (Ma-kro-dan'-tin)	Nitrofurantoin (Ni-tro-fur-an'-toin)
Mandelamine (Man-del'-a-meen)	Methenamine (Meth-en'-a-meen) Mandelate (Man'-deh-late)
Medihaler-Iso (Med-i-hail-er-I'-so)	Isoproterenol (I-so-pro-ter'-en-ol)
Mellaril (Mel'-la-ril)	Thioridazine (Thi-o-rid'-a-zeen)
Metamucil (Met-a-mu'-sil)	Psyllium (Sil'-e-um)
Metaprel (Meh'-ta-prel)	Metaproterenol (Meh'-ta-pro-ter'-eh-nol)
Methotrexate (Meth-o-treks'-ate)	Amethopterin (Ah-meth-op'-ter-in)
Milk of Magnesia	Same
Minipress (Min'-i-press)	Prazosin (Pra'-zo-sin)
Minocin (Min'-o-sin)	Minocycline (Mi-no-si'-kleen)
Monistat (Mon'-i-stat)	Miconazole (Mi-kon'-ah-zole)
Motrin (Mo'-trin)	Ibuprofen (I-bu'-pro-fen)
Myambutol (My-am'-bu-tol)	Ethambutol (Eth-am'-bu-tol)
Mycostatin (My-co-stat'-in)	Nystatin (Ny-stat'-in)
Mylanta (My-lan'-ta)	Aluminum (Ah-loo'-mi-num) and Magnesium (Mag-nee'-zee-um) Hydroxides and Simethicone (Si-meth'-i-kone)
Myleran (My-ler-an)	Busulfan (Bu-sul'-fan)
Mylicon (My'-li-kon)	Simethicone (Si-meth'-i-kone)
Mysoline (My'-so-leen)	Primidone (Pri'-mi-done)
Nalfon (Nal'-fon)	Fenoprofen (Fen-o-pro'-fen)
Naprosyn (Na'-pro-sin)	Naproxen (Na-prok'-sen)
Nembutal (Nem'-bu-tal)	Pentobarbital (Pen-to-barb'-i-tal)
Neosynephrine (Nee-o-sin-eh'-frin)	Phenylephrine (Fen-il-eh'-frin)
Nitrobid (Ni'-tro-bid)	Nitroglycerin (Ni-tro-gli'-ser-in)
Nitrol (Ni'-trol)	" "
Nitrostat (Ni-tro-stat)	" "
Noctec (Nok'-tek)	Chloral Hydrate (Klor'-al- Hy'-drate)
Norfiex (Nor'-fleks)	Orphenadrine Citrate (Or-fen'-a-dreen)
Norpace (Nor'-pace)	Disopyramide (Di-so-peer'-a-mide)

Trade Name	Generic Name
Novahistine (No-va-his'-teen) Expectorant	Guaifenesin (Gwi-fen'-eh-sin), Phenylpropanolamine (Fen-il-pro-pan-ol'-a-meen), and Codeine (Ko'-deen)
NTG	Nitroclycerin (Ni-tro-gli'-ser-in)
Nupercainal (New-per-kain'-al)	Dibucaine (Die'-bu-kain)
Oretic (O-ret'-ik)	Hydrochiorothiazide (Hy-dro-kior-thi'-a-zide)
Orinase (Or'-in-ase)	Tolbutamide (Tol-bu'-tah-mide)
Ornade (Or'-nade)	Chlorpheniramine (Klor-fen-ir'-a-meen), Triprolidine (Tri-pro-li-deen) and Pseudoephedrine (Su-do-eh-fed'-rin)
Parafon Forte (Pair'-a-fon For'-tay)	Chlorzoxazone (Klor-zok'-sa-zone)
Percodan (Per'-ko-dan)	Oxycodone (Ok-si-ko'-done)
Periactin (Per-ee-ak'-tin)	Cyproheptadine (Si-pro-hep'-tah-deen)
Persantine (Per-san'-teen)	Dipyridamole (Di-pi-rid'-ah-mole)
Phenobarbital (Feen-o-barb'-it-al)	Same
Phenylpropanolamine (Fen-il-pro-pan-ol'-a-meen)	Same
Pitocin (Pi-tow'-sin)	Oxytocin (Ok-see-tow'-sin)
Pontocaine (Pon'-to-kain)	Tetracaine (Teh'-tra-kain)
Povan (Po'-van)	Pyrvinium (Pire-vin'-ee-um)
Premarin (Prem'-ar-in)	Conjugated (Kon'-joo-gay-ted) Estrogens (Es-tro-jens)
Presamine (Press'-a-meen)	Imipramine (Im-ip'-rah-meen)
Primaquine (Pri'-mah-kwin)	Same
Probanthine (Pro-ban'-theen)	Propantheline (Pro-pan'-the-leen)
Pronestyl (Pro-nes'-til)	Procainamide (Pro-kain'-a-mide)
Prophylthiouracil (Pro-pil-thi-o-u'-rah-sil)	Same
Prostaphlin (Pro-staff'-lin)	Oxacillin (Oks'-ah-sil-in)
Provera (Pro-ver'-ah)	Medroxyprogesterone (Med-rok-see-pro-jes'-ter-one)
Pyridium (Pie-rid'-ee-um)	Phenazopyridine (Fen-ahs-o-per'-i-deen)
Quinidine (Kwin'-i-deen)	Same
Quinine (Kwie'-nine)	Same
Reserpine (Ree-ser'-peen)	Same
Retin A (Reh'-tin A)	Tretinoin (Tret'-i-noin)
Rifadin (Rie-fad'-in)	Rifampin (Rie-fam'-pin)
Riopan (Rie'-o-pan)	Magaidrate (Mag'-al-drate)

Trade Name	Generic Name
Rimactane (Rim-act'-ane)	Rifampin (Rie-fam'-pin)
Ritalin (Rit'-a-lin)	Methylphenidate (Meth-il-fen'-i-date)
Robaxin (Ro-bak'-sin)	Methocarbamol (Meth-o-kar'-ba-mol)
Robitussin (Row-i-tus'-sin)	Guaifenesin (Gwie-fen'-eh-sin)
Robitussin DM	Guiafenesin and Dextromethorphan (Dek-tro-meh-or'-fan)
Sansert (San'-sert)	Methysergide (Meth-ee-ser'-jide)
Seconal (Sek'-o-nal)	Secobarbital (Sek-o-bar'-bi-tal)
Selsun (Sel'-sun)	Selenium (Se-leh'-nee-um)
Septra (Sep'-tra)	Sulfamethoxazole (Sul-fah-meth-oks'-a-zole) and Trimethroprim (Tri-meth'-o-prim)
Serax (See'-raks)	Oxazepam (Oks-az'-eh-pam)
Silvadene (Sil'-va-deen)	Silver Sulfadiazine (Sul-fa-die'-a-zeen)
Sinemet (Si'-ne-met)	Levodopa (Le-vo-do'-pa)
Sinequan (Sin'-a-kwan)	Doxepin (Dok'-seh-pin)
Sorbitrate (Sor'-bi-trate)	Isosorbide (I-so-sor'-bide)
Stelazine (Stel'-a-zeen)	Trifluoperazine(Tri-floo-o-per'-a-zeen)
Sudafed (Soo'-da-fed)	Pseudophedrine (Soo-do-eh-feh'-drin)
Sulamyd (Sul'-a-mid)	Sulfacetamide (Sul-fah-set'-a-mide)
Sulfamylon (Sul-fa-mie'-lon)	Mafenide (Maf'-eh-nide)
Sultrin (Sul'-trin)	Sulfathiazole (Sul-fah-thi'-ah-zole) Sulfacetamide (Sul-fah-set'-ah-mide) and Sulfabenzamide (Sul-fah-benz'-ah-mide)
Surfak (Sur'-fak)	Dioctyl (Di-ok'-til) Calcium (Kal'-see-um) Sulfosuccinate (Sul-fo-suk'-si-nate)
Synalar (Sine'-a-lar)	Fluocinolone (Floo-o-sin'-o-lone)
Synthroid (Sin'-throid)	Levothyroxine (Lee-vo-thi-rok'-sin)
Tace (Tace)	Chlorotrianisene (Klor-o-tri-an'-I-seen)
Tagamet (Tag'-a-met)	Cimetidine (Si-met'-i-deen)
Talwin (Tal'-win)	Pentazocine (Pen-taz'-o-seen)
Tandearil (Tan'-da-ril)	Oxyphenbutazone (Ok-see-fen-bute'-a-zone)
Tegretol (Teg'-reh-tol)	Carbamazepine (Kar-ba-maz'-eh-peen)
Tessalon (Tess'-a-lon)	Benzonatate (Benz-on'-a-tate)
Tetracycline (Tet-ra-si'-kleen)	
Thorazine (Thor'-a-zeen)	Chlorpromazine (Klor-pro'-ma-zeen)
Thyroid (Thy'-roid)	Same
Tigan (Tie'-gan)	Trimethobenzamide (Tri-meth-o-benz'-a-mide)
Timoptic (Tim-op'-tic)	Timilol (Tim'-o-lol)

Trade Name	Generic Name
Tinactin (Tin-act'-in)	Tolnaftate (Tol-naf'-tate)
Titralac (Ti'-tra-lak)	Calcium (Kal-see-um) Carbonate (Kar'-bon-ate) and Glycine (Gly'-seen)
Tofranil (Toe'-fra-nil)	Imipramine (I-mip'-rah-meen)
Tolectin (Tow-lek'-tin)	Tolmetin (Tol-met'-in)
Triavil (Tri'-a-vil)	Perphenazine (Per-fen'-a-zeen) and Amitriptlyline (Am-i-trip'-ti-leen)
Trilafon (Try'-la-fon)	Perphenazine (Per-fen-a-zeen)
Tylenol (Tie'-leh-nol)	Acetaminophen (As-et-am'-ino-fen)
Tylenol #3	Acetaminophen and Codeine (Ko'-deen)
Unipen (U'-ni-pen)	Nafcillin (Naf-sil-lin)
Urecholine (Ur-eh-ko'-leen)	Bethanecol (Beth-an'-eh-kol)
Valisone (Val'-i-sone)	Betamethasone (Beh-tah-meth'-a-sone)
Valium (Val'-ee-um)	Diazepam (Die-aze-eh-pam)
Vermox (Ver'-moks)	Mebendazole (Meh-ben'-dah-zole)
Vibramycin (Vie-bra-my'-sin)	Doxycycline (Doks-see-si'-kleen)
Xylocaine (Zie'-low-kain)	Lidocaine (Lie-do-kain)
Zarontin (Zar-on'-tin)	Ethosuximide (Eh-tho-suks'-a-mide)
Zyloprim (Zie'-low-prim)	Allopurinol (Al-lo-pure'-in-ol)

End of Lesson 6 Annex

LESSON 7   Adrenergic Agents.

TEXT ASSIGNMENT   Paragraphs 7-1 through 7-6.

LESSON OBJECTIVES After completing this lesson, you should be able to:

7-1. Given a group of statements, select the mechanism(s) of action of drugs which stimulate the sympathetic nervous system.

7-2. Given the name of one of the receptor sites of the adrenergic nervous system and a list of effects, select the effect produced by the stimulation of that receptor site.

7-3. Given the name of a certain part of the body and a group of effects, select the effect produced on that part of the body by adrenergic stimulation.

7-4. Given a group of statements, select the best definition of the term adrenergic (sympathomimetic) drug.

7-5. Given the trade and/or generic name of an adrenergic (sympathomimetic) drug and a list of pharmacological effects, indications for use, cautions and warnings, or side effects, select the effect(s), use(s), caution(s) and warning(s), or side effect(s) for that drug.

7-6. Given the trade or generic name of an adrenergic (sympathomimetic) drug and a group of trade and/or generic names of drugs, select the appropriate trade or generic name for that drug.

SUGGESTION   After studying the assignment, complete the exercises at the end of this lesson. These exercises will help you to achieve the lesson objectives.

LESSON 7

ADRENERGIC AGENTS

7-1. BACKGROUND

The autonomic nervous system was discussed in lesson 6 of this subcourse. In that lesson, you learned of the sympathetic division of this nervous system. Specifically, it was stated that the sympathetic nervous system is frequently referred to as the adrenergic nervous system because of its transmitter epinephrine that is more commonly known by its trade name, "Adrenalin." The adrenergic nervous system prepares the body for stress situations. Stimulation of the adrenergic nervous system has the general effect of expending energy. When a person is scared, this system prepares the body for the fight or flight response.

7-2 MECHANISMS OF ACTION OF AGENTS WHICH STIMULATE SYMPATHETIC NERVOUS SYSTEM

Drugs that stimulate the sympathetic nervous system have a variety of mechanisms of action. These include:

    a.   Mimicking the action of the transmitter norepinephrine. See figure 7-1 for a diagrammatic representation of the sympathetic nervous system.

    b.   Rapidly displacing the transmitter from its storage site to activate the receptor.

    c.   Blocking the uptake of the transmitter into storage sites.

    d.   Inhibiting enzymes that break down the transmitter.

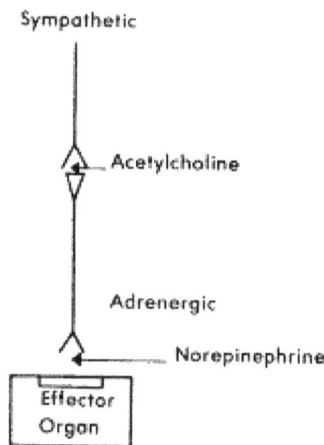

Figure 7-1. Diagrammatic representation of the sympathetic nervous system.

7-3. RECEPTOR SITE THEORY OF ADRENERGIC TRANSMISSION

Two types of receptor sites are theorized to explain adrenergic effects.

a. **Alpha-Receptors**. Alpha-receptors are associated mainly with increased contractibility of vascular smooth muscle and intestinal relaxation.

(1) Alpha$_1$. The alpha$_1$ is located at postsynaptic effector sites to stimulate transmitter release in smooth muscle. For example, the smooth muscle of peripheral blood vessels is contracted in alpha$_1$ stimulation.

(2) Alpha$_2$. The alpha$_2$ receptor site is located presynaptic on axon terminals to inhibit the release of norepinephrine (the transmitter). The effects of alpha$_2$ stimulation results in relaxation of the intestinal tract--motility and tone are decreased.

b. **Beta-Receptors**. Beta-receptors are associated with vasodilation and relaxation of nonintestinal smooth muscle and cardiac stimulation.

(1) Beta$_1$. Stimulation of beta$_1$ receptor sites results in cardiac stimulation and lipolysis.

(2) Beta$_2$. Stimulation of beta$_2$ receptor sites causes bronchodilation, relaxation of blood vessels (usually in skeletal muscles), and muscle glycogenolysis.

7-4. PHARMACOLOGICAL EFFECTS PRODUCED BY ADRENERGIC STIMULATION

a. **Certain Types of Smooth Muscle**. The adrenergic effect on certain types of smooth muscle--especially the blood vessels of the skin, mucous membranes, and salivary glands--is constriction. This is an alpha$_1$ effect.

b. **Other Types of Smooth Muscle**. The adrenergic effect on other types of smooth muscle varies according to the receptor site. The wall of the gut is relaxed through inhibition--this is an alpha$_2$ effect. The bronchial smooth muscle is dilated--this is a beta$_2$ effect. The blood vessels supplying skeletal muscle are dilated--this is a beta$_2$ effect.

c. **Cardiac Stimulation**. Cardiac stimulation is a beta$_1$ effect. Such stimulation results in increased heart rate and increased force of contraction by the heart.

d. **Metabolic Effects**. Beta$_2$ stimulation causes glycogenolysis in liver and muscle tissue. Beta$_1$ stimulation causes liberation of free fatty acids (lipolysis) from adipose tissue.

e. **Central Nervous System (CNS) Excitatory Actions**. Adrenergic stimulation results in respiratory stimulation, an increase in wakefulness, and in a reduction of appetite.

7-5. ADRENERGIC (SYMPATHOHIMETIC) DRUGS

Sympathomimetic drugs are agents which when administered will mimic (produce the same effects) normal adrenergic (sympathetic) stimulation. This normal adrenergic stimulation refers to the effects produced by epinephrine on the body. Two agents produce the adrenergic effects: epinephrine and norepinephrine. Epinephrine is the original model of the sympathomimetic agent. It has both Alpha and Beta activity. Figure 7-2 shows the chemical structure of epinephrine.

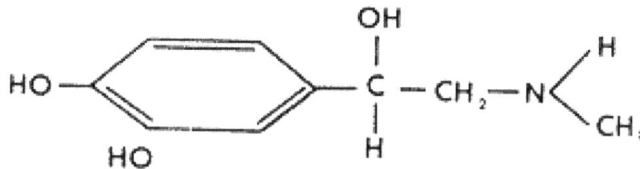

Figure 7-2. Chemical structure of epinephrine.

7-6. SPECIFIC ADRENERGIC (SYMPATHOMIMETIC) AGENTS

a. **Epinephrine (Adrenalin).**

(1) Pharmacological effects.

(a) Blood pressure. The blood pressure in the skin and mucosa is increased via vasopressor action of peripheral vessels.

(b) Vascular effects. Epinephrine constricts the blood vessels of mucosa and the skin (alpha$_1$ effect). Physiological doses (0.5-1.0 milligram) administered subcutaneously) causes dilatation of vessels in skeletal muscle tissue. This effect decreases peripheral resistance and overcomes the vasoconstriction of peripheral vessels so that blood pressure is not greatly affected (predominantly beta effect). Large doses of epinephrine increase blood pressure: Alpha-receptor stimulation in the skeletal muscles overcome beta stimulation and the blood pressure is increased.

(c) Cardiac effects. Epinephrine acts upon Beta$_1$ receptors to greatly increase heart rate and output.

(d) Smooth muscle. The effect upon smooth muscle by epinephrine varies according to the organ stimulated and the type of adrenergic receptor effected in the muscle.

(e)   Gastrointestinal (G.I.) tract. Epinephrine decreases the motility and tone of the gastrointestinal tract (alpha$_2$ and beta$_2$ effects).

(f)   Central nervous system (CNS). Epinephrine provides some stimulation; therefore, it may produce some restlessness, apprehension, headache, and tremor.

(2)   Indications for the use of epinephrine.

(a)   Relieve bronchospasm. Epinephrine is used to relieve bronchiospasm as is seen with patients who have asthma. It opens the breathing pathways and allows for easier breathing.

(b)   Prolong the action of local anesthetics. Epinephrine is sometimes combined with a local anesthetic (that is, lidocaine). Because epinephrine is a vasoconstrictor, it prolongs the effects of the local anesthetic by increasing the time the local anesthetic is in contact with the affected tissue (reduces blood flow to and from the area).

(c)   Restore cardiac rhythm in cardiac arrest. Because of its effects upon the heart, epinephrine is administered to increase cardiac output and rate in persons who experience cardiac arrest.

(d)   Stop bleeding on topical surfaces. Because it is a vasoconstrictor, epinephrine is sometimes applied to topical surfaces to reduce or stop bleeding.

(e)   Treat allergic reactions. Epinephrine is the drug of choice for the treatment of anaphylactic shock. It overcomes the physiological effects of histamine (substance which causes the anaphylactoid reaction). It should be noted that epinephrine is not an antihistamine. One, epinephrine reverses the drop in blood pressure caused by the vasodilatation effect of histamine because epinephrine produces vasoconstriction. Two, the epinephrine reverses the bronchoconstriction produced by the anaphylaxis.

(3)   Cautions and warnings associated with the use of epinephrine.

(a)   Epinephrine can cause anxiety, tenseness, headache, and an awareness of a forceful, rapid heart beat.

(b)   Epinephrine should be used cautiously in-patients who have hypertension (high blood pressure), hyperthyroidism, and heart disease (that is, angina).

b. **Norepinephrine, Levarterenol (Levophed®).** This adrenergic drug acts almost exclusively on alpha-receptors.

(1) Pharmacological effects.

(a) Peripheral vasoconstriction. Norephinephrine causes marked peripheral vasoconstriction.

(b) Constriction of blood vessels in skeletal muscles. Unlike epinephrine, norepinephrine produces constriction of blood vessels in skeletal muscles.

(c) Increase in blood pressure. Norepinephrine causes a net increase in blood pressure.

(2) Indication for the use of norepinephrine. Norepinephrine is used to restore blood pressure in selected hypotensive states (that is, when hypotension occurs during spinal anesthesia).

(3) Cautions and warnings associated with the use of norepinephrine.

(a) Norepinephrine can cause local necrosis due to vasoconstriction when it is injected intravenously. Therefore, it should be infused slowly into a rapidly flowing vein, and the site into which the drug solution is being administered should be changed every 12 hours.

(b) The drug can produce anxiety and transient headaches.

(c) Norepinephrine should be used cautiously with patients who have heart disease (that is, angina), hypertension, and hyperthyroidism.

c. **Isoproterenol (Isuprel®).** Isoproterenol produces a powerful action on both beta$_1$ and beta$_2$ receptors. It has no alpha activity. Injection or aerosol readily absorbs Isoproterenol; however, oral absorption of the drug is unreliable.

(1) Pharmacological effects.

(a) Cardiovascular effects. Isoproterenol produces increased cardiac output and decreased blood pressure. Beta$_2$ stimulation is responsible for the increase in heart rate and the increase in the force of contraction. Isoproterenol causes a reduction in blood pressure because of a decrease in peripheral resistance. Beta$_2$ receptors cause vasodilatation in skeletal muscle.

(b) Smooth muscle. Smooth muscle is relaxed by isoproterenol. This relaxation is most pronounced in the bronchi and gastrointestinal (G.I.) tract.

(c) Central nervous system (CNS). Isoproterenol produces some central nervous system stimulation.

(2) Indications for the use of isoproterenol. Isoproterenol is indicated in a variety of conditions. These include:

(a) Brochodilator in respiratory disorders.

(b) Cardiac stimulant in instances of heart block and cardiogenic shock following myocardial infarction or septicemia.

(3) Side effects associated with isoproterenol. Side effects associated with the use of isoproterenol include palpitation, tachycardia, headache, and flushing of the skin.

(4) Cautions and warnings associated with isoproterenol. Isoproterenol is contraindicated in-patients who have pre-existing cardiac arrhythmias associated with tachycardia.

d. **Dopamine (Intropin®).** Dopamine is a chemical compound in the body which is the immediate precursor (a substance from which another substance is formed) of norepinephrine.

(1) Pharmacological actions. Dopamine exerts both alpha and beta effects. When administered intravenously in doses of 1 to 10 micrograms per kilogram of body weight per minute, the drug acts primarily on beta and dopaminergic receptors. In higher doses, alpha-receptors are stimulated and the net effect of the drug is the result of alpha, beta, and dopaminergic stimulation. Dopaminergic receptors cause dilatation in renal and mesenteric vascular beds. $Beta_1$ effects result in an increase in cardiac output. Dopaminergic effects cause vasodilatation in mesenteric and renal beds.

(2) Indications for the use of dopamine. Dopamine is indicated in the treatment of shock syndrome, including cardiogenic shock, trauma, or hypovolemic shock.

(3) Cautions and warnings associated with the use of dopamine.

(a) Dopamine should not be used in the presence of uncorrected tachyarrhythmias or ventricular fibrillation.

(b) This drug should not be administered in the presence of hypovolemia (that is, to administer fluids).

(c) This drug should not be added to any alkaline dilution solution since the drug is inactivated in alkaline solutions.

e. **Metaproterenol (Alupent®).**

(1) Pharmacological actions. Because of its specificity for beta$_2$ receptors, metaproterenol causes a relaxation of the bronchi and uterus--little effect upon the heart is seen.

(2) Indication for the use of metaproterenol. Metaproterenol is used as a bronchodilator for bronchial asthma. It improves pulmonary function for a period of from 1 to 5 hours.

(3) Cautions and warnings associated with the use of metaproterenol:

(a) This drug is contraindicated with patients who have pre-existing cardiac arrhythmias associated with tachycardia.

(b) This drug is contraindicated in children under six years of age.

(4) Side effects associated with the use of this agent. Central nervous system (CNS) stimulation and muscle tremors are commonly seen in-patients who take this medication.

f. **Albuterol (Ventolin®).**

(1) Pharmacological actions. This drug is specific for beta$_2$ receptors and causes relaxation of the bronchi and uterus. It has a longer duration of action than metaproterenol

(2) Indications. Patients use albuterol as indicated for relief of broncho spasm with reversible obstructive airway disease and prevention of exercise-induced bronchospasm.

(3) Cautions and warnings.

(a) Safety and efficacy in children under age 12 have not been established.

(b) Use with caution in individuals with cardiovascular disorders.

(4) Side effects. Possible side effects associated with Albuterol include CNS stimulation and palpitations.

g. **Terbutaline (Brethine®, Bricanyl®).**

(1) Pharmacological actions. This drug is specific for beta$_2$ receptors with resultant relaxation of bronchial smooth muscle and uterus.

(2)   Indication. Terbutaline is indicated as a bronchodilator for persons who have bronchial asthma. Terbutaline is longer acting than metaproterenol

(3)   Cautions and warnings associated with terbutaline.

(a)   This drug is contraindicated in patients who have preexisting cardiac arrhythmias associated with tachycardia .

(b)   Terbutaline is not recommended for use with patients who are under 12 years of age.

(4)   Side effects. Central nervous system (CNS) stimulation and muscle tremors are commonly seen in patients who take this drug.

h.   **Amphetamine**.

(1)   Pharmacological actions. Amphetamine is a powerful central nervous system (CNS) stimulant with both alpha and beta activity.

(a)   CNS effects. Amphetamine causes the person to be awake and alert. Furthermore, the person feels a decreased sense of fatigue.

(b)   Cardiovascular effects. Amphetamine increases cardiac input and increases blood pressure.

NOTE: Overdosing or repeated dosing can reverse the effects of amphetamine. This occurs because amphetamine promotes the release of norepinephrine from its storage sites. Thus, large amounts of amphetamine deplete the stores of norepinephrine and results in diminished or in no effect being produced (tachyphylaxis).

(2)   Indications for the use of amphetamine derivatives. Amphetamine derivatives are used to treat a variety of conditions. They are as follows:

(a)   Obesity. Amphetamine derivatives are sometimes prescribed to help an individual lose weight.

(b)   Narcolepsy. Narcolepsy is a condition characterized by brief attacks of deep sleep. Amphetamine-like products are used to treat this condition because of their ability to stimulate the patient.

(c)   Hyperkinetic syndrome (attention deficient disorder) in children. Amphetamine derivatives normally stimulate adults; however, in children, it produces a paradoxical (unexpected) effect of calming the patient, decreasing hyperactivity, and prolonging attention span.

NOTE: Amphetamine derivatives are Note R (Schedule II).

  (3) Cautions and warnings.

    (a) Patients taking amphetamine derivatives develop tolerance and psychological dependence with chronic use.

    (b) Amphetamine derivatives should be used cautiously with patients who have arteriosclerosis, cardiovascular disease, glaucoma, hypertension, and hyperthyroid sin.

  (4) Side effects. Side effects commonly seen in patients who take amphetamine-like products are restlessness, tremor, hyperactive reflexes, irritability, insomnia, euphoria, and confusion.

  i. **Ephedrine.**

  (1) Pharmacological effects. Ephedrine directly stimulates both alpha and beta-receptors and indirectly stimulates Alpha-receptors by causing release of norepinephrine. Ephedrine is similar to epinephrine; however, it is longer acting and produces more effect on the central nervous system (CNS). Ephedrine produces cardiovascular effects similar to those produced by epinephrine. Finally, the bronchial muscle relaxation produced caused by ephedrine is less intense, but more sustained than that caused by epinephrine.

  (2) Indications. Ephedrine is most commonly used as a bronchodilator. It is also used as a nasal decongestant, as a treatment for narcolepsy, and as agent to control blood pressure in patients under the effects of spinal and epidural anesthesia.

  (3) Caution and warning. Ephedrine is contraindicated in patients who have severe hypertension and chronic heart disease.

  j. **Metaraminol (Aramine®).**

  (1) Pharmacological effects. Metaraminol produces alpha stimulation with $beta_1$ effects. The vasoconstriction produced by metaraminol is very pronounced. The $beta_1$ effects produced by metaraminol are similar to epinephrine. Overall, metaraminol produces less potent and longer duration with more gradual onset than the effects produced by norepinephrine.

  (2) Indications. Metaraminol is indicated in the treatment of hypotensive states (that is, shock); however, it must be used with caution because it increases the myocardium's demand of oxygen.

(3) Cautions and warnings. Metaraminol may induce arrhythmias in large doses. Furthermore, the drug should be used with caution with patients who have heart disease, thyroid disease, hypertension, or diabetes.

k. **Phenylephrine (Neo-Synephrine®).**

(1) Pharmacological effects. Phenylephrine is a powerful alpha stimulator with little or no effect on beta-receptors.

(2) Indications. Phenylephrine has a variety of uses. These include:

(a) Nasal decongestant.

(b) Vasopressor. The drug is used as a vasopressor for hypotension associated with spinal anesthesia and neurogenic shock.

(c) Mydriatic. The drug is used to produce mydriasis (dilatation of the pupil).

(3) Cautions and warnings. The drug is contraindicated in hypertension and existing ventricular tachycardia. Phenylephrine can induce cardiac irregularities.

l. **Tetrahydrozoline (Tyzine®).**

(1) Indications. This drug is used as a nasal decongestant.

(2) Caution and warning. Prolonged use of this agent as a nasal decongestant may produce chemical rhinitis.

(3) Side effects. Tetrahydrozoline may cause sneezing, stinging or burning of the mucous membranes, insomnia, or tachycardia.

NOTE: Agents listed in m and n, below, are referred to as incomplete sympathomimetics. They produce topical vasoconstriction of the nasal mucosa or conjunctiva. They have no direct effect on the myocardium or on the smooth muscle of the bronchioles. However, they do relax the intestine. Remember, although both the intestine and the bronchi are smooth muscles, they are affected by different receptors. Intestinal relaxation is moderated by $alpha_2$ receptors and bronchi relaxation by $beta_2$ receptors.

m. **Xylometazoline (Otrivin®).**

(1) Indications. Xylometazoline is used as a nasal decongestant.

(2) Caution and warning. No significant caution and warning is associated with the drug.

(3) <u>Side effects</u>. Side effects associated with this drug include stinging or burning of the mucous membranes, dry nose, and rebound congestion.

n. **Oxymetazoline (Afrin®).**

(1) <u>Indications</u>. Oxymetazoline is used as a nasal decongestant.

(2) <u>Caution and warning</u>. No significant caution and warning is associated with the drug.

(3) <u>Side effects</u>. Side effects associated with oxymetazoline include rebound congestion, dryness of the nose, and stinging or burning of the mucous membranes.

Continue with Exercises

EXERCISES, LESSON 7

INSTRUCTIONS: Answer the following exercises by marking the lettered response which best answers the question.

After you have completed all the exercises, turn to "Solutions to Exercises" at the end of the lesson, and check your answers. For each exercise answered incorrectly, reread the material referenced with the solution.

1. Select the mechanism(s) of action of drugs that stimulate the sympathetic nervous system.

    a. Mimicking the action of the transmitter acetylcholine.

    b. Rapidly displacing the transmitter from its storage site to activate the receptor.

    c. Increasing the uptake of transmitter into the storage sites.

    d. Helping the enzymes that break down the transmitter.

2. Stimulation of the beta2 receptor site results in:

    a. Intestinal relaxation.

    b. Decreased motility of the intestinal tract.

    c. Bronchodilation.

    d. Cardiac stimulation.

3. What is the effect upon the heart of adrenergic stimulation?

    a. No effect is known.

    b. Decreased cardiac output.

    c. Increased heart rate.

    d. Decreased force of contraction.

4. The pharmacological effect of epinephrine (Adrenalin®) upon the gastrointestinal (G.I.) tract is:

   a.   Increases motility and tone.

   b.   Decreases motility and tone.

   c.   Increases secretions.

   d.   None of the above.

5. What is the indication for the use of norepinephrine?

   a.   To prolong the action of local anesthetics.

   b.   To stop bleeding on topical surfaces.

   c.   To treat allergic reactions.

   d.   To restore blood pressure in selective hypotensive states.

6. Isoproterenol (Isuprel®) is used in a variety of conditions. It is used:

   a.   To restore blood pressure in selected hypotensive states.

   b.   As a bronchodilator in respiratory disorders.

   c.   To stop bleeding on topical surfaces.

   d.   As a local vasoconstrictor to prolong the effects of local anesthetics.

7. Metaproterenol (Alupent®) is indicated for use as a:

   a.   Bronchodilator for bronchial asthma.

   b.   Nasal decongestant.

   c.   Treatment for narcolepsy.

   d.   Cardiac stimulant.

8. Ephedrine is most commonly used as a (n):

    a. Cardiac stimulant.

    b. Bronchodilator.

    c. Peripheral vasoconstrictor.

    d. Intestinal stimulant.

9. Caution should be used if patients that use metaraminol have:

    a. Diabetes.

    b. Thyroid disease.

    c. Hypertension.

    d. All the above.

10. Tetrahydrozoline (Tyzine®) is commonly used as a:

    a. Nasal decongestant.

    b. Cardiac stimulant.

    c. Mydriatic.

    d. Vasopressor.

11. One side effect associated with oxymetazoline (Afrin®) is:

    a. Rebound congestion

    b. Loss of appetite.

    c. Cardiac arrhythmias.

    d. Hypertension.

12.   Match the trade or generic name in Column A with its appropriate trade or generic name in Column B.

Column A   Column B

_____Xylometazoline®   a. Otrivin®

_____Levophed®   b. Metaraminol

_____Intropin®   c. Metaproterenol

_____Epinephrine   d. Dopamine

_____Aramine®   e. Terbutaline

_____Brethine®   f. Adrenalin

_____Neo-Synephrine®   g. Phenylephrine

_____Alupent®   h. Levarterenol

Check Your Answers on Next Page

SOLUTIONS TO EXERCISES, LESSON 7

1. b   Rapidly displacing the transmitter from its storage site to activate the receptor. (para 7-2b)

2. c   Bronchodilation. (para 7-3b(2))

3. c   Increased heart rate. (para 7-4c)

4. b   Decreases motility and tone. (para 7-6a(1)(e))

5. d   To restore blood pressure in selective hypotensive states. (para 7-6b(2))

6. b   As a bronchodilator in respiratory disorders. (para 7-6c(2)(a))

7. a   A bronchodilator for bronchial asthma. (para 7-6e(2))

8. b   Bronchodilator. (para 7-6i(2))

9. d   All the above. (para 7-6j(3))

10. a   Nasal decongestant. (para 7-6l(1))

11. a   Rebound congestion. (para 7-6n(3))

12.
    a   Xylometazoline. (para 7-6m)

    h   Levophed®. (para 7-6b)

    d   Intropin®. (para 7-6d)

    f   Epinephrine. (para 7-6a)

    b   Aramine®. (para 7-6j)

    e   Brethine®. (para 7-6g)

    g   Neo-Synephrine®. (para 7-6k)

    c   Alupent®. (para 7-6e)

End of Lesson 6

ANNEX

DRUG PRONUNCIATION GUIDE

This Drug Pronunciation Guide was developed to help you to learn how the trade and generic names of commonly prescribed medications are frequently pronounced. Not all the drugs in the guide are discussed in this subcourse. Remember, it is not enough to be able to know the uses, indications, cautions and warnings, and contraindications for a drug--you must also know how to pronounce that drug's name.

Trade Name	*Generic Name*
Actifed (Ak'-ti-fed)	Triprolidine (Tri-pro'-li-deen) and Pseudoephedrine (Soo-do-e-fed'-rin)
Adapin (Ad'-a-pin)	Doxepin (Dok'-se-pin)
Sinequan (Sin'-a-kwan)	" "
Afrin (Af'-rin)	Oxymetazoline (Ok-see-met-az'-o-leen)
Aldactazide (Al-dak'-ta-zide)	Spironolactone (Spi-ro-no-lak'-tone) and Hydrochlorothiazide (Hy-dro-klor-thi'-a-zide)
Aldactone (Al-dak'-tone)	Spironolactone (Spi-ro-no-lak'-tone)
Aldomet (Al'-do-met)	Methyldopa (Meth-il-do'-pah)
Alupent (Al'-u-pent)	Metaproterenol (Met-a-pro-ter'-eh-nol)
Amoxil (Am-ok'-sil)	Amoxicillin (Ah-moks'-i-sil-in)
Amphojel (Am'-fo-jel)	Aluminum (Al-loo'-mi-num) Hydroxide (Hy-drok'-side)
Ampicillin (Amp'-I-sil-in)	Same
Antepar (Ab'-te-par)	Piperazine (Pi-per'-ah-zeen)
Anturane (An'-tu-rain)	Sulfinpyrazone (Sul-fin-pie'-ra-zone)
Anusol (An'-u-sol)	Pramoxine (Pram-ok'-seen)
Apresoline (A-press'-o-leen)	Hydralazine (Hy-dral'-ah-zeen)
Aralen (Ar'-a-len)	Chloroquine (Klor'-o-kwin)
Aristocort (A-ris'-to-cort)	Triamcinolone (Tri-am-sin'-o-lone)
Artane (Ar'-tane)	Trihexyphenidyl(Tri-hek-see-fen'-i-dil)
A.S.A.	Aspirin (As'-per-in)
Atromid S (A'-tro-mid)	Clofibrate (Klo-fi'-brate)
Avlosulfon (Av-lo-sul'-fon)	Dapsone (Dap'-sone)
Azolid (Az'-o-lid)	Phenylbutazone (Fen-il-bute'-a-zone)
Bactrim (Bak'-trim)	Sulfamethoxazole (Sul-fah-meth-oks'-ah-zole) and Trimethoprim (Tri-meth'-o-prim)
Bellergal (Bel'-er-gal)	Ergotamine (Er-got'-a-meen), Phenobarbital (Feen-o-bar'-bi-tal) and Belladonna (Bel-la-don'-na) Alkaloids
Benadryl (Ben'-a-dril)	Diphenhydramine (Di-fen-hy'-dra-meen)

Trade Name	Generic Name
Bendectin (Ben-dek'-tin)	Doxylamine (Dok-sil'-a-meen)
Benemid (Ben'-eh-mid)	Probenecid (Pro-ben'-eh-sid)
Bonine (Bo'-neen)	Meclizine (Mek'-li-zeen)
Cafergot (Kaf'-er-got)	Ergotamine (Er-got'-a-meen) and Caffeine (Kaf'-feen)
Calamine (Kal'-a-mine)	Same
Catapres (Kat'-a-press)	Clonidine (Klo'-ni-deen)
CeeNu (See'-new)	Lomustine (Lo-mus'-teen)
Chlor-Trimeton (Klo-tri '-meh-ton)	Chlorpheniramine (Klor-fen-it'-a-meen)
Clomid (Klo'-mid)	Clomiphene (Klo'-mi-feen)
Clonopin (Klo-o-pin)	Clonazepam (Klo-na'-ze-pam)
Codeine (Ko'-deen)	Same
Cogentin (Ko-jen'-tin)	Benztropine (Benz'-tro-peen)
Colace (Ko'-lace)	Dioctyl(Di-ok'-til) Sodium (So'-dee-um) Sulfosuccinate (Sul-fo-suk'-si-nate)
Colchicine (Kol'-chi-seen)	Same
Compazine (Kom'-pa-zeen)	Prochiorperazine (Pro-klor-per'-a-zeen)
Cordran (Kor'-dran)	Flurandrenolide (Floor-an-dren'-o-lide)
Coumadin (Koo'-mah-din)	Warfarin (War'-fah-rin)
CP	Cloroquine (Klor'-o-kwin) and Primaquine (Prim'-a-kwin)
Cyclogyl (Si'-klo-jel)	Cyclopentolate (Si-klo-pen'-to-late)
Cytomel (Si'-to-mel)	Liothyronine (Li-o-thy-ro-neen)
Cytoxan (Si-tok'-san)	Cyclophosphamide (Si-klo-fos'-fa-mide)
Dalmane (Dal '-mane)	Flurazepam (Floor-az'-e-pam)
Darvocet (Dar'-vo-set)	Propoxyphene (Pro-pok'-se-feen) and Acetaminopen (As-et-am'-ino-fen)
Darvon (Dar'-von)	Propoxyphene (Pro-pok-se-feen)
Decadron (Dek'-a-dron)	Dexamethasone (Dek-sa-meth'-ah-sone)
Deltasone (Del '-ta-sone)	Prednisone (Pred'-ni-sone)
Demerol (Dem'-er-ol)	Meperidine (Meh-pair'-i-deen)
Dexedrine (Deks '-eh-dreen)	Dextroamphetamine (Deks-tro-am-fet'-a-meen)
Diabinese (Di-ab'-i-nees)	Chlorpropamide (Klor-prop'-a-mide)
Diethylstilbestrol (Di-eth-il-stil-bes'-trol)	Same
Dilantin (Di-lan'-tin)	Phenytoin (Fen'-i-toin)
Dilaudid (Di-law'-did)	Hydromorphone (Hy-dro-more' -fon)
Dimetane (Di'-meh-tane)	Brompheniramine (Brom-fen-ir'-a-meen)

Trade Name	Generic Name
Dimetapp (Di'-meh-tap)	Brompheniramine (Brom-fen-ir'-a-meen) Phenylephrine (Fen-il-ef'-rin) and Phenylpropanolamine (Fen-il-pro-pan-ol'-a-meen)
Disophrol (Dice'-o-frol)	Dexbrompheniramine (Deks-brom-fen-ir'-a-meen) and Pseudoephedrine (Soo-do-e-fed'-rin)
Dolophine (Dol'-o-feen)	Methadone (Meth'-a-done)
Domeboro (Dome-bor'-o)	Aluminum (Ah-loo'-mi-num) Acetate (As'-e-tate)
Donnatal (Don'-na-tal)	Belladonna (Bel-la-don'-na) Alkaloids (Al'-ka-loids) and Phenobarbital (Feen-o-barb'-i-tal)
Doxidan (Dok'-si-dan)	Danthron (Dan'-thron) and Dicctyl (Di-ok'-til) Calcium (Kal'-see-um) Sulfosuccinate (Sul-fo-suk'-si-nate)
Drixoral (Driks'-or-al)	Dexbrompheniramine (Deks-brom-fen-ir'-a-meen) and Pseudoephedrine (Soo-do-e-fed'-rin)
Dulcolax (Dul'-ko-laks)	Bisacodyl (Bis-a'-ko-dil)
Dyazine (Di'-a-zide)	Triamterene (Tri-am'-ter-een) and Hydrochlorothiazide (Hy-dro-klor-o-thi'-a-zide)
Dymelor (Die'-meh-lor)	Acetohexamide (As-e-to-heks'-a-mide)
Dyrenium (Die-ren'-i-um)	Triamterene (Tri-am'-ter-een)
Efudex (Ef'-u-deks)	Fluorouracil (Floo-ro-ur'-ah-sil)
Elavil (El'-ah-vil)	Amitriptyline (Am-i-trip'-til-een)
Elixir Terpin (Ter'-pin) Hydrate	Same
Empirin (Em'-per-in)	Codeine (Ko'-deen) and Aspirin (As'-per-in)
E-Mycin (E-mie'-sin)	Erythromycin (E-rith-ro-mie'-sin)
Equanil (Ek'-wa-nil)	Meprobamate (Me-pro-bam'-ate)
Ergomar (Er'-go-mar)	Ergotamine (Er-got'-a-meen)
Ergotrate (Er'-go-trate)	Ergonovine (Er-go-no'-veen)
Erythrocin (Er-eeth'-ro-sin)	Erythromycin (Er-eeth-ro-my'-sin) Stearate (Stare'-rate)
Esidrix (Es'-i-driks)	Hyrochlorothiazide (Hy-dro-klor-o-thi'-a-zide)
Feosol (Fe'-o-sol)	Ferrous (Fer'-rus) Sulfate (Sul'-fate)
Fergon (Fer'-gon)	Ferrous (Fer'-rus) Gluconate (Glu'-con-ate)

Trade Name	Generic Name
Fiorinal (Fee-or'-i-nal)	Butalbi tal (Bu-tal'-bi-tal), Apririn, Phenacetin (Fen-ass'-eh-tin), and Caffeine (Kaf'-feen)
Flagyl (Fla'-jil)	Metronidazole (Me-tro-ni'-dah-zole)
Flexeril (Flek'-sa-ril)	Cyclobenzaprine (Si-klo-benz'-a-preen)
Fulvicin (Ful'-vi-sin)	Griseofulvin (Griz-e-o-ful'-vin)
Guantanol (Gan'-ta-nol)	Suiphamethoxazole (Sul-fah-meth-oks'-ah-zole)
Gantrisin (Gan'-tri-sin)	Sulfisoxazole (Sul-fi-sok'-sah-zole)
Gelusil (Jel'-u-sil)	Aluminum (Ah-loo'-mi-num) Hydroxide (Hy-drok'-side) and Magnesium (Mag-nee'-zee-um) Hydroxide
Grifulvin (Gri-ful'-vin)	Griseofulvin (Griz-e-o-ful'-vin)
Gynergen (Jin'-er-jen)	Ergotamine (Er-got'-a-meen)
Haldol (Hal'-dol)	Haloperidol (Hal-o-pair'-i-dol)
Halotestin (Hal-o-tes'-tin)	Fluoxymesterone (Floo-ok-see-mes-teh-rone)
Hexadrol (Hek'-sa-drol)	Dexamethasone (Dek-sa-meth'-a-sone)
Hydrodiuril (Hy-dro-di'-ur-il)	Hydroclorothiazide (Hy-dro-kior-thi'-a-zide)
Hygroton (Hy-grow'-ton)	Chiorthalidone (Kior-thal'-i-done)
Ilosone (I'-low-sone)	Erythromycin (Er-ith-ro-mi'-sin) Estolate (Es'-to-late)
Inderal (In'-der-al)	Propranolol (Pro-pran'-o-lol)
Indocin (In'-do-sin)	Indomethacin (In-do-meth'-a-sin)
INH	Isoniazid (I-so-ni'-a-zid)
Insulin (In'-sul-in)	Same
Intal	Cromolyn (Kro'-mo-lin)
Ismelin (Is'-meh-lin)	Guanethidine (Gwan-eth'-i-dine)
Isopto-Atropine (I-sop-to-at'-ro-peen)	Atropine (At'-ro-peen)
Isopto-Carpine (I-sop-to-car'-peen)	Pilocarpine (Pile-o-car'-peen)
Isordil (I'-sor-dil)	Isosorbide (I-so-sor'-bide)
Keflex (Kef'-lex)	Cephalexin (Sef-ah-lek'-sin)
Lanoxin (Lan-ok'-sin)	Digoxin (Di-jok'-sin)
Larodopa (Lar-o-do'-pa)	Levodopa (Le-o-do'-pa)
Larotid (Lar'-o-tid)	Amoxicillin (Ah-moks'-i-sil-in)
Lasix (La'-siks)	Furosemide (Fu-ro'-se-mide)
Leukeran (Lu'-ker-an)	Chlorambucil (Klor-ram'-bu-sil)
Librium (Lib'-ree-um)	Chlordiazepoxide (Klor-die-az-eh-pok'-side)

Trade Name	Generic Name
Lidex (Lie'-deks)	Fluocinoide (Floo-o-sin'-o-nide)
Lomotil (Lo'-mo-til)	Diphenoxylate (Die-fen-ok'-si-late)
Lopressor (Lo'-pres-sor)	Metoprolol (Met-o-pro'-lol)
Lotrimin (Lo'-tri-min)	Chlotrimazole (Klo-trim'-ah-zole)
Maalox (May'-loks)	Aluminum (Ah-loo'-mi-num) and Magnesium (Mag-nee'-zee-um) Hydroxides
Macrodanton (Ma-kro-dan'-tin)	Nitrofurantoin (Ni-tro-fur-an'-toin)
Mandelamine (Man-del'-a-meen)	Methenamine (Meth-en-'-a-meen) Mandelate (Man'-deh-late)
Medihaler-Iso (Med-i-hail-er-I'-so)	Isoproterenol (I-so-pro-ter'-en-ol)
Mellaril (Mel'-la-ril)	Thioridazine (Thi-o-rid'-a-zeen)
Metamucil (Met-a-mu'-sil)	Psyllium (Sil'-e-um)
Metaprel (Meh'-ta-prel)	Metaproterenol (Meh'-ta-pro-ter'-eh-nol)
Methotrexate (Meth-o-treks'-ate)	Amethopterin (Ah-meth-op'-ter-in)
Milk of Magnesia	Same
Minipress (Min'-i-press)	Prazosin (Pra'-zo-sin)
Minocin (Min'-o-sin)	Minocycline (Mi-no-si'-kleen)
Monistat (Mon'-i-stat)	Miconazole (Mi-kon'-ah-zole)
Motrin (Mo'-trin)	Ibuprofen (I-bu'-pro-fen)
Myambutol (My-am'-bu-tol)	Ethambutol (Eth-am'-bu-tol)
Mycostatin (My-co-stat'-in)	Nystatin (Ny-stat'-in)
Mylanta (My-lan'-ta)	Aluminum (Ah-loo'-mi-num) and Magnesium (Mag-nee'-zee-um) Hydroxides and Simethicone (Si-meth'-i-kone)
Myleran (My-ler-an)	Busulfan (Bu-sul'-fan)
Mylicon (My'-li-kon)	Simethicone (Si-meth'-i-kone)
Mysoline (My'-so-leen)	Primidone (Pri'-mi-done)
Nalfon (Nal'-fon)	Fenoprofen (Fen-o-pro'-fen)
Naprosyn (Na'-pro-sin)	Naproxen (Na-prok'-sen)
Nembutal (Nem'-bu-tal)	Pentobarbital (Pen-to-barb'-i-tal)
Neosynephrine (Nee-o-sin-eh'-frin)	Phenylephrine (Fen-il-eh'-frin)
Nitrobid (Ni'-tro-bid)	Nitroglycerin (Ni-tro-gli'-ser-in)
Nitrol (Ni'-trol)	" "
Nitrostat (Ni-tro-stat)	" "
Noctec (Nok'-tek)	Chloral Hydrate (Klor'-al- Hy'-drate)
Norfiex (Nor'-fleks)	Orphenadrine Citrate (Or-fen'-a-dreen)
Norpace (Nor'-pace)	Disopyramide (Di-so-peer'-a-mide)

Trade Name	Generic Name
Novahistine (No-va-his'-teen) Expectorant	Guaifenesin (Gwi-fen'-eh-sin), Phenylpropanolamine (Fen-il-pro-pan-ol'-a-meen), and Codeine (Ko'-deen)
NTG	Nitroclycerin (Ni-tro-gli'-ser-in)
Nupercainal (New-per-kain'-al)	Dibucaine (Die'-bu-kain)
Oretic (O-ret'-ik)	Hydrochiorothiazide (Hy-dro-kior-thi'-a-zide)
Orinase (Or'-in-ase)	Tolbutamide (Tol-bu'-tah-mide)
Ornade (Or'-nade)	Chlorpheniramine (Klor-fen-ir'-a-meen), Triprolidine (Tri-pro-li-deen) and Pseudoephedrine (Su-do-eh-fed'-rin)
Parafon Forte (Pair'-a-fon For'-tay)	Chlorzoxazone (Klor-zok'-sa-zone)
Percodan (Per'-ko-dan)	Oxycodone (Ok-si-ko'-done)
Periactin (Per-ee-ak'-tin)	Cyproheptadine (Si-pro-hep'-tah-deen)
Persantine (Per-san'-teen)	Dipyridamole (Di-pi-rid'-ah-mole)
Phenobarbital (Feen-o-barb'-it-al)	Same
Phenylpropanolamine (Fen-il-pro-pan-ol'-a-meen)	Same
Pitocin (Pi-tow'-sin)	Oxytocin (Ok-see-tow'-sin)
Pontocaine (Pon'-to-kain)	Tetracaine (Teh'-tra-kain)
Povan (Po'-van)	Pyrvinium (Pire-vin'-ee-um)
Premarin (Prem'-ar-in)	Conjugated (Kon'-joo-gay-ted) Estrogens (Es-tro-jens)
Presamine (Press'-a-meen)	Imipramine (Im-ip'-rah-meen)
Primaquine (Pri'-mah-kwin)	Same
Probanthine (Pro-ban'-theen)	Propantheline (Pro-pan'-the-leen)
Pronestyl (Pro-nes'-til)	Procainamide (Pro-kain'-a-mide)
Prophylthiouracil (Pro-pil-thi-o-u'-rah-sil)	Same
Prostaphlin (Pro-staff'-lin)	Oxacillin (Oks'-ah-sil-in)
Provera (Pro-ver'-ah)	Medroxyprogesterone (Med-rok-see-pro-jes'-ter-one)
Pyridium (Pie-rid'-ee-um)	Phenazopyridine (Fen-ahs-o-per'-i-deen)
Quinidine (Kwin'-i-deen)	Same
Quinine (Kwie'-nine)	Same
Reserpine (Ree-ser'-peen)	Same
Retin A (Reh'-tin A)	Tretinoin (Tret'-i-noin)
Rifadin (Rie-fad'-in)	Rifampin (Rie-fam'-pin)
Riopan (Rie'-o-pan)	Magaidrate (Mag'-al-drate)

Trade Name	Generic Name
Rimactane (Rim-act'-ane)	Rifampin (Rie-fam'-pin)
Ritalin (Rit'-a-lin)	Methylphenidate (Meth-il-fen'-i-date)
Robaxin (Ro-bak'-sin)	Methocarbamol (Meth-o-kar'-ba-mol)
Robitussin (Row-i-tus'-sin)	Guaifenesin (Gwie-fen'-eh-sin)
Robitussin DM	Guiafenesin and Dextromethorphan (Dek-tro-meh-or'-fan)
Sansert (San'-sert)	Methysergide (Meth-ee-ser'-jide)
Seconal (Sek'-o-nal)	Secobarbital (Sek-o-bar'-bi-tal)
Selsun (Sel'-sun)	Selenium (Se-leh'-nee-um)
Septra (Sep'-tra)	Sulfamethoxazole (Sul-fah-meth-oks'-a-zole) and Trimethroprim (Tri-meth'-o-prim)
Serax (See'-raks)	Oxazepam (Oks-az'-eh-pam)
Silvadene (Sil'-va-deen)	Silver Sulfadiazine (Sul-fa-die'-a-zeen)
Sinemet (Si'-ne-met)	Levodopa (Le-vo-do'-pa)
Sinequan (Sin'-a-kwan)	Doxepin (Dok'-seh-pin)
Sorbitrate (Sor'-bi-trate)	Isosorbide (I-so-sor'-bide)
Stelazine (Stel'-a-zeen)	Trifluoperazine(Tri-floo-o-per'-a-zeen)
Sudafed (Soo'-da-fed)	Pseudophedrine (Soo-do-eh-feh'-drin)
Sulamyd (Sul'-a-mid)	Sulfacetamide (Sul-fah-set'-a-mide)
Sulfamylon (Sul-fa-mie'-lon)	Mafenide (Maf'-eh-nide)
Sultrin (Sul'-trin)	Sulfathiazole (Sul-fah-thi'-ah-zole) Sulfacetamide (Sul-fah-set'-ah-mide) and Sulfabenzamide (Sul-fah-benz'-ah-mide)
Surfak (Sur'-fak)	Dioctyl (Di-ok'-til) Calcium (Kal'-see-um) Sulfosuccinate (Sul-fo-suk'-si-nate)
Synalar (Sine'-a-lar)	Fluocinolone (Floo-o-sin'-o-lone)
Synthroid (Sin'-throid)	Levothyroxine (Lee-vo-thi-rok'-sin)
Tace (Tace)	Chlorotrianisene (Klor-o-tri-an'-I-seen)
Tagamet (Tag'-a-met)	Cimetidine (Si-met'-i-deen)
Talwin (Tal'-win)	Pentazocine (Pen-taz'-o-seen)
Tandearil (Tan'-da-ril)	Oxyphenbutazone (Ok-see-fen-bute'-a-zone)
Tegretol (Teg'-reh-tol)	Carbamazepine (Kar-ba-maz'-eh-peen)
Tessalon (Tess'-a-lon)	Benzonatate (Benz-on'-a-tate)
Tetracycline (Tet-ra-si'-kleen)	
Thorazine (Thor'-a-zeen)	Chlorpromazine (Klor-pro'-ma-zeen)
Thyroid (Thy'-roid)	Same
Tigan (Tie'-gan)	Trimethobenzamide (Tri-meth-o-benz'-a-mide)
Timoptic (Tim-op'-tic)	Timilol (Tim'-o-lol)

Trade Name	Generic Name
Tinactin (Tin-act'-in)	Tolnaftate (Tol-naf'-tate)
Titralac (Ti'-tra-lak)	Calcium (Kal-see-um) Carbonate (Kar'-bon-ate) and Glycine (Gly'-seen)
Tofranil (Toe'-fra-nil)	Imipramine (I-mip'-rah-meen)
Tolectin (Tow-lek'-tin)	Tolmetin (Tol-met'-in)
Triavil (Tri'-a-vil)	Perphenazine (Per-fen'-a-zeen) and Amitriptlyline (Am-i-trip'-ti-leen)
Trilafon (Try'-la-fon)	Perphenazine (Per-fen-a-zeen)
Tylenol (Tie'-leh-nol)	Acetaminophen (As-et-am'-ino-fen)
Tylenol #3	Acetaminophen and Codeine (Ko'-deen)
Unipen (U'-ni-pen)	Nafcillin (Naf-sil-lin)
Urecholine (Ur-eh-ko'-leen)	Bethanecol (Beth-an'-eh-kol)
Valisone (Val'-i-sone)	Betamethasone (Beh-tah-meth'-a-sone)
Valium (Val'-ee-um)	Diazepam (Die-aze-eh-pam)
Vermox (Ver'-moks)	Mebendazole (Meh-ben'-dah-zole)
Vibramycin (Vie-bra-my'-sin)	Doxycycline (Doks-see-si'-kleen)
Xylocaine (Zie'-low-kain)	Lidocaine (Lie-do-kain)
Zarontin (Zar-on'-tin)	Ethosuximide (Eh-tho-suks'-a-mide)
Zyloprim (Zie'-low-prim)	Allopurinol (Al-lo-pure'-in-ol)

End of Lesson 7 Annex

LESSON 8   Adrenergic Blocking Agents.

TEXT ASSIGNMENT   Paragraphs 8-1 through 8-5.

LESSON OBJECTIVES   After completing this lesson, you should be able to:

8-1. Given a group of statements, select the statement that best describes one of the mechanisms of actions of adrenergic blocking agents.

8-2. Given one of the following categories of drugs: alpha-blockers or beta-blockers and a group of statements, select the statement that best describes the mechanism by which that category of drugs produces its effects.

8-3. Given the trade and/or generic name of an adrenergic blocking agent, classify that agent as either an alpha or beta blocker.

8-4. Given the trade and/or generic name of an adrenergic blocking agent and a group of pharmacological actions, indications/uses, and side effects, select the action(s), indication(s)/use(s), and side effect(s) associated with that agent.

8-5. Given the trade or generic name of an adrenergic blocking agent and a group of trade and generic names of drugs, select the appropriate trade or generic name for the stated drug.

SUGGESTION   After studying the assignment, complete the exercises at the end of this lesson. These exercises will help you to achieve the lesson objectives.

LESSON 8

ADRENERGIC BLOCKING AGENTS

8-1. INTRODUCTION TO ADRENERGIC BLOCKING AGENTS

a. In the last lesson, the topic of adrenergic (sympathomimetic) agents was discussed. As you will recall, this group of drugs produces effects like those produced by epinephrine.

b. This lesson will focus on the topic of adrenergic blocking agents. This group of agents blocks or interferes with the types of responses typically caused by the transmitters of the adrenergic (sympathetic) nervous system. Adrenergic blocking agents are sometimes referred to as sympatholytic agents.

8-2. GENERAL MECHANISMS OF ACTION OF ADRENERGIC BLOCKING AGENTS

There are two basic categories of mechanisms of action demonstrated by adrenergic blocking agents.

a. Some adrenergic blocking agents inhibit the synthesis, storage, or release of norepinephrine. Therefore, less norepinephrine is available to the receptors to produce its effects (adrenergic stimulation).

b. Other adrenergic blocking agents inhibit the reaction between norepinephrine and the receptor.

8-3. PRINCIPAL TYPES OF ADRENERGIC RECEPTORS

a. **Alpha-Receptors.** Alpha-receptors produce salivation, sweating, and contraction of smooth muscle (except in the gastrointestinal tract).

b. **Beta-Receptors**. Beta-receptors increase the frequency and strength of the heartbeat and cause relaxation of smooth muscle (except In the gastrointestinal tract).

8-4. ALPHA ADRENERGIC BLOCKING AGENTS

Effects produced by these agents occur because the alpha-receptors are blocked while beta-receptors are still capable of producing their effects.

a. **Phentolamine (Regitine®).**

(1) Pharmacological actions.

(a) Phentolamine causes blockage of the $alpha_1$ receptors. This causes vasodilatation that results in decreased blood pressure.

(b) Phentolamine also causes blockage of $alpha_2$ receptors. This causes a release of norepinephrine. Since the normal effect of norepinephrine is blocked at the $alpha_2$ receptor, the effect of epinephrine on the cardiac beta-receptors occurs.

(2) Indication/use. Phentolamine is used to prevent or treat dermal necrosis and sloughing caused by the extravasation (administration outside the vein) of norepinephrine (levarterenol).

(3) Side effects. Phentolamine can cause side effects such as tachycardia, flushing, cardiac arrhythmias, and orthostatic hypotension.

b. **Prazosin (Minipress®).**

(1) Pharmacological actions. Prazosin is an antihypertensive agent that selectively blocks $alpha_1$ receptors. This drug produces vasodilation and reduces peripheral resistance, but it produces little effect upon cardiac output.

(2) Indications/uses. Prazosin is an antihypertensive agent.

(3) Cautions and warnings. This agent should be used caution with patients who have severe cardiac disease or a history of mental depression.

(4) Side effects. Side effects associated with the use of prazosin include dizziness, sudden fainting, drowsiness, and lack of energy.

c. Other alpha blockers include terazosin (Hytrin®) and doxazosin (Cardura®). They are used for hypertension.

8-5. BETA-ADRENERGIC BLOCKING AGENTS

Beta-adrenergic blocking agents block beta effects--cardiac rate and force of contraction, vasodilatation in skeletal muscles, hyperglycemia, and bronchodilatation.

a. **Propranolol (Inderal®).**

(1) Pharmacological action. Propranolol blocks both $beta_1$ and $beta_2$ receptors.

(2) Indications/uses. Propranolol is used to treat a variety of conditions. Its uses are listed below:

(a) Antianginal agent. It lessens the heart's need for oxygen because it slows the heart rate. With a slower heart rate, there is decreased need for oxygen and the angina pain diminishes.

(b) Antiarrhythmic agent.

(c) Antihypertensive agent.

(d) Suppressant agent (in the treatment of migraine headaches)

(3) Cautions and warnings. Propranolol should not be administered to patients who have bronchial asthma, cardiogenic shock, or sinus bradycardia. It should be used in caution with patients who have a history of allergies, diabetes mellitus, congestive heart failure, and emphysema. It is important to note that the abrupt withdrawal of this agent with patients who have heart disease (that is, angina) can cause arrhythmias or myocardial infarction (heart attack). This occurs because the sympathetic tone is adjusted to the blockage (probably by producing extra amounts of norepinephrine); thus, when the blockage is withdrawn, the heart cannot tolerate the extra norepinephrine that is present.

(4) Side effects. Side effects that can be produced by propranolol include dizziness or lightheadedness, very slow pulse, mental confusion or depression, cold hands, and numbness of the toes or fingers.

b. **Metoprolol Tartrate (Lopressor®).**

(1) Pharmacological actions. Metoprolol is a somewhat selective beta1 blocker.

(2) Indication. Metoprolol is used as an antihypertensive agent.

(3) Side effects. Side effects associated with this agent include dizziness or drowsiness, mental depression, and hallucinations.

c.   **Atenolol (Tenormin®).**

(1)   <u>Pharmacological actions</u>. Atenolol is a selective beta1 blocker; its long half-life permits once daily dosing.

(2)   <u>Indications.</u> Atenolol is used as an antihypertensive agent and for the treatment of angina pectoris because of coronary atherosclerosis.

(3)   <u>Side effects.</u> Side effects include dizziness, drowsiness, and some mental depression, but less than that of other agents.

d.   **Timolol (Timoptic®).**

(1)   <u>Pharmacological actions</u>. Timolol has both beta1 and beta2 blocking activity.

(2)   <u>Indications</u>. The oral tablets are used as an anti-hypertensive agent. The eye drops are used for glaucoma.

(3)   <u>Side effects.</u> Possible side effects include dizziness, drowsiness, hallucinations, fatigue, slow pulse, confusion, depression, and cold hands and feet.

Continue with Exercises

EXERCISES, LESSON 8

INSTRUCTIONS: Answer the following exercises by marking the lettered response which best answers the question.

After you have completed all the exercises, turn to "Solutions to Exercises" at the end of the lesson and check your answers. For each exercise answered incorrectly, reread the material referenced with the solution.

1. Which of the following statements best describes one of the mechanisms of action of adrenergic blocking agents?

   a. The production of excessive levels of acetylcholinesterase.

   b. The inhibition of the reaction between norepinephrine and the receptor.

   c. The inhibition of the synthesis, storage, or release of acetylcholine.

   d. The production of substances that produce physiological effects the opposite of norepinephrine.

2. Select the statement that best describes how alpha-adrenergic blocking agents produce their effects.

   a. The alpha-receptors are blocked and this allows the parasympathetic nervous system to produce its effects.

   b. The alpha-receptors are blocked while the beta-receptors still produce their effects.

   c. The alpha-receptors as well as the beta1 receptors are blocked, but the beta2 receptors still produce their effects.

   d. The alpha-receptors are blocked and the effects of the beta-receptors are antagonized.

3. Prazosin is used as:

   a. An antianginal agent.

   b. A suppressant agent (in the treatment of migraine headaches).

   c. An antihypertensive agent.

   d. A vasodilator.

4. Side effect(s) commonly associated with phentolamine (Regitine®) include:

   a. Bradycardia.

   b. Cardiac arrhythmias.

   c. Sudden fainting.

   d. Extremely slow pulse rate.

5. Select the side effect(s) commonly associated with propranolol.

   a. Very slow pulse.

   b. Mental confusion.

   c. Dizziness.

   d. All the above.

6. Metoprolol tartrate is used as a(n):

   a. Antianginal agent.

   b. Antihypertensive.

   c. Means to prevent or treat dermal necrosis and sloughing caused by the extravasation of norepinephrine.

   d. Suppressant agent (in the treatment of migraine headaches).

7. The drug prazosin is classified as a(n):

a. Alpha-blocker.

b. Beta-blocker.

8. The trade name of prazosin is:

a. Minipress®.

b. Inderal®.

c. Lopressor®.

d. Prapressor®.

Check Your Answers on Next Page

SOLUTIONS TO EXERCISES, LESSON 8

1. b The inhibition of the reaction between norepinephrine and the receptor. (para 8-2)

2. b The alpha-receptors are blocked while the beta-receptors still produce their effects. (para 8-4)

3. c An antihypertensive agent. (para 8-4)

4. b Cardiac arrhythmias. (para 8-4a(3))

5. d All the above. (para 8-5a(4))

6. b Antihypertensive. (para 8-5b(2))

7. a Alpha-blocker. (para 8-4b)

8. a Minipress®. (para 8-4b)

End of Lesson 8

ANNEX

DRUG PRONUNCIATION GUIDE

This Drug Pronunciation Guide was developed to help you to learn how the trade and generic names of commonly prescribed medications are frequently pronounced. Not all the drugs in the guide are discussed in this subcourse. Remember, it is not enough to be able to know the uses, indications, cautions and warnings, and contraindications for a drug--you must also know how to pronounce that drug's name.

Trade Name	*Generic Name*
Actifed (Ak'-ti-fed)	Triprolidine (Tri-pro'-li-deen) and Pseudoephedrine (Soo-do-e-fed'-rin)
Adapin (Ad'-a-pin)	Doxepin (Dok'-se-pin)
Sinequan (Sin'-a-kwan)	" "
Afrin (Af'-rin)	Oxymetazoline (Ok-see-met-az'-o-leen)
Aldactazide (Al-dak'-ta-zide)	Spironolactone (Spi-ro-no-lak'-tone) and Hydrochlorothiazide (Hy-dro-klor-thi'-a-zide)
Aldactone (Al-dak'-tone)	Spironolactone (Spi-ro-no-lak'-tone)
Aldomet (Al'-do-met)	Methyldopa (Meth-il-do'-pah)
Alupent (Al'-u-pent)	Metaproterenol (Met-a-pro-ter'-eh-nol)
Amoxil (Am-ok'-sil)	Amoxicillin (Ah-moks'-i-sil-in)
Amphojel (Am'-fo-jel)	Aluminum (Al-loo'-mi-num) Hydroxide (Hy-drok'-side)
Ampicillin (Amp'-I-sil-in)	Same
Antepar (Ab'-te-par)	Piperazine (Pi-per'-ah-zeen)
Anturane (An'-tu-rain)	Sulfinpyrazone (Sul-fin-pie'-ra-zone)
Anusol (An'-u-sol)	Pramoxine (Pram-ok'-seen)
Apresoline (A-press'-o-leen)	Hydralazine (Hy-dral'-ah-zeen)
Aralen (Ar'-a-len)	Chloroquine (Klor'-o-kwin)
Aristocort (A-ris'-to-cort)	Triamcinolone (Tri-am-sin'-o-lone)
Artane (Ar'-tane)	Trihexyphenidyl(Tri-hek-see-fen'-i-dil)
A.S.A.	Aspirin (As'-per-in)
Atromid S (A'-tro-mid)	Clofibrate (Klo-fi'-brate)
Avlosulfon (Av-lo-sul'-fon)	Dapsone (Dap'-sone)
Azolid (Az'-o-lid)	Phenylbutazone (Fen-il-bute'-a-zone)
Bactrim (Bak'-trim)	Sulfamethoxazole (Sul-fah-meth-oks'-ah-zole) and Trimethoprim (Tri-meth'-o-prim)
Bellergal (Bel'-er-gal)	Ergotamine (Er-got'-a-meen), Phenobarbital (Feen-o-bar'-bi-tal) and Belladonna (Bel-la-don'-na) Alkaloids
Benadryl (Ben'-a-dril)	Diphenhydramine (Di-fen-hy'-dra-meen)

Trade Name	Generic Name
Bendectin (Ben-dek'-tin)	Doxylamine (Dok-sil'-a-meen)
Benemid (Ben'-eh-mid)	Probenecid (Pro-ben'-eh-sid)
Bonine (Bo'-neen)	Meclizine (Mek'-li-zeen)
Cafergot (Kaf'-er-got)	Ergotamine (Er-got'-a-meen) and Caffeine (Kaf'-feen)
Calamine (Kal'-a-mine)	Same
Catapres (Kat'-a-press)	Clonidine (Klo'-ni-deen)
CeeNu (See'-new)	Lomustine (Lo-mus'-teen)
Chlor-Trimeton (Klo-tri '-meh-ton)	Chlorpheniramine (Klor-fen-it'-a-meen)
Clomid (Klo'-mid)	Clomiphene (Klo'-mi-feen)
Clonopin (Klo-o-pin)	Clonazepam (Klo-na'-ze-pam)
Codeine (Ko'-deen)	Same
Cogentin (Ko-jen'-tin)	Benztropine (Benz'-tro-peen)
Colace (Ko'-lace)	Dioctyl(Di-ok'-til) Sodium (So'-dee-um) Sulfosuccinate (Sul-fo-suk'-si-nate)
Colchicine (Kol'-chi-seen)	Same
Compazine (Kom'-pa-zeen)	Prochlorperazine (Pro-klor-per'-a-zeen)
Cordran (Kor'-dran)	Flurandrenolide (Floor-an-dren'-o-lide)
Coumadin (Koo'-mah-din)	Warfarin (War'-fah-rin)
CP	Cloroquine (Klor'-o-kwin) and Primaquine (Prim'-a-kwin)
Cyclogyl (Si'-klo-jel)	Cyclopentolate (Si-klo-pen'-to-late)
Cytomel (Si'-to-mel)	Liothyronine (Li-o-thy-ro-neen)
Cytoxan (Si-tok'-san)	Cyclophosphamide (Si-klo-fos'-fa-mide)
Dalmane (Dal '-mane)	Flurazepam (Floor-az'-e-pam)
Darvocet (Dar'-vo-set)	Propoxyphene (Pro-pok'-se-feen) and Acetaminopen (As-et-am'-ino-fen)
Darvon (Dar'-von)	Propoxyphene (Pro-pok-se-feen)
Decadron (Dek'-a-dron)	Dexamethasone (Dek-sa-meth'-ah-sone)
Deltasone (Del '-ta-sone)	Prednisone (Pred'-ni-sone)
Demerol (Dem'-er-ol)	Meperidine (Meh-pair'-i-deen)
Dexedrine (Deks '-eh-dreen)	Dextroamphetamine (Deks-tro-am-fet'-a-meen)
Diabinese (Di-ab'-i-nees)	Chlorpropamide (Klor-prop'-a-mide)
Diethylstilbestrol (Di-eth-il-stil-bes'-trol)	Same
Dilantin (Di-lan'-tin)	Phenytoin (Fen'-i-toin)
Dilaudid (Di-law'-did)	Hydromorphone (Hy-dro-more' -fon)
Dimetane (Di'-meh-tane)	Brompheniramine (Brom-fen-ir'-a-meen)

Trade Name	Generic Name
Dimetapp (Di'-meh-tap)	Brompheniramine (Brom-fen-ir'-a-meen) Phenylephrine (Fen-il-ef'-rin) and Phenylpropanolamine (Fen-il-pro-pan-ol'-a-meen)
Disophrol (Dice'-o-frol)	Dexbrompheniramine (Deks-brom-fen-ir'-a-meen) and Pseudoephedrine (Soo-do-e-fed'-rin)
Dolophine (Dol'-o-feen)	Methadone (Meth'-a-done)
Domeboro (Dome-bor'-o)	Aluminum (Ah-loo'-mi-num) Acetate (As'-e-tate)
Donnatal (Don'-na-tal)	Belladonna (Bel-la-don'-na) Alkaloids (Al'-ka-loids) and Phenobarbital (Feen-o-barb'-i-tal)
Doxidan (Dok'-si-dan)	Danthron (Dan'-thron) and Dicctyl (Di-ok'-til) Calcium (Kal'-see-um) Sulfosuccinate (Sul-fo-suk'-si-nate)
Drixoral (Driks'-or-al)	Dexbrompheniramine (Deks-brom-fen-ir'-a-meen) and Pseudoephedrine (Soo-do-e-fed'-rin)
Dulcolax (Dul'-ko-laks)	Bisacodyl (Bis-a'-ko-dil)
Dyazine (Di'-a-zide)	Triamterene (Tri-am'-ter-een) and Hydrochlorothiazide (Hy-dro-klor-o-thi'-a-zide)
Dymelor (Die'-meh-lor)	Acetohexamide (As-e-to-heks'-a-mide)
Dyrenium (Die-ren'-i-um)	Triamterene (Tri-am'-ter-een)
Efudex (Ef'-u-deks)	Fluorouracil (Floo-ro-ur'-ah-sil)
Elavil (El'-ah-vil)	Amitriptyline (Am-i-trip'-til-een)
Elixir Terpin (Ter'-pin) Hydrate	Same
Empirin (Em'-per-in)	Codeine (Ko'-deen) and Aspirin (As'-per-in)
E-Mycin (E-mie'-sin)	Erythromycin (E-rith-ro-mie'-sin)
Equanil (Ek'-wa-nil)	Meprobamate (Me-pro-bam'-ate)
Ergomar (Er'-go-mar)	Ergotamine (Er-got'-a-meen)
Ergotrate (Er'-go-trate)	Ergonovine (Er-go-no'-veen)
Erythrocin (Er-eeth'-ro-sin)	Erythromycin (Er-eeth-ro-my'-sin) Stearate (Stare'-rate)
Esidrix (Es'-i-driks)	Hyrochlorothiazide (Hy-dro-klor-o-thi'-a-zide)
Feosol (Fe'-o-sol)	Ferrous (Fer'-rus) Sulfate (Sul'-fate)
Fergon (Fer'-gon)	Ferrous (Fer'-rus) Gluconate (Glu'-con-ate)

Trade Name	Generic Name
Fiorinal (Fee-or'-i-nal)	Butalbi tal (Bu-tal'-bi-tal), Apririn, Phenacetin (Fen-ass'-eh-tin), and Caffeine (Kaf'-feen)
Flagyl (Fla'-jil)	Metronidazole (Me-tro-ni'-dah-zole)
Flexeril (Flek'-sa-ril)	Cyclobenzaprine (Si-klo-benz'-a-preen)
Fulvicin (Ful'-vi-sin)	Griseofulvin (Griz-e-o-ful'-vin)
Guantanol (Gan'-ta-nol)	Suiphamethoxazole (Sul-fah-meth-oks'-ah-zole)
Gantrisin (Gan'-tri-sin)	Sulfisoxazole (Sul-fi-sok'-sah-zole)
Gelusil (Jel'-u-sil)	Aluminum (Ah-loo'-mi-num) Hydroxide (Hy-drok'-side) and Magnesium (Mag-nee'-zee-um) Hydroxide
Grifulvin (Gri-ful'-vin)	Griseofulvin (Griz-e-o-ful'-vin)
Gynergen (Jin'-er-jen)	Ergotamine (Er-got'-a-meen)
Haldol (Hal'-dol)	Haloperidol (Hal-o-pair'-i-dol)
Halotestin (Hal-o-tes'-tin)	Fluoxymesterone (Floo-ok-see-mes-teh-rone)
Hexadrol (Hek'-sa-drol)	Dexamethasone (Dek-sa-meth'-a-sone)
Hydrodiuril (Hy-dro-di'-ur-il)	Hydroclorothiazide (Hy-dro-kior-thi'-a-zide)
Hygroton (Hy-grow'-ton)	Chiorthalidone (Kior-thal'-i-done)
Ilosone (I'-low-sone)	Erythromycin (Er-ith-ro-mi'-sin) Estolate (Es'-to-late)
Inderal (In'-der-al)	Propranolol (Pro-pran'-o-lol)
Indocin (In'-do-sin)	Indomethacin (In-do-meth'-a-sin)
INH	Isoniazid (I-so-ni'-a-zid)
Insulin (In'-sul-in)	Same
Intal	Cromolyn (Kro'-mo-lin)
Ismelin (Is'-meh-lin)	Guanethidine (Gwan-eth'-i-dine)
Isopto-Atropine (I-sop-to-at'-ro-peen)	Atropine (At'-ro-peen)
Isopto-Carpine (I-sop-to-car'-peen)	Pilocarpine (Pile-o-car'-peen)
Isordil (I'-sor-dil)	Isosorbide (I-so-sor'-bide)
Keflex (Kef'-lex)	Cephalexin (Sef-ah-lek'-sin)
Lanoxin (Lan-ok'-sin)	Digoxin (Di-jok'-sin)
Larodopa (Lar-o-do'-pa)	Levodopa (Le-o-do'-pa)
Larotid (Lar'-o-tid)	Amoxicillin (Ah-moks'-i-sil-in)
Lasix (La'-siks)	Furosemide (Fu-ro'-se-mide)
Leukeran (Lu'-ker-an)	Chlorambucil (Klor-ram'-bu-sil)
Librium (Lib'-ree-um)	Chlordiazepoxide (Klor-die-az-eh-pok'-side)

Trade Name	Generic Name
Lidex (Lie'-deks)	Fluocinoide (Floo-o-sin'-o-nide)
Lomotil (Lo'-mo-til)	Diphenoxylate (Die-fen-ok'-si-late)
Lopressor (Lo'-pres-sor)	Metoprolol (Met-o-pro'-lol)
Lotrimin (Lo'-tri-min)	Chlotrimazole (Klo-trim'-ah-zole)
Maalox (May'-loks)	Aluminum (Ah-loo'-mi-num) and Magnesium (Mag-nee'-zee-um) Hydroxides
Macrodanton (Ma-kro-dan'-tin)	Nitrofurantoin (Ni-tro-fur-an'-toin)
Mandelamine (Man-del'-a-meen)	Methenamine (Meth-en'-a-meen) Mandelate (Man'-deh-late)
Medihaler-Iso (Med-i-hail-er-I'-so)	Isoproterenol (I-so-pro-ter'-en-ol)
Mellaril (Mel'-la-ril)	Thioridazine (Thi-o-rid'-a-zeen)
Metamucil (Met-a-mu'-sil)	Psyllium (Sil'-e-um)
Metaprel (Meh'-ta-prel)	Metaproterenol (Meh'-ta-pro-ter'-eh-nol)
Methotrexate (Meth-o-treks'-ate)	Amethopterin (Ah-meth-op'-ter-in)
Milk of Magnesia	Same
Minipress (Min'-i-press)	Prazosin (Pra'-zo-sin)
Minocin (Min'-o-sin)	Minocycline (Mi-no-si'-kleen)
Monistat (Mon'-i-stat)	Miconazole (Mi-kon'-ah-zole)
Motrin (Mo'-trin)	Ibuprofen (I-bu'-pro-fen)
Myambutol (My-am'-bu-tol)	Ethambutol (Eth-am'-bu-tol)
Mycostatin (My-co-stat'-in)	Nystatin (Ny-stat'-in)
Mylanta (My-lan'-ta)	Aluminum (Ah-loo'-mi-num) and Magnesium (Mag-nee'-zee-um) Hydroxides and Simethicone (Si-meth'-i-kone)
Myleran (My-ler-an)	Busulfan (Bu-sul'-fan)
Mylicon (My'-li-kon)	Simethicone (Si-meth'-i-kone)
Mysoline (My'-so-leen)	Primidone (Pri'-mi-done)
Nalfon (Nal'-fon)	Fenoprofen (Fen-o-pro'-fen)
Naprosyn (Na'-pro-sin)	Naproxen (Na-prok'-sen)
Nembutal (Nem'-bu-tal)	Pentobarbital (Pen-to-barb'-i-tal)
Neosynephrine (Nee-o-sin-eh'-frin)	Phenylephrine (Fen-il-eh'-frin)
Nitrobid (Ni'-tro-bid)	Nitroglycerin (Ni-tro-gli'-ser-in)
Nitrol (Ni'-trol)	" "
Nitrostat (Ni-tro-stat)	" "
Noctec (Nok'-tek)	Chloral Hydrate (Klor'-al- Hy'-drate)
Norfiex (Nor'-fleks)	Orphenadrine Citrate (Or-fen'-a-dreen)
Norpace (Nor'-pace)	Disopyramide (Di-so-peer'-a-mide)

Trade Name	Generic Name
Novahistine (No-va-his'-teen) Expectorant	Guaifenesin (Gwi-fen'-eh-sin), Phenylpropanolamine (Fen-il-pro-pan-ol'-a-meen), and Codeine (Ko'-deen)
NTG	Nitroclycerin (Ni-tro-gli'-ser-in)
Nupercainal (New-per-kain'-al)	Dibucaine (Die'-bu-kain)
Oretic (O-ret'-ik)	Hydrochiorothiazide (Hy-dro-kior-thi'-a-zide)
Orinase (Or'-in-ase)	Tolbutamide (Tol-bu'-tah-mide)
Ornade (Or'-nade)	Chlorpheniramine (Klor-fen-ir'-a-meen), Triprolidine (Tri-pro-li-deen) and Pseudoephedrine (Su-do-eh-fed'-rin)
Parafon Forte (Pair'-a-fon For'-tay)	Chlorzoxazone (Klor-zok'-sa-zone)
Percodan (Per'-ko-dan)	Oxycodone (Ok-si-ko'-done)
Periactin (Per-ee-ak'-tin)	Cyproheptadine (Si-pro-hep'-tah-deen)
Persantine (Per-san'-teen)	Dipyridamole (Di-pi-rid'-ah-mole)
Phenobarbital (Feen-o-barb'-it-al)	Same
Phenylpropanolamine (Fen-il-pro-pan-ol'-a-meen)	Same
Pitocin (Pi-tow'-sin)	Oxytocin (Ok-see-tow'-sin)
Pontocaine (Pon'-to-kain)	Tetracaine (Teh'-tra-kain)
Povan (Po'-van)	Pyrvinium (Pire-vin'-ee-um)
Premarin (Prem'-ar-in)	Conjugated (Kon'-joo-gay-ted) Estrogens (Es-tro-jens)
Presamine (Press'-a-meen)	Imipramine (Im-ip'-rah-meen)
Primaquine (Pri'-mah-kwin)	Same
Probanthine (Pro-ban'-theen)	Propantheline (Pro-pan'-the-leen)
Pronestyl (Pro-nes'-til)	Procainamide (Pro-kain'-a-mide)
Prophylthiouracil (Pro-pil-thi-o-u'-rah-sil)	Same
Prostaphlin (Pro-staff'-lin)	Oxacillin (Oks'-ah-sil-in)
Provera (Pro-ver'-ah)	Medroxyprogesterone (Med-rok-see-pro-jes'-ter-one)
Pyridium (Pie-rid'-ee-um)	Phenazopyridine (Fen-ahs-o-per'-i-deen)
Quinidine (Kwin'-i-deen)	Same
Quinine (Kwie'-nine)	Same
Reserpine (Ree-ser'-peen)	Same
Retin A (Reh'-tin A)	Tretinoin (Tret'-i-noin)
Rifadin (Rie-fad'-in)	Rifampin (Rie-fam'-pin)
Riopan (Rie'-o-pan)	Magaidrate (Mag'-al-drate)

Trade Name	Generic Name
Rimactane (Rim-act'-ane)	Rifampin (Rie-fam'-pin)
Ritalin (Rit'-a-lin)	Methylphenidate (Meth-il-fen'-i-date)
Robaxin (Ro-bak'-sin)	Methocarbamol (Meth-o-kar'-ba-mol)
Robitussin (Row-i-tus'-sin)	Guaifenesin (Gwie-fen'-eh-sin)
Robitussin DM	Guiafenesin and Dextromethorphan (Dek-tro-meh-or'-fan)
Sansert (San'-sert)	Methysergide (Meth-ee-ser'-jide)
Seconal (Sek'-o-nal)	Secobarbital (Sek-o-bar'-bi-tal)
Selsun (Sel'-sun)	Selenium (Se-leh'-nee-um)
Septra (Sep'-tra)	Sulfamethoxazole (Sul-fah-meth-oks'-a-zole) and Trimethroprim (Tri-meth'-o-prim)
Serax (See'-raks)	Oxazepam (Oks-az'-eh-pam)
Silvadene (Sil'-va-deen)	Silver Sulfadiazine (Sul-fa-die'-a-zeen)
Sinemet (Si'-ne-met)	Levodopa (Le-vo-do'-pa)
Sinequan (Sin'-a-kwan)	Doxepin (Dok'-seh-pin)
Sorbitrate (Sor'-bi-trate)	Isosorbide (I-so-sor'-bide)
Stelazine (Stel'-a-zeen)	Trifluoperazine(Tri-floo-o-per'-a-zeen)
Sudafed (Soo'-da-fed)	Pseudophedrine (Soo-do-eh-feh'-drin)
Sulamyd (Sul'-a-mid)	Sulfacetamide (Sul-fah-set'-a-mide)
Sulfamylon (Sul-fa-mie'-lon)	Mafenide (Maf'-eh-nide)
Sultrin (Sul'-trin)	Sulfathiazole (Sul-fah-thi'-ah-zole) Sulfacetamide (Sul-fah-set'-ah-mide) and Sulfabenzamide (Sul-fah-benz'-ah-mide)
Surfak (Sur'-fak)	Dioctyl (Di-ok'-til) Calcium (Kal'-see-um) Sulfosuccinate (Sul-fo-suk'-si-nate)
Synalar (Sine'-a-lar)	Fluocinolone (Floo-o-sin'-o-lone)
Synthroid (Sin'-throid)	Levothyroxine (Lee-vo-thi-rok'-sin)
Tace (Tace)	Chlorotrianisene (Klor-o-tri-an'-I-seen)
Tagamet (Tag'-a-met)	Cimetidine (Si-met'-i-deen)
Talwin (Tal'-win)	Pentazocine (Pen-taz'-o-seen)
Tandearil (Tan'-da-ril)	Oxyphenbutazone (Ok-see-fen-bute'-a-zone)
Tegretol (Teg'-reh-tol)	Carbamazepine (Kar-ba-maz'-eh-peen)
Tessalon (Tess'-a-lon)	Benzonatate (Benz-on'-a-tate)
Tetracycline (Tet-ra-si'-kleen)	
Thorazine (Thor'-a-zeen)	Chlorpromazine (Klor-pro'-ma-zeen)
Thyroid (Thy'-roid)	Same
Tigan (Tie'-gan)	Trimethobenzamide (Tri-meth-o-benz'-a-mide)
Timoptic (Tim-op'-tic)	Timilol (Tim'-o-lol)

Trade Name	Generic Name
Tinactin (Tin-act'-in)	Tolnaftate (Tol-naf'-tate)
Titralac (Ti'-tra-lak)	Calcium (Kal-see-um) Carbonate (Kar'-bon-ate) and Glycine (Gly'-seen)
Tofranil (Toe'-fra-nil)	Imipramine (I-mip'-rah-meen)
Tolectin (Tow-lek'-tin)	Tolmetin (Tol-met'-in)
Triavil (Tri'-a-vil)	Perphenazine (Per-fen'-a-zeen) and Amitriptlyline (Am-i-trip'-ti-leen)
Trilafon (Try'-la-fon)	Perphenazine (Per-fen-a-zeen)
Tylenol (Tie'-leh-nol)	Acetaminophen (As-et-am'-ino-fen)
Tylenol #3	Acetaminophen and Codeine (Ko'-deen)
Unipen (U'-ni-pen)	Nafcillin (Naf-sil-lin)
Urecholine (Ur-eh-ko'-leen)	Bethanecol (Beth-an'-eh-kol)
Valisone (Val'-i-sone)	Betamethasone (Beh-tah-meth'-a-sone)
Valium (Val'-ee-um)	Diazepam (Die-aze-eh-pam)
Vermox (Ver'-moks)	Mebendazole (Meh-ben'-dah-zole)
Vibramycin (Vie-bra-my'-sin)	Doxycycline (Doks-see-si'-kleen)
Xylocaine (Zie'-low-kain)	Lidocaine (Lie-do-kain)
Zarontin (Zar-on'-tin)	Ethosuximide (Eh-tho-suks'-a-mide)
Zyloprim (Zie'-low-prim)	Allopurinol (Al-lo-pure'-in-ol)

End of Lesson Annex

LESSON 9   Cholinergic Agents.

TEXT ASSIGNMENT   Paragraphs 9-1 through 9-6.

LESSON OBJECTIVES   After completing this lesson, you should be able to:

9-1. Given a group of statements, select the statement that best describes the term cholinergic agent.

9-2. Given a group of chemical transmitters, select the name of the chemical transmitter that acts at both the preganglionic synapse and the effector organ in relation to the cholinergic nervous system.

9-3. Given the name of a part of the body and a group of effects, select the effect(s) produced on that part of the body by the cholinergic nervous system.

9-4. Given the name of one of the types of cholinergic agents and a group of statements, select the statement that best describes that type of agent.

9-5. From a group of statements, select the statement that best describes the difference between reversible cholinesterase inhibitors and irreversible cholinesterase inhibitors.

9-6. Given the trade and/or generic name of a cholinergic agent and a group of indications/uses cautions and warnings, side effects, or patient warning statements, select the indication/use, caution and warning, side effect, or patient warning statement that applies to that drug.

9-7. Given the trade or generic name of a cholinergic drug and a group of trade and/or generic names of drugs, select the trade or generic name of the given drug.

SUGGESTION   After studying the assignment, complete the exercises at the end of this lesson. These exercises will help you to achieve the lesson objectives.

LESSON 9

CHOLINERGIC AGENTS

9-1. INTRODUCTION

Cholinergic (parasympathomimetic) agents are drugs which when administered will mimic the action of acetylcholine or normal parasympathetic stimulation. As you will remember (lesson 6), the parasympathetic nervous system is responsible for bringing the body back to normal after the fight or flight response. The parasympathetic (cholinergic) nervous system is responsible for maintaining the daily functions performed within the body. This division of the autonomic nervous system serves to conserve energy.

9-2. REVIEW OF THE PHYSIOLOGY OF THE CHOLINERGIC PARASYMPATHETIC) NERVOUS SYSTEM

The cholinergic (parasympathetic) nervous system is stimulated by the hypothalamus. This nervous system has long preganglionic fibers and short postganglionic fibers (see Figure 9-1). The short postganglionic fibers are usually located within the effector organ.

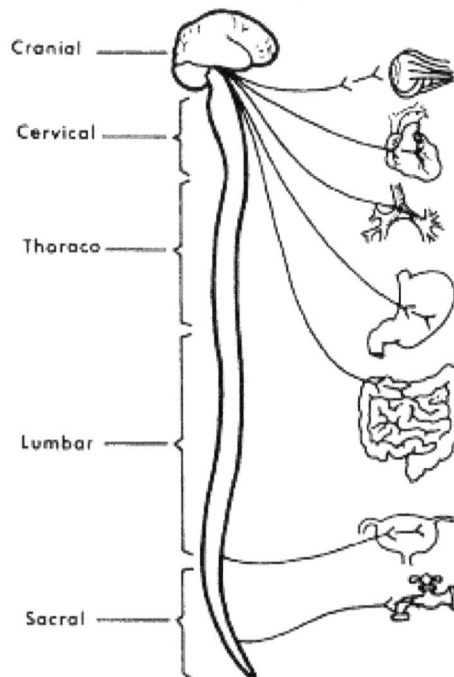

Figure 9-1. The cholinergic (parasympathetic) nervous system.

9-3. CHEMICAL TRANSMISSION IN THE CHOLINERGIC (PARASYMPATHETIC) NERVOUS SYSTEM

The chemical transmitter at both the preganglionic synapse and at the effector organ is acetylcholine. Transmission of impulses is terminated by the destruction of acetylcholine by the enzyme acetylcholinesterase.

9-4. EFFECTS PRODUCED BY THE CHOLINERGIC NERVOUS SYSTEM

The general effects of parasympathetic stimulation are conservation and restoration of energy. The specific effects of the cholinergic nervous system are listed below:

a. **Eye (Pupil).** Contraction of the pupil (miosis) is produced by cholinergic stimulation.

b. **Heart.** A decrease in the heart rate and a slight increase in the contraction strength of the heart are cholinergic effects.

c. **Bronchi.** The bronchi are contracted by cholinergic stimulation.

d. **Blood Vessels.** The blood vessels of the skin and mucosa and skeletal muscles are dilated by stimulation by the cholinergic nervous system.

e. **Salivary Glands.** Cholinergic stimulation of the salivary glands leads to profuse, watery secretions.

f. **Stomach.** Cholinergic stimulation of the stomach leads to increased motility and tone and relaxed (usually) sphincters.

g. **Intestines.** Increased intestinal motility and tone and stimulated secretion of intestinal fluids are products of cholinergic stimulation.

h. **Urinary Bladder.** Contraction of the bladder wall and relaxation of the sphincter are products of cholinergic stimulation. The result is that urination is stimulated.

9-5. THERAPEUTIC USE OF CHOLINERGIC AGENTS

The cholinergic (parasympathomimetic) agents mimic the action of acetylcholine. These drugs represent a relatively small class of therapeutic agents with very specific clinical indications. For the most part, cholinergic agents are used in the treatment of glaucoma (see lesson 5) and in the treatment of certain urinary tract disorders (they help produce urination and the emptying of the bladder).

9-6. TYPES OF CHOLINERGIC AGENTS

a. **Direct Acting Agents.** Direct acting drugs have molecules that resemble acetylcholine molecules; thus, they have a direct action on the acetylcholine receptor sites of the postganglionic synapse. These drugs are usually specific in their site of action. An example of a direct acting agent is pilocarpine hydrochloride (Isopto-Carpine®).

(1) <u>Pilocarpine hydrochloride (Isopto-Carpine®).</u> Pilocarpine hydrochloride is a direct acting parasympathomimetic. It is used in the treatment of glaucoma. It causes the contraction of the iris sphincter muscle; this results in miosis (pupil constriction). Pilocarpine can produce the following side effects: muscle tremors, unusual increase in perspiration, unusual watering of the mouth, blurred vision, and eye pain. The patient instilling this medication into the eye should be informed that the drug could cause a change in his near or distant vision. Therefore, he should ensure that his vision is clear before he drives or does any jobs that require him to see well.

(2) <u>Bethanecol chloride (Urecholine®).</u> Bethanecol chloride is a direct acting parasympathomimetic. It is used in the treatment of non-obstructive urinary retention. Bethanecol can produce side effects such as shortness of breath, blurred vision, and dizziness. This drug should not be administered to patients who have bronchial asthma. Patients should be instructed to take the drug on an empty stomach (one or two hours before meals) in order to decrease the probability of having stomach upset.

b. **Indirect Acting Agents**. Indirect acting agents alter or inhibit the activity of acetylcholinesterase. Since the activity of acetylcholinesterase is inhibited or altered, the acetylcholine levels will increase causing cholinergic activity. The indirect acting agents form a complex with acetylcholinesterase. Based upon the type of complex they form, the agents are placed into two groups:

(1) <u>Reversible cholinesterase inhibitors</u>. These agents form a temporary complex with acetylcholinesterase.

(a) Neostigmine (Prostigmin®). Neostigmine is a reversible indirect acting acetylcholinesterase inhibitor. This drug is used in the treatment of myasthenia gravis, a condition characterized by muscle weakness and fatigue. The drug is also used to treat urinary bladder atony. Side effects associated with this agent are diarrhea, abdominal cramps, increased salivation, and increased bronchial secretions.

(b) Physostigmine (Eserine®). Physostigmine is a reversible indirect acting acetylcholinesterase inhibitor. It is used in the treatment of glaucoma. Side effects associated with the use of physostigmine include loss of bladder control, muscle weakness, unusual increase in perspiration, blurred vision or change in distant vision, and headache. The patient using this medication should be warned that it can cause a change in near or distant vision; therefore, the patient should ensure that his vision is clear before he drives or performs any job which requires that he see well.

(2) Irreversible cholinesterase inhibitors. These agents form a stable complex with acetylcholinesterase.

(a) Echothiophate Iodide (Phospholine Iodide®). Echothiophate iodide is an irreversible indirect acting acetylcholinesterase inhibitor. It is used in the treatment of glaucoma. The side effects associated with echothiophate include loss of bladder control, muscle weakness, and shortness of breath. You should note that this medication is supplied as a dry powder with diluent. The diluent and the dry powder must be mixed just before you dispense it. The shelf life of the prepared solution can be extended by refrigeration. Since echothiophate may cause changes in the patient's vision, the patient should be warned to insure his vision is clear before he drives or performs any job that requires him to have clear vision.

(b) Demecarium bromide (Humorsol®). Demecarium bromide is an irreversible, indirect acting acetylcholinesterase inhibitor. It is used in the treatment of glaucoma. Side effects that can occur while taking this medication include loss of bladder control, muscle weakness, and shortness of breath. Since this medication may cause changes in the patient's vision, the patient should be warned to ensure his vision is clear before he drives or performs any job which requires him to have clear vision.

Continue with Exercises

EXERCISES, LESSON 9

INSTRUCTIONS: Answer the following exercises by marking the lettered response which best answers the question.

After you have completed all the exercises, turn to "Solutions to Exercises" at the end of the lesson and check your answers. For each exercise answered incorrectly, reread the material referenced with the solution.

1. Which statement best describes the term cholinergic agent?

    a. Drugs which when administered will mimic the action of epinephrine or normal parasympathetic stimulation.

    b. Drugs which when administered will mimic the action of acetylcholine or normal parasympathetic stimulation.

    c. Drugs that produce the same effects as the adrenergic blocking drug.

    d. Drugs that antagonize the effects of the adrenergic nervous system.

2. Select the effect of cholinergic stimulation upon the eye (pupil).

    a. No effect.

    b. Mydriasis.

    c. Miosis.

3. Select the effect of cholinergic stimulation on the bronchi.

    a. No effect.

    b. Dilation.

    c. Contraction.

4. Select the effect of cholinergic stimulation on the urinary bladder.

   a. No effect.

   b. Urination is stimulated.

   c. Urination is suppressed.

5. Which statement best describes direct acting cholinergic agents?

   a. These agents alter or inhibit the activity of acetylcholinesterase.

   b. These agents form a complex with acetylcholinesterase thus producing cholinergic activity.

   c. These agents reduce the activity of epinephrine in order to enhance the effects of cholinergic stimulation.

   d. These agents have molecules that resemble acetylcholine molecules and produce action on the acetylcholine receptor sites of the postganglionic synapse.

6. Pilocarpine hydrochloride is used in the treatment of:

   a. Nonobstructive urinary retention.

   b. Glaucoma.

   c. Myasthenia gravis.

   d. Obstructive urinary retention.

7. Neostigmine (Prostigmine®) is used in the treatment of:

   a. Nonobstructive urinary retention.

   b. Glaucoma.

   c. Myasthenia gravis.

   d. Obstructive urinary retention.

8. Select the side effect(s) associated with the use of physostigmine.

    a. Loss of bladder control.

    b. Unusual decrease in perspiration.

    c. Dryness of the mouth and other mucous membranes.

    d. All the above.

9. Match the trade or generic name in Column A with its appropriate trade or generic name in Column B.

Column A	Column B
_____ Urecholine®	a. Physostigmine
_____ Demecarium bromide	b. Echothiophate iodide
_____ Phospholine iodide®	c. Bethanecol chloride
_____ Eserine®	d. Floropryl®
	e. Humorsol®
	f. Pilocarpine hydrochloride
	g. Isopto-Carpine®

Check Your Answers on Next Page

SOLUTIONS TO EXERCISES, LESSON 9

1. b   Drugs which when administered will mimic the action of acetylcholine or normal parasympathetic stimulation. (para 9-1)

2. c   Miosis. (para 9-4a)

3. c   Contraction. (para 9-4c)

4. b   Urination is stimulated. (para 9-4h)

5. d   These agents have molecules which resemble acetylcholine molecules and produce action on the acetylcholine receptor sites of the postganglionic synapse. (para 9-6a)

6. b   Glaucoma. (para 9-6a(1))

7. c   Myasthenia gravis. (para 9-6b(1)(a))

8. a   Loss of bladder control. (para 9-6b(1)(b))

9. c   Urecholine®. (para 9-6a(2))

   e   Demecarium bromide. (para 9-6b(2)(b))

   b   Phospholine iodide®. (para 9-6b(2)(a))

   a   Eserine®. (para 9-6b(1)(b))

End of Lesson 9

ANNEX

DRUG PRONUNCIATION GUIDE

This Drug Pronunciation Guide was developed to help you to learn how the trade and generic names of commonly prescribed medications are frequently pronounced. Not all the drugs in the guide are discussed in this subcourse. Remember, it is not enough to be able to know the uses, indications, cautions and warnings, and contraindications for a drug--you must also know how to pronounce that drug's name.

Trade Name	*Generic Name*
Actifed (Ak'-ti-fed)	Triprolidine (Tri-pro'-li-deen) and Pseudoephedrine (Soo-do-e-fed'-rin)
Adapin (Ad'-a-pin)	Doxepin (Dok'-se-pin)
Sinequan (Sin'-a-kwan)	" "
Afrin (Af'-rin)	Oxymetazoline (Ok-see-met-az'-o-leen)
Aldactazide (Al-dak'-ta-zide)	Spironolactone (Spi-ro-no-lak'-tone) and Hydrochlorothiazide (Hy-dro-klor-thi'-a-zide)
Aldactone (Al-dak'-tone)	Spironolactone (Spi-ro-no-lak'-tone)
Aldomet (Al'-do-met)	Methyldopa (Meth-il-do'-pah)
Alupent (Al'-u-pent)	Metaproterenol (Met-a-pro-ter'-eh-nol)
Amoxil (Am-ok'-sil)	Amoxicillin (Ah-moks'-i-sil-in)
Amphojel (Am'-fo-jel)	Aluminum (Al-loo'-mi-num) Hydroxide (Hy-drok'-side)
Ampicillin (Amp'-I-sil-in)	Same
Antepar (Ab'-te-par)	Piperazine (Pi-per'-ah-zeen)
Anturane (An'-tu-rain)	Sulfinpyrazone (Sul-fin-pie'-ra-zone)
Anusol (An'-u-sol)	Pramoxine (Pram-ok'-seen)
Apresoline (A-press'-o-leen)	Hydralazine (Hy-dral'-ah-zeen)
Aralen (Ar'-a-len)	Chloroquine (Klor'-o-kwin)
Aristocort (A-ris'-to-cort)	Triamcinolone (Tri-am-sin'-o-lone)
Artane (Ar'-tane)	Trihexyphenidyl(Tri-hek-see-fen'-i-dil)
A.S.A.	Aspirin (As'-per-in)
Atromid S (A'-tro-mid)	Clofibrate (Klo-fi'-brate)
Avlosulfon (Av-lo-sul'-fon)	Dapsone (Dap'-sone)
Azolid (Az'-o-lid)	Phenylbutazone (Fen-il-bute'-a-zone)
Bactrim (Bak'-trim)	Sulfamethoxazole (Sul-fah-meth-oks'-ah-zole) and Trimethoprim (Tri-meth'-o-prim)
Bellergal (Bel'-er-gal)	Ergotamine (Er-got'-a-meen), Phenobarbital (Feen-o-bar'-bi-tal) and Belladonna (Bel-la-don'-na) Alkaloids
Benadryl (Ben'-a-dril)	Diphenhydramine (Di-fen-hy'-dra-meen)

Trade Name	Generic Name
Bendectin (Ben-dek'-tin)	Doxylamine (Dok-sil'-a-meen)
Benemid (Ben'-eh-mid)	Probenecid (Pro-ben'-eh-sid)
Bonine (Bo'-neen)	Meclizine (Mek'-li-zeen)
Cafergot (Kaf'-er-got)	Ergotamine (Er-got'-a-meen) and Caffeine (Kaf'-feen)
Calamine (Kal'-a-mine)	Same
Catapres (Kat'-a-press)	Clonidine (Klo'-ni-deen)
CeeNu (See'-new)	Lomustine (Lo-mus'-teen)
Chlor-Trimeton (Klo-tri '-meh-ton)	Chlorpheniramine (Klor-fen-it'-a-meen)
Clomid (Klo'-mid)	Clomiphene (Klo'-mi-feen)
Clonopin (Klo-o-pin)	Clonazepam (Klo-na'-ze-pam)
Codeine (Ko'-deen)	Same
Cogentin (Ko-jen'-tin)	Benztropine (Benz'-tro-peen)
Colace (Ko'-lace)	Dioctyl(Di-ok'-til) Sodium (So'-dee-um) Sulfosuccinate (Sul-fo-suk'-si-nate)
Colchicine (Kol'-chi-seen)	Same
Compazine (Kom'-pa-zeen)	Prochiorperazine (Pro-klor-per'-a-zeen)
Cordran (Kor'-dran)	Flurandrenolide (Floor-an-dren'-o-lide)
Coumadin (Koo'-mah-din)	Warfarin (War'-fah-rin)
CP	Cloroquine (Klor'-o-kwin) and Primaquine (Prim'-a-kwin)
Cyclogyl (Si'-klo-jel)	Cyclopentolate (Si-klo-pen'-to-late)
Cytomel (Si'-to-mel)	Liothyronine (Li-o-thy-ro-neen)
Cytoxan (Si-tok'-san)	Cyclophosphamide (Si-klo-fos'-fa-mide)
Dalmane (Dal '-mane)	Flurazepam (Floor-az'-e-pam)
Darvocet (Dar'-vo-set)	Propoxyphene (Pro-pok'-se-feen) and Acetaminopen (As-et-am'-ino-fen)
Darvon (Dar'-von)	Propoxyphene (Pro-pok-se-feen)
Decadron (Dek'-a-dron)	Dexamethasone (Dek-sa-meth'-ah-sone)
Deltasone (Del '-ta-sone)	Prednisone (Pred'-ni-sone)
Demerol (Dem'-er-ol)	Meperidine (Meh-pair'-i-deen)
Dexedrine (Deks '-eh-dreen)	Dextroamphetamine (Deks-tro-am-fet'-a-meen)
Diabinese (Di-ab'-i-nees)	Chlorpropamide (Klor-prop'-a-mide)
Diethylstilbestrol (Di-eth-il-stil-bes'-trol)	Same
Dilantin (Di-lan'-tin)	Phenytoin (Fen'-i-toin)
Dilaudid (Di-law'-did)	Hydromorphone (Hy-dro-more' -fon)
Dimetane (Di'-meh-tane)	Brompheniramine (Brom-fen-ir'-a-meen)

Trade Name	Generic Name
Dimetapp (Di'-meh-tap)	Brompheniramine (Brom-fen-ir'-a-meen) Phenylephrine (Fen-il-ef'-rin) and Phenylpropanolamine (Fen-il-pro-pan-ol'-a-meen)
Disophrol (Dice'-o-frol)	Dexbrompheniramine (Deks-brom-fen-ir'-a-meen) and Pseudoephedrine (Soo-do-e-fed'-rin)
Dolophine (Dol'-o-feen)	Methadone (Meth'-a-done)
Domeboro (Dome-bor'-o)	Aluminum (Ah-loo'-mi-num) Acetate (As'-e-tate)
Donnatal (Don'-na-tal)	Belladonna (Bel-la-don'-na) Alkaloids (Al'-ka-loids) and Phenobarbital (Feen-o-barb'-i-tal)
Doxidan (Dok'-si-dan)	Danthron (Dan'-thron) and Dicctyl (Di-ok'-til) Calcium (Kal'-see-um) Sulfosuccinate (Sul-fo-suk'-si-nate)
Drixoral (Driks'-or-al)	Dexbrompheniramine (Deks-brom-fen-ir'-a-meen) and Pseudoephedrine (Soo-do-e-fed'-rin)
Dulcolax (Dul'-ko-laks)	Bisacodyl (Bis-a'-ko-dil)
Dyazine (Di'-a-zide)	Triamterene (Tri-am'-ter-een) and Hydrochlorothiazide (Hy-dro-klor-o-thi'-a-zide)
Dymelor (Die'-meh-lor)	Acetohexamide (As-e-to-heks'-a-mide)
Dyrenium (Die-ren'-i-um)	Triamterene (Tri-am'-ter-een)
Efudex (Ef'-u-deks)	Fluorouracil (Floo-ro-ur'-ah-sil)
Elavil (El'-ah-vil)	Amitriptyline (Am-i-trip'-til-een)
Elixir Terpin (Ter'-pin) Hydrate	Same
Empirin (Em'-per-in)	Codeine (Ko'-deen) and Aspirin (As'-per-in)
E-Mycin (E-mie'-sin)	Erythromycin (E-rith-ro-mie'-sin)
Equanil (Ek'-wa-nil)	Meprobamate (Me-pro-bam'-ate)
Ergomar (Er'-go-mar)	Ergotamine (Er-got'-a-meen)
Ergotrate (Er'-go-trate)	Ergonovine (Er-go-no'-veen)
Erythrocin (Er-eeth'-ro-sin)	Erythromycin (Er-eeth-ro-my'-sin) Stearate (Stare'-rate)
Esidrix (Es'-i-driks)	Hyrochlorothiazide (Hy-dro-klor-o-thi'-a-zide)
Feosol (Fe'-o-sol)	Ferrous (Fer'-rus) Sulfate (Sul'-fate)
Fergon (Fer'-gon)	Ferrous (Fer'-rus) Gluconate (Glu'-con-ate)

Trade Name	Generic Name
Fiorinal (Fee-or'-i-nal)	Butalbital (Bu-tal'-bi-tal), Apririn, Phenacetin (Fen-ass'-eh-tin), and Caffeine (Kaf'-feen)
Flagyl (Fla'-jil)	Metronidazole (Me-tro-ni'-dah-zole)
Flexeril (Flek'-sa-ril)	Cyclobenzaprine (Si-klo-benz'-a-preen)
Fulvicin (Ful'-vi-sin)	Griseofulvin (Griz-e-o-ful'-vin)
Guantanol (Gan'-ta-nol)	Suiphamethoxazole (Sul-fah-meth-oks'-ah-zole)
Gantrisin (Gan'-tri-sin)	Sulfisoxazole (Sul-fi-sok'-sah-zole)
Gelusil (Jel'-u-sil)	Aluminum (Ah-loo'-mi-num) Hydroxide (Hy-drok'-side) and Magnesium (Mag-nee'-zee-um) Hydroxide
Grifulvin (Gri-ful'-vin)	Griseofulvin (Griz-e-o-ful'-vin)
Gynergen (Jin'-er-jen)	Ergotamine (Er-got'-a-meen)
Haldol (Hal'-dol)	Haloperidol (Hal-o-pair'-i-dol)
Halotestin (Hal-o-tes'-tin)	Fluoxymesterone (Floo-ok-see-mes-teh-rone)
Hexadrol (Hek'-sa-drol)	Dexamethasone (Dek-sa-meth'-a-sone)
Hydrodiuril (Hy-dro-di'-ur-il)	Hydroclorothiazide (Hy-dro-kior-thi'-a-zide)
Hygroton (Hy-grow'-ton)	Chiorthalidone (Kior-thal'-i-done)
Ilosone (I'-low-sone)	Erythromycin (Er-ith-ro-mi'-sin) Estolate (Es'-to-late)
Inderal (In'-der-al)	Propranolol (Pro-pran'-o-lol)
Indocin (In'-do-sin)	Indomethacin (In-do-meth'-a-sin)
INH	Isoniazid (I-so-ni'-a-zid)
Insulin (In'-sul-in)	Same
Intal	Cromolyn (Kro'-mo-lin)
Ismelin (Is'-meh-lin)	Guanethidine (Gwan-eth'-i-dine)
Isopto-Atropine (I-sop-to-at'-ro-peen)	Atropine (At'-ro-peen)
Isopto-Carpine (I-sop-to-car'-peen)	Pilocarpine (Pile-o-car'-peen)
Isordil (I'-sor-dil)	Isosorbide (I-so-sor'-bide)
Keflex (Kef'-lex)	Cephalexin (Sef-ah-lek'-sin)
Lanoxin (Lan-ok'-sin)	Digoxin (Di-jok'-sin)
Larodopa (Lar-o-do'-pa)	Levodopa (Le-o-do'-pa)
Larotid (Lar'-o-tid)	Amoxicillin (Ah-moks'-i-sil-in)
Lasix (La'-siks)	Furosemide (Fu-ro'-se-mide)
Leukeran (Lu'-ker-an)	Chlorambucil (Klor-ram'-bu-sil)
Librium (Lib'-ree-um)	Chlordiazepoxide (Klor-die-az-eh-pok'-side)

Trade Name	Generic Name
Lidex (Lie'-deks)	Fluocinoide (Floo-o-sin'-o-nide)
Lomotil (Lo'-mo-til)	Diphenoxylate (Die-fen-ok'-si-late)
Lopressor (Lo'-pres-sor)	Metoprolol (Met-o-pro'-lol)
Lotrimin (Lo'-tri-min)	Chlotrimazole (Klo-trim'-ah-zole)
Maalox (May'-loks)	Aluminum (Ah-loo'-mi-num) and Magnesium (Mag-nee'-zee-um) Hydroxides
Macrodanton (Ma-kro-dan'-tin)	Nitrofurantoin (Ni-tro-fur-an'-toin)
Mandelamine (Man-del'-a-meen)	Methenamine (Meth-en'-a-meen) Mandelate (Man'-deh-late)
Medihaler-Iso (Med-i-hail-er-I'-so)	Isoproterenol (I-so-pro-ter'-en-ol)
Mellaril (Mel'-la-ril)	Thioridazine (Thi-o-rid'-a-zeen)
Metamucil (Met-a-mu'-sil)	Psyllium (Sil'-e-um)
Metaprel (Meh'-ta-prel)	Metaproterenol (Meh'-ta-pro-ter'-eh-nol)
Methotrexate (Meth-o-treks'-ate)	Amethopterin (Ah-meth-op'-ter-in)
Milk of Magnesia	Same
Minipress (Min'-i-press)	Prazosin (Pra'-zo-sin)
Minocin (Min'-o-sin)	Minocycline (Mi-no-si'-kleen)
Monistat (Mon'-i-stat)	Miconazole (Mi-kon'-ah-zole)
Motrin (Mo'-trin)	Ibuprofen (I-bu'-pro-fen)
Myambutol (My-am'-bu-tol)	Ethambutol (Eth-am'-bu-tol)
Mycostatin (My-co-stat'-in)	Nystatin (Ny-stat'-in)
Mylanta (My-lan'-ta)	Aluminum (Ah-loo'-mi-num) and Magnesium (Mag-nee'-zee-um) Hydroxides and Simethicone (Si-meth'-i-kone)
Myleran (My-ler-an)	Busulfan (Bu-sul'-fan)
Mylicon (My'-li-kon)	Simethicone (Si-meth'-i-kone)
Mysoline (My'-so-leen)	Primidone (Pri'-mi-done)
Nalfon (Nal'-fon)	Fenoprofen (Fen-o-pro'-fen)
Naprosyn (Na'-pro-sin)	Naproxen (Na-prok'-sen)
Nembutal (Nem'-bu-tal)	Pentobarbital (Pen-to-barb'-i-tal)
Neosynephrine (Nee-o-sin-eh'-frin)	Phenylephrine (Fen-il-eh'-frin)
Nitrobid (Ni'-tro-bid)	Nitroglycerin (Ni-tro-gli'-ser-in)
Nitrol (Ni'-trol)	" "
Nitrostat (Ni-tro-stat)	" "
Noctec (Nok'-tek)	Chloral Hydrate (Klor'-al- Hy'-drate)
Norfiex (Nor'-fleks)	Orphenadrine Citrate (Or-fen'-a-dreen)
Norpace (Nor'-pace)	Disopyramide (Di-so-peer'-a-mide)

Trade Name	Generic Name
Novahistine (No-va-his'-teen) Expectorant	Guaifenesin (Gwi-fen'-eh-sin), Phenylpropanolamine (Fen-il-pro-pan-ol'-a-meen), and Codeine (Ko'-deen)
NTG	Nitroclycerin (Ni-tro-gli'-ser-in)
Nupercainal (New-per-kain'-al)	Dibucaine (Die'-bu-kain)
Oretic (O-ret'-ik)	Hydrochiorothiazide (Hy-dro-kior-thi'-a-zide)
Orinase (Or'-in-ase)	Tolbutamide (Tol-bu'-tah-mide)
Ornade (Or'-nade)	Chlorpheniramine (Klor-fen-ir'-a-meen), Triprolidine (Tri-pro-li-deen) and Pseudoephedrine (Su-do-eh-fed'-rin)
Parafon Forte (Pair'-a-fon For'-tay)	Chlorzoxazone (Klor-zok'-sa-zone)
Percodan (Per'-ko-dan)	Oxycodone (Ok-si-ko'-done)
Periactin (Per-ee-ak'-tin)	Cyproheptadine (Si-pro-hep'-tah-deen)
Persantine (Per-san'-teen)	Dipyridamole (Di-pi-rid'-ah-mole)
Phenobarbital (Feen-o-barb'-it-al)	Same
Phenylpropanolamine (Fen-il-pro-pan-ol'-a-meen)	Same
Pitocin (Pi-tow'-sin)	Oxytocin (Ok-see-tow'-sin)
Pontocaine (Pon'-to-kain)	Tetracaine (Teh'-tra-kain)
Povan (Po'-van)	Pyrvinium (Pire-vin'-ee-um)
Premarin (Prem'-ar-in)	Conjugated (Kon'-joo-gay-ted) Estrogens (Es-tro-jens)
Presamine (Press'-a-meen)	Imipramine (Im-ip'-rah-meen)
Primaquine (Pri'-mah-kwin)	Same
Probanthine (Pro-ban'-theen)	Propantheline (Pro-pan'-the-leen)
Pronestyl (Pro-nes'-til)	Procainamide (Pro-kain'-a-mide)
Prophylthiouracil (Pro-pil-thi-o-u'-rah-sil)	Same
Prostaphlin (Pro-staff'-lin)	Oxacillin (Oks'-ah-sil-in)
Provera (Pro-ver'-ah)	Medroxyprogesterone (Med-rok-see-pro-jes'-ter-one)
Pyridium (Pie-rid'-ee-um)	Phenazopyridine (Fen-ahs-o-per'-i-deen)
Quinidine (Kwin'-i-deen)	Same
Quinine (Kwie'-nine)	Same
Reserpine (Ree-ser'-peen)	Same
Retin A (Reh'-tin A)	Tretinoin (Tret'-i-noin)
Rifadin (Rie-fad'-in)	Rifampin (Rie-fam'-pin)
Riopan (Rie'-o-pan)	Magaidrate (Mag'-al-drate)

Trade Name	Generic Name
Rimactane (Rim-act'-ane)	Rifampin (Rie-fam'-pin)
Ritalin (Rit'-a-lin)	Methylphenidate (Meth-il-fen'-i-date)
Robaxin (Ro-bak'-sin)	Methocarbamol (Meth-o-kar'-ba-mol)
Robitussin (Row-i-tus'-sin)	Guaifenesin (Gwie-fen'-eh-sin)
Robitussin DM	Guiafenesin and Dextromethorphan (Dek-tro-meh-or'-fan)
Sansert (San'-sert)	Methysergide (Meth-ee-ser'-jide)
Seconal (Sek'-o-nal)	Secobarbital (Sek-o-bar'-bi-tal)
Selsun (Sel'-sun)	Selenium (Se-leh'-nee-um)
Septra (Sep'-tra)	Sulfamethoxazole (Sul-fah-meth-oks'-a-zole) and Trimethroprim (Tri-meth'-o-prim)
Serax (See'-raks)	Oxazepam (Oks-az'-eh-pam)
Silvadene (Sil'-va-deen)	Silver Sulfadiazine (Sul-fa-die'-a-zeen)
Sinemet (Si'-ne-met)	Levodopa (Le-vo-do'-pa)
Sinequan (Sin'-a-kwan)	Doxepin (Dok'-seh-pin)
Sorbitrate (Sor'-bi-trate)	Isosorbide (I-so-sor'-bide)
Stelazine (Stel'-a-zeen)	Trifluoperazine(Tri-floo-o-per'-a-zeen)
Sudafed (Soo'-da-fed)	Pseudophedrine (Soo-do-eh-feh'-drin)
Sulamyd (Sul'-a-mid)	Sulfacetamide (Sul-fah-set'-a-mide)
Sulfamylon (Sul-fa-mie'-lon)	Mafenide (Maf'-eh-nide)
Sultrin (Sul'-trin)	Sulfathiazole (Sul-fah-thi'-ah-zole) Sulfacetamide (Sul-fah-set'-ah-mide) and Sulfabenzamide (Sul-fah-benz'-ah-mide)
Surfak (Sur'-fak)	Dioctyl (Di-ok'-til) Calcium (Kal'-see-um) Sulfosuccinate (Sul-fo-suk'-si-nate)
Synalar (Sine'-a-lar)	Fluocinolone (Floo-o-sin'-o-lone)
Synthroid (Sin'-throid)	Levothyroxine (Lee-vo-thi-rok'-sin)
Tace (Tace)	Chlorotrianisene (Klor-o-tri-an'-l-seen)
Tagamet (Tag'-a-met)	Cimetidine (Si-met'-i-deen)
Talwin (Tal'-win)	Pentazocine (Pen-taz'-o-seen)
Tandearil (Tan'-da-ril)	Oxyphenbutazone (Ok-see-fen-bute'-a-zone)
Tegretol (Teg'-reh-tol)	Carbamazepine (Kar-ba-maz'-eh-peen)
Tessalon (Tess'-a-lon)	Benzonatate (Benz-on'-a-tate)
Tetracycline (Tet-ra-si'-kleen)	
Thorazine (Thor'-a-zeen)	Chlorpromazine (Klor-pro'-ma-zeen)
Thyroid (Thy'-roid)	Same
Tigan (Tie'-gan)	Trimethobenzamide (Tri-meth-o-benz'-a-mide)
Timoptic (Tim-op'-tic)	Timilol (Tim'-o-lol)

Trade Name	Generic Name
Tinactin (Tin-act'-in)	Tolnaftate (Tol-naf'-tate)
Titralac (Ti'-tra-lak)	Calcium (Kal-see-um) Carbonate (Kar'-bon-ate) and Glycine (Gly'-seen)
Tofranil (Toe'-fra-nil)	Imipramine (I-mip'-rah-meen)
Tolectin (Tow-lek'-tin)	Tolmetin (Tol-met'-in)
Triavil (Tri'-a-vil)	Perphenazine (Per-fen'-a-zeen) and Amitriptlyline (Am-i-trip'-ti-leen)
Trilafon (Try'-la-fon)	Perphenazine (Per-fen-a-zeen)
Tylenol (Tie'-leh-nol)	Acetaminophen (As-et-am'-ino-fen)
Tylenol #3	Acetaminophen and Codeine (Ko'-deen)
Unipen (U'-ni-pen)	Nafcillin (Naf-sil-lin)
Urecholine (Ur-eh-ko'-leen)	Bethanecol (Beth-an'-eh-kol)
Valisone (Val'-i-sone)	Betamethasone (Beh-tah-meth'-a-sone)
Valium (Val'-ee-um)	Diazepam (Die-aze-eh-pam)
Vermox (Ver'-moks)	Mebendazole (Meh-ben'-dah-zole)
Vibramycin (Vie-bra-my'-sin)	Doxycycline (Doks-see-si'-kleen)
Xylocaine (Zie'-low-kain)	Lidocaine (Lie-do-kain)
Zarontin (Zar-on'-tin)	Ethosuximide (Eh-tho-suks'-a-mide)
Zyloprim (Zie'-low-prim)	Allopurinol (Al-lo-pure'-in-ol)

End of Lesson 9 Annex

LESSON 10   Cholinergic Blocking Agents (Anticholinergic Agents).

TEXT ASSIGNMENT   Paragraphs 10-1--10-4.

LESSON OBJECTIVES   After completing this lesson, you should be able to:

10-1. From a list of statements, select the statement that best describes how the cholinergic blocking agents produce their effects.

10-2. Given a group of drug categories, select the alternate name sometimes given to cholinergic blocking agents.

10-3. Given the name of a part of the body and a list of pharmacological effects, select the effect of the cholinergic blocking agents on that part.

10-4. Given a list of clinical uses, select the clinical use(s) of the cholinergic blocking agents.

10-5. Given the trade and/or generic name of cholinergic blocking agent and a group of uses, side effects, cautions and warnings, or instructions to the patient, select the use(s), side effect(s), caution(s) and warning(s), and instruction(s) to the patient which are specific to the given drug.

10-6. Given the trade or generic name of a cholinergic blocking agent and a list of trade and/or generic names of drugs, select the trade or generic name for the given drug.

SUGGESTION   After studying the assignment, complete the exercises at the end of this lesson. These exercises will help you to achieve the lesson objectives.

LESSON 10

CHOLINERGIC BLOCKING AGENTS (ANTICHOLINERGIC AGENTS)

10-1. INTRODUCTION

In the last lesson, the topic of cholinergic agents was discussed. Now the topic of cholinergic blocking agents (anticholinergic agents) will be discussed. Cholinergic blocking agents block or reduce normal parasympathetic innervation at the postganglionic synapse (see Figure 10-1). Drugs in this category are sometimes referred to as parasympatholytics.

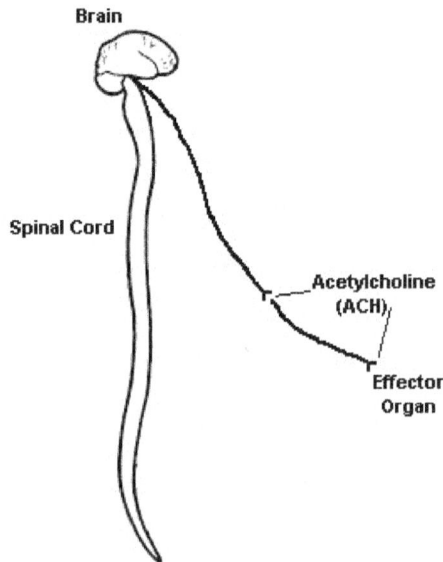

Figure 10-1. The postganglionic synapse--the site of action of the cholinergic blocking agents.

10-2. PHARMACOLOGICAL EFFECTS OF THE CHOLINERGIC BLOCKERS

The cholinergic blockers produce specific effects on certain organs in the body. These effects are:

a. **Stomach/Intestines**. The effect of the cholinergic blockers on the stomach and intestines is decreased activity.

b. **Salivary Glands**. The cholinergic blockers produce a drying effect.

c. **Eye (Pupil).** The cholinergic blockers produce dilation of the pupil (mydriasis).

d. **Urinary Bladder**. The cholinergic blockers produce urinary retention.

e. **Heart**. Increased heart rate is the effect produced on the heart by the cholinergic blockers.

f. **Bronchi.** The cholinergic blockers dilate the bronchi.

10-3. CLINICAL USES OF THE CHOLINERGIC BLOCKERS

The clinical uses of these drugs are based upon their normal pharmacological actions. Their most common clinical uses are listed below:

a. **Antispasmodics**. Antispasmodics are used to slow the motility of the gastrointestinal (GI) tract and reduce gastric secretions. Antispasmodics are commonly prescribed with other types of medications for patients who have ulcers or other GI disorders.

b. **Mydriatics/Cycloplegics.** These agents are used to produce pupil dilation (mydriasis) and to paralyze the muscles of accommodation (cycloplegia). In other words, these drugs prevent the eye from focusing. Medications used for these purposes are commonly used following ocular surgery and for certain types of eye examinations.

c. **Antiparkinsonism Agents**. These drugs are used to treat Parkinsonism, a condition characterized by excessive cholinergic activity in the brain. This condition results in an inability to perform fine motor movements.

d. **Cold Preparations**. Many over-the-counter and legend cold preparations contain cholinergic blocking agents. These cholinergic blockers help to dry secretions (that is, help to "dry" a runny nose).

e. **Antidote for Nerve Gas Poisoning**. Some cholinergic blocking drugs are used as antidotes for persons who have been poisoned by nerve gases (irreversible cholinesterase inhibitors). Certain cholinergic blocking agents are also used as antidotes for certain insecticides (irreversible cholinesterase inhibitors).

f. **Treatment of Bradycardia (Slow Heart Rate).** Atropine sulfate, a cholinergic blocker, is sometimes administered to a patient following cardiac arrest to increase the heart rate. By blocking cholinergic innervation to the heart, sympathetic nerves are allowed to override and increase the rate of the heart.

g. **Preoperative Medication**. Certain cholinergic blockers are administered to patients immediately before their undergoing a surgical procedure. In this case, the cholinergic blockers help to dry secretions in the mucous membranes.

10-4. EXAMPLES OF CHOLINERGIC BLOCKING AGENTS

a. **Atropine**. Atropine is a classic example of the cholinergic blockers. It is found alone and in combination with a wide-variety of other drugs. As an ophthalmic preparation (Isopto-Atropine®), it is used as a cycloplegic and as a mydriatic. Side effects associated with the use of atropine are unsteadiness, hallucinations, unusual dryness of mouth, and increased sensitivity of eyes to light. Patients who have glaucoma should use caution when using this preparation.

b. **Scopolamine.** Scopolamine is another classic example of the cholinergic blockers. Like atropine, scopolamine is found in a variety of medications. It is found in some over-the-counter cold medications. It is present in these products because of the drying effect it produces. In its ophthalmic form it is used as a mydriatic and as a cycloplegic. Side effects that can be caused by this drug include unsteadiness, fever, flushing, or redness of the face, hallucinations, and increased sensitivity of the eyes to light. Patients who have glaucoma should use this preparation with caution.

c. **Homatropine Hydrobomide (Isopto-Homatropine®).** This ophthalmic preparation is used as a mydriatic and as a cycloplegic. The side effects associated with this drug are the same as those associated with atropine and scopolamine (above). Patients who have glaucoma should use this preparation with caution.

d. **Cyclopentolate (Cyclogyl®).** This cholinergic blocker is used as a mydriatic and as a cycloplegic. Cyclopentolate can produce side effects such as unsteadiness, fever, redness of the face, hallucinations, or increased thirst. Patients who have glaucoma should use Cyclopentolate with caution.

e. **Belladonna Alkaloids with Phenobarbital (Donnatal®).** This preparation is used as an antispasmodic. Side effects associated with this agent are eye pain (from increased intraocular pressure), constipation, drowsiness, and dryness of the mouth. Patients taking this preparation should be informed of several things. Do not drink alcohol while taking Donnatal® (because of central nervous system depression). Never take this preparation within one hour of taking antacid (the effectiveness of the Donnatal® will be reduced). This drug may cause drowsiness in some patients; therefore, know how the drug will affect him before he drives or performs any job that requires alertness. Belladonna alkaloids sometimes make patients perspire less (this results in increased body temperature); therefore, do not become overheated because of excessive exercise or hot weather.

f. **Propantheline Bromide (Pro-Banthine®).** This agent is used in the treatment of peptic ulcers. Side effects associated with this drug include constipation, difficult urination (because of decreased muscle tone of the urinary bladder), eye pain (from increased intraocular pressure), and dizziness. Patients taking this medication should be informed of several things. Propantheline can produce drowsiness in some patients; therefore, they should ensure they know how the medicine will affect them before they drive or perform activities that require mental alertness. Sometimes patients taking this medication perspire less; therefore, they should ensure they do not become overheated because of excessive exercise or hot weather. Patients that have glaucoma or severe heart disease should use this drug with caution.

g. **Belladonna Tincture**. This preparation is used for its antispasmodic effect on the gastrointestinal tract (effect produced chiefly by its atropine content). Side effects associated with this agent include dryness of the mouth, dizziness, and constipation.

h. **Dicyclomine (Bentyl®)**. This preparation is used to relieve smooth muscle spasm of the gastrointestinal tract. Side effects that can be caused by this drug include constipation (caused by decreased peristalsis), difficult urination, and dizziness. Persons taking this drug should be cautioned against taking alcohol or other central nervous system (CNS) depressants.

i. **Trihexyphenidyl (Artane®)**. This drug is used in the treatment of parkinsonism. Side effects that can be caused by trihexyphenidyl include constipation, difficult urination, dizziness, dry mouth, and reduced perspiration. Patients taking this preparation should be told several things. Do not take with alcohol or other central nervous system depressants. Some patients perspire less; therefore do not become overheated because of exercise or hot weather.

j. **Benztropine (Cogentin®)**. Benztropine is used in the treatment of parkinsonism. The side effects and patient instructions for trihexyphenidyl (Artane®), above, also apply to benztropine.

IMPORTANT NOTE: Sometimes trihexyphenidyl (Artane®) and benztropine (Cogentin®) will be prescribed with certain phenothiazine tranquilizers to help reduce some of the centrally induced side effects produced by the tranquilizers.

NOTE: Drugs listed in k and l below are both antiparkinsonism drugs; however, they are NOT cholinergic blockers.

k. **Levodopa (Larodopa®)**. This drug is used in the treatment of parkinsonism. Side effects associated with this agent include depression, difficult urination, unusual and uncontrolled movements of the body (that is, face, tongue, and arms), and mood changes. Patients taking this drug should be informed of several things. Take this medication with solid food to decrease the possibility of stomach upset. This drug may cause drowsiness in some patients; therefore, know how the drug will affect him before he drives or performs any job that requires alertness). This drug may cause dizziness or fainting in some patients; therefore, persons taking the drug should get up slowly from a lying or sitting position.

l. **Carbidopa and Levodopa (Sinemet®).** This preparation is used in the treatment of parkinsonism. Side effects that can be caused by this medication include mental depression) mood changes, unusual and uncontrolled movements of the body (that is, face, tongue, arms), and difficult urination. Patients taking this product should be informed of several things. Patients need to take this medication with solid food to decrease the possibility of stomach upset. This drug may cause drowsiness in some patients; therefore, know how the drug will affect him before he drives or performs any job that requires alertness. This drug may cause dizziness or fainting, persons taking the drug should get up slowly from a lying or sitting position.

Continue with Exercises

EXERCISES, LESSON 10

INSTRUCTIONS: Answer the following exercises by marking the lettered response which best answers the question.

After you have completed all the exercises, turn to "Solutions to Exercises" at the end of the lesson and check your answers. For each exercise answered incorrectly, reread the material referenced with the solution.

1. The cholinergic blocking agents produce their effects by:

   a. Forming a stable complex with acetylcholine.

   b. Blocking or reducing normal parasympathetic innervation at the postganglionic synapse.

   c. Increasing the level of epinephrine or norepinephrine at the receptor site.

   d. Preventing the acetylcholinesterase from destroying the acetylcholine at the receptor site.

2. What other name is sometimes given to the cholinergic blocking agents?

   a. Parasympathomimetics.

   b. Para-adrenerolytics.

   c. Parasympatholytics.

   d. Paracholinomimetics.

3. The effect of the cholinergic blockers on the urinary bladder is:

   a. Urinary concentration.

   b. Urinary stimulation.

   c. Urinary retention.

4. The effect of the cholinergic blockers on the eye (pupil) is:

    a.   Miosis (contraction of the pupil).

    b.   Mydriasis (dilation of the pupil).

5. Select the clinical use(s) for the cholinergic blocking agents.

    a.   Drying agents (in cold preparations).

    b.   Antiparkinsonism agents.

    c.   Antispasmodics.

    d.   All the above.

6. Select the clinical use of Isopto-Atropine®.

    a.   Antispasmodic.

    b.   Cycloplegic.

    c.   Treatment of peptic ulcer.

    d.   Treatment of parkinsonism.

7. Persons who take belladonna alkaloids with phenobarbital (Donnatal®) should be cautioned:

    a.   Not to take the medication within one hour of taking antacid.

    b.   Not to exercise while taking the drug.

    c.   Not to take the medication with food or milk.

    d.   Not to take other medications while they are taking this product.

8. The product Bentyl® (dicyclomine) is used in the treatment of:

    a. Peptic ulcers.

    b. Glaucoma.

    c. Parkinsonism.

    d. Muscle spasms in the GI tract.

9. Select the side effect(s) associated with the use of trihexphenidyl.

    a. Loss of bladder control.

    b. Unusual increase in perspiration.

    c. Dry mouth.

    d. Muscle weakness.

10. Persons taking levodopa (Larodopa®) should be informed that:

    a. They should arise slowly from a sitting or lying position since the drug may cause fainting.

    b. They should take the drug on an empty stomach (one or two hours before meals) to decrease the likelihood of stomach upset.

    c. They should not take the drug with milk or antacid.

11. Match the trade or generic name of Column A with its appropriate trade or generic name in Column B.

Column A	Column B
_____ Trihexyphenidyl	a. Cyclopentolate
_____ Bentyl®	b. Carbidopa and levodopa
_____ Cyclogyl®	c. Cogentin®
_____ Benztropine	d. Dicyclomine
_____ Sinemet®	e. Artane®

Check Your Answers on Next Page

SOLUTIONS TO EXERCISES, LESSON 10

1. b Blocking or reducing normal parasympathetic innervation at the postganglionic synapse. (para 10-1)

2. c Parasympatholytics. (para 10-1)

3. c Urinary retention. (para 10-2d)

4. b Mydriasis (dilation of the pupil). (para 10-2c)

5. d All the above. (paras 10-3a, c, and d)

6. b Cycloplegic. (para 10-4a)

7. a Not to take the medication within one hour of taking antacid. (para 10-4e)

8. d Muscle spasms in the G.I tract. (para 10-4h)

9. c Dry mouth. (para 10-4i)

10. a They should arise slowly from a sitting or lying position since the drug may cause fainting. (para 10-4k)

11. e Trihexyphenidyl (para 10-4i)

    d Bentyl® (para 10-4h)

    a Cyclogyl® (para 10-4d)

    c Benztropine. (para 10-4j)

    b Sinemet®. (para 10-4l)

End of Lesson 10

ANNEX

DRUG PRONUNCIATION GUIDE

This Drug Pronunciation Guide was developed to help you to learn how the trade and generic names of commonly prescribed medications are frequently pronounced. Not all the drugs in the guide are discussed in this subcourse. Remember, it is not enough to be able to know the uses, indications, cautions and warnings, and contraindications for a drug--you must also know how to pronounce that drug's name.

Trade Name	*Generic Name*
Actifed (Ak'-ti-fed)	Triprolidine (Tri-pro'-li-deen) and Pseudoephedrine (Soo-do-e-fed'-rin)
Adapin (Ad'-a-pin)	Doxepin (Dok'-se-pin)
Sinequan (Sin'-a-kwan)	" "
Afrin (Af'-rin)	Oxymetazoline (Ok-see-met-az'-o-leen)
Aldactazide (Al-dak'-ta-zide)	Spironolactone (Spi-ro-no-lak'-tone) and Hydrochlorothiazide (Hy-dro-klor-thi'-a-zide)
Aldactone (Al-dak'-tone)	Spironolactone (Spi-ro-no-lak'-tone)
Aldomet (Al'-do-met)	Methyldopa (Meth-il-do'-pah)
Alupent (Al'-u-pent)	Metaproterenol (Met-a-pro-ter'-eh-nol)
Amoxil (Am-ok'-sil)	Amoxicillin (Ah-moks'-i-sil-in)
Amphojel (Am'-fo-jel)	Aluminum (Al-loo'-mi-num) Hydroxide (Hy-drok'-side)
Ampicillin (Amp'-I-sil-in)	Same
Antepar (Ab'-te-par)	Piperazine (Pi-per'-ah-zeen)
Anturane (An'-tu-rain)	Sulfinpyrazone (Sul-fin-pie'-ra-zone)
Anusol (An'-u-sol)	Pramoxine (Pram-ok'-seen)
Apresoline (A-press'-o-leen)	Hydralazine (Hy-dral'-ah-zeen)
Aralen (Ar'-a-len)	Chloroquine (Klor'-o-kwin)
Aristocort (A-ris'-to-cort)	Triamcinolone (Tri-am-sin'-o-lone)
Artane (Ar'-tane)	Trihexyphenidyl(Tri-hek-see-fen'-i-dil)
A.S.A.	Aspirin (As'-per-in)
Atromid S (A'-tro-mid)	Clofibrate (Klo-fi'-brate)
Avlosulfon (Av-lo-sul'-fon)	Dapsone (Dap'-sone)
Azolid (Az'-o-lid)	Phenylbutazone (Fen-il-bute'-a-zone)
Bactrim (Bak'-trim)	Sulfamethoxazole (Sul-fah-meth-oks'-ah-zole) and Trimethoprim (Tri-meth'-o-prim)
Bellergal (Bel'-er-gal)	Ergotamine (Er-got'-a-meen), Phenobarbital (Feen-o-bar'-bi-tal) and Belladonna (Bel-la-don'-na) Alkaloids
Benadryl (Ben'-a-dril)	Diphenhydramine (Di-fen-hy'-dra-meen)

Trade Name	Generic Name
Bendectin (Ben-dek'-tin)	Doxylamine (Dok-sil'-a-meen)
Benemid (Ben'-eh-mid)	Probenecid (Pro-ben'-eh-sid)
Bonine (Bo'-neen)	Meclizine (Mek'-li-zeen)
Cafergot (Kaf'-er-got)	Ergotamine (Er-got'-a-meen) and Caffeine (Kaf'-feen)
Calamine (Kal'-a-mine)	Same
Catapres (Kat'-a-press)	Clonidine (Klo'-ni-deen)
CeeNu (See'-new)	Lomustine (Lo-mus'-teen)
Chlor-Trimeton (Klo-tri '-meh-ton)	Chlorpheniramine (Klor-fen-it'-a-meen)
Clomid (Klo'-mid)	Clomiphene (Klo'-mi-feen)
Clonopin (Klo-o-pin)	Clonazepam (Klo-na'-ze-pam)
Codeine (Ko'-deen)	Same
Cogentin (Ko-jen'-tin)	Benztropine (Benz'-tro-peen)
Colace (Ko'-lace)	Dioctyl(Di-ok'-til) Sodium (So'-dee-um) Sulfosuccinate (Sul-fo-suk'-si-nate)
Colchicine (Kol'-chi-seen)	Same
Compazine (Kom'-pa-zeen)	Prochiorperazine (Pro-klor-per'-a-zeen)
Cordran (Kor'-dran)	Flurandrenolide (Floor-an-dren'-o-lide)
Coumadin (Koo'-mah-din)	Warfarin (War'-fah-rin)
CP	Cloroquine (Klor'-o-kwin) and Primaquine (Prim'-a-kwin)
Cyclogyl (Si'-klo-jel)	Cyclopentolate (Si-klo-pen'-to-late)
Cytomel (Si'-to-mel)	Liothyronine (Li-o-thy-ro-neen)
Cytoxan (Si-tok'-san)	Cyclophosphamide (Si-klo-fos'-fa-mide)
Dalmane (Dal '-mane)	Flurazepam (Floor-az'-e-pam)
Darvocet (Dar'-vo-set)	Propoxyphene (Pro-pok'-se-feen) and Acetaminopen (As-et-am'-ino-fen)
Darvon (Dar'-von)	Propoxyphene (Pro-pok-se-feen)
Decadron (Dek'-a-dron)	Dexamethasone (Dek-sa-meth'-ah-sone)
Deltasone (Del '-ta-sone)	Prednisone (Pred'-ni-sone)
Demerol (Dem'-er-ol)	Meperidine (Meh-pair'-i-deen)
Dexedrine (Deks '-eh-dreen)	Dextroamphetamine (Deks-tro-am-fet'-a-meen)
Diabinese (Di-ab'-i-nees)	Chlorpropamide (Klor-prop'-a-mide)
Diethylstilbestrol (Di-eth-il-stil-bes'-trol)	Same
Dilantin (Di-lan'-tin)	Phenytoin (Fen'-i-toin)
Dilaudid (Di-law'-did)	Hydromorphone (Hy-dro-more' -fon)
Dimetane (Di'-meh-tane)	Brompheniramine (Brom-fen-ir'-a-meen)

Trade Name	Generic Name
Dimetapp (Di'-meh-tap)	Brompheniramine (Brom-fen-ir'-a-meen) Phenylephrine (Fen-il-ef'-rin) and Phenylpropanolamine (Fen-il-pro-pan-ol'-a-meen)
Disophrol (Dice'-o-frol)	Dexbrompheniramine (Deks-brom-fen-ir'-a-meen) and Pseudoephedrine (Soo-do-e-fed'-rin)
Dolophine (Dol'-o-feen)	Methadone (Meth'-a-done)
Domeboro (Dome-bor'-o)	Aluminum (Ah-loo'-mi-num) Acetate (As'-e-tate)
Donnatal (Don'-na-tal)	Belladonna (Bel-la-don'-na) Alkaloids (Al'-ka-loids) and Phenobarbital (Feen-o-barb'-i-tal)
Doxidan (Dok'-si-dan)	Danthron (Dan'-thron) and Dicctyl (Di-ok'-til) Calcium (Kal'-see-um) Sulfosuccinate (Sul-fo-suk'-si-nate)
Drixoral (Driks'-or-al)	Dexbrompheniramine (Deks-brom-fen-ir'-a-meen) and Pseudoephedrine (Soo-do-e-fed'-rin)
Dulcolax (Dul'-ko-laks)	Bisacodyl (Bis-a'-ko-dil)
Dyazine (Di'-a-zide)	Triamterene (Tri-am'-ter-een) and Hydrochlorothiazide (Hy-dro-klor-o-thi'-a-zide)
Dymelor (Die'-meh-lor)	Acetohexamide (As-e-to-heks'-a-mide)
Dyrenium (Die-ren'-i-um)	Triamterene (Tri-am'-ter-een)
Efudex (Ef'-u-deks)	Fluorouracil (Floo-ro-ur'-ah-sil)
Elavil (El'-ah-vil)	Amitriptyline (Am-i-trip'-til-een)
Elixir Terpin (Ter'-pin) Hydrate	Same
Empirin (Em'-per-in)	Codeine (Ko'-deen) and Aspirin (As'-per-in)
E-Mycin (E-mie'-sin)	Erythromycin (E-rith-ro-mie'-sin)
Equanil (Ek'-wa-nil)	Meprobamate (Me-pro-bam'-ate)
Ergomar (Er'-go-mar)	Ergotamine (Er-got'-a-meen)
Ergotrate (Er'-go-trate)	Ergonovine (Er-go-no'-veen)
Erythrocin (Er-eeth'-ro-sin)	Erythromycin (Er-eeth-ro-my'-sin) Stearate (Stare'-rate)
Esidrix (Es'-i-driks)	Hyrochlorothiazide (Hy-dro-klor-o-thi'-a-zide)
Feosol (Fe'-o-sol)	Ferrous (Fer'-rus) Sulfate (Sul'-fate)
Fergon (Fer'-gon)	Ferrous (Fer'-rus) Gluconate (Glu'-con-ate)

Trade Name	Generic Name
Fiorinal (Fee-or'-i-nal)	Butalbi tal (Bu-tal'-bi-tal), Apririn, Phenacetin (Fen-ass'-eh-tin), and Caffeine (Kaf'-feen)
Flagyl (Fla'-jil)	Metronidazole (Me-tro-ni'-dah-zole)
Flexeril (Flek'-sa-ril)	Cyclobenzaprine (Si-klo-benz'-a-preen)
Fulvicin (Ful'-vi-sin)	Griseofulvin (Griz-e-o-ful'-vin)
Guantanol (Gan'-ta-nol)	Suiphamethoxazole (Sul-fah-meth-oks'-ah-zole)
Gantrisin (Gan'-tri-sin)	Sulfisoxazole (Sul-fi-sok'-sah-zole)
Gelusil (Jel'-u-sil)	Aluminum (Ah-loo'-mi-num) Hydroxide (Hy-drok'-side) and Magnesium (Mag-nee'-zee-um) Hydroxide
Grifulvin (Gri-ful'-vin)	Griseofulvin (Griz-e-o-ful'-vin)
Gynergen (Jin'-er-jen)	Ergotamine (Er-got'-a-meen)
Haldol (Hal'-dol)	Haloperidol (Hal-o-pair'-i-dol)
Halotestin (Hal-o-tes'-tin)	Fluoxymesterone (Floo-ok-see-mes-teh-rone)
Hexadrol (Hek'-sa-drol)	Dexamethasone (Dek-sa-meth'-a-sone)
Hydrodiuril (Hy-dro-di'-ur-il)	Hydroclorothiazide (Hy-dro-kior-thi'-a-zide)
Hygroton (Hy-grow'-ton)	Chiorthalidone (Kior-thal'-i-done)
Ilosone (I'-low-sone)	Erythromycin (Er-ith-ro-mi'-sin) Estolate (Es'-to-late)
Inderal (In'-der-al)	Propranolol (Pro-pran'-o-lol)
Indocin (In'-do-sin)	Indomethacin (In-do-meth'-a-sin)
INH	Isoniazid (I-so-ni'-a-zid)
Insulin (In'-sul-in)	Same
Intal	Cromolyn (Kro'-mo-lin)
Ismelin (Is'-meh-lin)	Guanethidine (Gwan-eth'-i-dine)
Isopto-Atropine (I-sop-to-at'-ro-peen)	Atropine (At'-ro-peen)
Isopto-Carpine (I-sop-to-car'-peen)	Pilocarpine (Pile-o-car'-peen)
Isordil (I'-sor-dil)	Isosorbide (I-so-sor'-bide)
Keflex (Kef'-lex)	Cephalexin (Sef-ah-lek'-sin)
Lanoxin (Lan-ok'-sin)	Digoxin (Di-jok'-sin)
Larodopa (Lar-o-do'-pa)	Levodopa (Le-o-do'-pa)
Larotid (Lar'-o-tid)	Amoxicillin (Ah-moks'-i-sil-in)
Lasix (La'-siks)	Furosemide (Fu-ro'-se-mide)
Leukeran (Lu'-ker-an)	Chlorambucil (Klor-ram'-bu-sil)
Librium (Lib'-ree-um)	Chlordiazepoxide (Klor-die-az-eh-pok'-side)

Trade Name	Generic Name
Lidex (Lie'-deks)	Fluocinoide (Floo-o-sin'-o-nide)
Lomotil (Lo'-mo-til)	Diphenoxylate (Die-fen-ok'-si-late)
Lopressor (Lo'-pres-sor)	Metoprolol (Met-o-pro'-lol)
Lotrimin (Lo'-tri-min)	Chlotrimazole (Klo-trim'-ah-zole)
Maalox (May'-loks)	Aluminum (Ah-loo'-mi-num) and Magnesium (Mag-nee'-zee-um) Hydroxides
Macrodanton (Ma-kro-dan'-tin)	Nitrofurantoin (Ni-tro-fur-an'-toin)
Mandelamine (Man-del'-a-meen)	Methenamine (Meth-en'-a-meen) Mandelate (Man'-deh-late)
Medihaler-Iso (Med-i-hail-er-I'-so)	Isoproterenol (I-so-pro-ter'-en-ol)
Mellaril (Mel'-la-ril)	Thioridazine (Thi-o-rid'-a-zeen)
Metamucil (Met-a-mu'-sil)	Psyllium (Sil'-e-um)
Metaprel (Meh'-ta-prel)	Metaproterenol (Meh'-ta-pro-ter'-eh-nol)
Methotrexate (Meth-o-treks'-ate)	Amethopterin (Ah-meth-op'-ter-in)
Milk of Magnesia	Same
Minipress (Min'-i-press)	Prazosin (Pra'-zo-sin)
Minocin (Min'-o-sin)	Minocycline (Mi-no-si'-kleen)
Monistat (Mon'-i-stat)	Miconazole (Mi-kon'-ah-zole)
Motrin (Mo'-trin)	Ibuprofen (I-bu'-pro-fen)
Myambutol (My-am'-bu-tol)	Ethambutol (Eth-am'-bu-tol)
Mycostatin (My-co-stat'-in)	Nystatin (Ny-stat'-in)
Mylanta (My-lan'-ta)	Aluminum (Ah-loo'-mi-num) and Magnesium (Mag-nee'-zee-um) Hydroxides and Simethicone (Si-meth'-i-kone)
Myleran (My-ler-an)	Busulfan (Bu-sul'-fan)
Mylicon (My'-li-kon)	Simethicone (Si-meth'-i-kone)
Mysoline (My'-so-leen)	Primidone (Pri'-mi-done)
Nalfon (Nal'-fon)	Fenoprofen (Fen-o-pro'-fen)
Naprosyn (Na'-pro-sin)	Naproxen (Na-prok'-sen)
Nembutal (Nem'-bu-tal)	Pentobarbital (Pen-to-barb'-i-tal)
Neosynephrine (Nee-o-sin-eh'-frin)	Phenylephrine (Fen-il-eh'-frin)
Nitrobid (Ni'-tro-bid)	Nitroglycerin (Ni-tro-gli'-ser-in)
Nitrol (Ni'-trol)	" "
Nitrostat (Ni-tro-stat)	" "
Noctec (Nok'-tek)	Chloral Hydrate (Klor'-al- Hy'-drate)
Norfiex (Nor'-fleks)	Orphenadrine Citrate (Or-fen'-a-dreen)
Norpace (Nor'-pace)	Disopyramide (Di-so-peer'-a-mide)

Trade Name	Generic Name
Novahistine (No-va-his'-teen) Expectorant	Guaifenesin (Gwi-fen'-eh-sin), Phenylpropanolamine (Fen-il-pro-pan-ol'-a-meen), and Codeine (Ko'-deen)
NTG	Nitroclycerin (Ni-tro-gli'-ser-in)
Nupercainal (New-per-kain'-al)	Dibucaine (Die'-bu-kain)
Oretic (O-ret'-ik)	Hydrochiorothiazide (Hy-dro-kior-thi'-a-zide)
Orinase (Or'-in-ase)	Tolbutamide (Tol-bu'-tah-mide)
Ornade (Or'-nade)	Chlorpheniramine (Klor-fen-ir'-a-meen), Triprolidine (Tri-pro-li-deen) and Pseudoephedrine (Su-do-eh-fed'-rin)
Parafon Forte (Pair'-a-fon For'-tay)	Chlorzoxazone (Klor-zok'-sa-zone)
Percodan (Per'-ko-dan)	Oxycodone (Ok-si-ko'-done)
Periactin (Per-ee-ak'-tin)	Cyproheptadine (Si-pro-hep'-tah-deen)
Persantine (Per-san'-teen)	Dipyridamole (Di-pi-rid'-ah-mole)
Phenobarbital (Feen-o-barb'-it-al)	Same
Phenylpropanolamine (Fen-il-pro-pan-ol'-a-meen)	Same
Pitocin (Pi-tow'-sin)	Oxytocin (Ok-see-tow'-sin)
Pontocaine (Pon'-to-kain)	Tetracaine (Teh'-tra-kain)
Povan (Po'-van)	Pyrvinium (Pire-vin'-ee-um)
Premarin (Prem'-ar-in)	Conjugated (Kon'-joo-gay-ted) Estrogens (Es-tro-jens)
Presamine (Press'-a-meen)	Imipramine (Im-ip'-rah-meen)
Primaquine (Pri'-mah-kwin)	Same
Probanthine (Pro-ban'-theen)	Propantheline (Pro-pan'-the-leen)
Pronestyl (Pro-nes'-til)	Procainamide (Pro-kain'-a-mide)
Prophylthiouracil (Pro-pil-thi-o-u'-rah-sil)	Same
Prostaphlin (Pro-staff'-lin)	Oxacillin (Oks'-ah-sil-in)
Provera (Pro-ver'-ah)	Medroxyprogesterone (Med-rok-see-pro-jes'-ter-one)
Pyridium (Pie-rid'-ee-um)	Phenazopyridine (Fen-ahs-o-per'-i-deen)
Quinidine (Kwin'-i-deen)	Same
Quinine (Kwie'-nine)	Same
Reserpine (Ree-ser'-peen)	Same
Retin A (Reh'-tin A)	Tretinoin (Tret'-i-noin)
Rifadin (Rie-fad'-in)	Rifampin (Rie-fam'-pin)
Riopan (Rie'-o-pan)	Magaidrate (Mag'-al-drate)

Trade Name	Generic Name
Rimactane (Rim-act'-ane)	Rifampin (Rie-fam'-pin)
Ritalin (Rit'-a-lin)	Methylphenidate (Meth-il-fen'-i-date)
Robaxin (Ro-bak'-sin)	Methocarbamol (Meth-o-kar'-ba-mol)
Robitussin (Row-i-tus'-sin)	Guaifenesin (Gwie-fen'-eh-sin)
Robitussin DM	Guiafenesin and Dextromethorphan (Dek-tro-meh-or'-fan)
Sansert (San'-sert)	Methysergide (Meth-ee-ser'-jide)
Seconal (Sek'-o-nal)	Secobarbital (Sek-o-bar'-bi-tal)
Selsun (Sel'-sun)	Selenium (Se-leh'-nee-um)
Septra (Sep'-tra)	Sulfamethoxazole (Sul-fah-meth-oks'-a-zole) and Trimethroprim (Tri-meth'-o-prim)
Serax (See'-raks)	Oxazepam (Oks-az'-eh-pam)
Silvadene (Sil'-va-deen)	Silver Sulfadiazine (Sul-fa-die'-a-zeen)
Sinemet (Si'-ne-met)	Levodopa (Le-vo-do'-pa)
Sinequan (Sin'-a-kwan)	Doxepin (Dok'-seh-pin)
Sorbitrate (Sor'-bi-trate)	Isosorbide (I-so-sor'-bide)
Stelazine (Stel'-a-zeen)	Trifluoperazine(Tri-floo-o-per'-a-zeen)
Sudafed (Soo'-da-fed)	Pseudophedrine (Soo-do-eh-feh'-drin)
Sulamyd (Sul'-a-mid)	Sulfacetamide (Sul-fah-set'-a-mide)
Sulfamylon (Sul-fa-mie'-lon)	Mafenide (Maf'-eh-nide)
Sultrin (Sul'-trin)	Sulfathiazole (Sul-fah-thi'-ah-zole) Sulfacetamide (Sul-fah-set'-ah-mide) and Sulfabenzamide (Sul-fah-benz'-ah-mide)
Surfak (Sur'-fak)	Dioctyl (Di-ok'-til) Calcium (Kal'-see-um) Sulfosuccinate (Sul-fo-suk'-si-nate)
Synalar (Sine'-a-lar)	Fluocinolone (Floo-o-sin'-o-lone)
Synthroid (Sin'-throid)	Levothyroxine (Lee-vo-thi-rok'-sin)
Tace (Tace)	Chlorotrianisene (Klor-o-tri-an'-I-seen)
Tagamet (Tag'-a-met)	Cimetidine (Si-met'-i-deen)
Talwin (Tal'-win)	Pentazocine (Pen-taz'-o-seen)
Tandearil (Tan'-da-ril)	Oxyphenbutazone (Ok-see-fen-bute'-a-zone)
Tegretol (Teg'-reh-tol)	Carbamazepine (Kar-ba-maz'-eh-peen)
Tessalon (Tess'-a-lon)	Benzonatate (Benz-on'-a-tate)
Tetracycline (Tet-ra-si'-kleen)	
Thorazine (Thor'-a-zeen)	Chlorpromazine (Klor-pro'-ma-zeen)
Thyroid (Thy'-roid)	Same
Tigan (Tie'-gan)	Trimethobenzamide (Tri-meth-o-benz'-a-mide)
Timoptic (Tim-op'-tic)	Timilol (Tim'-o-lol)

Trade Name	Generic Name
Tinactin (Tin-act'-in)	Tolnaftate (Tol-naf'-tate)
Titralac (Ti'-tra-lak)	Calcium (Kal-see-um) Carbonate (Kar'-bon-ate) and Glycine (Gly'-seen)
Tofranil (Toe'-fra-nil)	Imipramine (I-mip'-rah-meen)
Tolectin (Tow-lek'-tin)	Tolmetin (Tol-met'-in)
Triavil (Tri'-a-vil)	Perphenazine (Per-fen'-a-zeen) and Amitriptlyline (Am-i-trip'-ti-leen)
Trilafon (Try'-la-fon)	Perphenazine (Per-fen-a-zeen)
Tylenol (Tie'-leh-nol)	Acetaminophen (As-et-am'-ino-fen)
Tylenol #3	Acetaminophen and Codeine (Ko'-deen)
Unipen (U'-ni-pen)	Nafcillin (Naf-sil-lin)
Urecholine (Ur-eh-ko'-leen)	Bethanecol (Beth-an'-eh-kol)
Valisone (Val'-i-sone)	Betamethasone (Beh-tah-meth'-a-sone)
Valium (Val'-ee-um)	Diazepam (Die-aze-eh-pam)
Vermox (Ver'-moks)	Mebendazole (Meh-ben'-dah-zole)
Vibramycin (Vie-bra-my'-sin)	Doxycycline (Doks-see-si'-kleen)
Xylocaine (Zie'-low-kain)	Lidocaine (Lie-do-kain)
Zarontin (Zar-on'-tin)	Ethosuximide (Eh-tho-suks'-a-mide)
Zyloprim (Zie'-low-prim)	Allopurinol (Al-lo-pure'-in-ol)

End of Lesson 10 Annex

This page intentionally left blank.

Pharmacology III

Subcourse MD0806

This page intentionally left blank.

U. S. ARMY MEDICAL DEPARTMENT CENTER AND SCHOOL
FORT SAM HOUSTON, TEXAS 78234

PHARMACOLOGY III

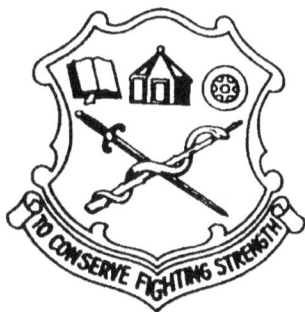

SUBCOURSE MD0806

EDITION 100

DEVELOPMENT

This subcourse is approved for resident and correspondence course instruction. It reflects the current thought of the Academy of Health Sciences and conforms to printed Department of the Army doctrine as closely as currently possible. Development and progress render such doctrine continuously subject to change.

The instructional systems specialist for the revision of this version of the subcourse was: Mr. John Arreguin; AMEDDC&S, ATTN: MCCS-HCP, 3151 Scott Road, Fort Sam Houston, TX 78234; DSN 471-8958; john.arreguin@amedd.army.mil.

The subject matter expert responsible for the revision of this version of the subcourse was: MAJ Jennifer R. Styles, MCCS-HCP, Pharmacy Branch, Department of Clinical Support Services.

ADMINISTRATION

Students who desire credit hours for this correspondence subcourse must meet eligibility requirements and must enroll through the Nonresident Instruction Branch of the U.S. Army Medical Department Center and School (AMEDDC&S).

Application for enrollment should be made at the Internet website: http://www.atrrs.army.mil. You can access the course catalog in the upper right corner. Enter School Code 555 for medical correspondence courses. Copy down the course number and title. To apply for enrollment, return to the main ATRRS screen and scroll down the right side for ATRRS Channels. Click on SELF DEVELOPMENT to open the application and then follow the on screen instructions.

In general, eligible personnel include enlisted personnel of all components of the U.S. Army who hold an AMEDD MOS or MOS 18D. Officer personnel, members of other branches of the Armed Forces, and civilian employees will be considered eligible based upon their AOC, NEC, AFSC or Job Series which will verify job relevance. Applicants who wish to be considered for a waiver should submit justification to the Nonresident Instruction Branch at e-mail address: accp@amedd.army.mil.

For comments or questions regarding enrollment, student records, or shipments, contact the Nonresident Instruction Branch at DSN 471-5877, commercial (210) 221-5877, toll-free 1-800-344-2380; fax: 210-221-4012 or DSN 471-4012, e-mail accp@amedd.army.mil, or write to:

NONRESIDENT INSTRUCTION BRANCH
AMEDDC&S
ATTN: MCCS-HSN
2105 11TH STREET SUITE 4191
FORT SAM HOUSTON TX 78234-5064

TABLE OF CONTENTS

TABLE OF CONTENTS (Cont)

TABLE OF CONTENTS (Cont)

LIST OF ILLUSTRATIONS

CORRESPONDENCE COURSE OF THE
U.S. ARMY MEDICAL DEPARTMENT CENTER AND SCHOOL

SUBCOURSE MD0806

PHARMACOLOGY III

Drugs that act upon the respiratory system, cardiovascular system, or urinary system are frequently dispensed in both military and civilian pharmacies. This is because conditions that affect these systems (that is, hypertension affecting the cardiovascular system) affect many people. Consequently, it is imperative that you have an understanding of these systems and the drugs that act on them.

As with MD0804, Pharmacology I, and MD0805, Pharmacology II, anatomy, physiology, and pharmacology are presented in a combined perspective in this subcourse. This is done in order to help you to understand and remember the actions, uses, side effects, and patient warnings associated with the drugs included in the lessons.

You should remember that this subcourse is not intended to replace accepted references in anatomy, physiology, or pharmacology. Instead, it is designed to help you gain a background in these areas so that you may continue learning in a self-directed manner. You are encouraged to read pertinent journals, study pharmacology texts, and talk to fellow health-care professionals in order to learn more about the topics presented in this subcourse.

This subcourse consists of 9 lessons and an examination as follows:

Lesson 1. Respiratory System and Respiratory System Drugs.

Lesson 2. The Human Cardiovascular and Lymphatic Systems.

Lesson 3. Cardiac Drugs.

Lesson 4. Vasodilator Drugs.

Lesson 5. Drugs Acting on the Hematopoietic System.

Lesson 6. The Human Urogenital Systems.

Lesson 7. Antihypertensive Agents.

Lesson 8. Diuretic and Antidiuretic Agents.

Lesson 9. Toxicology and Poison Control.

Credit Awarded:

Upon successful completion of this subcourse, you will be awarded 14 credit hours.

<u>Materials Furnished</u>:

Materials provided include this booklet, an examination answer sheet, and an envelope. Answer sheets are not provided for individual lessons in this subcourse because you are to grade your own lessons. Exercises and solutions for all lessons are contained in this booklet. <u>You must furnish a #2 pencil.</u>

<u>Procedures for Subcourse Completion</u>:

You are encouraged to complete the subcourse lesson by lesson. When you have completed all of the lessons to your satisfaction, fill out the examination answer sheet and mail it to the AMEDDC&S along with the Student Comment Sheet in the envelope provided. *Be sure that your name, rank, social security number, and return address is on all correspondence sent to the AMEDDC&S.* You will be notified by return mail of the examination results. Your grade on the examination will be your rating for the subcourse.

<u>Study Suggestions</u>:

Here are some suggestions that may be helpful to you in completing this subcourse:

Read and study each lesson carefully.

Complete the subcourse lesson by lesson. After completing each lesson, work the exercises at the end of the lesson, marking your answers in this booklet.

After completing each set of lesson exercises, compare your answers with those On the solution sheet, that follows the exercises. If you have answered an exercise Incorrectly, check the reference cited after the answer on the solution sheet to determine why your response was not the correct one.

As you successfully complete each lesson, go on to the next. When you have Completed all of the lessons, complete the examination. Mark your answers in this Booklet, then transfer your responses to the examination answer sheet using a #2 pencil.

<u>Student Comment Sheet</u>:

Be sure to provide us with your suggestions and criticisms by filling out the Student Comment Sheet (found at the back of this booklet) and returning it to us with your examination answer sheet. Please review this comment sheet before studying this subcourse. In this way, you will help us to improve the quality of this subcourse.

LESSON ASSIGNMENT

LESSON 1   The Respiratory System and Respiratory System Drugs.

LESSON ASSIGNMENT   Paragraphs 1-1--1-20.

TASKS   081-824-0001, Perform Initial Screening of a Prescription.

081-824-0026, Evaluate a Prescription.

081-824-0002/3, Fill a Prescription For a Controlled/Non-Controlled Drug.

081-824-0027, Evaluate a Completed Prescription.

081-824-0028, Issue Outpatient Medications.

LESSON OBJECTIVES   After you finish this lesson you should be able to:

1-1.   Given a group of statements and one of the following terms: respiration, external respiration, or internal respiration, select the statement which best defines the given term.

1-2.   Given a diagram of the human respiratory system and a list of names of the parts of the human respiratory system, match the name of its part with its proper location.

1-3.   Given the name of one of the components of the human respiratory system and a group of statements, select the statement that best describes that component or its function.

1-4.   From a group of statements, select the statement which best describes either costal (thoracic) or diaphragmatic (abdominal) breathing.

1-5.   Given the name of a condition affecting the respiratory system and a group of statements, select the statement that best describes the given condition.

1-6.   Given the name of a type of respiratory system drug (that is, antitussive agent) and a group of statements, select the statement that best describes that type of agent.

1-7.   Given the trade or generic name of a respiratory system drug and a group of indications, uses, side effects, or patient precautionary statements, select the indication(s), use(s), side effect(s), or patient precautionary statement(s) for the given drug name.

1-8.   Given the trade or generic name of a respiratory system drug and a group of trade and/or generic names, select the given drug's corresponding trade or generic name.

SUGGESTION

After completing the assignment, complete the exercises at the end of this lesson. These exercises will help you to achieve the lesson objectives.

LESSON 1

THE RESPIRATORY SYSTEM AND RESPIRATORY SYSTEM DRUGS

Section I. THE RESPIRATORY SYSTEM

1-1. INTRODUCTION

a. **Respiration.** Respiration is the exchange of gases between the atmosphere and the cells of the body. It is a physiological process. There are two types of respiration-external and internal. External respiration is the exchange of gases between the air in the lungs and blood. Internal respiration is the exchange of gases between the blood and the individual cells of the body.

b. **Breathing**. Breathing is the process that moves air into and out of the lungs. It is a mechanical process. There are two types of breathing in humans--costal (thoracic) and diaphragmatic (abdominal). In costal breathing, the major structure causing the movement of the air is the rib cage. In diaphragmatic breathing, interaction between the diaphragm and the abdominal wall causes the air to move into and out of the lungs.

1-2. COMPONENTS AND SUBDIVISIONS OF THE HUMAN RESPIRATORY SYSTEM

NOTE: See Figure 1-1 for an illustration of the human respiratory system.

a. **Components**. The components of the human respiratory system consist of air passageways and two lungs. Air moves from the outside of the body into tiny sacs in the lungs called alveoli (pronounced al-VE-oh-lie).

b. **Main Subdivisions**. The main subdivisions of the respiratory system may be identified by their relationship to the voice box or larynx. Thus, the main subdivisions are as follows:

SUBDIVISION	FUNCTION
(1) SUPRALARYNGEAL STRUCTURES (su-prah-lah-RIN-je-al)	cleanse, warm, moisten, and test inflowing air
(2) LARYNX (voice-box) (LARE-inks)	controls the volume of inflowing air; produces selected pitch (vibration frequency) in the moving column of air

(3) <u>INFRALARYNGEAL STRUCTURES</u>
(in-frah-lah-RIN-je-al)

distribute air to the alveoli
of the lung where the actual
external respiration takes
place

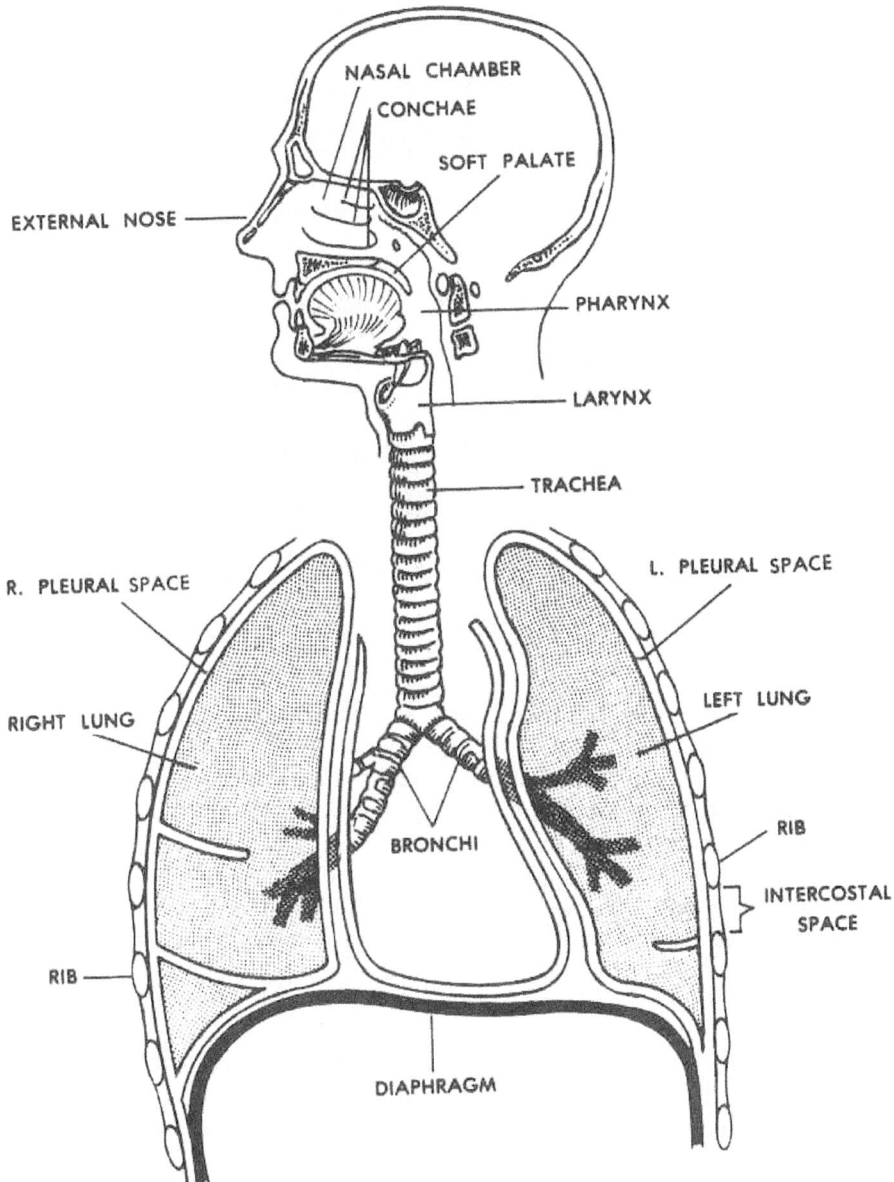

Figure 1-1. The human respiratory system.

1-3. SUPRALARYNGEAL STRUCTURES (See Figure 1-2.)

a. **External Nose**. The external nose is the portion projecting from the face. Primarily cartilages support it. It has a midline divider called the nasal septum, which extends from the internal nose. Paired openings (nostrils lead to paired spaces (vestibules). Guard hairs in the nostrils filter inflowing air.

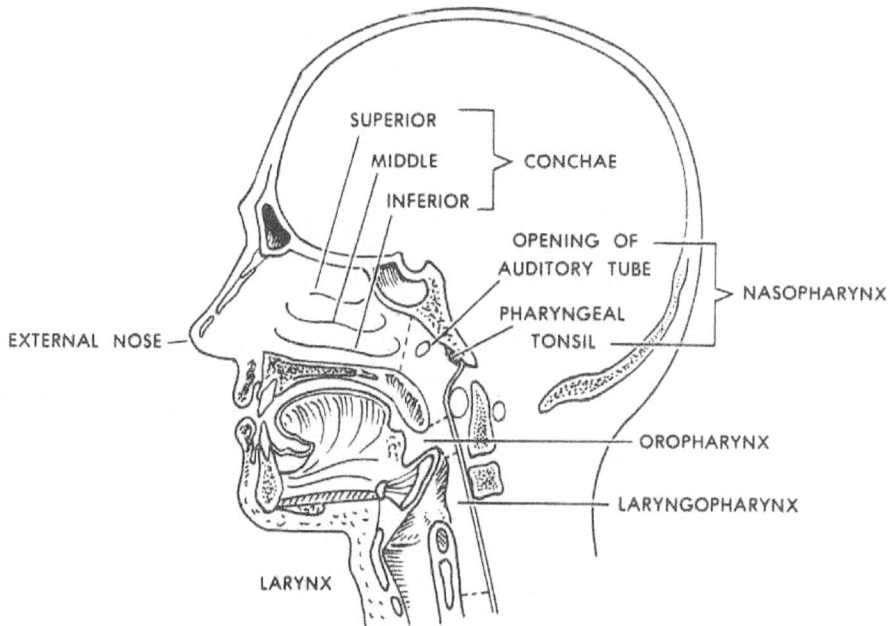

Figure 1-2. Supralaryngeal structures.

b. **Nasal Chambers (Internal Nose)**. Behind each vestibule of the external nose is a nasal chamber. The two nasal chambers together form the internal nose. These chambers too are separated by the nasal septum.

(1) Mucoperiosteum. The walls of the nasal chambers are lined with a thick mucous-type membrane known as the mucoperiosteum. It has a ciliated epithelial surface and a rich blood supply, which provides warmth and moisture. At times, it may become quite swollen.

CILIATED = Provided with cilia (hair like projections that move
fluids to the rear)

(2) Conchae. The lateral wall of each chamber has three scroll-like extensions into the nasal chamber, which help to increase the surface area exposed to the inflowing air. These scroll-like extensions are known as conchae.

CONCHA =sea shell   CONCHA (singular), CONCHAE (plural)
(pronounced KON -kah)

(3) Olfactory epithelium. The sense of smell is because of special nerve endings located in the upper areas of the nasal chambers. The epithelium containing the sensory endings is known as the olfactory epithelium.

(4) Paranasal sinuses. There are air "cells" or cavities in the skull known as paranasal sinuses. The paranasal sinuses are connected with the nasal chambers and are lined with the same ciliated mucoperiosteum. Thus, these sinuses are extensions of the nasal chambers into the skull bones. For this reason, they are known as paranasal sinuses.

c. **Pharynx.** The pharynx (FAIR-inks) is the common posterior space for the respiratory and digestive systems.

(1) Nasopharynx. That portion of the pharynx specifically related to the respiratory system is the nasopharynx. It is the portion of the pharynx above the soft palate. The two posterior openings (nares) of the nasal chambers lead into the single space of the nasopharynx. The auditory (eustachian) tubes also open into the nasopharynx. The auditory tubes connect the nasopharynx with the middle ears (to equalize the pressure between the outside and inside of the eardrum). Lying in the upper posterior wall of the nasopharynx are the pharyngeal tonsils (adenoids). The soft palate floor of the nasopharynx is a trap door that closes off the upper respiratory passageways during swallowing.

(2) Oropharynx. The portion of the pharynx closely related to the digestive system is the oropharynx. It is the portion of the pharynx below the soft palate and above the upper edge of the epiglottis. (The epiglottis is the flap that prevents food from entering the larynx (discussed below) during swallowing.)

(3) Laryngopharynx. That portion of the pharynx that is common to the respiratory a digestive systems is the laryngopharynx. It is the portion of the pharynx below the upper edge of the epiglottis. Thus, the digestive and respiratory systems lead into it from above, and lead off from it below.

1-4. LARYNX

The larynx, also called the Adam's apple or voice box, connects the pharynx with the trachea. The larynx, located in the anterior neck region, has a box-like shape. See Figure 1-3 for an illustration. Since the voice box of the male becomes larger and heavier during puberty, the voice deepens. The adult male's voice box tends to be located lower in the neck; in the female, the larynx remains higher and smaller and the voice is of a higher pitch.

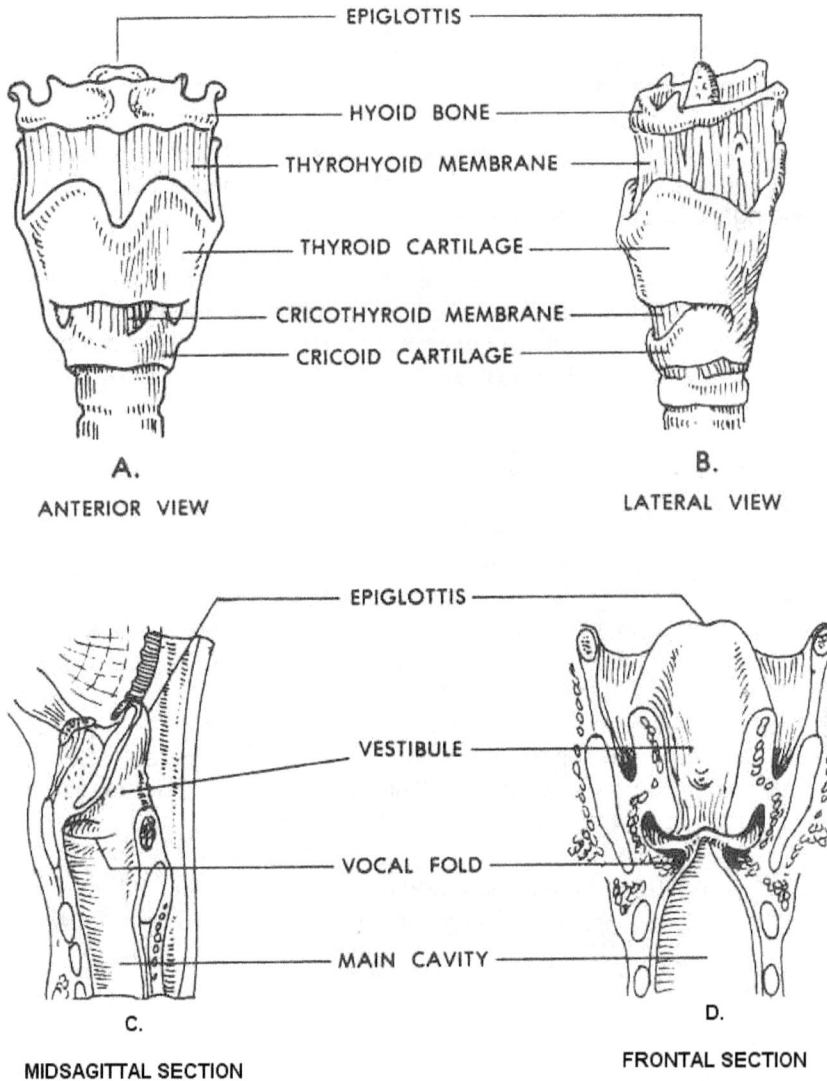

EPIGLOTTIS

HYOID BONE

THYROHYOID MEMBRANE

THYROID CARTILAGE

CRICOTHYROID MEMBRANE

CRICOID CARTILAGE

A.
ANTERIOR VIEW

B.
LATERAL VIEW

EPIGLOTTIS

VESTIBULE

VOCAL FOLD

MAIN CAVITY

C.
MIDSAGITTAL SECTION

D.
FRONTAL SECTION

Figure 1-3. The larynx.

a. **Parts and Spaces**. The larynx has a vestibule ("entrance hallway") that can be covered over by the epiglottis. The glottis itself is the hole between the vocal cords. Through the glottis, air passes from the vestibule into the main chamber of the larynx (below the cords) and then into the trachea. The skeleton of the larynx is made up of a series of cartilages.

b. **Muscles.** The larynx serves two functions and there are two sets of muscles- -one for each function.

(1)   One set controls the size of the glottis. Thus, it regulates the volume of air passing through the trachea.

(2)   The other set controls the tension of the vocal cords. Thus, it produces vibrations of selected frequencies (variations in pitch) of the moving air to be used in the process of speaking.

1-5. INFRALARYNGEAL STRUCTURES

a. **Trachea and Bronchi.** The respiratory tree (Figure 1-4) is the set of tubular structures that carry the air from the larynx to the alveoli of the lungs. Looking at a person UPSIDE DOWN, the trachea is the trunk of the tree and the bronchi are the branches. These tubular parts are held open (made patent) by rings of cartilage. Their lining is ciliated to remove mucus and other materials that get into the passageway.

b. **Alveoli.** The alveoli (alveolus, singular) are tiny spherical (balloon-like) sacs that are connected to the larger tubes of the lungs by tiny tubes known as alveolar ducts and bronchioles. The alveoli are so small that there are millions in the adult lungs. This very small size produces a maximum surface area through which external respiration takes place. External respiration is the actual exchange of gases between the air in the alveolar spaces and the adjacent blood capillaries through their walls.

c. **Lungs**. A lung is an individual organ composed of tubular structures and alveoli, bound together by fibrous connective tissue (FCT). In the human, there are two lungs, right and left. Each lung is supplied by a primary or mainstem bronchus leading off from the trachea. The right lung is larger in volume than the left lung. The left lung must leave room for the heart. The right lung is divided into 3 pulmonary lobes (upper, middle and lower) and 10 bronchopulmonary segments (2 + 3 + 5). The left lung is divided into 2 pulmonary lobes upper and lower) and 8 bronchopulmonary segments (4 + 4). A pulmonary lobe is a major subdivision of a lung marked by fissures (deep folds. Each lobe is further partitioned into bronchopulmonary segments. Each lobe is supplied by a secondary or lobar bronchus. A tertiary or segmental bronchus, a branch of the lobar bronchus supplies each segment.

d. **Pleural Cavities.** Each serous cavity has inner and outer membranes. In the case of the lungs, the inner membrane, is known as the visceral pleura which very closely covers the surface of the lungs. The outer membrane is known as the parietal pleura, forming the outer wall of the space. The pleural spaces are the potential spaces between the inner and outer membranes. The opening between the pleural layers contains a slick fluid called pleural fluid. The pleural fluid serves as a lubricant and allows the lungs to move freely with a minimum of friction.

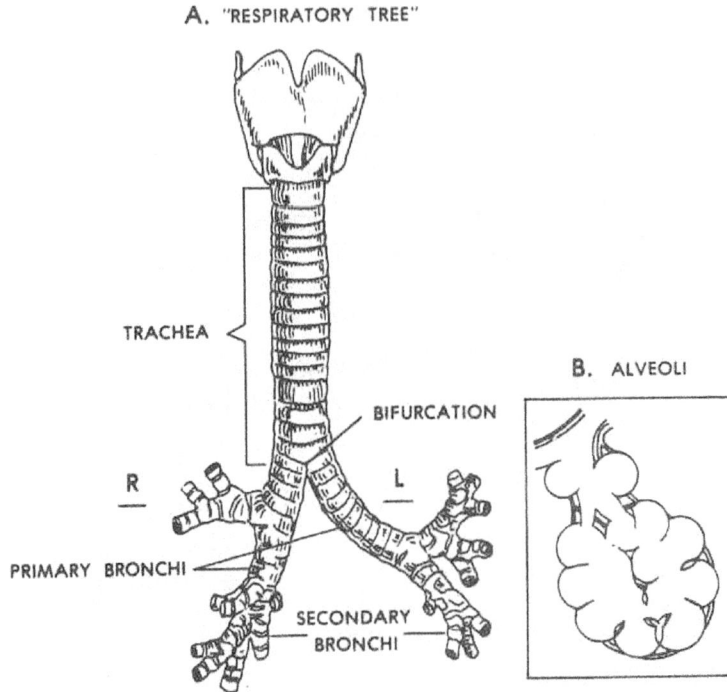

Figure 1-4. Infralaryngeal structures.

Section II. BREATHING AND BREATHING MECHANISMS IN HUMANS

1-6. INTRODUCTION

a. Boyle's law tells us that as the volume (V) of a gas-filled container increases, the pressure (P) inside decreases; as the volume (V) of a closed container decreases, the pressure (P) inside increases. When two connected spaces of air have different pressures, the air moves from the space with greater pressure to the one with lesser pressure. In regard to breathing, we can consider the air pressure around the human body to be constant. The pressure inside the lungs may be greater or less than the pressure outside the body. Thus, a greater internal pressure causes air to flow out; a greater external pressure causes air to flow in.

b. We can compare the human trunk to a hollow cylinder. This cylinder is divided into upper and lower cavities by the diaphragm. The upper is the thoracic cavity and is essentially gas-filled. The lower is the abdominopelvic cavity and is essentially water-filled.

1-7. COSTAL (THORACIC) BREATHING

a. **Inhalation**. Muscles attached to the thoracic cage raise the rib cage. A typical rib might be compared to a bucket handle, attached at one end to the sternum (breastbone) and at the other end to the vertebral column. The "bucket handle" is lifted by the overall movement upward and outward of the rib cage. These movements increase the thoracic diameters from right to left (transverse) and from front to back (A-P). Thus, the intrathoracic volume increases. Recalling Boyle's law, the increase in volume leads to a decrease in pressure. The air-pressure outside the body then forces air into the lungs and inflates them.

b. **Exhalation.** The rib cage movements and pressure relationships are reversed for exhalation. Thus, intrathoracic volume decreases. The intrathoracic pressure increases and forces air outside the body.

1-8. DIAPHRAGMATIC (ABDOMINAL) BREATHING

The diaphragm is a thin, but strong, dome-shaped muscular membrane that separates the abdominal and thoracic cavities. The abdominal wall is elastic in nature. The abdominal cavity is filled with soft, watery tissues.

a. **Inhalation**. As the diaphragm contracts, the dome flattens and the diaphragm descends. This increases the depth (vertical diameter) of the thoracic cavity and thus increases its volume. This decreases air pressure within the thoracic cavity. The greater air pressure outside the body then forces air into the lungs.

b. **Exhalation**. As the diaphragm relaxes, the elastic abdominal wall forces the diaphragm back up by pushing the watery tissues of the abdomen against the underside of the relaxed diaphragm. The dome extends upward. The process of inhalation is thus reversed.

Section III. CONDITIONS AFFECTING THE RESPIRATORY SYSTEM

1-9. INTRODUCTION

Many conditions affect the respiratory system. Some of the conditions are life-threatening, while many are chronic conditions which affect thousands of patients. Many of the patients who suffer from these conditions will be standing in front of the outpatient pharmacy in order to receive prescriptions to obtain some relief.

1-10. PNEUMONIA

Pneumonia is caused by an infection of the lung. This infection is caused by either bacteria (like the pneumococcus bacterium) or viruses. In pneumonia the walls of the alveoli become inflamed and filled with fluid and the air spaces in the alveoli become filled with blood and fluid. As you might expect, the exchange of gases in the alveoli becomes impaired. Death can result from pneumonia.

1-11. ASTHMA

Asthma, a condition usually caused by allergic reactions to substances in the environment, affects many people. The allergic reactions cause the bronchioles to spasm. Hence, the flow of air into and out of the lungs becomes impaired. For some unknown reason, the flow of air out of the lungs is more impeded than the flow of air into the lungs. Hence, the person with asthma often finds it more difficult to expire (expel the air) than to inspire. Furthermore, such labored breathing, after many years, often results in the asthma-sufferer having a barrel-shaped chest.

1-12. STATUS ASTHMATICUS

Status asthmaticus is a very sudden, continuous, and intense asthmatic attack.

1-13. EMPHYSEMA

Emphysema is a condition in which the patient has large portions of the alveolar walls destroyed. Consequently, the patient finds it necessary to breathe faster and more deeply in order to obtain the oxygen needed to live. Emphysema is often associated with smoking. Emphysema may also be referred to as Chronic Obstructive Pulmonary Disease (COPD).

I-14. PULMONARY EDEMA

Pulmonary edema is a condition in which fluid collects in the interstitial spaces of the lungs and in the alveoli. Obviously, the exchange of gases in the alveoli becomes impaired. Pulmonary edema is usually caused when the left side of the heart fails to pump efficiently; when this happens blood backs up into the pulmonary circulation and causes fluid in the lungs.

Section IV. RESPIRATORY SYSTEM DRUGS

1-15. INTRODUCTION

Drugs affecting the respiratory system have been in use for years. In the first part of this century, for example, various members of the morphine family (that is, heroin) were used in the treatment of coughs. In the 1980s, people are using both legend and over-the-counter cough preparations. At certain times of the year you will see many prescriptions for cough medicines and expectorants. You have probably seen such increases when winter arrives. This section of the subcourse will discuss some respiratory systems medications commonly seen in the pharmacy.

1-16. ANTITUSSIVE AGENTS

a. **Background**. Antitussives are agents that relieve or prevent coughing. These agents, in general, act on the central nervous system to depress the cough reflex center in the medulla of the brain. Antitussives are used to reduce respiratory irritation. Such reduction of respiratory irritation results in the patient's being able to rest better at night because he is not kept awake by his coughing.

b. **Antitussive Agents**.

(1) Codeine. Codeine is considered to be the most useful narcotic antitussive agent. Codeine aids in relieving the pain (that is, producing analgesia) associated with a hacking cough. The main side effects associated with codeine include drowsiness, nausea, vomiting, and constipation. When a preparation containing codeine is dispensed to a patient that patient should be told that the product may cause drowsiness, and that he should not drink alcohol while taking the medication. Codeine is a Note R drug alone and cannot be refilled. It is a Note Q item when it is found in combination products (for example: Robitussin A-C Syrup). The usual oral dosage of codeine alone is 15 milligrams (1/4 grain) every 4 to 6 hours as needed for cough. The dosage can be increased but should not exceed 120 milligrams in 24 hours because of its central nervous system (CNS) depressant effects.

(2) Benzonatate (Tessalon®). Benzonatate is a nonnarcotic antitussive that produces its effect through a CNS depressant effect similar to codeine. Furthermore, it produces a local anesthetic effect on the stretch receptors in the lower respiratory tract, which control coughing. Benzonatate is usually given in 100 milligram doses--three to six times daily. This drug has few side effects except that it will numb the mouth, tongue, and pharynx if the capsules are chewed (this is because of its topical anesthetic effect). Benzonatate is available in the form of 100 milligram capsules.

(3) Dextromethorphan, DM (Pertussin CS®). Dextromethorphan is another non-narcotic antitussive. It is found alone or in combination--usually with expectorants. The most common side effect associated with this drug is gastrointestinal (G.I.) upset. Dextromethorphan is a non-legend drug, which may be written as a prescription drug or as a hand-out item depending on the local policy of your hospital. The usual oral dosage of this drug is 10 to 30 milligrams, every four to eight hours. Do not exceed 120mg in 24 hours. There are many products on the market, which contain dextromethorphan in combination. Examples of such products include Robitussin-DM® and Baytussin-DM®.

1-17. EXPECTORANT AGENTS

a. **Background**. Expectorants are agents, which facilitate the removal of secretions of the bronchopulmonary mucous membrane. Most of the expectorants discussed below act reflexively by irritating the gastric mucosa. This, in turn, stimulates secretions in the respiratory tract. Expectorants are used to remove bronchial secretions which are purulent (containing pus), viscid (thick), or excessive. The loosened material is then moved toward the pharynx through ciliary motion and coughing.

b. **Expectorant Agents**.

(1) Guaifenesin (Robitussin®, Baytussin®). Guaifenesin is the most commonly used expectorant today. This nonlegend drug has the side effect of gastrointestinal (G.I.) upset. Guaifenesin may be found alone as a syrup (100 milligrams per 5 milliliters), tablet 600 mg (Humibid® L.A.), or in many combination products such as Robitussin-DM®.

(2) Saturated Solution of Potassium Iodide. Saturated Solution of Potassium Iodide (SSKI) is an expectorant administered as 300 milligrams (10 drops) in a glass of water or fruit juice every three or four times daily. SSKI has a very unpleasant taste. Overdoses of this product may lead to a condition known as iodism that produces an acne-type rash, fever, and rhinitis or runny nose. Patient compliance with this product may be low because of its unpleasant taste. Consequently, when the medication is dispensed you should tell the patient to place the required amount of SSKI in fruit juice in order to mask its taste. This drug is available in a saturated solution of 1 gram per milliliter in 30 milliliter containers.

(3) Elixir of Terpin Hydrate. Elixir of Terpin Hydrate (ETH) is an expectorant, which works directly on the bronchial secretory cells in the lower respiratory tract to facilitate the removal of bronchial secretions. It is usually given in doses, which range from 85 to 170 milligrams (1 or 2 teaspoonsful) 3 or 4 times daily. The side effects of this drug are related to its alcohol content (42 percent or 84 proof). If enough ETH is consumed it will produce significant CNS depression. Even with the high alcohol content, ETH is an Over the Counter (OTC) product. It is available as a syrup (85 milligrams per 5 milliliters) in 120 milliliter containers.

NOTE: Terpin Hydrate is no longer approved for use as an expectorant; it is used mainly as a vehicle for cough mixtures.

1-18. ANTITUSSIVE-EXPECTORANT COMBINATION PRODUCTS

The antitussive-expectorant combinations are used for a hyperactive nonproductive cough. The side effects of these drugs, or course, will be dependent on the antitussive-expectorant combination used. Some typical combination products used by the military are Robitussin-DM®, Robitussin® A-C Syrup, and Novahistine® Expectorant Liquid.

1-19. MUCOLYTICS

a. **Background.** Mucolytics are respiratory drugs that dissolve mucous in the respiratory tract. They are used by inhalation in an attempt to reduce the viscosity (thickness) of respiratory tract fluid. The loosened material can then be moved toward the pharynx more easily by ciliary motion and coughing. Like the expectorants, the mucolytics are used in the treatment of respiratory disorders in which the secretions are purulent (contain pus), viscid, or excessive. Consequently, the mucolytics represent an alternative to the oral use of expectorants.

b. **Mucolytic Agents**.

(1) Acetylcysteine (Mucomyst®). This is a mucolytic given by inhalation or nebulization. Nebulization is treatment by spray. Two to twenty milliliters of a 10 percent drug solution or 1 to 10 milliliters of a 20 percent Mucomyst® solution is nebulized into a face mask or mouth piece every two to six hours daily. Acetylcysteine has an unpleasant (like rotten eggs) smell. Side effects associated with this agent include nausea and vomiting and broncho-spasms with higher concentrations (with the 20 percent solution). This medication is only dispensed for inpatient use--usually to the respiratory therapy clinic or to the nursing station. The sterile solution should be covered, refrigerated, and used within 96 hours after the vial is opened. It is available in 10 percent and 20 percent solutions in containers of 4, 10, or 30 milliliters.

(2) Sodium Chloride Solution U.S.P. (0.9 percent sodium chloride solution). This agent is used alone or in combination with other mucolytic agents. Sodium chloride solution increases the respiratory fluid volume by osmosis, which tends to decrease the viscosity of the respiratory fluid. It is also administered by inhalation in a nebulized form as a dense mist in a tent or delivered through a face mask or mouth piece. The main side effect seen with sodium chloride solution occurs after prolonged inhalation. This will cause localized irritation of the bronchial mucosa. Sodium chloride solution for this purpose is for inpatient use by respiratory therapy personnel or by nursing personnel. Concentrated Sodium Chloride (23.4%) is used by respiratory therapy to induce sputum production (sputum induction procedure).

1-20. BRONCHODILATOR AGENTS

a. **Background**. The bronchodilators are agents that cause expansion of the air passages of the lungs. This allows the patient to breathe more easily and are of value in overcoming acute bronchospasms. They are employed as adjuncts in prophylactic and symptomatic treatment of the individual complications of obstructive pulmonary diseases such as asthma, bronchitis, and emphysema. Most of these agents have been discussed in other lessons of the pharmacology series.

b. **Bronchodilator Agents (Sympathomimetics).** Sympathomimetic bronchodilators act by relaxing contractions of the smooth muscle of the bronchioles. These agents are often referred to as "Beta agonists".

(1) Albuterol (Proventil®, Ventolin®). Albuterol is a short acting beta-agonist or bronchodilator. It is used in the relief and prevention of bronchospasm and in the prevention of exercise-induced bronchospasm. Albuterol is available as an inhalation aerosol, inhalation solution, inhalation capsules, regular and sustained release tablets, and syrup. Other than the sustained release products, it is prescribed every 4 to 6 hours. Albuterol is often used as "rescue therapy" due to its quick onset of action.

(2) Salmeterol (Serevent®). Salmeterol is indicated for the same conditions as albuterol, however its distinct advantage is that it is administered twice daily. It is available as an inhalation aerosol. Salmeterol CANNOT be used for "rescue therapy"; a short acting beta agonist such as albuterol must be used.

(3) (Epinephrine (Adrenalin®). Epinephrine is used as a bronchodilator because of its beta effects on the bronchi and a pharmacologic antagonist of histamine. Epinephrine is employed for the treatment of acute attacks of bronchospasms associated with emphysema, bronchitis, or anaphylaxis. The inhalation route is not the preferred route of administration, however, it may be used. Epinephrine is usually administered subcutaneously when used and is fairly effective at reducing bronchospasms.

(4) Metaproterenol (Alupent®, Metaprel®). This is an adrenergic agent that has primary beta2 activity. That is, its main effect is to relax the bronchioles. It has the same indications as epinephrine. It may be used for the prevention of bronchospasms associated with chronic obstructive pulmonary diseases. Inhalation of metaproterenol may be used in the treatment of mild bronchospasm attacks. Metaproterenol is somewhat more effective than inhaled isoproterenol. Metaproterenol's duration of action is substantially longer than that of isoproterenol.

(5) Ephedrine. Ephedrine has actions of those similar to those of epinephrine. Ephedrine is not frequently used because of the availability of other more suitable agents. Ephedrine is administered orally. It is used to treat mild bronchospasm attacks and prophylactically to prevent bronchospasm attacks. Ephedrine is not as suitable as epineprhine for the treatment of severe attacks of bronchial asthma because its bronchodilator action is weaker.

(6) Isoproterenol (Isuprel®). Isoproterenol is an adrenergic agent used to treat asthma, bronchitis, and emphysema. Like metaproterenol, isoproterenol is administered by inhalation for the treatment of mild bronchospasms. Isoproterenol may be administered intravenously with great caution to treat status asthmaticus.

(7) Other sympathomimetic bronchodilators include terbutaline (Brethine®), pirbuterol (Maxair®), and bitolterol mesylate (Tornalate®).

c. **Bronchodilator Agents (Xanthine derivatives).** The methylxanthines (theophylline and derivatives) directly relax the smooth muscle of the bronchi and pulmonary blood vessels. They may also reduce the fatigability and thereby improve contractility in patients with chronic obstructive airway disease. Xanthine derivatives are often used in the treatment of apnea and bradycardia of prematurity in infants.

(1) Aminophylline. Aminophylline is a xanthine derivative containing ~80% theophylline. It is prescribed as a bronchodilator to treat asthma. It will also relieve bronchospasms associated with emphysema and bronchitis. Aminophylline may be administered orally or rectally to prevent severe attacks of bronchial asthma but is generally administered intravenously (I.V.) to relieve acute bronchospasms or status asthmaticus resistant to adrenergic drugs.

(2) Theophylline (Theolair®, Slo-Phyllin®, Theodur®). Theophylline is often prescribed as the xanthine of choice for oral administration (tablets, capsules, elixir, syrup, or solution). One must take care when dispensing theophylline products. Each different brand varies in the actual amount of theophylline contained in the product and in the duration of action. Theophylline is a drug with a very narrow therapeutic index (the treatment dose is very close to the toxic dose). For this reason, patients should have their theophylline blood levels monitored on a routine basis.

d. **Miscellaneous Respiratory Agents.**

(1) Cromolyn (Intal®). Cromolyn is a unique product that works by inhibiting the release of histamine and other spasm-causing compounds from mast cells located in the lungs and prevents bronchoconstriction. It is used mainly for the treatment or prevention of mild bronchospasms associated with asthma. It is available as an inhalation aerosol and nebulization solution.

(2) Leukotriene modifiers. The production of leukotrienes (immunologic proteins) and the binding of leukotriene receptors appears to be responsible for airway edema, smooth muscle constriction and altered inflammatory processes contributing to the signs and symptoms of asthma. For this reason, several new agents have been developed.

(a) Zafirlukast (Accolate®), montelukast (Singulair®). Both of these agents are leukotriene receptor antagonists which cause inhibition of bronchoconstriction. Zafirlukast is available as a tablet prescribed twice daily. Montelukast is prescribed as a once daily tablet.

(b) Ziluton (Zyflo®), Ziluton works a little differently in that it inhibits the formation of leukotrienes to prevent bronchoconstriction. Ziluton is administered four times daily.

Continue with Exercises

EXERCISES, LESSON 1

REQUIREMENT: The following exercises are to be answered by marking the lettered response that best answers the question; or by completing the incomplete statement; or by writing the answer in the space provided at the end of the question.

After you have completed all the exercises, turn to "Solutions to Exercises", at the end of the lesson, and check your answers with the solutions.

1. External respiration is _____.

    a. The exchange of gases between the atmosphere and the cells of the body.

    b. The exchange of gases between the blood and the individual cells of the body.

    c.   The exchange of gases between the air in the lungs and blood.

    d.   The aeration of the lungs.

2. Bronchi are _____.

    a. Tubes that lead from the larynx to the lungs.

    b. Tubes that warm and humidify the air as it enters the lungs.

    c. Tubes that extend into the nasal chamber in order to increase the surface area exposed to inflowing air.

    d. Tubes that lead from the trachea to the lungs.

3. Select the statement that best describes the paranasal sinuses.

    a. Air cells or cavities in the skull that are connected with the nasal chambers and lined with ciliated mucoperiosteum.

    b. Special nerve endings located in the upper areas of the nasal chambers.

    c. The portion of the pharynx that is common to both the respiratory and digestive systems.

    d. The vestibules that are covered by the epiglottis.

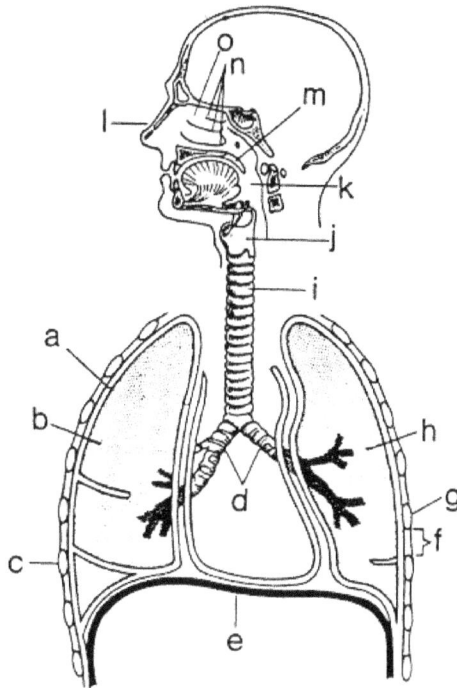

The human respiratory system.

4. Which letter in the illustration above refers to the bronchi?

    a. a

    b. b

    c. c

    d. d

5. Which letter in the illustration above refers to the pleural space?

    a. a

    b. b

    c. c

    d. d

6. Which of the statements below best describes abdominal breathing?

    a. Breathing which occurs because of the contractions of the small intestine and other abdominal organs.

    b. Breathing which occurs because of changes in the intrathoracic volume.

    c. Breathing which occurs because of the contraction and relaxation of the diaphragm.

    d. Breathing which occurs because of changes in the position of the rib cage.

7. Pneumonia is best described as _____.

    a. A condition in which fluid collects in the interstitial spaces of the lungs caused by the left heart's inability to pump efficiently.

    b. An infection of the lungs caused by bacteria or viruses in which the walls of the alveoli become inflamed.

    c. A condition in which the patient has large portions of the walls of the alveoli destroyed.

    d. A state of impaired breathing caused by spasms of the bronchi.

8. Mucolytic agents are drugs which _____.

    a. Relieve bronchospasms.

    b. Dissolve mucous in the respiratory tract.

    c. Are used to irritate the gastric mucosa.

    d. Relieve or prevent coughing.

9. Acetylcysteine is used as a(n) _____.

    a. Antitussive agent.

    b. Mucolytic agent.

    c. Expectorant agent.

    d. Bronchodilator.

10. Elixir of Terpin Hydrate is used as a(n) _____.

    a. Expectorant.

    b. Antitussive.

    c. Mucolytic.

    d. Bronchodilator.

11. Match the drug name in Column A with its corresponding trade name in Column B.

Column A	Column B
_____Acetylcysteine.	a. Isuprel®.
_____Metaproterenol.	b. Alupent®.
_____Guaifenesin.	c. Tessalon®
_____Cromolyn.	d. Mucomyst®.
_____Isoproterenol.	e. Intal®.
_____Benzonatate.	f. Baytussin®.

Check Your Answers on Next Page

SOLUTIONS TO EXERCISES, LESSON 1

1. c   The exchange of gases between the air in the lungs and blood. (para 1-1a)

2. d   Tubes which lead from the trachea to the lungs. (para 1-5a)

3. a   Air cells or cavities in the skull which are connected with the nasal chambers and lined with ciliated mucoperiosteum. (para 1-3b(4))

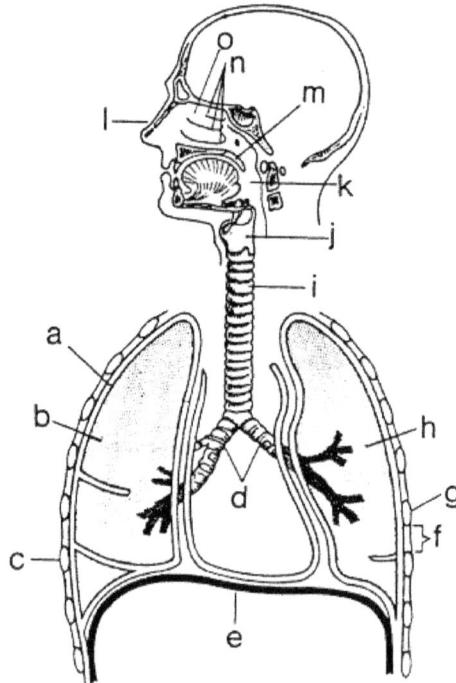

4. d   (Figure 1-1)

5. a   (Figure 1-1)

6. c   Breathing which occurs because of the contraction and relaxation of the diaphragm. (para 1-8)

7. b   An infection of the lungs caused by bacteria or viruses in which the walls of the alveoli become inflamed. (para 1-10)

8. b   Dissolve mucous in the respiratory tract. (para 1-19a)

9. b   Mucolytic agent. (para 1-19b(1))

10. a   Expectorant. (para 1-17b(3))

11.   COLUMN A   COLUMN B

    __d__   Acetylcysteine. (para 1-19b(1))   a. Isuprel®.

    __b__   Metaproterenol. (para 1-20b(4))   b. Alupent®.

    __f__   Guaifenesin. (para 1-17b(1))   c. Tessalon®.

    __e__   Cromolyn. (para 1-20d(1))   d. Mucomyst®.

    __a__   Isoproterenol. (para 1-20b(6))   e. Intal®.

    __c__   Benzonatate. (para 1-16b(2))   f. Baytussin®.

End of Lesson 1

LESSON ASSIGNMENT

LESSON 2   The Human Cardiovascular and Lymphatic Systems.

LESSON ASSIGNMENT   Paragraphs 2-1--2-22.

TASKS   081-824-0001, Perform Initial Screening of a Prescription.

                                     081-824-0026, Evaluate a Prescription.

                                     081-824-0002/3, Fill a Prescription for a Controlled/Non-Controlled Drug.

                                     081-824-0027, Evaluate a Completed Prescription.

                                     081-824-0028, Issue Outpatient Medications.

LESSON OBJECTIVES   After you finish this lesson you should be able to:

2-1.   Given a group of statements, select the statement that best explains the need for circulatory systems.

2-2.   Given a group of systems, select the two circulatory systems in the human body.

2-3.   Given the name of one of the major components of the human circulatory system and a group of statements, select the statement that best describes that component.

2-4.   Given a group of components, select the components of blood.

2-5.   From a group of statements, select the statement that best describes either the plasma or the formed elements of the blood.

2-6.   Given a group of statements and the names of one of the formed elements of the blood, select the statement that best describes the given formed elements.

2-7.   From a group of functions, select the function(s) of the blood.

2-8.   Given a group of statements and one of the types of blood vessels, select the statement that best describes that type of blood vessel.

2-9.   Given the steps of blood clotting in an unsequential order and several selections of varying sequence, select the sequence of blood clotting as the steps actually occur.

2-10.   From a group of statements, select the definition of the term blood pressure, systolic blood pressure, and diastolic blood pressure.

2-11.   Given a group of medical problems and one of the following conditions: hypertension and hypotension, select the medical problem(s) associated with the given condition.

2-12.   Given a group of statements and the name of a disorder which may affect the circulatory system, select the statement that best describes the disorder.

2-13.   Given a drawing of either the anterior or the interior view of the human heart and a list of names of parts of the heart, match the name of each part of the heart with its location.

2-14.   From a group of statements, select the statement that best describes the property of inherent rhythmicity.

2-15.   Given one of the following: sinoatrial node, atrioventricular node, Bundle of HIS, or Purkinje fibers and a group of statements; select the statement that best describes the role of the given heart structure in the heartbeat.

2-16.   Given one of the following electrolytes: sodium, potassium, or calcium and a group of statements, select the statement which best describes the effect(s) of abnormal amounts of that electrolyte on the myocardium.

2-17. Given the name of a cardiac disorder and a group of statements, select the statement that best describes that disorder.

2-18. Given the name of one of the structures of the human lymphatic system and a group of statements, select the statement that best describes that structure.

SUGGESTION

After completing the assignment, complete the exercises at the end of this lesson. These exercises will help you to achieve the lesson objectives.

LESSON 2

THE HUMAN CARDIOVASCULAR AND LYMPHATIC SYSTEMS

Section I. INTRODUCTION

2-1. NEED FOR CIRCULATORY SYSTEMS

    a. The need for circulatory systems is based on two criteria:

    (1) <u>Number of cells</u>. Multicellular animals are animals with great numbers of cells.

    (2) <u>Size</u>. In larger animals, most cells are too far away from sources of food and oxygen for simple diffusion to provide sufficient amounts. Also, distances are too great for simple removal of wastes.

    b. Because of these criteria, we need a system (or systems) to carry materials to all cells. To get food and oxygen to the cells and to remove waste products, we need a <u>transport</u> system, or <u>circulatory</u> system. Human circulatory systems are so effective that few cells are more than the width of two cells away from a capillary.

2-2. BASIC COMPONENTS OF ANY CIRCULATORY SYSTEM

    The four basic components of any circulatory system are a vehicle, conduits, a motive force, and exchange areas.

    a. **Vehicle.** The <u>vehicle</u> is the substance that actually carries the materials being transported.

    b. **Conduits**. A <u>conduit</u> is a channel, pipe, or tube through which a vehicle travels.

    c. **Motive Force**. If we say that a force is <u>motive</u>, we mean that it produces movement. Systems providing a motive force are often known as <u>pumps</u>.

    d. **Exchange Areas**. Since the materials being transported must eventually be exchanged with a part of the body, special areas are developed for this purpose. They are called <u>exchange areas</u>.

2-3. CIRCULATORY SYSTEMS IN THE HUMAN BODY

    a. The <u>cardiovascular system</u> is the circulatory system involving the heart and blood vessels.

b. The lymphatic system is a drainage-type circulatory system involved with the clear fluid known as lymph.

c. There are other minor circulatory systems in the human body, such as the one involved with cerebrospinal fluid.

Section II. THE HUMAN CARDIOVASCULAR SYSTEM

2-4. GENERAL

The human cardiovascular system is a collection of interacting structures designed to supply oxygen and nutrients to living cells and to remove carbon dioxide and other wastes. Its major components are the:

a. **Blood**. Blood is the vehicle for oxygen, nutrients, and wastes.

b. **Blood Vessels**. Blood vessels are the conduits, or channels, through which the blood is moved.

c. **Heart**. The heart is the pump that provides the primary motive force.

d. **Capillaries**. The capillaries, minute (very small) vessels, provide exchange areas. For example, in the capillaries of the lungs, oxygen is added and carbon dioxide is removed from the blood.

2-5. BLOOD

Blood is the vehicle for the human cardiovascular system. Its major subdivisions are the plasma, a fluid containing proteins, and the formed elements, including red blood cells, white blood cells, and platelets.

a. **Plasma.**

(1) Plasma makes up about 55 percent of the total blood volume. It is mainly composed of water. A variety of materials are dissolved in plasma. Among the most important of these are proteins.

(2) After the blood clots, the clear fluid remaining is called serum. Serum does not contain the proteins used for clotting. Otherwise, it is very similar to plasma.

b. **Formed Elements**. The formed elements make up about 45 percent of the total blood volume. The formed elements are cellular in nature. While the red blood cells (RBCs) and white blood cells (WBCs) are cells, the platelets are only fragments of cells.

(1) Red blood cells (erythrocytes). Red blood cells (RBCs) are biconcave discs. That is, they are shaped something like an inner tube from an automobile tire, but with a thin middle portion instead of a hole. There are approximately 5,000,000 RBCs in a cubic millimeter of normal adult blood. Red blood cells contain hemoglobin, a protein that carries most of the oxygen transported by the blood.

(2) White blood cells (leukocytes). There are various types of WBCs, but the most common are neutrophils and lymphocytes. Neutrophils phagocytize (swallow up) foreign particles and organisms, and digest them. Lymphocytes produce antibodies and serve other functions in immunity. In normal adults, there are about 5,000 to 11,000 WBCs per cubic millimeter of blood.

(3) Platelets. Platelets are about half the size of erythrocytes. They are fragments of cells. Since they are fragile, they last only about 3-5 days. Their main function is to aid in clotting by clumping together and by releasing chemical factors relating to clotting. There are 150,000-350,000 platelets in a cubic millimeter of normal blood.

c. **Some General Functions of the Blood**.

(1) Blood serves as a vehicle for oxygen nutrients, carbon dioxide and other wastes, hormones, antibodies, heat, and so forth.

(2) Blood aids in temperature control. Beneath the skin, there is a network of vessels that functions much like a radiator. To avoid accumulation of excess heat in the body, the flow of blood to these vessels can be increased greatly. Here, aided by the evaporative cooling provided by the sweat glands, large amounts of heat can be rapidly given off. The flow of blood also keeps the outer parts of the body from becoming too cold.

(3) The blood aids in protecting our bodies by providing immunity. Some WBCs phagocytize (swallow up) foreign particles and microorganisms. Other WBCs produce antibodies. The blood transports antibodies throughout the body.

(4) Blood clotting is another function of blood. Not only does this prevent continued blood loss; it also helps prevent invasion of the body by microorganisms and viruses by sealing the wound opening.

2-6. BLOOD VESSELS

The blood is conducted or carried through the body by tubular structures known as blood vessels. Since at no time does the whole blood ever leave a blood vessel of some sort, we refer to this system as a closed system.

a. **General Construction**. The blood vessels in general are tubular and have a three-layered wall.

(1) Intima. A layer of smooth epithelium known as the intima lines the lumen (hollow central cavity).

(2) Media. A middle layer of smooth muscle tissue is called the media.

(3) Adventitia. The adventitia is the outer layer of fibrous connective tissue that holds everything together.

b. Types of Blood Vessels. See Figure 2-1 for a diagram of the human circulatory system. We recognize three types of blood vessels:

(1) The arteries carry blood away from the chambers of the heart.

(2) The veins carry blood to the chambers of the heart.

(3) Capillaries are extremely thin-walled vessels having only the intimal layer through which exchanges can take place between the blood and the tissue cells.

c. **Relationships.** Arteries and veins are largest where they are closest to the heart. Away from the heart, they branch into smaller and smaller and more numerous vessels. The branching continues until the smallest arteries (arterioles) empty into the capillaries. The capillaries in turn are drained by the venules of the venous system.

d. **Valves**. Within the heart and the veins are structures known as valves. Valves function to insure that the blood flows in only one direction.

2-7. BLOOD CLOTTING

Blood clotting is a process that is dependent on several different factors. This process is also known as hemostasis. There are three general mechanisms involved in blood clotting: vascular spasm, the platelet plug, and the clotting mechanism.

a. **Vascular Spasm**. When a blood vessel is cut, the vascular spasm causes rapid constriction of the cut blood vessel. This decreases the amount of blood lost. The mechanism by which this mechanism occurs is not fully known, but it appears to be a reflex response initiated by pain. It is interesting to note that when a vessel is cut by crushing, the vascular spasm response seems to occur more rapidly and more intensely than if the vessel is quickly cut (as with a knife). After the vascular spasm has occurred, the second mechanism involved with the clotting process--the platelet plug--occurs.

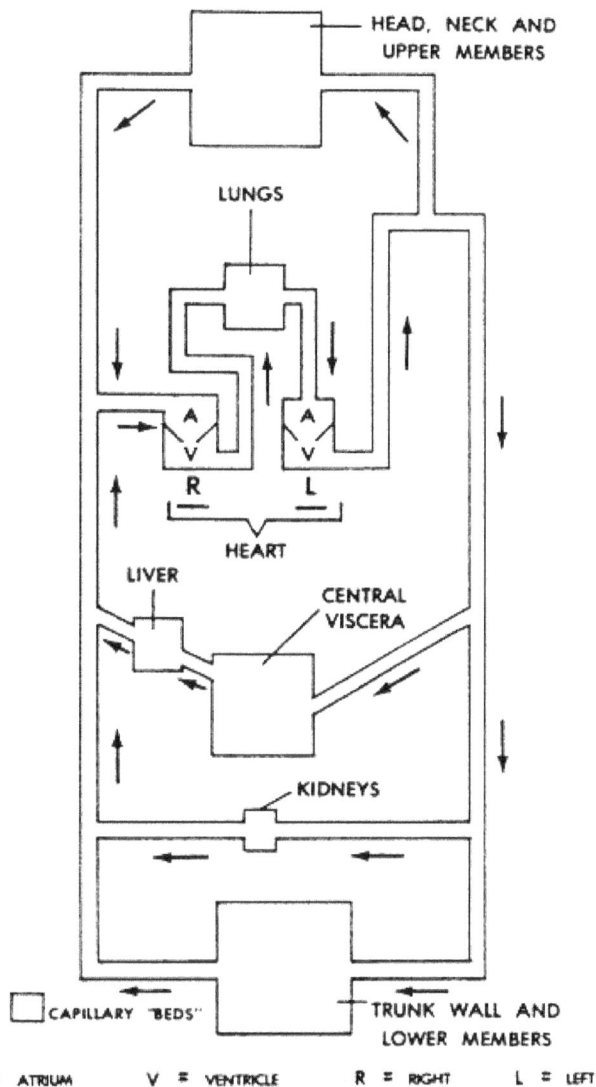

Figure 2-1. Diagram of the human circulatory system.

    b. **Platelet Plug**. The blood platelets circulate freely in the blood until they reach a blood vessel that has been severed. Platelets then adhere to the ruptured point of the blood vessel. After a period of time, the platelets partially plug the severed vessel.

    c. **Clotting Mechanism**. The third mechanism involves the formation of the blood clot. The clot forms within three to six minutes after the rupturing of the blood vessel. In about 30 minutes the clot shrinks; thus pulling the end of the severed vessel in to close the diameter of the vessel even further.

2-8. MECHANISMS OF BLOOD CLOTTING

The actual clotting mechanisms involve several steps--each step is essential to clotting:

STEP 1: The blood platelets release a substance that is known as thromboplastin.

STEP 2: Thromboplastin reacts with calcium and another substance, prothrombin, to form thrombin. Vitamin K is necessary for the proper formation of prothrombin.

STEP 3: The thrombin formed acts as an enzyme to convert fibrinogen to fibrin threads that eventually form the blood clot.

NOTE: For a more in-depth discussion of blood clotting you should locate and read a physiology text that is appropriate to your level of understanding.

2-9. BLOOD PRESSURE

a. **Introduction**. Blood pressure is the force exerted by the blood as it is pumped throughout the circulatory system. Blood pressure is needed by the body for the perfusion and distribution of nutrients throughout the body. Blood pressure is expressed in numerical values with the use of an instrument such as the sphygmomanometer. Blood pressure is expressed as systolic blood pressure over diastolic blood pressure (for example, 120/70). Systolic blood pressure is the pressure of blood as it is being pumped from the heart. When the heart contracts, it is said to be in systole. Diastolic pressure is the residual pressure of the blood because of the elasticity of the blood vessels (when the heart is at rest).

b. **Regulation**. In order to regulate blood pressure to meet the immediate needs of the body, the body is equipped with various systems that can change the blood pressure both by a change in the size of the openings of the various blood vessels and by a change in the volume of the blood (that is, blood plasma).

(1) Baroreceptors. Baroreceptors are located in the aortic arch of the aorta and in the internal carotid arteries. Baroreceptors are really a series of specialized neurons that function as rapidly acting blood pressure regulators. They sense changes in blood pressure and act in a reflex manner to change both the rate and force of the contraction of the heart and the size of the openings of the blood vessels.

(2) Chemoreceptors. Chemoreceptors are receptors which sense changes in the oxygen content of the blood. They are located in high numbers in the aortic arch

and internal carotid arteries. The chemoreceptors have a dual purpose in that they help to regulate blood pressure in addition to the regulation of blood pressure. The change in blood pressure they produce is due mainly to the change in heart rate. Working in conjunction with the chemoreceptors is a mechanism known as the CNS ischemic response. The CNS ischemic response senses an increase in carbon dioxide and lactic acid (both waste products of metabolism) in the blood and reacts to increase or decrease heart rate to maintain these products within normal amounts. The CNS ischemic response generally decreases the heart rate so that blood spends a longer time in the lungs thereby allowing for an increased exchange of oxygen and carbon dioxide.

   c.   **Correction of Blood Pressure**. Blood pressure is corrected by changing blood vessel tone and cardiac output. The baroreceptors eventually adapt to whatever pressure level to which they are exposed. Therefore, prolonged regulation of arterial pressure requires other control systems. Kidney malfunctions, fluid shifts, and electrolyte imbalances will eventually occur if this condition is not corrected. These are also known as long term regulators.

   d.   **Renal Fluid-Volume Mechanism.** The renal fluid-volume mechanism is one of the long-term regulators located in the kidneys. This mechanism works by causing changes in the amount of water reabsorbed by the kidneys. An increase in water reabsorption leads to an increase in blood pressure and a decrease in water reabsorption leads to a corresponding decrease in the blood pressure. The secretion of certain hormones also affects blood pressure. Aldosterone, a hormone secreted by the adrenal cortex, leads to an increase in sodium retention. This increase in sodium retention leads to a corresponding increase in water retention with an overall effect of higher blood pressure.

2-10.   ABNORMAL BLOOD PRESSURE

   a.   **Hypertension.** Hypertension is characterized by a persistent increase in blood pressure. It should be noted that there are always periodic increases in blood pressure due to times of stress or physical exertion. However, if the blood pressure remains at these high levels serious complications could result. Some of the effects of hypertension on the body are frequent nosebleeds, strokes, hypertrophy of the myocardium, and arteriosclerosis. Hypertension is one of the easiest disorders to treat if it is detected early. Drug therapy consists of diuretics and other antihypertensives. It is essential for the patient who has controlled his blood pressure by the use of medication to continue to take that medication even after the outward signs and symptoms subside.

   b.   **Hypotension**. Hypotension is defined as persistent and abnormal low blood pressure. This condition is not usually fatal in itself; however, the hypotensive patient is much more susceptible to shock in case of a rapid loss of blood. Many times low blood pressure is observed in persons who exercise a great deal. When hypotension becomes serious, it can be treated by drug therapy. Effects of hypotension on the body include general fatigue and weakness and decreased kidney function. An increase in the susceptibility to orthostatic hypotension (that is, the patient faints when arising too quickly from a bed or chair) or fainting is also seen.

2-11. DISORDERS WHICH AFFECT THE BLOOD SYSTEM

As with any other system of the body, some disorders may affect the blood system. Usually these disorders are types of anemias, but there are other disorders involved.

a. **Iron Deficiency Anemia.** Iron deficiency anemia is due to a deficiency of elemental iron in the blood. Iron is essential for the proper functioning of hemoglobin. In iron deficiency anemia, the blood cannot transport as much oxygen. Therefore, the tissues of the body are deprived of the much-needed oxygen. Furthermore, the presence of iron deficiency anemia affects the formulation of blood cells. Treatment of iron deficiency anemia requires the administration of iron either orally or parenterally.

b. **Hemolytic Anemia.** Hemolytic anemia is a general term referring to anemias caused by weakened red blood cell membranes. There are several types of hemolytic anemias that are often classified according to their cause. Some of the causes of hemolytic anemia are drugs (such as primaquine or the sulfonamides), heredity, or lack of either vitamin B_{12} or folic acid. In hemolytic anemia, the red blood cells are weak and lyse (break apart) as they squeeze through the small capillaries or spleen. The treatment of the hemolytic anemias is obviously dependent on the particular cause. Splenectomies, discontinuance of the causative agent, or the administration of folic acid or vitamin B_{12} are some of the treatment possibilities.

c. **Sickle Cell Anemia.** Sickle cell anemia is a serious anemia that is predominant in people of black race. The erythrocytes of a person who has sickle cell anemia become sickle-shaped and, therefore, are not efficient carriers of gases or nutrients. The sickle-shaped cells also increase the viscosity of the blood that leads to decreased circulation in the small arteries and capillaries. Symptoms of sickle-cell anemia include pain of certain organs, bone and joint pain, fever, and cerebral thrombosis. The spleen is not usually enlarged. Complications associated with sickle cell anemia are leg ulcers, osteomyelitis, and occasionally, cardiac enlargement. The treatment for sickle cell anemia is usually symptomatic as the actual cause of the condition is unknown. Blood transfusions are usually involved in most treatment regimens.

d. **Aplastic Anemia.** Aplastic anemia is a very serious and usually fatal condition that affects about four out of every one million people. It is characterized by a progressive degeneration of the bone marrow that is rarely reversible. The usual cause appears to be toxins or drugs and excessive use of X-rays. The prognosis of this severe bone marrow depression is generally poor.

e.   **Hemophilia**. Hemophilia is usually a hereditary disease characterized by a lack of one of the factors necessary for the clotting of the blood. Hemophilia is a disease that occurs more commonly in men than women. Patients who have hemophilia do not usually develop massive hemorrhages, but rather slow oozing or trickling of blood. The primary danger with hemophiliac patients is trauma involving severe bleeding. In these cases, the patient may soon die because of a severe loss of blood that will occur if the missing clotting factor is not soon administered.

f.   **Leukemia**. Leukemia is a disease of the white blood cell forming tissue. It is characterized by an abnormally high white blood cell count. During the progression of the disease, the white blood cells gradually crowd out the erythrocytes and in some cases the leukocytes phagocytize (engulf) the red blood cells.

g.   **Mononucleosis**. Mononucleosis is an extremely contagious disease **characterized** by an abnormally large number of one type of white blood cells (the monocytes). The disease affects the lymph tissue and is characterized by fever, sore throat, and inflamed lymph nodes. The spleen may become enlarged and lassitude (general tired feeling) on the part of the patient is not uncommon. Mononucleosis is thought to be a disease of viral origin that usually strikes people between the ages of ten and thirty-five. The treatment of mononucleosis is symptomatic. The disease usually runs its complete course in about four to six weeks.

h.   **Pernicious Anemia**. Pernicious anemia is caused by the inability of the body to absorb vitamin B_{12} from the intestine. This failure to absorb vitamin B_{12} is caused by a lack of the intrinsic factor that is normally secreted by the parietal cells in the stomach. The presence of this intrinsic factor is needed in order to absorb vitamin B_{12}. Perncious anemia rarely affects persons under the age of thirty-five. It is more common in persons of English, Scandinavian, and Irish descent. It may be difficult to detect this condition because there are few outwardly visible signs associated with it. As with all anemias, fatigability is usually the first noticeable symptom. The red blood cells are large and oval. The treatment of pernicious anemia centers on the parenteral administration of vitamin B_{12} (cyanocobalamin) which must be continued for the remainder of the patient's life.

2-12.   DISORDERS ASSOCIATED WITH THE CIRCULATORY SYSTEM

NOTE: Two rather acute disorders that affect the circulatory system are a thrombus and an embolus. They are not considered diseases, but acute disorders.

a.   **Thrombus**. A thrombus is a clot formed in a blood vessel that remains attached to the wall of the vessel. A thrombus can conceivably occur in any blood vessel. However, they are of primary concern when they occur in vessels serving vital organ systems such as the liver, kidneys, brain, and heart. Thrombi frequently get larger within the vessel and, if untreated, may eventually lead to complete blockage of the vessel. Such a blockage could lead to an infarction, an area of necrosis in a tissue or organ that results from the obstruction of circulation to that area.

b. **Embolus**. If the thrombus becomes dislodged from the wall of the vessel, it becomes an embolus. The usual treatment for an embolus is anticoagulant therapy in an effort to decrease the possibility of any future clotting. If necessary, certain enzymes may be administered to the patient in order to dissolve the existing clot. Treatment of an embolus is nearly impossible until it becomes an embolism. When the embolism has been identified, the treatment usually involves bed rest, anticoagulant therapy, and the possible administration of fibrinolytic enzymes.

2-13. VASCULAR DISORDERS

Vascular disorders comprise some of the most common disorders in humans. Usually symptoms of vascular disorders are not seen until the condition reaches a point where it is considered serious. Several vascular disorders are discussed below:

a. **Arteriosclerosis.** A loss of elasticity or hardening of the arterial walls characterizes arteriosclerosis. The result is a decrease in the ability of these arteries to change their diameter. A complication that usually accompanies arteriosclerosis is atherosclerosis. Atherosclerosis is a condition in which lipid (fat) deposits form on the inside of the arteries causing a decrease in the flow of blood through the arteries. Both these conditions show a higher incidence in diabetics and in overweight individuals. Surgery and antihyperlipidemic drugs are used to treat these conditions.

b. **Varicose Veins**. A varicose vein is a condition that is probably because of excessively prolonged pooling of blood in the lower extremities (for example: legs). Varicose veins are especially common in people who are required to stand for prolonged periods of time with little or no exercise.

c. **Peripheral Vascular Disease**. Peripheral vascular disease is characterized by vasoconstriction of the arteries (especially in the extremities). Decreased blood flow to the extremities and corresponding hypothermia are some of the usual signs of this condition.

2-14. BONE MARROW DEPRESSION

Bone marrow depression is a condition characterized by a decrease in the function of the bone marrow that leads to a reduction in the cellular components of the blood. The overall effect of bone marrow depression is anemia and susceptibility to infection. The most common cause of bone marrow depression seems to be the toxicity of drugs. If detected early, the reversal of the disease may be accomplished by the removal of the causative agent (for example, the drug).

Section III. THE HEART AND THE SYSTEMIC CIRCULATION OF BLOOD

2-15. THE HEART

Through the action of its very muscular walls, the heart produces the primary motive force to drive the blood through the arterial system. In humans, the heart is located just above the diaphragm, in the middle of the thorax, and extending slightly to the left. It is said that the heart of an average individual is about the size of that individual's clenched fist.

a. **General Construction of the Human Heart**. See Figure 2-2 for an illustration of the human heart.

(1) <u>Chambers</u>. The heart is divided into four cavities known as the <u>chambers</u>. The upper two chambers are known as the atria, right and left. Each atrium has an ear-like projection known as an auricle. The lower two chambers are known as <u>ventricles</u>, right and left. Between the two atria is a common wall known as the <u>interatrial septum</u>. Between the two ventricles is a common wall known as the <u>interventricular</u> septum.

ATRIUM	=	hall
AURICLE	=	ear-like flap
VENTER	=	belly
SEPTUM	=	fence

(2) <u>Wall layers</u>. The walls of the chambers are in three general layers. Lining the cavity of each chamber is a smooth epithelium known as the <u>endocardium.</u> (Endocarditis is an inflammation of the endocardium.) The middle layer is made up of cardiac muscle tissue and is known as the <u>myocardium</u>. The outer layer of the heart is another epithelium known as the <u>epicardium</u>.

(3) <u>Relationship of wall thickness to required pressure levels.</u> A cross-section of the chambers shows that the atrial walls are relatively thin. The right ventricular wall is much thicker. The left ventricular wall is three to five times thicker than that of the right. These differences in wall thickness reflect the amount of muscle tissue needed to produce the amount of pressure required of each chamber.

A. ANTERIOR VIEW

B. INTERIOR VIEW

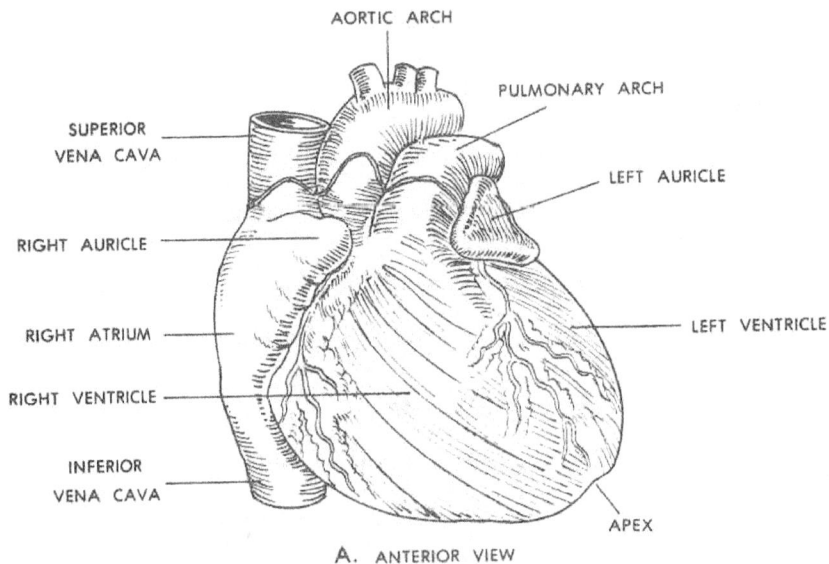

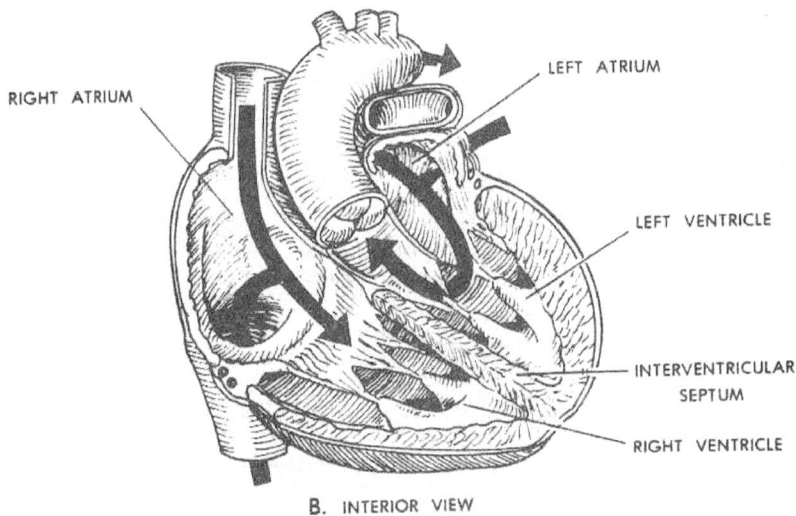

Figure 2-2. The human heart.

(4) <u>Cardiac valves (Figure 2-3)</u>.

(a) Between the atrium and ventricle of each side is the atrioventricular (A-V) <u>valve</u>. Each A-V valve prevents the blood from going back into the atrium from the ventricle of the same side. The right A-V valve is known as the <u>tricuspid valve</u>. The left A-V valve is known as the <u>mitral valve</u>. ("Might is never right."). The mitral valve is sometimes called the bicuspid valve. The leaflets (flaps) of the A-V valves are prevented from being pushed back into the atria by fibrous cords. These fibrous cords are attached to the undersides (the ventricular side) of the leaflets and are called chordae tendineae. At their other ends, the chordae tendineae are attached to the inner walls of the ventricles by papillary muscles.

(b)   A major artery leads away from each ventricle: the pulmonary trunk from the right ventricle and the aortic arch from the left ventricle. A semilunar valve is found at the base of each of the pulmonary trunk and the aortic arch. These semilunar valves prevent blood from flowing back into the ventricles. The pulmonary (semilunar) valve and the aortic (semilunar) valve are each made up of three semilunar ("pocket-like") cusps.

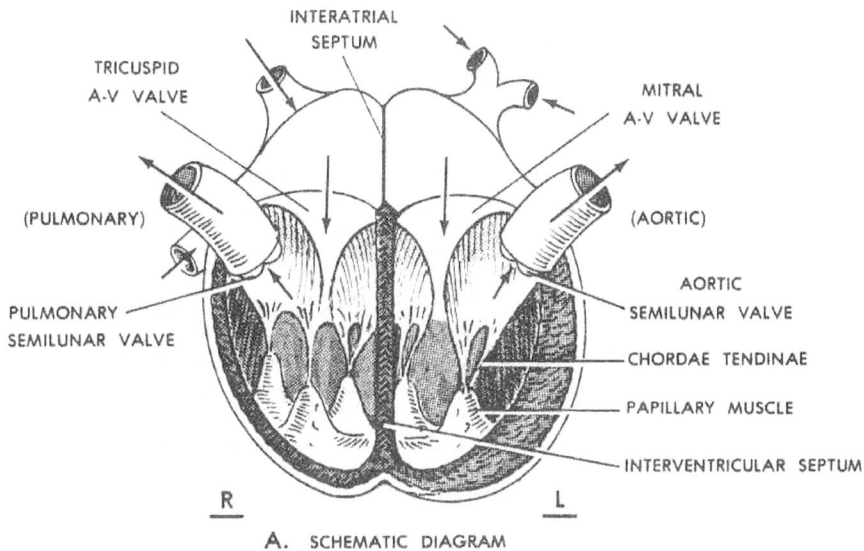

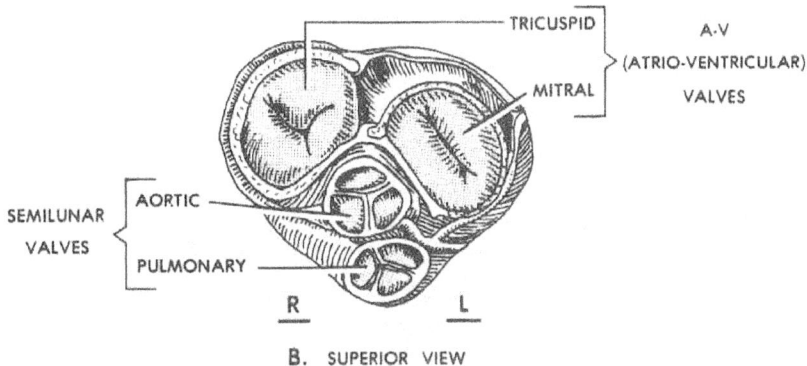

Figure 2-3. Scheme of heart valves.

    b. **Coronary Arteries and Cardiac Veins.** We may say that the heart deals with two different kinds of blood flow: "functional" blood and "nutritive" blood. "Functional" blood is the blood that the heart works on, or pushes with its motive force. However, the walls of the heart require nutrition that they cannot get directly from the blood within the chambers. "Nutritive" blood is supplied to these walls by the coronary arteries, right and left. The coronary arteries arise from the base of the aortic arch and are distributed over the surface of the heart. This blood is collected by the cardiac veins and empties into the right atrium of the heart. Should a coronary artery, or one of its branches, become closed for whatever reason, that part of the heart wall formerly supplied nutrient blood by the closed vessel will very likely die.

    c. **Pericardial Sac**. The average heart contracts in what is known as a heart beat, about 70-80 times a minute. To reduce the frictional forces that would be applied to its moving surfaces, the heart is enclosed in a special serous sac known as the pericardium ("around the heart").

2-16. THE PROPERTY OF INHERENT RHYTHMICITY

    a. The heart muscle (myocardium), like other muscles, is dependent upon electrical energy for its proper contraction. One property of cardiac muscle that cannot be found in any other muscle is inherent rhythmicity. Inherent rhythmicity is the property of the cardiac muscle that allows cardiac muscle cells to beat separately without any stimulation. If a cardiac muscle cell is placed in a saline (salt) bath containing the required amount of essential electrolytes the muscle cell will contract and relax rhythmically with no external stimulation. Furthermore, if another cardiac cell is placed in the same bath it, too, will beat at its own separate rate. It is interesting that when the two cardiac cells are placed together (in contact) the two cells will begin to beat as a unit. The property of inherent rhythmicity allows the myocardium to beat together with a minimal amount of nervous stimulation.

    b. Instead of initiating the contractile process, nervous stimulation functions rather to govern the rate of the heartbeat. The property of inherent rhythmicity appears to be embryonic in origin. That is, the heart begins beating and systemic circulation occurs before any nervous tissue is formed.

2-17. THE HEARTBEAT

    a. Initiation of the Cardiac Impulse. The initiation of the cardiac impulse begins in a highly specialized node of nervous tissue known as the sinoatrial node (also known as the SA node). As the name implies, the sino-atrial node is located in one of the atria-specifically the right atrium. The SA node initiates the electrical impulse that spreads out over both the atria causing the atrial muscles to contract. The fact that the SA node is located within the right atrium explains why the right atrium contracts 0.08 seconds before the left atrium contracts--although the contraction of the atria can still be considered to be simultaneous. As the atrial, muscle contracts the impulse travels through the atrial muscle to the atrioventricular (AV).node

b. **Atrioventricular Node.** The AV node is located between the right atrium and the right ventricle. The AV node is responsible for the contraction of both the ventricles. From the atrioventricular node, the impulse travels through the <u>Bundle of HIS</u> to the <u>purkinje fibers</u> of the ventricles.

c. **Bundle of HIS.** The Bundle of HIS is a collection of cardiac fibers through which the impulse travels on its way to the Purkinje fiber system. The Bundle of HIS is located at the uppermost portion of the ventricular septum. The ventricular septum is the thick muscular membrane that separates the right ventricle from the left ventricle.

d. **Purkinje Fibers.** The Purkinje fibers transverse and branch off within the ventricular septum branching to supply both ventricles near the bottom of the septum. By branching close to the bottom of the ventricular septum, the contractions of the ventricles go in an upward direction that is necessary for proper blood flow. Consequently, the contraction of the ventricles forces the blood upward to the aorta and pulmonary arteries.

e. **Control of the SA Node and AV Node**. Both the SA and the AV node are controlled by the autonomic nervous system. Parasympathetic stimulation, supplied by the <u>vagus nerve</u> tends to decrease both the rate and force of contraction of the heart. Sympathetic stimulation, from the cervical sympathetic ganglia, serves to increase both the rate and force of contraction of the heart. The predominant sympathetic receptor is a beta-receptor although it has been shown that a small amount of alpha-receptors are present in the heart.

2-18. ELECTROLYTES OF SIGNIFICANCE IN HEART FUNCTIONING

As with all muscle and nervous tissue, a proper concentration of electrolytes is essential for normal heart function. The three electrolytes essential for proper cardiac function are potassium, calcium, and sodium.

a. **Potassium**. An increase in the level of potassium in the extra-cellular fluid causes a decrease in the heart rate as well as a decrease in the force of contraction. The heart becomes dilated and flaccid. An extremely large increase in potassium can block nervous conduction through the atrioventricular bundle. If potassium levels are increased two or three times above normal, the atrioventricular blockade is usually so severe that death occurs. Potassium depletion also causes a decrease in the heart rate and an increase in the force of contraction. This is of concern, especially in the patient who has been taking digitalis. As you will remember, digitalis is valuable in the treatment of heart failure because it decreases the heart rate as well as increases the force of contraction, thus the efficiency of the heart is increased. If potassium levels are depleted at too great a degree, digitalis intoxication can result in which case the heart rate might decrease to too slow a rate.

b. **Calcium**. Calcium is primarily involved with the contractile processes of the myocardium. An increase in calcium levels may cause over contraction of the heart and a decrease in calcium levels may cause cardiac flaccidity. It should be noted that calcium level alterations rarely reach the point where these effects can be seen.

c. **Sodium**. Sodium is another essential electrolyte involved in cardiac function. However, sodium imbalances are usually manifested in some of the other systems before cardiac problems arise. If sodium levels are increased above normal depressed cardiac function occurs. Sodium levels are of concern in congestive heart failure because of the edema that can certainly aggravate congestive heart failure. Persons having congestive heart failure must carefully monitor their sodium intake in that too much sodium can cause an excessive fluid accumulation in the tissues. This fluid accumulation causes the heart to work harder in order to compensate for the water.

d. **Magnesium.** Magnesium is an essential electrolyte involved as a cofactor in many enzyme systems. It is also closely linked to regulating intracellular potassium and calcium content. High magnesium levels may affect heart rate, cardiac conduction, and blood pressure. Hypotension, vasodilation, bradycardia, heart block, and cardiac arrest can occur with increasing levels. Low magnesium may cause cardiac arrhythmias and may play an important role in atypical ventricular tachycardia (torsades de pointes). Attempting to replace potassium is difficult if an existing magnesium or calcium deficiency is also present.

2-19. CARDIAC DISORDERS

Cardiac disorders are some of the top killers in the United States. A variety of medications are used in the treatment of these conditions.

a. **Bradycardia**. Bradycardia is a slow heart rate. Generally, bradycardia refers to a heart rate less than 60 beats per minute. This condition is sometimes referred to as sinus bradycardia because the decrease in heart rate is usually attributed to a decrease in the activity of the sinoatrial node. An increase in vagal tone is probably the cause of most cases of bradycardia. In most cases, bradycardia is not serious. Bradycardia is often observed in sleeping persons and in young athletes. There are no symptoms of bradycardia unless it is severe. For simple bradycardia, no treatment is usually needed; however, severe bradycardia may be treated with atropine.

b. **Tachycardia**. Tachycardia means a rapid heart rate. Generally, tachycardia refers to a heart rate more than 100 beats per minute. Tachycardia can be caused by a number of disorders (for example, hyperthyroidism, vagal suppression, sympathetic nervous system stimulation, emotional responses, and exercise). The usual treatment of tachycardia is aimed at removing its cause.

c. **Arrhythmia.** Arrhythmia is a term that is used to refer to any abnormal heartbeat (that is, missed beats or extra beats). There are two types of arrhythmias that will be discussed in this subcourse: flutter and fibrillation.

(1) <u>Flutter</u>. Flutter is a very rapid heart rate with rhythm present. Usually the heart rate is much faster than in simple tachycardia (between 200 to 400 beats per minute).

(2) <u>Fibrillation</u>. Fibrillation is a term which refers to an extremely rapid heart rate with no rhythm. This condition is treated with an electric defibrillator that reverses fibrillation with the use of an electric shock.

d. **Angina Pectoris**. Angina pectoris is an acute condition in which one or more of the coronary arteries becomes blocked. A sharp burning pain in the chest that may be felt also in the neck and left arm characterizes angina. The coronary arteries may become partially occluded (closed) by an embolism or thrombus, or a simple increase in oxygen demand when exercising, but is usually attributed to be a result of atherosclerotic obstruction of the coronary arteries. The heart muscle cells are thus deprived of oxygen because of the decreased flow of blood and death of the myocardial cells may result if the condition is not remedied. Acute management of angina pectoris is usually achieved with the use of a rapid acting vasodilator such as nitroglycerin or amyl nitrite.

e. **Myocardial Infarction**. A myocardial infarction is similar to angina pectoris, but it is usually more serious. During angina pectoris the coronary arteries are usually only partially blocked; however, during a myocardial infarction complete blockage of one of the coronary arteries results. The symptoms are essentially the same as angina pectoris, but are not usually relieved by vasodilators. Complete bed rest is essential for the patient. Death of cardiac muscle cells often results unless another vessel is able to carry blood to the affected area.

f. **Congestive Heart Failure**. Congestive heart failure is defined as a decrease in the efficiency of the pumping of the heart. This condition usually leads to pulmonary edema, a complication attributed to the fluid back up. Because of decreased blood flow, there is a decrease in renal circulation that can further aggravate the associated edema because of both decreased glomerular filtration rate and increased sodium retention. Vasodilators that belong to a class of drugs called Angiotensin Converting Enzyme Inhibitors (ACE inhibitors) are the first line drug of choice for treatment of congestive heart failure. If a patient cannot tolerate ACE inhibitors, they may be placed on a nitrate (Isordil®) and hydralazine instead. As heart failure worsens and edema increases, diuretics are used to decrease edema. Digitalis glycosides (digoxin) used to be the drug of choice for heart failure, however due to many drug-drug interactions and narrow therapeutic index, it is reserved for acute symptomatic heart failure or in patients with heart failure and atrial fibrillation. Digoxin works by increasing the efficiency of the heart as a pump by decreasing both the size of the heart and the rate of the heart while at the same time increasing the force of contraction. As heart failure worsens, treatment may involve the addition of beta-adrenergic blockers (carvedilol, metoprolol) and spironolactone (potassium-sparing diuretic).

g. **Cardiac Arrest**. A cardiac arrest is simply the sudden cessation (stoppage) of the heartbeat. The cause of the stoppage may or may not be known. Treatment of the cardiac arrest is dependent upon the cause of the arrest.

h. **Rheumatic Fever**. Rheumatic fever is a streptococcal infection which many times attacks the valves of the heart. The result is a deformed or weakened valve that results in a heart murmur.

i. **Endocarditis**. Endocarditis is an inflammation of the membrane that lines the heart. Bacteria that repeatedly enter the bloodstream usually cause endocarditis. The bacteria which causes the endocarditis may enter the bloodstream following a tooth extraction and, on occasion, is associated with unsanitary intravenous injection techniques. Diagnosis of endocarditis usually involves the presence of a low fever and a soft, muffled heart murmur. The valves of the heart are also affected and if not detected and treated early endocarditis may cause irreversible damage. The treatment of endocarditis usually centers on bed rest and long term (4-6 weeks) antibiotic therapy.

j. **Heart Block**. A heart block is defined as a condition in which the cardiac excitation is slowed or interrupted somewhere in the normal pathway where conduction takes place. The two primary types of heart block usually seen are the SA or sinoatrial block and the atrioventricular or AV block. The term "heart block" is somewhat ambiguous. Usually the block only occurs occasionally and the result is manifested in only a skipped beat. Generally, the SA block requires no treatment; however, the prognosis is dependent on the cause and frequency of the block. During the AV block several or all impulses from the SA node are delayed or blocked in the AV node or bundle. Obviously, this type of block is much more serious than the SA block. Treatment of AV block depends upon the cause and the severity of the block. Digitalis toxicity may cause AV block on occasion.

2-20. CARDIOVASCULAR CIRCULATORY PATTERNS

See Figure 2-4 for an illustration depicting cardiovascular circulatory patterns.

a. **General**. The human cardiovascular system is described as a closed, two-cycle system.

(1) It is closed because at no place is the blood as whole blood ever outside the system.

(2) It is two-cycle because the blood passes through the heart twice with each complete circuit of the body. In the pulmonary cycle, the blood passes from the right heart, through the lungs, and to the left heart. In the systemic cycle, the blood passes from the left heart, through the body in general, and returns to the right heart.

(3) It is common for an area of the body to be supplied by more than one blood vessel, so that if one is damaged, the others will continue the supply. This is

known as collateral circulation. However, there are situations, such as in the heart and the brain, where a single artery supplies a specific part of a structure. Such an artery is called an end artery. When an end artery is damaged, that area supplied by it will usually die, as in the case of the coronary artery above, or the cause of a "stroke" in the brain.

   b.   **Pulmonary Cycle**. The pulmonary cycle begins in the right ventricle of the heart. Contraction of the right ventricular wall applies pressure to the blood. This forces the tricuspid valve closed, and the closed valve prevents blood from going back into the right atrium. The pressure forces blood past the semilunar valve into the pulmonary trunk. Upon relaxation of the right ventricle, backpressure of the blood in the pulmonary trunk closes the pulmonary semilunar valve. The blood then passes into the lungs through the pulmonary arterial system. Gases are exchanged between the alveoli. This blood, now saturated with oxygen, is collected by the pulmonary veins and carried to the left atrium of the heart. This completes the pulmonary cycle.

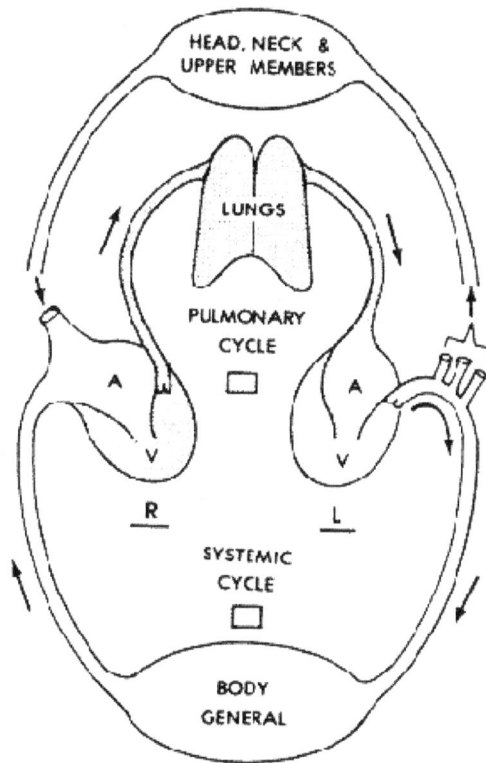

Figure 2-4. Cardiovascular circulatory pattern.

c. **Systemic Cycle**.

(1) Left ventricle of the heart. The oxygen-saturated blood is moved from the left atrium into the left ventricle. When the left ventricular wall contracts, the pressure closes the mitral valve, which prevents blood from returning to the left atrium. The contraction of the left ventricular wall therefore forces the blood through the aortic semilunar valve into the aortic arch. Upon relaxation of the left ventricular valve, the back pressure of the aortic arch forces the aortic semilunar valve closed.

(2) Arterial distributions. The blood then passes through the various arteries to the tissues of the body. See Figure 2-5 for an illustration of the main arteries of the human body.

(a) The carotid arteries supply the head. The neck and upper members are supplied by the subclavian arteries.

(b) The aortic arch continues as a large single vessel known as the aorta passing down through the trunk of the body in front of the vertebral column. It gives off branches to the trunk wall and to the contents of the trunk.

(c) At the lower end of the trunk, the aorta divides into right and left iliac arteries, supplying the pelvic region and lower members.

(3) Capillary beds of the body tissues. In the capillary beds of the tissues of the body, materials (such as food, oxygen, and waste products) are exchanged between the blood and the cells of the body.

(4) Venous tributaries. See Figure 2-6 for an illustration of the main veins of the human body.

(a) The blood from the capillaries among the tissues is collected by a venous system parallel to the arteries. This system of deep veins returns the blood back to the right atrium of the heart.

(b) In the subcutaneous layer, immediately beneath the skin, is a network of superficial veins draining the skin areas. These superficial veins collect, and then join the deep veins in the axillae (armpits) and the inguinal region (groin).

(c) The superior vena cava collects the blood from the head, neck, and upper members. The inferior vena cava collects the blood from the rest of the body. As the final major veins, the venae cavae empty the returned blood into the right atrium of the heart.

(d) The veins are generally supplied with valves to assist in making the blood flow toward the heart. It is of some interest to note that the veins from the head do not contain valves.

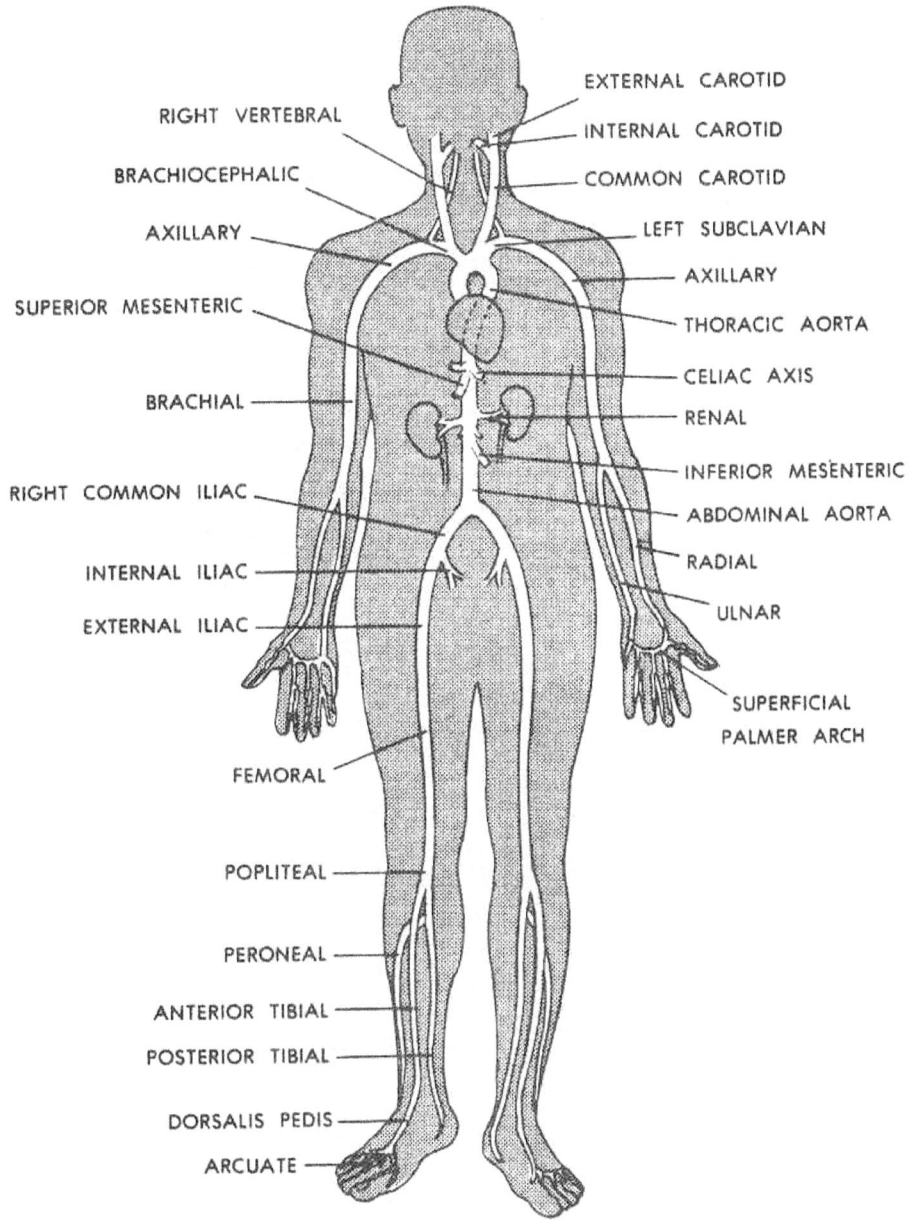

Figure 2-5. Main arteries of the human body.

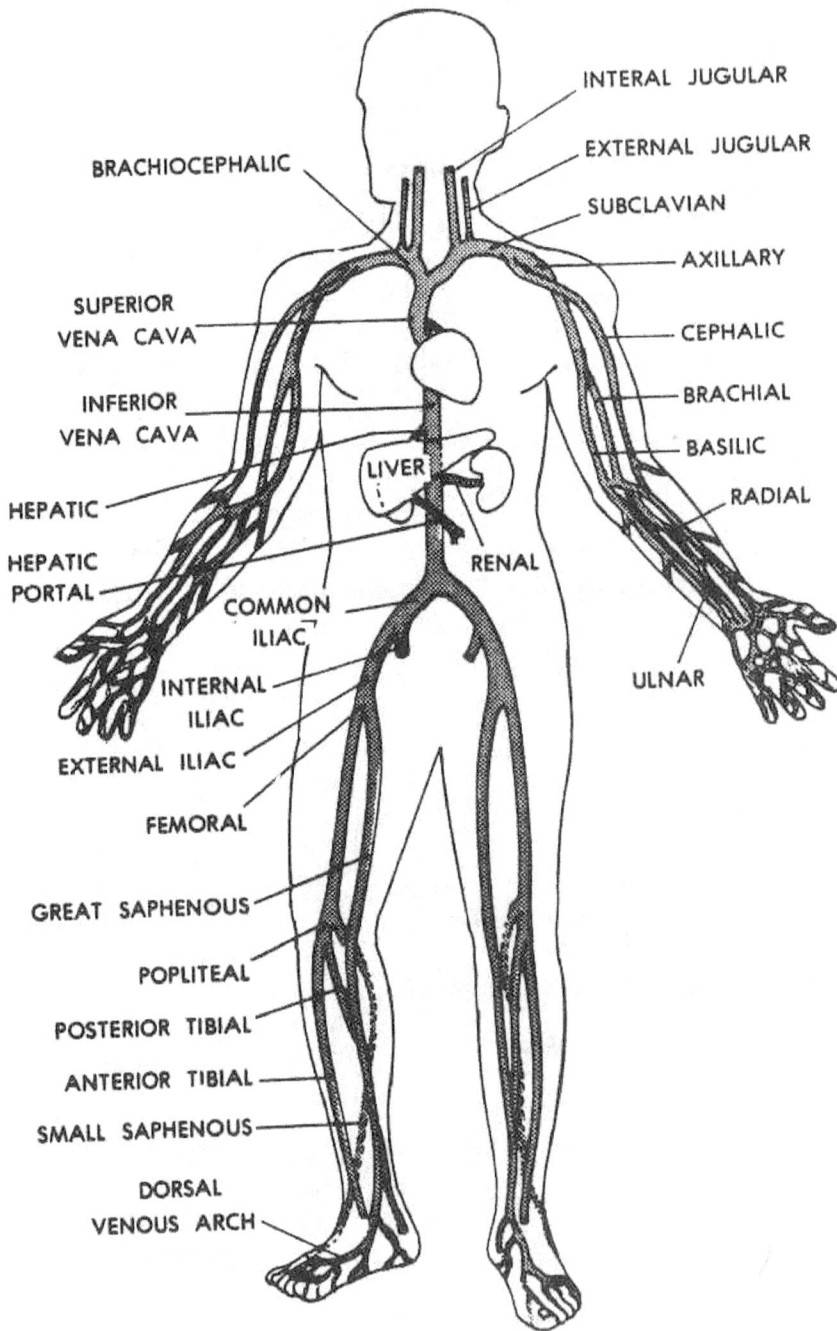

Figure 2-6. Main veins of the human body.

(e)   From that portion of the gut where materials are absorbed through the walls into the capillaries, the blood receives a great variety of substances. While most of these substances are useful, some may be harmful to the body. The blood carrying these substances is carried directly to the liver by the hepatic portal venous system. This blood is specially treated and conditioned in the liver before it is returned to the general circulation by way of the hepatic veins.

Section IV. THE HUMAN LYMPHATIC SYSTEM

2-21.   GENERAL

Between the cells of the body are spaces filled with fluid. This is the interstitial (or tissue) fluid, often referred to as intercellular fluid. There are continuous exchanges between the intracellular fluid, the interstitial fluid, and the plasma of the blood. The lymphatic system returns to the bloodstream the excess interstitial fluid, which includes proteins and fluid derived from the blood.

2-22.   STRUCTURES OF THE HUMAN LYMPHATIC SYSTEM

See Figure 2-7 for an illustration of the human lymphatic system.

a.   **Lymphatic Capillaries**. Lymphatic capillaries are located in the interstitial spaces. Here, they absorb the excess fluids.

b.   **Lymph Vessels.** A tributary system of vessels collects these excess fluids, now called lymph. Like veins, lymphatic vessels are supplied with valves to help maintain a flow of lymph in one direction only. The lymphatic vessels, to a greater or lesser extent, parallel the venous vessels along the way. The major lymph vessel in the human body is called the thoracic duct. The thoracic duct passes from the abdomen up through the thorax and into the root of the neck in front of the vertebral column. The thoracic duct empties into the junction of the left subclavian and jugular veins.

c.   **Lymph Nodes**. Along the way, lymphatic vessels are interrupted by special structures known as lymph nodes. These lymph nodes serve as special filters for the lymph fluid passing through.

d.   **Tonsils**. Tonsils are special collections of lymphoid tissue, very similar to a group of lymph nodes. These are protective structures and are located primarily at the entrances of the respiratory and digestive systems.

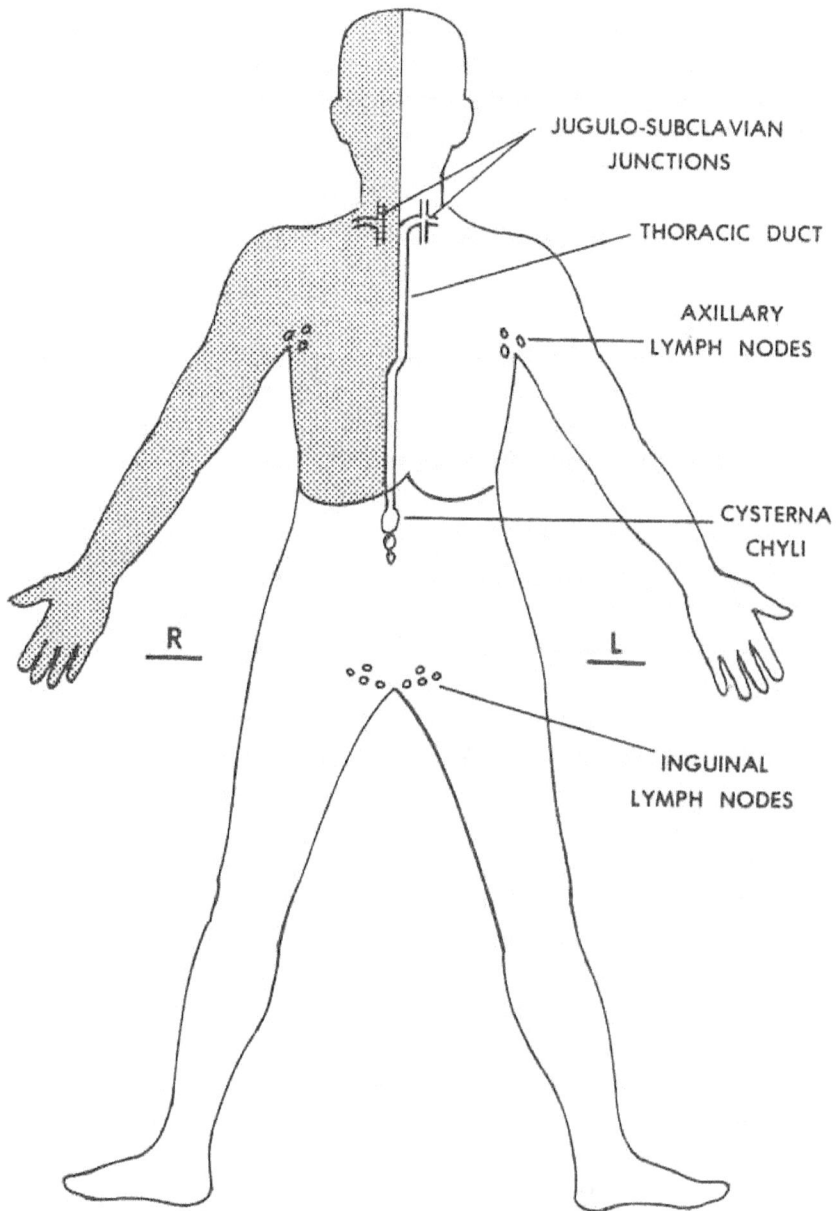

Figure 2-7. The human lymphatic system.

Continue with Exercises

EXERCISES, LESSON 2

REQUIREMENT: The following exercises are to be answered by marking the lettered response that best answers the question; or by completing the incomplete statement; or by writing the answer in the space provided at the end of the question.

After you have completed all the exercises, turn to "Solutions to Exercises," at the end of the lesson, and check your answers with the solutions.

1. Which of the following statements best explain the need for circulatory systems?

    a.   To protect the body from invading bacteria.

    b.   To get food and oxygen to the cells.

    c.   To remove waste products from the cells.

    d.   To provide a means of cell reproduction.

2. Which of the following are circulatory systems in the human body?

    a.   The sinoatrial system.

    b.   The lymphatic system.

    c.   The diastolic system.

    d.   The cardiovascular system.

3. Capillaries are best described as _____

    a.   Vehicles for nutrients, oxygen, and wastes.

    b.   Very large conduits or channels through which the blood is moved.

    c.   Very small vessels that provide exchange areas.

    d.   The component of the cardiovascular system that serves as the primary motive force of blood movement.

4. Select the components of the blood.

    a. Plasma.

    b. Formed elements (red blood cells, white blood cells, and platelets).

    c. Both a and b.

5. Plasma is best described as _____

    a. The protein material that carries dissolved oxygen in the blood.

    b. The liquid portion of the blood that is responsible for blood clotting.

    c. The clear fluid that remains after the blood has clotted.

    d. The clear fluid portion of the blood that accounts for approximately 55 percent of the total blood volume.

6. Red blood cells (RBCs) are best described as _____

    a. Fragments of cells that aid in the clotting of blood by clumping together and by releasing certain chemical factors related to clotting.

    b. The formed elements of the blood that phagocytize (swallow up) foreign particles and organisms.

    c. Biconcave discs that contain hemoglobin, a protein responsible for carrying most of the oxygen transported by the blood.

    d. The formed elements of the blood that produce antibodies and serve other functions in immunity.

7. Which of the following statements best describes veins?

    a. The blood vessels that carry blood to the chambers of the heart.

    b. The blood vessels that carry blood away from the chambers of the heart.

    c. Extremely thin-walled blood vessels that act as exchange areas.

    d. Blood vessels that always carry deoxygenated blood.

8.   Below are the steps involved in the clotting of blood. Select the arrangement of steps that best reflects their sequential order in the clotting process.

>   I.   Thromboplastin reacts with calcium and another substance, prothrombin, to form thrombin.
>
>   II. The blood platelets release a substance that is known as thromboplastin.
>
>   III. The thrombin formed acts as an enzyme to convert fibrinogen to fibrin threads that eventually form the blood clot.

>   a.   I, II, and III.
>
>   b.   III, II, and I.
>
>   c.   II, III, and I.
>
>   d.   II, I, and III.

9.   Blood pressure is best described as _____.

>   a.   The residual pressure of the blood due to the elasticity of the blood vessels.
>
>   b.   The force exerted by the blood as it is pumped throughout the circulatory system.
>
>   c.   The pressure the blood exerts as it is pumped from the heart.
>
>   d.   The pressure the blood exerts when the heart is resting.

10. Select the medical problems associated with high blood pressure.

>   a.   Frequent nosebleeds.
>
>   b.   Arteriosclerosis.
>
>   c.   Strokes.
>
>   d.   Hypertrophy of the myocardium.
>
>   e.   All of the above.

11. Hemophilia is _____.

   a.   A very serious type of anemia characterized by a progressive degeneration of the bone marrow.

   b.   A hereditary disease characterized by a lack of one of the factors necessary for the clotting of the blood.

   c.   A general term that refers to a group of anemias caused by weakened red blood cell membranes.

   d.   A type of anemia caused by a deficiency of elemental iron in the blood.

12. Leukemia is _____.

   a.   A very serious and usually fatal condition characterized by the excessive production of red blood cells.

   b.   A serious type of anemia predominant in older people because they tend to have red blood cells with weakened membranes.

   c.   A disease of the white blood cell forming tissue characterized by an abnormally high white blood cell count.

   d.   A disease of the red blood cell forming tissue which results in the production of excessive numbers of red blood cells which phagocytize the other cells in the blood.

13. Arteriosclerosis is _____.

   a.   A condition characterized by a loss of elasticity or hardening of the arterial walls.

   b.   A condition characterized by vasoconstriction of the arteries in the extremities.

   c.   A condition that occurs when a clot is formed in a blood vessel.

   d.   A serious condition that affects the arteries and causes them to lose vital fluids.

14. Which of the following statements best describes the property inherent rhythmicity?

     a.   The property of cardiac cells which allows them to beat without the presence of any electrolytes.

     b.   The property of the heart cells that allows them to initiate each contractile process instead of requiring them to govern the rate of the heart beat.

     c.   The property of the myocardium to continue pumping blood after the individual has died.

     d.   The property of the cardiac muscle that allows cardiac muscle cells to beat separately without any stimulation.

15. Match the name of each part of the heart with its respective structure.

   _____ Left atrium.

   _____ Right atrium.

   _____ Left ventricle.

   _____ Right ventricle.

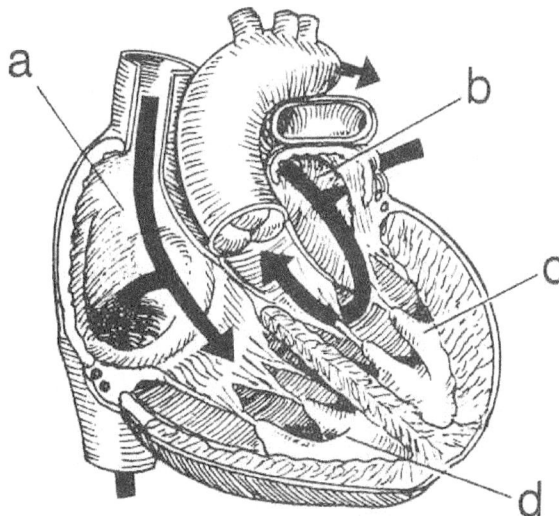

16. Which statement best describes the role of the Bundle of HIS in the heartbeat?

     a.   The Bundle of HIS is responsible for the contraction of both the ventricles.

     b.   The Bundle of HIS is a collection of cardiac fibers through which the impulse travels on its way to the Purkinje fibers.

     c.   The Bundle of HIS provides nervous stimulation so that the ventricles go in a downward direction, which is necessary for proper blood flow.

     d.   The Bundle of HIS is responsible for initiating the cardiac impulse.

17. Select the effect of excessive levels of calcium in the extracellular fluid.

     a.   Cardiac flaccidity.

     b.   Cardiac edema.

     c.   Spastic condition of the heart.

     d.   A decrease in the force of contraction of the heart beat.

18. Congestive heart failure is best described as _____.

     a.   An acute condition in which one or more of the coronary arteries become blocked.

     b.   A complete blockage of one or more of the coronary arteries which results in damage to the cardiac muscle.

     c.   An inflammation of the membrane that lines the heart.

     d.   A decrease in the efficiency of the pumping of the heart which usually leads to pulmonary edema.

19. A lymph node is _____.

    a.   A special structure that filters the lymph fluid.

    b.   A structure located in the interstitial spaces which absorbs excess extracellular fluids.

    c.   The major lymph vessel in the body.

    d.   A special collection of lymphoid tissue which serves as the major site of red blood cell destruction in the body.

Check Your Answers on Next Page

SOLUTIONS TO EXERCISES, LESSON 2

1. b   To get food and oxygen to the cells. (para 2-1b)
    c   To remove waste products from the cells. (para 2-1b)

2. b   The lymphatic system. (para 2-3b)
    d   The cardiovascular system. (para 2-3a)

3. c   Very small vessels that provide exchange areas. (para 2-4d)

4. c   Both a and b. (para 2-5)

5. d   The clear fluid portion of the blood which accounts for approximately
        55 percent of the total blood volume. (para 2-5a)

6. c   Biconcave discs which contain hemoglobin, a protein responsible
        for carrying most of the oxygen transported by the blood.
        (para 2-5b(1))

7. a   The blood vessels which carry blood to the chambers of the
        heart. (para 2-6b(2))

8. d   II, I, and III. (para 2-8)

9. b   The force exerted by the blood as it is pumped throughout the
        circulatory system. (para 2-9a)

10. e   All the above. (para 2-10a)

11. b   A hereditary disease characterized by a lack of one of the
        factors necessary for the clotting of the blood. (para 2-11e)

12. c   A disease of the white blood cell forming tissue characterized
        by an abnormally high white blood cell count. (para 2-11f)

13. a   A condition characterized by a loss of elasticity or hardening
        of the arterial walls. (para 2-13a)

14. d   The property of the cardiac muscle which allows cardiac muscle
        cells to beat separately without any stimulation. (para 2-16a)

15. _____b_____Left atrium. (Figure 2-2)

_____a_____Right atrium. (Figure 2-2)

_____c_____Left ventricle. (Figure 2-2)

_____d_____Right ventricle. (Figure 2-2)

16. b   The Bundle of HIS is a collection of cardiac fibers through which the impulse travels on its way to the Purkinje fibers. (para 2-17c)

17. c   Spastic condition of the heart. (para 2-18b)

18. d   A decrease in the efficiency of the pumping of the heart, which usually leads to pulmonary edema. (para 2-19f)

19. a   A special structure which filters the lymph fluid. (para 2-22c)

End of Lesson 2

LESSON ASSIGNMENT

LESSON 3	Cardiac Drugs.
LESSON ASSIGNMENT	Paragraphs 3-1--3-15.
TASKS	081-824-0001, Perform Initial Screening of a Prescription.
	081-824-0026, Evaluate a Prescription.
	081-824-0002/3, Fill a Prescription For a Controlled/Non-Controlled Drug.
	081-824-0027, Evaluate a Completed Prescription.
	081-824-0028, Issue Outpatient Medications.
OBJECTIVES	After you finish this lesson you should be able to:

3-1.   From a group of statements, select the best description of congestive heart failure.

3-2.   Given a group of statements, select the statement which best describes the primary pharmacological property of digitalis and related cardiac glycosides.

3-3.   Given a group of statements, select the statement which best describes digitalizing dose.

3-4.   From a group of statements, select the statement that best describes the difference between the <u>digitalizing dose</u> and the maintenance dose of digitalis.

3-5.   Given the trade and/or generic name of a cardiac drug and a group of uses, side effects, or patient precautionary statements, select the use(s), side effect(s), or patient precautionary statement(s) for that drug.

3-6.   Given the trade or generic name of a cardiac agent and a group of drug names (trade and/or generic), select the corresponding trade or generic name for the given drug.

3-7.   Given a group of statements and one of the following terms: cardiac arrhythmia flutter or fibrillation, select the statement which best defines the given term.

SUGGESTION

After completing the assignment, complete the exercises at the end of this lesson. These exercises will help you to achieve the lesson objectives.

LESSON 3

CARDIAC DRUGS

Section I. CONGESTIVE HEART FAILURE AND ITS TREATMENT

3-1. INTRODUCTION

Heart disease is the number one killer in the United States today. Two people succumb to conditions related to heart disease every minute of the day. However, it must be remembered that heart disease can be treated. Discoveries of new ways to use existing drugs and improved surgical techniques translate into longer and more productive lives for persons who have heart disease. In lesson 2 of this subcourse, various disease states that can affect the circulatory system were discussed. In this lesson, some of these conditions will be reviewed. The primary focus of this lesson will be the drug used to treat these conditions.

3-2. REVIEW OF CONGESTIVE HEART FAILURE

Congestive heart failure may be defined as nonefficient pumping of the heart. This inefficiency in pumping the heart leads to an increase in the size of the heart and an increase in the heart rate. This increase in heart size and heart rate result because of the heart's attempt to compensate for the poor efficiency in pumping blood to other parts of the body. Consequently, the kidneys improperly function. Improperly functioning kidneys result in edema of the extremities due to improper excretion (removal) of sodium and waste products in the urine. If a patient's congestive heart failure becomes acute, he may have pulmonary edema due to poor kidney function.

3-3. TREATMENT OF CONGESTIVE HEART FAILURE

Rest and restriction of sodium (that is, sodium chloride) intake are important aspects of the non-pharmacologic treatment of congestive heart failure. Drug treatment includes ACE Inhibitors, diuretics (see Lesson 8), digitalis and the related cardiac glycosides, beta adrenergic blockers, and spironolactone.

3-4. ANGIOTENSIN-CONVERTING ENZYME INHIBITORS (ACE INHIBITORS)

a. Angiotensin-converting enzyme inhibitors (ACE inhibitors) belong to a unique class of vasodilators. ACE inhibitors block a specific enzyme (angiotensin converting enzyme) that converts angiotensin I to angiotensin II. Angiotensin II is one of the most potent vasodilators in the body. The mechanism of action of ACE inhibitors in the treatment of congestive heart failure relies on the ability to cause both arterial and venous vasodilation through this inhibition, thereby decreasing the workload on the heart. Hemodynamic effects associated with long term use include increased cardiac function and decreased blood pressure and heart rate. Significant improvements are seen in exercise tolerance and left ventricular size. ACE inhibitors are well tolerated and have been shown to decrease hospitalizations and deaths. For these reasons, agents in this class are first line pharmacologic treatment for congestive heart failure.

b. ACE Inhibitors are often initiated immediately after a heart attack or when a patient still has mild symptoms of heart failure. The starting dose is low and titrated (gradually increased) up to the maximum tolerated dose (based on heart rate and blood pressure). The most bothersome side effect is a dry cough which develops in some patients. Other side effects include angioedema (facial swelling) and elevated potassium levels.

c. Agents included in this class include captopril (Capoten®), enalapril (Vasotec®), lisinopril (Prinivil®, Zestril®), and ramipril (Altace®)

3-5. DIGITALIS AND THE RELATED GLYCOSIDES

a. The mechanisms of action of digitalis and related cardiac glycosides in the treatment of congestive heart failure are not fully understood. The main pharmacological property of these drugs is their ability to increase the force of myocardial contraction (the heart muscle's contraction) by a direct action on the ventricular heart muscles. Conduction is also slowed somehow between the SA node and the AV node, resulting in a decrease in heart rate. Because of the slower heart rate and increase in the force of the myocardial contraction, the heart has more time to adequately fill with venous blood. The secondary changes seen as a result of the first three mechanisms of action will be a <u>decrease</u> in heart size and a decrease in heart rate due to more efficient pumping of the heart. Because of the slower heart rate, cardiac glycosides are also used in the treatment of atrial flutter or atrial fibrillation.

b. Because of improved circulation to the kidneys, an increase in urinary output (diuresis) within 24 to 48 hours following administration of cardiac glycosides will also be seen. Digitalis toxicity is enhanced in patients who have low serum potassium (hypokalemia), so potassium supplements may be given based upon periodic blood test analysis.

c. Digitalis and related glycosides have very narrow therapeutic indices (the treatment dose is very close to the toxic dose) and many drug-drug interactions. The dose must also be adjusted in renal failure, which is common in CHF patients. For these reasons digitalis is reserved for acute symptomatic heart failure or in those patients with CHF and atrial fibrillation.

3-6. DIGITALIZING DOSE

a. The digitalizing dose of a cardiac glycoside is the initial large dose of the drug that is given to the patient in order to relieve the symptoms of congestive heart failure or to render the patient asymptomatic as it is commonly referred to. Often the digitalization is accomplished by administering relatively large doses of digitalis preparations within a

18-24 hours to the patient. This type of intensive administration of "loading" doses can cause toxic reactions since digitalis preparations have only a moderate safety margin.

b. Although a patient's condition may have responded to digitalization, he may have to continue to take a digitalis product for a long period. The physician must determine the amount of drug the patient must take on a daily basis in order for the patient's heart to perform at its optimal level. Maintenance doses are ordered which are just enough to replace the amount of digitalis eliminated since the administration of the last dose. The maintenance dose is then taken each day to maintain the quantity of drug required to keep the patient's heart beating efficiently. Although these daily maintenance doses are much lower than the original digitalizing doses, the risk of toxicity remains.

3-7. DIGITALIS PRODUCTS

a. **Digoxin (Lanoxin®).** Digoxin is the most common cardiac glycoside used to treat congestive heart failure. The drug is usually administered intravenously (IV) for digitalization in a total dosage of from 1 to 1.5 milligrams. This drug may be given orally if the physician desires. The maintenance dose ranges from 0.125 milligram to 0.5 milligram daily, but normally 0.25 milligram of digoxin is given each day to the patient. The side effects of digoxin include anorexia (loss of appetite), arrhythmias, nausea and vomiting, and yellowish-green vision. Digoxin should be used with caution in patients who have kidney problems because the kidneys are the primary route of excretion for this agent. This drug should be used with caution in patients who have low serum potassium. Digoxin is available in 0.125 milligram, 0.25 milligram, and 0.5 milligram tablets; 0.05 milligram, 0.1 milligram and 0.2 mg liquid filled capsules; or in an injectable solution of 0.1 milligram per milliliter in 1 milliliter containers and 0.25 milligram per milliliter in 2 milliliter containers. It is also available in a 0.05 milligram per milliliter pediatric elixir. The bioavailability is improved with the liquid filled capsules such that 0.1mg of the capsule is equivalent to 0.125 mg of the tablet. Many times the physician will prescribe the pediatric elixir with directions for the patient to take a certain total daily dose (e.g., 0.125 milligram). You must interpret this as milliliters (or cubic centimeters-cc's) in order for the patient to dose himself with the calibrated dropper supplied with the preparation. As you probably realize, you might have to use your pharmaceutical calculation skills to calculate the dose of the drug solution.

b. **Digitoxin (Crystodigin®).** Digitoxin is another cardiac glycoside obtained from Digitalis purpurea. Although rarely used, you must be aware of this agent as it can be confused with digoxin. This product must be used with caution in patients with liver problems since this drug is excreted primarily in the bile and consequently, has a long half-life (5 to 7 days). The drug is available as a 0.1 mg and 0.2 mg tablet.

3-8. OTHER AGENTS USED IN CONGESTIVE HEART FAILURE

a. **Beta Adrenergic Blocking Agents.** The stimulation of beta-1 receptors in cardiac tissue causes an increased heart rate often causing an increase in workload of the heart. As heart failure worsens, the body compensates by stimulating beta receptors to make the heart pump faster and faster. Consequently, the faster the heart pumps, the less time the ventricles have to fill and pump efficiently. Beta adrenergic blocking agents work by blocking this stimulation and allowing less work by the heart by decreasing the heart rate. Doses are initiated very low and titrated very slowly (over weeks to months). Large initial doses of beta blockers will actually worsen and produce heart failure. The most common agents used in the treatment of heart failure include carvedilol (Coreg®) and metoprolol (Lopressor®).

b. **Spironolactone (Aldactone®).** Spironolactone is a potassium sparing diuretic that works by inhibiting aldosterone and causing diuresis. It is useful in the treatment of edema common in CHF patients.

c. **Amiodarone (Cordarone®).** Amiodarone is an agent used in the treatment of atrial and ventricular arrhythmias. However, when used in patients who have CHF and arrhythmias, it has been shown to improve exercise tolerance, decrease hospitalizations, and improve pump function.

Section II. THE ANTIARRHYTHMIC AGENTS

3-9. REVIEW OF CARDIAC ARRHYTHMIAS

Disorders of impulse information, impulse conduction, or a combination of these factors produces cardiac arrhythmias (or abnormal heartbeats). These are two types of arrhythmias that we will consider: flutter and fibrillation.

a. **Flutter**. Flutter is a very rapid heart rate with rhythm present. Usually the heart rate is much faster in flutter than it is in simple tachycardia. In flutter, the heart can beat from 200 to 400 beats per minute.

b. **Fibrillation**. Fibrillation occurs when there is a very rapid heart beat with no rhythm.

3-10. THE USE OF ANTIARRHYTHMIC DRUGS

The term antiarrhythmic drugs refer to the agents that suppress abnormal beats or restore normal cardiac rhythm by depressing various properties of the myocardium (heart muscle). This is a general mechanism of action for all these drugs. The toxicity of the drugs will be discussed with each individual drug since it varies with each agent.

3-11. SPECIFIC ANTIARRHYTHMIC DRUGS

a. **Quinidine (Quiniglute®, Quinidex®).** Quinidine is an antiarrhythmic agent used in the treatment of atrial fibrillation and ventricular arrhythmias. It is given orally in a usual dose of 200 to 400 milligrams every 6-8 hours. The side effects associated with quinidine include hypersensitivity reactions, gastrointestinal (GI) disturbances (nausea, vomiting, and diarrhea) and a group of symptoms known as cinchonism. Some symptoms associated with cinchonism are tinnitus (ringing in the ears), vertigo (dizziness), and headaches.

b. **Procainamide (Pronestyl®).** Procainamide is used in the treatment of atrial and ventricular arrhythmias in an oral dosage range of from 250 to 500 milligrams four times daily. Procainamide is similar in chemical structure to procaine. It retains the quinidine like actions of procaine, but it is not rapidly hydrolyzed and its action persists long enough so that it is active even after oral as well as parenteral administration. Pharmacologically, procainamide is equivalent to quinidine. Procainamide may cause anorexia, nausea and vomiting, and drug hypersensitivity.

c. **Propranolol (Inderal®).** Propranolol is an agent that is used in the treatment of hypertension, angina pectoris, and cardiac arrhythmias. It is especially useful in the treatment of ventricular arrhythmias. The normal dosage of this drug for antiarrhythmic purposes is 10 to 40 milligrams given three or four times daily. As you might expect, the dose of the drug can be adjusted to meet the individual needs of the patient. The side effects associated with propranolol include bradycardia, bronchoconstriction, and congestive heart failure (CHF). These arise because of the beta blocking effects of the drug. The drug should be used with caution in persons who have asthma. Other beta blocking agents commonly used include Metoprolol (Lopressor®) and Atenolol (Tenormin®) and Sotalol (Betapace®).

d. **Phenytoin (Dilantin®).** Phenytoin is an agent that may be administered intravenously to reverse digitalis-induced arrhythmias. Rapid intravenous administration may cause bradycardia, hypotension, and cardiac arrest (rarely).

e. **Lidocaine (Xylocaine®).** Lidocaine is an agent that may be given intravenously in the treatment of ventricular arrhythmias. Large intravenous doses may produce convulsions, coma, and respiratory depression. You should be aware that not all lidocaine solutions are to be administered intravenously. Lidocaine for intravenous use is clearly marked as such on the container.

f. **Amiodarone (Cordarone®).** Amiodarone is an agent that is used to treat life- threatening ventricular arrhythmias and occassionally atrial arrhythmias. It is administered as an IV loading dose over 24 hours followed by oral maintenance. Use of amiodarone is associated with hepatic, ophthalmic, thyroid, and pulmonary side effects.

g. **Diltiazem (Cardizem®).** Diltiazem is used intravenously (5-20 mg/hr) to control ventricular rate in atrial flutter or fibrillation. The oral dosage is 240 mg to 320 mg per day in divided doses 1 to 4 times daily. Side effects include hypotension, bradycardia, congestive heart failure (CHF), edema, and dermatitis.

Section III. ANTIHYPERLIPIDEMIC AGENTS

3-12. REVIEW OF ATHEROSCLEROSIS

Atherosclerosis is a condition in which lipid (fat) deposits form on the inside of the arteries causing a decrease in the flow of blood through the arteries. The make up of these deposits is mostly cholesterol as a consequence of genetic and dietary factors which result in too much cholesterol. The arteries of most concern are the coronary arteries (those that supply the heart) and the carotid arteries (those that supply the brain). Hyperlipidemia is a condition of high levels of cholesterol, triglycerides, and /or lipoprotein in the blood. The higher the levels in the blood, the greater the risk that they will deposit on the inside of arteries. Several studies have shown a correlation between cholesterol levels and premature heart disease. Studies have shown that each 1% reduction in serum cholesterol correlates with a 2% decline in the risk of myocardial infarction. For example, a 25% reduction in cholesterol will reduce the risk of myocardial infarction by 50%. Diet, exercise, antihyperlipidemic drugs, and surgery are the most common treatments. If a patient has high cholesterol only, and no evidence of atherosclerosis, the treatment of the hyperlipidemia is referred to as primary prevention. If the patient already has atherosclerosis, treatment is known as secondary prevention.

3-13. DEFINITIONS

a. **Cholesterol:** A fat-related compound. It is a normal constituent of bile and a principal constituent of gallstones. In body metabolism cholesterol is important as a precursor of various steroid hormones such as sex hormones and adrenal corticoids. Cholesterol is synthesized by the liver. It is widely distributed in nature, especially in animal tissue such as glandular meats and egg yolk.

b. **Triglyceride (TG):** A compound of three fatty acids esterified to glycerol. A neutral fat, synthesized from carbohydrate, stored in adipose tissue. It releases free fatty acids into the blood on being hydrolyzed by enzymes.

c. **Lipoproteins:** Fat with protein. Major carrier of lipids in the plasma.

(1) Chylomicron: Particle of fat - lipoproteins - appearing in the lymph and blood after a meal rich in fat. These particles are composed largely of triglycerides with lesser amounts of phospholipids, cholesterol, esters, and protein. About 2 to 3 hours after a fat meal, the chylomicrons cause lactescene (milkiness) in the blood plasma; this is termed alimentary lipemia.

(2) Very low-density Lipoprotein (VLDL): Still carries a large lipid (TG) content but includes about 10% to 15% cholesterol; formed in the liver from endogenous fat sources.

(3) Intermediate-density Lipoprotein (IDL): Continues the delivery of endogenous TG to cells and carries about 30% cholesterol.

(4) Low-density Lipoprotein (LDL): Carries in addition to other lipids about two thirds or more of the total plasma cholesterol; formed in the serum from catabolism of VLDL. Because LDL carries cholesterol to the cells for deposit in the tissues, it is considered the main agent of concern in elevated serum cholesterol levels.

(5) High-density Lipoprotein (HDL): Carries less total lipid and more protein; it is also formed in the liver from endogenous fat sources. Because HDL carries cholesterol from the tissues to the liver for catabolism and excretion, higher serum levels are considered protective against cardiovascular disease.

3-14. RISK FACTORS

Although high cholesterol levels are a risk factor for the development of atherosclerosis, it is not the only risk factor. How aggressively the health care provider decides to treat hyperlipidemia depends on the patient's overall risk for developing atherosclerosis (heart disease). In addition to hyperlipidemia, the following are significant risk factors:

a. **Uncontrollable Risk Factors.** These include age (greater than 45 for males and greater than 55 for females), sex (male), and family history of premature coronary heart disease (MI, stroke, or sudden death before age 55 in a male parent or sibling, 65 in a female parent or sibling).

b. **Controllable Risk Factors.** These include active tobacco smoking, hypertension (treated or untreated), diabetes, severe obesity (>30% overweight), physical inactivity, and Type A personality traits.

NOTE: A high HDL (>60 mg/dl) is actually considered a *negative risk factor.* This means one positive risk factor may be subtracted in overall risk assessment. When determining treatment, two or more risk factors are considered significant.

3-15. TREATMENT

The treatment of hyperlipidemia depends on two factors: 1) whether that patient has existing atherosclerosis and 2) the patient's other risk factors for atherosclerosis. The treatment goal is usually expressed at the Low-density Lipoprotein (LDL) goal as this is the major carrier of cholesterol in the blood.

Treatment goals:

Category	LDL-Cholesterol Goal
No atherosclerosis & < 2 risk factors	<160 mg/dl
No atherosclerosis & 2 or more risk factors	<130 mg/dl
Existing atherosclerosis	<100 mg/dl

a. **Diet and Exercise**. Diet and exercise are considered lifestyle modifications which may lower cholesterol levels to goal. Diet changes reduce intake of cholesterol and fat, especially saturated fat. Exercise may involve aerobic exercise for at least 20-30 minutes, 3-5 times weekly. Whether a patient is on medication to lower their cholesterol or not, diet and exercise should always be a part of the treatment regimen.

b. **Drug therapy** – Medications are often prescribed for hyperlipidemia when diet and exercise fail to normalize LDL levels. Agents may prevent cholesterol synthesis or promote the breakdown of internal cholesterol.

(1) Statins - also called HMG CoA **(hydro-methylglutaryl Coenzyme A)** Reductase Inhibitors. HMG CoA is needed to produce mevalonic acid in the body, which is used to produce many products, among them cholesterol. As cholesterol synthesis is inhibited, LDL receptor site production is increased to draw cholesterol from serum. All of the statins work the same but may differ in potency (degree to which they decrease cholesterol levels). The more potent statins may significantly reduce triglycerides as well as LDL; some agents may increase HDL (this is good!). Because our liver makes most of our cholesterol at night, these agents work best when administered at bedtime. The most common side effects include muscle aches and weakness, diarrhea, constipation, and headache. Generalized muscle aches (over the entire body) must be reported immediately as this may indicate a more serious condition. Common statins include cerivastatin (Baycol®), simvastatin (Zocor®), atorvastatin (Lipitor®), and pravastatin (Pravachol®).

(2) Resins. Resins, also known as bile acid sequestrants, bind to bile acids in the GI tract and cause us to break down our internally produced cholesterol and thus lowering our cholesterol levels. Resins may increase triglyceride levels so must be used with caution in patients that have high triglycerides. Resins are very effective, however patients express poor compliance with these agents due to the side effects of heatburn, nausea, flatulence, constipation; dosing regimens; and significant drug-drug interactions. Resins are positively charged and many medications that carry a negative charge will bind with them. Medications such as digoxin, thiazide diuretics, betablockers, warfarin, thyroxine, and fat soluble vitamins (A, D, K, and folic acid) should not be taken after these agents. If a patient is prescribed a resin, he/she should take other medications 2 hours before or 4 hours after the resin. These agents are in

the form of a powder (must be mixed with juice) or very large tablet. Commonly prescribed resins include colestipol (Colestid®) and cholestyramine (Questran®).

(3) Fibrates. Fibrates are used primarily to treat high triglyceride levels. They also increase HDL significantly and their effect on LDL varies. Side effects include nausea, flatulence, abdominal pain, and diarrhea. While on this medication there is 2% to 4% increase in the risk of developing gallstones. This medication should not be taken with HMG CoA Enzyme Inhibitors as there is the potential for development of severe muscle aches and weakness (myopathy). Fibrates include gemfibrozil (Lopid®) and fenofibrate (Tricor®).

(4) Nicotinic Acid Derivatives (Niacin, vitamin B_3). Nicotinic acid derivatives are used for reducing high LDLs and triglycerides. They are also useful for treating low HDL levels. As with fibrates, HMG CoA Reductase Inhibitors should be avoided as the combination will lead to a serum increase of HMG CoA and myopathy. The classic side effect of niacin is facial redness and flushing. Often aspirin is administered 30 minutes prior to the niacin dose or niacin is initiated at low doses and gradually increased to reduce this side effect. Other side effects include headache, gastrointestinal upset, and dizziness. Only about 50-60% of patients can tolerate niacin because of its side effects. Some other side effects other than those listed are itching, rashes, hepatotoxicity, elevated glucose levels, and gout. Niacin is relatively contraindicated in diabetics, patients with gout, and patients with peptic ulcer disease.

Continue with Exercises

EXERCISES, LESSON 3

REQUIREMENT: The exercises that follow require you to read a question and select the response that best answers that question.

After you have answered all the questions, turn to "Solutions to Exercises," at the end of the lesson, and check your answers with the solutions.

1. From the statements below, select the statement that best describes congestive heart failure (CHF).

    a.   Congestive heart failure is nonefficient pumping of the heart that leads to an increase in the heart size and heart rate.

    b.   Congestive heart failure is a condition in which there is a build-up of edema in the extremities because of too forceful contractions of the myocardium.

    c.   Congestive heart failure is a condition in which the heart fills with fluid after each contraction.

    d.   Congestive heart failure is a state in which the heart valves open and close at inappropriate times resulting in backflow into the lungs.

2. Which of the following statements best describes the term <u>digitalizing dose</u>?

    a.   The dose of digitalis required on a daily basis to prevent the patient from having the signs and symptoms of congestive heart failure.

    b.   The large dose of digitalis which is first given to the patient in order to prevent cardiac arrhythmias.

    c.   The digitalizing dose is the large initial dose of the drug that is given to the patient in order to relieve the symptoms of congestive heart failure.

    d.   The large doses of digitalis that are frequently administered to patients who have acute cases of congestive heart failure.

3. The primary difference between the digitalizing dose and the maintenance dose of digitalis is _____

    a.   The digitalizing dose is the first and largest dose given to the patient, while the maintenance dose is the amount of drug given to the patient on a daily basis.

    b.   The digitalizing dose is always smaller than the daily maintenance dose that is given to the patient.

    c.   The digitalizing dose is the amount of digitalis given to the patient during the first three weeks of therapy, while the maintenance dose is given thereafter.

    d.   The digitalizing dose is given to patients, who have acute CHF, while the maintenance dose is given to only those patients who must continue to take digitalis for the rest of their lives.

4. Phenytoin can be administered intravenously (IV) to treat _____.

    a.   Congestive heart failure.

    b.   Digitalis induced arrhythmias.

    c.   Cinchonism.

    d.   Anorexia.

5. Inderal® is an agent used in the treatment of hypertension, angina pectoris, and _____

    a.   Cinchonism.

    b.   Cardiac arrhythmias.

    c.   Urine retention.

    d.   Diarrhea.

6. Amiodarone is used in the treatment of _____

    a.   Cinchonism.

    b.   Anorexia.

    c.   Ventricular arrhythmias.

    d.   Hypertension.

7. A side effect associated with the use of Zestril® is _____

    a.   Edema of the left ventricle.

    b.   Localized analgesia.

    c.   Dry cough.

    d.   Postural hypotension.

8. One of the side effects associated with large initial doses of beta blocking agents is _____

    a.   Anemia.

    b.   Hypertension.

    c.   Ventricular arrhythmias.

    d.   Congestive heart failure.

9. Flutter is best described as _____

    a.   A rapid heart beat with no rhythm.

    b.   A rapid heart rate of at least 200 to 400 beats per minute.

    c.   A type of cardiac arrest characterized by pain in the right shoulder.

    d.   A very rapid heart beat with rhythm present.

10. Hyperlipidemia is best described as_____

    a. Elevated levels of cholesterol, triglycerides, and/or lipoproteins in the blood.

    b. Reduced levels of cholesterol in the blood.

    c. Reduced levels of triglycerides in the blood.

    d. Elevated levels of triglycerides in the blood.

11. The following are acceptable treatments for hyperlipidemia:

    a. Diet and exercise

    b. Drug therapy

    c. Surgical intervention.

    d. All of the above.

12. Match the generic in Column A with its corresponding trade name in Column B.

Column A		Column B
____Digoxin.	a.	Coreg®
____Enalapril.	b.	Xylocaine®
____Diltiazem.	c.	Lanoxin®
____Carvedilol.	d.	Cardizem®
____Metoprolol.	e.	Vasotec®
____Lidocaine.	f.	Lopressor®
____Simvastatin.	g.	Lopid®
____Gemfibrozil.	h.	Zocor®

Check Your Answers on Next Page

SOLUTIONS TO EXERCISES, LESSON 3

1. a Congestive heart failure is nonefficient pumping of the heart that leads to an increase in the heart size and heart rate. (para 3-2)

2. c The digitalizing dose is the large initial dose of the drug that is given to the patient in order to relieve the symptoms of congestive heart failure. (para 3-6a)

3. a The digitalizing dose is the first and largest dose given to the patient, while the maintenance dose is the amount of drug given to the patient on a daily basis. (para 3-6)

4. b Digitalis-induced arrhythmias. (para 3-11d)

5. b Cardiac arrhythmias. (para 3-11c)

6. c Ventricular arrhythmias. (para 3-11f)

7. c Dry cough. (para 3-4b)

8. d Congestive heart failure. (para 3-11c)

9. d A very rapid heart beat with rhythm present. (para 3-9a)

10. a Elevated levels of cholesterol, triglycerides, and/or lipoproteins in the blood. (para 3-12)

11. d All of the above (para 3-12, 3-15(a))

12.

Column A	Column B
__c__ Digoxin. (para 3-7a)	a. Coreg®
__e__ Enalapril. (para 3-4c)	b. Xylocaine®
__d__ Diltiazem. (para 3-11g)	c. Lanoxin®
__a__ Carvedilol. (para 3-8a)	d. Cardizem®
__f__ Metoprolol. (para 3-11c)	e. Vasotec®
__b__ Lidocaine. (para 3-11e)	f. Lopressor®
__h__ Simvastatin. (para 3-15b(1))	g. Lopid®
__g.__ Gemfibrozil. (para 3-15b(3))	h. Zocor®

End of Lesson 3

LESSON ASSIGNMENT

LESSON 4   Vasodilator Drugs.

LESSON ASSIGNMENT   Paragraphs 4-1--4-5.

TASKS   081-824-0001, Perform Initial Screening of a Prescription.

081-824-0026, Evaluate a Prescription.

081-824-0002/3, Fill a Prescription For a Controlled/Non-Controlled Drug.

081-824-0027, Evaluate a Completed Prescription.

081-824-0028, Issue Outpatient Medications.

LESSON OBJECTIVES   After completing this lesson you will be able to:

4-1.   Given one of the following terms: vasodilator, orthostatic hypotension, angina pectoris, arteriosclerosis, antherosclerosis, or peripheral vascular disease and a group of statements, select the statement that best defines the given term.

4-2.   Given the trade or generic name of a vasodilator and a list of trade and/or generic names of drugs, select the trade or generic name that corresponds to the given trade or generic name.

4-3.   Given the trade or generic name of a vasodilator and a list of indications, uses, side effects, patient precautionary statements, or dispensing statements, select the indication(s), use(s), side effect(s), patient precautionary statement(s), or dispensing statement for the given drug name.

SUGGESTION   After completing the assignment, complete the exercises at the end of this lesson. These exercises will help you to achieve the lesson objectives.

LESSON 4

VASODILATOR DRUGS

Section I. DEFINITIONS

4-1. INTRODUCTION

Visualize a man walking down a hallway. He pauses at the foot of a stairway. From his pocket, he takes a small bottle containing some very small white tablets and he places one of these tablets under his tongue. After waiting a few seconds, he proceeds up the stairs. What was this scene? It was a man preparing his body-- especially his heart--for the extra work required for walking up the stairs. This man, suffering from a condition called angina pectoris, used one of the vasodilators that will be discussed in this subcourse lesson. Without this drug, he would be unable to perform many of the energy expending tasks required for everyday life. In this lesson, you will be given the opportunity to broaden your background in some cardiovascular diseases as well as learn more about various vasodilators.

4-2. IMPORTANT TERMS AND THEIR DEFINITIONS

You have already been introduced to some of the terms below in another lesson in this subcourse. Some of the terms below might be new to you. In any event, each term applies to vasodilator agents.

a. **Vasodilator.** A vasodilator is a drug that dilates blood vessels with a resultant increase in blood flow.

b. **Orthostatic Hypotension.** Orthostatic hypotension is a condition characterized by fainting or dizziness because of inadequate blood supply to the brain because the blood has been pooled elsewhere in the body. Vasodilator agents may cause this condition. You may have experienced this condition before. Have you ever arisen quickly from a lying position to find that you are light-headed and dizzy? This is orthostatic hypotension.

c. **Angina Pectoris**. Angina pectoris is a condition manifested by excruciating chest pain sometimes radiating down the left arm. The pain probably arises from ischemia (lack of oxygen) in the heart caused by the increased demand for or decreased supply of oxygen.

d. **Arteriosclerosis**. Arteriosclerosis is characterized by thickening, hardening, and loss of elasticity of the walls of blood vessels.

e. **Atherosclerosis.** Atherosclerosis is a form of arteriosclerosis characterized by localized accumulation of lipids (fats), leading to a narrowing of the arteries and possible occlusion (blockage) of the vessels.

f. **Peripheral Vascular Disease**. Peripheral vascular disease (PVD) is a condition characterized by a narrowing or occlusion of peripheral arterioles leading to limited circulation to the extremities such as toes, fingers, and shoulders. You have probably seen elderly patients who wear extra clothing during hot weather. The cold feeling they have, even in hot weather, is probably due to lack of adequate circulation.

Section II. VASODILATOR DRUGS

4-3. INTRODUCTION

Now that you have some background in some cardiovascular disease, you will review some general categories of vasodilators and some of the specific agents that belong to each group.

4-4. SMOOTH MUSCLE RELAXANT VASODILATORS

Although the agents in this category affect almost all smooth muscle, our concern here is only with their relaxant effect upon the smooth muscle of the coronary vessels as well as peripheral (to the heart) blood vessels.

a. **Amyl Nitrite**. Amyl nitrite is a vasodilator administered only by inhalation. It is rapidly absorbed from the lungs. This product is supplied in perles (like many ammonia inhalants). When a person suffering from angina pectoris feels an attack about to occur, he will crush an amyl nitrite perle and inhale its vapors. The attack of angina pectoris is warded off or aborted in from one to two minutes. Because amyl nitrite perles may explode when stored above normal room temperature, it is very difficult for the patient to carry them in his pocket. This adverse situation normally prohibits their use in the treatment of angina pectoris. The side effects associated with amyl nitrite are usually attributed to the relaxation of all smooth muscle causing vasodilation. Headache and dizziness are very common side effects associated with amyl nitrite. Amyl nitrite does have an additional use, which is the treatment of cyanide poisoning.

b. **Glyceryl Trinitrate (Nitroglycerin).** Glyceryl trinitrate is the most common smooth muscle relaxant vasodilator used in the treatment of acute angina pectoris. This drug is the product described in the introductory remarks of this subcourse lesson when the man placed the small tablet under his tongue. Sublingual nitroglycerin tablets may be used to allow a person who has angina to do extra work or to alleviate an acute angina attack. Nitroglycerin's sublingual onset of action is from 1 to 3 minutes with duration of action of from 9 to 11 minutes. Side effects associated with this drug include headache, dizziness, and orthostatic hypotension. The vasodilating effect of the drug may be so sudden that circulating blood pools in vascular (vessel) beds. This may cause the patient to become unconscious because of a lack of blood to the brain. Falling to the floor in a faint allows the immediate return of that blood flow to the brain and consciousness returns. Besides the sublingual form of nitroglycerin, sustained release capsules (Nitro-Bid Plateau Caps®) with 5 to 20 milligrams of drug taken daily in divided doses, topical ointments (Nitrol®, Nitro-Bid®), and transdermal patches (Nitro-Dur®) are available. The ointment is applied using special paper every 6 hours. The transdermal system patches are applied to the chest wall each morning and removed after 12 hours. The patches offer the advantage of once daily dosing and less side effects for the patient. Each of these dosage forms is used for the prevention of angina attacks. Nitroglycerin sublingual tablets are volatile. They will lose their potency quickly when they are incorrectly stored. Therefore, the tablets must be dispensed in their original container (light-resistant container). The patient should also be instructed not to remove the tablets from the original glass container (that is, to place the tablets in a fancy pillbox). Federal law requires that all nitroglycerin products should be dispensed in their original containers (that is, glass, light resistant, and not child-resistant packaging). Another problem area with the nitroglycerin prescription is the dose. Normally physicians prescribe them in grains using 1/100 grain, 1/150 grain, or 1/200-grain tablets. We should be able to convert these to micrograms or milligrams. Intravenous nitroglycerin is used in patients that present with unstable angina (persisting chest pain) or possible myocardial infarction. The physician normally orders the nitroglycerin as a drip (mcg/min) and titrates (adjusts) the dose to pain relief.

    c.   **Isosorbide Dinitrate (Isordil®, Sorbitrate®).** Isosorbide dinitrate is thought to be effective in the prophylactic treatment of angina pectoris, as well as the treatment of acute angina attacks. The side effects associated with this drug are headache and dizziness. Isordil® is supplied in many different dosage forms to include sublingual, chewable, compressed, and sustained action tablets and capsules (Tembids®). The sublingual tablets are used in the acute angina attacks in a dose of from 2.5 to 10 milligrams. The usual oral dose is from 15 to 80 milligrams daily in divided doses. These products should be dispensed in their original containers. Isosorbide mononitrate (Ismo®, Imdur®) is another product often prescribed.

NOTE: Tolerance develops to nitrate products. For the agents to maintain effectiveness, the patient must have a "nitrate-free" interval as part of the dosing regimen. Nitroglycerin patches are generally applied in the morning and removed in the evening (12-hours on/ 12-hours off); isosorbide products are administer in the morning, usually at 7am or 8 am with the second dose 7 hours later (2pm-3pm). No additional doses are administered so that the patient has a nitrate-free interval.

    d.   **Hydralazine (Apresoline®) and Minoxidil (Loniten®).** Hydralazine and minoxidil are direct acting peripheral vasodilators used in the treatment of hypertension. Hydralazine may be prescribed in combination with an oral nitrate in the treatment of congestive heart failure. The addition of hydralazine further dilates peripheral vessels and decreases workload on the heart.

4-5. AUTONOMIC NERVOUS SYSTEM VASODILATORS

The agent discussed in this paragraph is thought to dilate blood vessels supplying blood to skeletal muscles.

Isoxsuprine (Vasodilan®). Isoxsuprine is sometimes used in the treatment of various conditions causing peripheral vascular disease. Dilating blood vessels to skeletal muscles allows greater blood flow to peripheral areas of the body. Such increased blood flow alleviates some of the symptoms normally associated with peripheral vascular disease (for example: numbness or tingling sensations in the toes and fingers or a feeling of never being warm enough regardless of the atmospheric temperature). The effectiveness of this agent has not been supported by objective studies. The side effects associated with isoxsuprine therapy are severe rash (with some patients), tachycardia, and nausea and vomiting. Vasodilan® is supplied as 10 milligram and 20 milligram tablets. The usual daily dosage is 30 milligrams to 80 milligrams in 4 divided doses.

Continue with Exercises

EXERCISES, LESSON 4

REQUIREMENTS: The following exercises are to be answered by marking the lettered response that best answers the question; or by completing the incomplete statement; or by writing the answer in the space provided at the end of the question.

After you have completed all the exercises, turn to "Solutions to Exercises," at the end of the lesson, and check your answers with the solutions.

1.   A vasodilator is a drug which _____.

     a.   Dilates blood vessels with a resultant increase in blood flow.

     b.   Removes deposits of fat and calcium from the inside of vessels in order to increase blood flow.

     c.   Causes the heart to beat faster causing an increase in blood flow to the brain and to the peripheral areas.

     d.   Counteracts inadequate blood flow to the brain and peripheral areas by causing the arteries and veins to become more elastic.

2.   Orthostatic hypotension is a condition characterized by _____.

     a.   Dizziness, fainting, or vertigo caused by a rupture of blood vessels of the brain.

     b.   Dizziness or fainting caused by excessive flow of blood to the semicircular canals of the inner ear.

     c.   Fainting or dizziness because of inadequate blood supply to the brain.

     d.   Fainting or dizziness caused by lack of adequate exercise.

3. Atherosclerosis is best defined as _____.

    a.   A condition characterized by thickening, hardening, and a loss of elasticity of the walls of the blood vessels.

    b.   A condition manifested by excruciating chest pain caused by lack of oxygen in the heart.

    c.   A form of arteriosclerosis characterized by localized accumulation of fats in the arteries.

    d.   A form of angina pectoris in which the vessels of the heart are occluded by fats and carbohydrates.

4. Amyl nitrite is a vasodilator that is used in the treatment of _____.

    a.   Angina pectoris.

    b.   Frostbite.

    c.   Cyanide poisoning.

    d.   a and b.

    e.   a and c.

5. Isoxsuprine is used in the treatment of _____.

    a.   Tachycardia.

    b.   Various conditions causing peripheral vascular disease.

    c.   Orthostatic hypotension.

    d.   Irregular heartbeat and muscle tension.

6. Select the side effects associated with nitroglycerin.

    a. Irregular heartbeat and tachycardia.

    b. Orthostatic hypertension and sedation.

    c. Acute angina attacks and flushing of the face.

    d. Headache and dizziness.

7. Hydralazine is used in _____.

    a. The treatment of hypertension and congestive heart failure.

    b. The treatment of night leg cramps and frostbite.

    c. The treatment of atherosclerosis.

    d. The prophylactic treatment of angina pectoris.

8. Which of the following best describes the concept of "nitrate-free" interval associated with the use of nitrates?

    a. Nitrates prescribed day on/day off, to reduce side effects.

    b. Nitrates prescribed 8-12 hours per day, followed by a 12-16 hours drug free interval to decrease tolerance and side effects.

    c. Nitrates prescribed every 6-8 hours and instructed to skip every other dose.

    d. Nitrates prescribed week on/week off, to reduce tolerance and side effects.

9. Match the drug name listed in Column A with its corresponding name listed in Column B.

<u>COLUMN A</u>   <u>COLUMN B</u>

_____ Minoxidil.   a. Sorbitrate®

_____ Isosorbide dinitrate.   b. Nitroglycerin

_____ Isoxsuprine.   c. Loniten®

_____ Isosorbide mononitrate.   d. Imdur®

_____ Glyceryl trinitrate.   e. Vasodilan®

Check Your Answers on Next Page

SOLUTIONS TO EXERCISES, LESSON 4

1. a Dilates blood vessels with a resultant increase in blood flow.
(para 4-2a)

2. c Fainting or dizziness because of inadequate blood supply to the brain.
(para 4-2b)

3. c A form of arteriosclerosis characterized by localized accumulation
of fats in the arteries. (para 4-2e)

4. e a and c, (Angina pectoris and cyanide poisoning). (para 4-4a)

5. b Various conditions causing peripheral vascular disease.
(para 4-5)

6. d Headache and dizziness. (para 4-4b)

7. a The treatment of hypertension and congestive heart failure.
(para 4-4d)

8. b Nitrates prescribed 8-12 hours per day, followed by a 12-16 hours drug
free interval to decrease tolerance and side effects. (para 4-4c)

9. COLUMN A   COLUMN B

_c_ Minoxidil.   a. Sorbitrate®
(para 4-4d)

_a_ Isosorbide dinitrate.   b. Nitroglycerin
(para 4-4c)

_e_ Isoxsuprine.   c. Loniten®
(para 4-5)

_d_ Isosorbide mononitrate.   d. Imdur®
(para 4-4c)

_b_ Glyceryl trinitrate.   e. Vasodilan®
(para 4-4b)

End of Lesson 4

LESSON ASSIGNMENT

LESSON 5   Drugs Acting on the Hematopoietic System.

LESSON ASSIGNMENT   Paragraphs 5-1--5-10.

TASKS   081-824-0001, Perform Initial Screening of a
                             Prescription.

                             081-824-0026, Evaluate a Prescription.

                             081-824-0002/3, Fill a Prescription For a
                             Controlled/Non-Controlled Drug.

                             081-824-0027, Evaluate a Completed Prescription.

                             081-824-0028, Issue Outpatient Medications.

LESSON OBJECTIVES   After completing this lesson you will be able to:

                             5-1.   Given a group of statements, select the
                             statement which best describes hematopoietic drugs.

                             5-2.   Given one of the following terms: coagulant,
                             anticoagulant, hematinic, or growth factors, and a
                             group of statements, select the statement that best
                             defines the given term.

                             5-3.   Given a list of the steps involved in the clotting
                             of blood and a group of sequences of those steps,
                             select the proper sequence of those steps required for
                             clotting of the blood.

                             5-4.   Given the trade or generic name of a drug that
                             acts on the hematopoietic and a list of other trade and
                             generic names, select the trade or generic name that
                             corresponds to the given name.

                             5-5.   Given the trade and/or generic name of a drug
                             that acts on the hematopoietic system and a list of
                             indications, uses, side effects, or precautionary
                             statements, select the indication(s), use(s), side
                             effect(s), or precautionary statement(s) for that
                             drug.

5-6. Given a group of statements, select the statement which should be communicated to each patient to whom an anticoagulant is dispensed.

SUGGESTION

After completing the assignment, complete the exercises at the end of this lesson. These exercises will help you to achieve the lesson objectives.

LESSON 5

DRUGS ACTING ON THE HEMATOPOIETIC SYSTEM

Section I. DEFINITIONS

5-1. INTRODUCTION

The word hematopoietic means, "blood producing." Therefore, drugs acting on the hematopoietic system would pertain to drugs that act on the blood producing system of the body. As you might expect, these drugs are potentially dangerous because they can affect blood production in the body.

5-2. DEFINITIONS

a. **Coagulant**. A coagulant is a drug that stimulates the clotting of the blood. Coagulants can be of great aid in an emergency in which the patient may be losing a large volume of blood.

b. **Anticoagulant**. An anticoagulant is a drug that prevents the clotting of the blood. Anticoagulants are used in various types of surgery as well as in everyday use in order to control blood clots.

c. **Hematinic**. A hematinic is a drug that stimulates the formation of red blood cells. Hematinics are used in the treatment of anemias.

d. **Stimulating Factors.** A stimulating factor is an agent that stimulates the formation of specific blood cells (red blood cells, white blood cells, or platelets).

Section II. COAGULANTS

5-3. REVIEW OF THE CLOTTING PROCESS (FIGURE 5-1)

The area of blood clotting was discussed in paragraphs 2-7 and 2-8 of this subcourse. The actual clotting of blood involves several steps. Each step is essential to clotting.

STEP 1: The blood platelets release a substance that is known as thromboplastin.

STEP 2: Thromboplastin reacts with calcium and another substance, prothrombin, to form thrombin. Vitamin K is necessary for the proper formation of prothrombin.

STEP 3: The thrombin formed acts as an enzyme to convert fibrinogen to fibrin threads that eventually form the blood clot.

NOTE: For a more in-depth discussion of blood clotting you should locate and read a physiology text that is appropriate to your level of understanding.

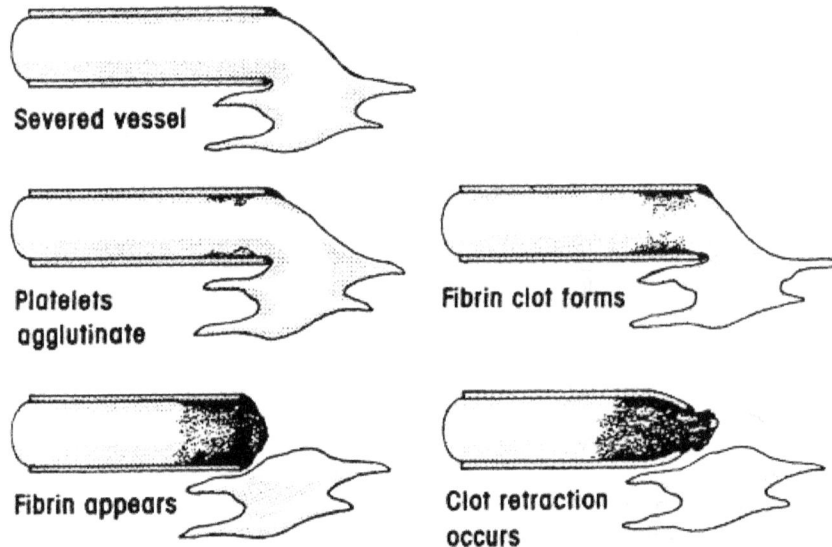

Severed vessel

Platelets agglutinate

Fibrin clot forms

Fibrin appears

Clot retraction occurs

Figure 5-1. The blood clotting process.

STEP 4: Clot breakdown. Plasminogen binds to fibrin as the clot forms. In response to thrombin formation and venous stasis (clot), plasminogen activators convert plasminogen to plasmin. Plasmin digests fibrin and dissolves the clot.

5-4. COAGULANTS (PROMOTING CLOT FORMATION)

There are several drugs that affect the clotting process at different stages to promote coagulation. Vitamin K derivatives and coagulation factors work by enhancing the formation or increasing the amount of circulating clotting factors and promoting the coagulation process (steps 2 and 3 above). Drugs that inhibit plasminogen or plasmin result in coagulation by preventing the breakdown of clots (step 4 above).

a. **Phytonadione (Mephyton®, Aqua-Mephyton®, Vitamin K₁)**. Phytonadione or vitamin K is the most commonly prescribed coagulant and antidote for warfarin overdose. As a coagulant, the usual dose is 0.5 to 1.0 milligram given intramuscularly

(IM) to infants at birth to prevent infant hemorrhagic disease. Infants are administered this medication because at birth they lack the normal intestinal flora required to produce enough Vitamin K to play its role in blood clotting. When phytonadione is used for its anticoagulant effects, the dosage is based on the level of warfarin anticoagulation in the patient. This level of anticoagulation is determined by blood sample and expressed as the International Normalized Ratio (INR) by the laboratory. Doses may be as small as 0.5-1 mg (oral) up to 10 mg administered subcutaneously. The initial effects of vitamin K take up to 6 hours with maximum effects in 2-3 days. If a patient is actively bleeding, the coagulant of choice may be fresh frozen plasma or a blood transfusion. Side effects associated with this agent include "flushing" sensations and peculiar sensations of taste. The injectable form of this agent is used only on an inpatient basis (that, in the hospital or emergency room), and it should be remembered that it should only be administered subcutaneously--severe reactions (including death) have been reported when the product was given intravenously (IV). Phytonadione will not counteract the anticoagulant action of heparin.

b. **Vitamin K$_3$, Menadione.** Menadione is another coagulant prescribed in patients who have bleeding problems. The only side effect of real concern with menadione is hepatomegaly. Hepatomegaly is a condition in which the liver becomes enlarged because of an excess of fat soluble vitamins stored in the lipid tissue. This agent is commonly supplied in tablet form.

c. **Menadiol (Synkayvite®).** Menadiol (observe its similiarity to menadione) is a synthetic Vitamin K$_3$. Menadiol is also used as a coagulant available in a tablet and injectable form.

d. **Specific Clotting Factors.** In patients that have an acquired or hereditary clotting factor deficiency, specific clotting factors are available. Factor VIII and Factor IX are available as concentrates often stocked within the pharmacy. The agents are available for minor procedures or surgery in select patients with these deficiencies.

e. **Desmopressin Acetate (DDAVP®).** Desmopresin is a synthetic analog of vasopressin, the naturally occurring human antidiuretic hormone. It has the unique activity of producing a dose-related increase in circulating Factor VIII and von Willdebrand's factor levels. Both of these factors are essential to normal human coagulation. This agent is used in individuals with Hemophilia A (lacking factor VIII) or von Willdebrand's disease. Desmopressin will maintain homeostasis in these patients during surgery and post-operatively. Desmopressin may also be prescribed for uncontrolled bleeding related to surgery in patients without a coagulation dysfunction.

f. **Aminocaproic Acid (Amicar®).** Aminocaproic acid is an agent that inhibits fibrinolysis (clot breakdown) by inhibiting plasminogen activators. Consequently, it stabilizes clots in excessive bleeding. Aminocaproic acid is given either intravenously or orally. Individuals with bleeding dysfunction (hemophilia) may take this product 12-24 hours prior to a dental procedure or surgery. It is often prescribed with desmopressin.

g. **Tranexamic Acid (Cyklokapron®) and Aprotinin (Trasylol®).** Tranexamic acid is a competitve inhibitor of plasminogen activation. Its action is similar to aminocaproic acid but approximately 10x more potent. It is used in hemophiliacs undergoing invasive procedures. Apotinin is a natural protease inhibitor that inhibits plasmin. It is used prophylactically in patients undergoing coronary artery bypass surgery to prevent peri-operative blood loss.

NOTE: The administration of blood products (whole blood, fresh frozen plasma, or cryoprecipitate) may be used in place of any or all of the above agents to correct excess bleeding. They are often the fastest means of correcting excess anticoagulation. Although each of the drugs discussed above has side effects, the risk/benefit of a transfusion must be weighed in each patient.

Section III. ANTICOAGULANTS

5-5. INTRODUCTION

Just as there are conditions of excess bleeding (anticoagulation), so are there conditions in which excess clotting (coagulation) may be detrimental to the patient. The major components that promote excess clot formation are: 1) venous stasis (altered or decreased blood flow to the deep veins of the lower extremities) which occurs with impaired mobility (traumatic injury, obesity); 2) vascular injury which occurs as the result of mechanical or chemical trauma causing an inflammation of the vessel; and 3) hypercoagulability which results from a deficiency of natural anticoagulants (antithrombin III, protein C, protein S) or a specific disease state (cancer).

Anticoagulants are essential to correcting the propensity to clot. However, they are a potentially dangerous class of drugs. One reason for their dangerous status is that anticoagulants interact with a variety of medications (over the counter and legend). Second, there is always a risk of uncontrolled bleeding when you inhibit a process that promotes clotting. One of the most important interactions to remember is the combination of anticoagulants with other drugs--especially salicylates (aspirin) or non-steroidal antiinflammatory drugs (ibuprofen, naproxen). These products can potentiate the effects of the anticoagulants by inhibiting platelet aggregation which is the first line of defense to stop bleeding.

5-6. IMPORTANT WARNING ASSOCIATED WITH THE ANTICOAGULANTS

There is one warning common to all anticoagulants. When you dispense an anticoagulant to a patient you should tell the person that they should not take any other medication--over the counter or legend--without first consulting the physician who prescribed the anticoagulant. Emphasize that over-the-counter products such as aspirin and ibuprofen are also classified as medications.

5-7. ANTICOAGULANT AGENTS

a. **Anti-platelet agents.** Anti-platelet agents are used to prevent a clot from forming (step I) or prevent the clot from getting larger and occluding the entire vessel. All patients must be warned of the increased risk of bleeding when taking these drugs.

(1) Aspirin. Aspirin is the most widely used anti-platelet drug. It inhibits platelet aggregation for the life of the platelet (7-10 days). Because of this effect, aspirin is prescribed in the setting of acute myocardial infarction and prophylactically to prevent reinfarction. Always ask the patient if he/she has an allergy to aspirin.

(2) Clopidogrel (Plavix®) and Ticlopidine (Ticlid®). Clopidogrel and ticlopidine work by inhibiting platelet aggregation. They are often prescribed for patients that have an aspirin allergy or are intolerant of aspirin (usually stomach upset). Both agents may be used in patients with atherosclerotic disease to prevent heart attacks, prevent stokes, and prevent coronary artery closure in patient undergoing angioplasty. Ticlopidine is administered twice daily and is associated with a risk of decreased white blood cells (neutropenia). Clopidogrel is administered once daily and has a much lower risk of neutropenia. Both agents can cause a rash.

(3) Dipyridomole (Persantine®). Dipyridomole works by inhibiting platelets from adhering to the injured cell wall. Although not used extensively, it may be prescribed in combination with other anticoagulants. The combination product of dipyridomole and aspirin is called Aggrenox®.

(4) Abciximab (ReoPro®), Tirofiban (Aggrastat®), and Eptifibatide (Integrelin®). The following agents are known as glycoprotein IIb/IIIa inhibitors. The GP IIb/IIIa receptor is the major receptor on the platelet responsible for platelets adhering to each other and forming the initial clot. These drugs are administered intravenously in patients with acute coronary syndromes (unstable angina) or in patients undergoing angioplasty with or without stent placement in the cardiac catheterization lab. The agents prevent clots from forming in the coronary arteries of the heart. The agents are not interchangeable and differ in their respective half-lives and infusion schedules. The major side effect is thrombocytopenia (low platelet count) occasionally requiring a platelet transfusion.

b. **Heparin products.** Heparin is used to prevent the clotting of blood in the patient and in laboratory samples by inhibiting certain clotting factors (Thrombin/Factor IIa and Factor Xa). Like anti-platelet drugs, heparin will not dissolve a clot but prevents it from getting larger. The dosage of this agent is based upon the needs of the patient (prophylactic vs. treatment doses). It may be administered subcutaneously or intravenous (IV Push or IV continuous infusion). The major side effect associated with heparin is possible hemorrhage. Protamine sulfate is used to treat heparin overdose. Although protamine sulfate is also an anticoagulant, it counteracts the effects of heparin by binding with the heparin. The net result is removing the effects of the heparin. The primary side effects associated with protamine sulfate are temporary hypotension, bradycardia, and dyspnea.

(1)   Heparin Sodium, Heparin Calcium. Commerical heparin (unfractionated heparin) comes from beef lung or pork intestinal mucosa. It is dosed in "units" and measured in the lab by the partial thromboplastin time (PTT). Although some heparin is administered in a "fixed dose" for prophylaxis against clots, it is more often administered in a "wt-based" fashion for prophylaxis and treatment of clots. Therapeutic dose goals are 1.2-1.5x the PTT control. Doses, especially for continuous infusion are adjusted to meet this goal. Heparin may be administered in a very small fixed dose (10-100 units) to clear intravenous ports in patients with long term IV lines. This dose is called a "heparin flush". The absorption of subcutaneous heparin is unpredictable.

(2)   Enoxaparin (Lovenox®), Dalteparin (Fragmin®). Enoxaparin and dalteparin are two of several "low molecular weight heparins (LMWH)" (fractionated heparin). They differ from unfractionated heparin by having more predictable subcutaneous absorption, a longer duration of action, and primarily inhibit only one clotting factor (Factor Xa). Either agent may be administered once or twice daily (SC) usually for 7-10 days. The primary use for these agents is in the prevention and treatment of deep vein thrombosis (leg clots) and pulmonary embolus (lung clots). The sides effects are the same as with unfractionated heparin however they offer distinct advantages in that the patient can self-administer these agents (discharged from the hospital sooner), they do not require monitoring of the PTT, and are just as effective as standard heparin. The major disadvantages are pain at the injection site and high cost.

c.   **Coumarin products**. Coumarin products inhibit coagulation by interfering with the incorporation of vitamin K into vitamin-K dependent clotting factors (Factors II, VII, IX, and X). Their initial and maximum effect is based on the half-lives of each of these factors. For example, Factor VII has a half-life of 6 hours so the effect of coumarin on this factor will increase the bleeding to a certain degree within 6 hours, however Factor II and X exhibit half-lives of 48-72 hours, so the maximum effect of coumarin is not seen until 3 days after initiation or dose change. It does not matter whether the drug is given orally or intravenously, it takes the same amount of time to reach the maximum effect (essentially you cannot load a patient on coumarin agents). Coumarin products do not dissolve clots but prevent clots from forming (prophylaxis) and getting larger. The degree of anticoagulation is measured by a blood sample and expressed as the prothrombin time (PT) or the International Normalized Ratio (INR). The INR is the international standard. The therapeutic INR is generally between 2-3.5 which correlates with a 30-50% inhibition of vitamin K dependent clotting factors. Ideally, the patient should have his/her INR checked every 4-6 weeks while on this medication.

Warfarin sodium (Coumadin®). Warfarin sodium is one of the most commonly used anticoagulants (coumarins). It is used to prevent the extension of blood clots in phlebitis or deep vein thrombosis and as a prophylactic agent in patients that have mechanical heart valves (life-long therapy). The main side effect associated with the use of warfarin sodium is hemorrhaging. This product is available in both oral and injectable forms. This agent has over 50 documented drug-drug interactions. You must research this drug carefully against the patient profile before dispensing.

d. **"Clot Busters".** As discussed above, we can administer aspirin, heparin, or warfarin to prevent clots or stop clots from getting bigger. But none of these drugs can dissolve a clot that is already established. In many cases we cannot wait for the body to reabsorb these clots back into the lining of the vessel (4-6 months); we need to dissolve the clot immediately. This is the case for the patient having heart attacks and strokes. "Clot busters" do just that—by acting as tissue plasminogen activator and converting plasminogen to plasmin or mimicking fibrinolytic enzymes, they break down the clot. These agents are always administered intravenously and require close observation for bleeding in the patient. They are most effective when administered as close to onset of symptoms as possible (ideally within 3-6 hours).

(1) Streptokinase (Streptase®), Urokinase ((Abbokinase®). Streptokinase and urokinase were some of the first clot busters developed and act as fibrinolytic enzymes. Streptokinase comes from streptococcus species so patients with strept antibodies may have an allergic reaction to this agent. Urokinase comes from human kidney cells so the incidence of side effects is less. Both agents are administered via continuous IV infusion (12-24 hours) and are rarely used with the advent of recombinant products.

(2) Alteplase (Activase®). Alteplase, also known as tPA (tissue plasminogen activator) was the first recombinant product developed. It offers the advantage of short infusion time (1 hour) and is more effective than streptokinase. It is used for heart attacks (within 4-6 hours of symptoms) and strokes (within 3 hours of symptoms). Alteplase (2 mg) is also used to dissolve clots in IV lines. Reteplase (Retavase®) and anistreplase (Eminase®) are other clot busters.

Section IV. HEMATINICS

5-8. INTRODUCTION

Hematinics are drugs used to stimulate the formation of red blood cells. These agents are used primarily in the treatment of certain types of anemias. Some of these preparations are routinely given to women during pregnancy.

5-9. HEMATINIC AGENTS

a. **Ferrous Gluconate (Fergon®) Ferrous Sulfate (Feosol®).** Ferrous gluconate and ferrous sulfate are used to treat iron deficiency anemia. The usual dosage given is 1-4 times daily. Side effects associated with these agents include gastrointestinal upset, constipation, and black stools. Warn the patient about these possible side effects.

b. **Iron Dextran (InFed®).** This drug is also used to treat iron deficiency anemia. Side effects associated with this agent include gastrointestinal upset, constipation, and black stools. Extreme caution should be observed with this product because it is administered parenterally and some patients have demonstrated an anaphylactic type reaction to the drug. This product is used on an inpatient basic and is administered by injection. Iron dextran should not be administered concurrently with oral iron preparation because the side effects mentioned above will be potentiated.

c. **Cyanocobalamin, Vitamin B$_{12}$ (Rubesol-1000®).** Cyanocobalamin is used in the treatment of pernicious anemia. Pernicious anemia is a condition characterized by a progressive decrease in the number and an increase in the size of red blood cells. Patients who have this condition are usually very weak and have various gastro-intestinal disturbances. This condition results from a lack of Vitamin B$_{12}$. This occurs because of the lack of intrinsic factor, an element that is needed in the intestine in order to effectively absorb Vitamin B$_{12}$. Thus, cyanocobalamin is used to replace the Vitamin B$_{12}$ that was not absorbed. Cyanocobalamin should be protected from light. It is available in injectable or tablet form.

d. **Folic Acid (Folate®).** Folic acid is used in combination with other drugs to treat pernicious anemia because it causes an increase in the number of red blood cells. If the drug is administered alone to treat pernicious anemia, it will mask the symptoms of that condition. This is potentially dangerous because if the symptoms are masked, the condition might flourish and cause irreversible neurologic damage. Folic acid is available in both tablet and injectable dosage forms.

e. **Erythropoetin; EPO; Epoten alfa (Epogen®, Procrit®).** Erythropoetin is a protein naturally produced in the kidney that stimulates red blood cell production. It is administered in a variety of chronic anemia states (cancer, renal failure, dialysis, and HIV infection). It may also be used prophylactically to reduce the need for a blood transfusion in patients scheduled for major surgery. The major side effect of erythropoetin is hypertension, especially if the hematocrit rises above 36%. Erythropoetin is administered subcutaneously 1-3 times weekly. Single dose vials MUST be disposed of immediately after use. Multidose vials are discarded 21 days after initial entry. Erythopoetin requires refrigeration.

Section V. STIMULATING FACTORS

5-10. INTRODUCTION

Stimulating factors are naturally occurring substances which promote the proliferation of blood components. Similar to the effects of erythropoetin, stimulating the production of red blood cells, the stimulating factors discussed below affect the production of white blood cells and platelets.

a. **Granulocyte Colony Stimulating Factor; G-CSF; Filgrastim (Neupogen®).** Filgrastim stimulates the growth of white blood cells, specifically the granulocytes (neutrophils). It is used in the treatment of neutropenia (low neutrophils) from chemotherapy or bone marrow transplant patients. The most common complaints associated with use are nausea, vomiting, and joint aches. Filgrastim is administered subcutaneously 5-10 mcg/kg/day until neutrophil counts rise to normal. Filgrastim is available as an injection without preservative; it requires refrigeration.

b. **Granulocyte Macrophage Colony Stimulating Factor; GM-CSF; Sargramostim (Leukine®).** Sargramostim is used to stimulate the proliferation of granulocytes and macrophages in patients with leukemia and/or undergoing bone marrow transplant. This agent is administered 250 mcg/m^2/day via IV infusion over 2-4 hours until neutrophil recovery. The side effects are similar to filgrastim. Sargramostim must be refrigerated.

Continue with Exercises

EXERCISES, LESSON 5

REQUIREMENTS: The following exercises are to be answered by marking the lettered response that best answers the question; or by completing the incomplete statement; or by writing the answer in the space provided at the end of the question.

After you have completed all the exercises, turn to "Solutions to Exercises," at the end of the lesson, and check your answers with the solutions.

1. Which of the following statements best describes hematopoietic system drugs?

    a. Drugs that produce pernicious anemia or mask its effects on the body.

    b. Drugs that clot the blood.

    c. Drugs that act on the blood producing system of the body.

    d. Drugs that decrease the clotting capability of the blood.

2. Hematinic drugs _____.

    a. Stimulate the formation of red blood cells.

    b. Stimulate the clotting of the blood.

    c. Stimulate the production of hematin in the body.

    d. Stimulate the mechanism responsible for preventing the clotting of the blood.

3.   Immediately below are the three steps involved in blood clotting. Select the sequence of steps that reflects the proper sequence of steps required for blood clotting.

      I. Thromboplastin reacts with calcium and prothrombin to form thrombin. Vitamin K is necessary for the proper formation of prothrombin.

      II. The thrombin formed acted acts as an enzyme to convert fibrinogen to fibrin threads that eventually form the blood clot.

      III. The blood platelets release a substance which is know as thromboplastin.

    a.   II, I, and III.

    b.   II, III, and I.

    c.   III, I, and II.

4.   Heparin sodium is used to _____.

    a.   Stimulate the formation of red blood cells.

    b.   Stimulate the clotting of the blood in people with clotting difficulties.

    c.   Prevent Vitamin K from being formed and absorbed in the body.

    d.   Prevent the clotting of blood in the patient and in laboratory examples.

5.   Select the side effect(s) associated with ferrous gluconate.

    a.   Pernicious anemia.

    b.   Black stools.

    c.   Phlebitis.

    d.   Hepatomegaly.

6. Select the side effect(s) associated with enoxaparin.

   a. Black stools.

   b. Phelebitis.

   c. Pernicious anemia.

   d. Hemorrhaging.

7. All of the following classes of drugs are used for anticoagulation EXCEPT:

   a. Clot busters such as alteplase.

   b. Anti-platelets such as aspirin.

   c. Vitamin K derivatives such as phytonadione.

   d. Heparin derivatives such as dalteparin.

8. Folic acid can mask the symptoms of _____ if it is administered alone.

   a. Pernicious anemia.

   b. Iron deficiency anemia.

   c. Hepatomegaly.

   d. Phlebitis.

9. Clot busters are agents used to_____

   a. Prevent platelets from adhering to each other.

   b. Block certain clotting factors to prevent blood from clotting.

   c. Stimulate the production of certain blood components.

   d. Dissolve clots that have already formed.

10. Match the generic in Column A with its corresponding trade name in Column B.

COLUMN A

___ Ferrous gluconate.

___ Enoxaparin.

___ Iron Dextran.

___ Phytonadione.

___ Warfarin sodium.

___ Desmopressin acetate

___ Abciximab

___ Clopidogrel

___ Aprotinin

___ Erythropoetin

___ Alteplase

___ Filgrastim

COLUMN B

a. Aqua-Mephyton®.

b. ReoPro®

c. DDAVP®.

d. Activase®.

e. Fergon®.

f. Neupogen®

g. InFed®.

h. Lovenox®

i. Procrit®

j. Coumadin®.

k. Trasylol®

l. Plavix®

Check Your Answers on Next Page

SOLUTIONS TO EXERCISES, LESSON 5

1. c Drugs that act on the blood producing system of the body. (para 5-l)

2. a Stimulate the formation of red blood cells. (para 5-2c)

3. c III, I, and II. (para 5-3)

4. d Prevent the clotting of blood in the patient and in laboratory samples.
       (para 5-7b)

5. b Black stools. (para 5-9a)

6. d Hemorrhaging. (para 5-7b)

7. c Vitamin K derivatives such as phytonadione. (para 5-4)

8. a Pernicious anemia. (para 5-9d)

9. d Dissolve clots that have already formed. (para 5-7d)

10.   COLUMN A   COLUMN B

     e   Ferrous gluconate. (para 5-9a)   a.   Aqua-Mephyton®

     h   Enoxaparin. (para 5-7b(2))   b.   ReoPro®

     g   Iron Dextran. (para 5-9b)   c.   DDAVP®

     a   Phytonadione. (para 5-4a)   d.   Activase®

     j   Warfarin sodium. (para 5-7c)   e.   Fergon®

     c   Desmopressin acetate. (para 5-4e)   f.   Neupogen®

     b   Abciximab. (para 5-7a(4))   g.   InFed®

     l   Clopidogrel. (para 5-7a(2))   h.   Lovenox®

     k   Aprotinin. (para 5-4g)   i.   Procrit®

     i   Erythropoetin (para 5-9e)   j.   Coumadin®

     d   Alteplase (para 5-7d(2))   k.   Trasylol®

     f   Filgrastim   (para 5-10a)   l.   Plavix®

End of Lesson 5

LESSON ASSIGNMENT

LESSON 6	The Human Urogenital Systems.
LESSON ASSIGNMENT	Paragraphs 6-1--6-20.
TASKS	081-824-0001, Perform Initial Screening of a Prescription.
	081-824-0026, Evaluate a Prescription.
	081-824-0002/3, Fill a Prescription For a Controlled/Non-Controlled Drug.
	081-824--0027, Evaluate a Completed Prescription.
	081-824-0028, Issue Outpatient Medications.
LESSON OBJECTIVES	After completing this lesson you will be able to:

6-1.   Given a group of components, select the two components of the human urogenital system.

6-2.   Given a group of functions, select the specialized function of the urinary system.

6-3.   Given a group of components, select the major components of the human urinary system.

6-4.   Given a drawing of the human urinary system and a group of names of the major components of the urinary system, match the name of each major component with its location on the drawing.

6-5.   From a group of names of structures, select the name of the functional unit of the human kidney.

6-6.   From a list of functions, select the functions(s) of the nephron.

6-7.   Given a drawing of a nephron and a list of the names of the parts of a nephron, match the name of each part with its location on the drawing.

6-8. Given the name of one of the parts of the nephron and a group of statements, select the statement that best describes the role of the part in the production of urine.

6-9. Given the name of one of the hormones involved in the formation of urine and a group of statements, select the statement that best describes the role of that hormone in the formation of urine.

6-10. Given the name of a part of the urinary system and a group of statements, select the statement that best describes that part of the urinary system.

6-11. Given the name of a urinary tract disorder and a group of statements, select the statement that best describes the disorder.

6-12. From a list of organs, select the primary sex organ in the human female.

6-13. Given the name of a secondary sex organ in the human female and a group of statements, select the statement that best describes the secondary sex organ.

6-14. Given a list of organs, select the primary sex organ in the human male.

6-15. From a group of statements, select the function(s) of the testis.

6-16. Given the name of a secondary sex organ in the human male and a group of statements, select the statement that best describes the secondary sex organ.

SUGGESTION

After completing the assignment, complete the exercises at the end of this lesson. These exercises will help you to achieve the lesson objectives.

LESSON 6

THE HUMAN UROGENTIAL SYSTEM

Section I. OVERVIEW OF THE UROGENITAL SYSTEMS

6-1. INTRODUCTION

The human <u>urogenital systems</u> are made up of the <u>urinary organs,</u> which produce the fluid called urine, and the <u>genital</u> or <u>reproductive</u> organs, organs of male and female humans, which together can produce a new human being.

6-2. DISCUSSION OF LESSON CONTENT

This lesson will focus on the human urinary and reproductive systems. The urinary system will be discussed first.

Section II. THE HUMAN URINARY SYSTEM

6-3. INTRODUCTION

The urinary system is one of the major systems of your body. When something goes wrong with this system, medical assistance must quickly be obtained. An understanding of the anatomy and physiology of the urinary system will help you as you study such drug categories as diuretics (those drugs which increase urine output).

6-4. THE HUMAN URINARY SYSTEM

a. **Proteins.** Proteins are one of the basic foodstuffs that humans consume. When the body uses proteins, residue or waste products can be poisonous (toxic) if allowed to accumulate in large amounts. The urinary system of the human body is specialized to remove these nitrogenous waste products from the circulating blood.

b. **Major Parts.** See Figure 6-1 for the major parts of the human urinary system. This system includes <u>two kidneys</u>, two <u>ureters</u> (one connecting each kidney to the <u>urinary bladder</u>), the <u>urinary bladder</u>, and the <u>urethra</u>.

6-5. THE KIDNEY

a. **General.**

(1)   The kidneys have the same shape and color as kidney beans, but are about 8-10 cm (3"-3 1/2") in length.

(2)   Each kidney has a fibrous capsule. On the concave, medial side of each kidney, there is a notch called the hilus. Through the hilus, pass the ureter and the NAVL (nerve, artery, vein, and lymphatic), which service the kidney.

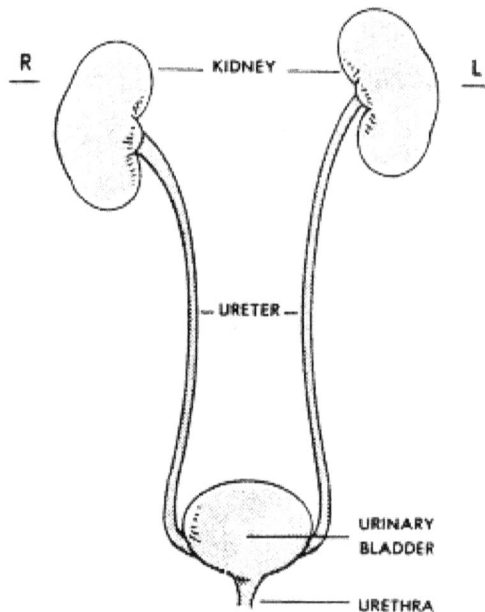

Figure 6-1. The human urinary system.

(3)   Each kidney is attached to the posterior wall of the abdominal cavity, just above the waistline level. Each is held in place by special fascia and fat.

b.   **Gross Internal Structure.** If we compare the structure of the kidney with that of a cantaloupe (muskmelon), the renal cortex would correspond to the hard rind, the renal medulla would correspond with the edible flesh of the melon, while the renal sinus would correspond to the hollow center (after the seeds have been removed. The medulla consists of pyramids with their bases at the cortex and forming peaks, papillae, which empty into the sinus.

PAPILLA = pimple, nipple

See Figure 6-2 for a section of the kidney showing the inner structure.

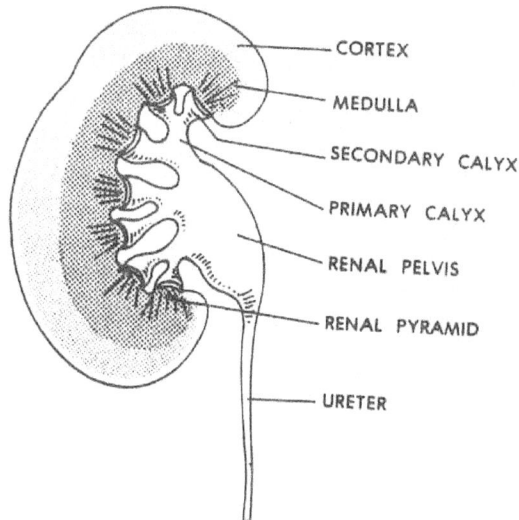

Figure 6-2. A section of a human kidney.

    c. **The Nephron.** (See Figure 6-3 for an illustration of a nephron.) Nephrons are the functional units of the human kidney. Their primary function is to remove the wastes of protein usage from the blood. In addition, they serve to conserve water and other materials for continued use by the body. The result of nephron function is more or less concentrated fluid called <u>urine</u>. The kidneys contain great numbers of nephrons, about a million for each kidney. The main subdivisions of a nephron are the renal corpuscle and a tubular system.

       (1) <u>Renal corpuscle</u>. The renal corpuscle has a hollow double walled sac called the <u>renal capsule</u> ("Bowman's capsule"). Leading into the capsule is a very small artery called the <u>afferent arteriole</u>. Within the capsule, this artery becomes a mass of capillaries known as the <u>glomerulus</u>. An <u>efferent arteriole</u> drains the blood away from the capsule. The capsule and the glomerulus together are known as the <u>renal corpuscle.</u>

       (2) <u>Tubules</u>. Each renal capsule is drained by a renal tubule. The first part of this tubule runs quite a distance in a coiled formation and is called the <u>proximal convoluted tubule</u>. A long loop, the <u>renal loop</u> (of Henle) extends down into the medulla with two straight parts and a sharp bend at the bottom. As the tube returns to the cortex layer, it becomes coiled once more and here is known as the <u>distal convoluted tubule</u>.

       (3) <u>Filtration/reabsorption</u>. Except for the blood cells and the larger proteins, the fluid portion of the blood passes through the walls of the glomerulus into the cavity between the two layers of the renal capsule. This fluid is called the <u>glomerular filtrate</u>. By a process of taking back (resorption), the majority of the fluid is removed from the tubules and the concentrated fluid is called urine.

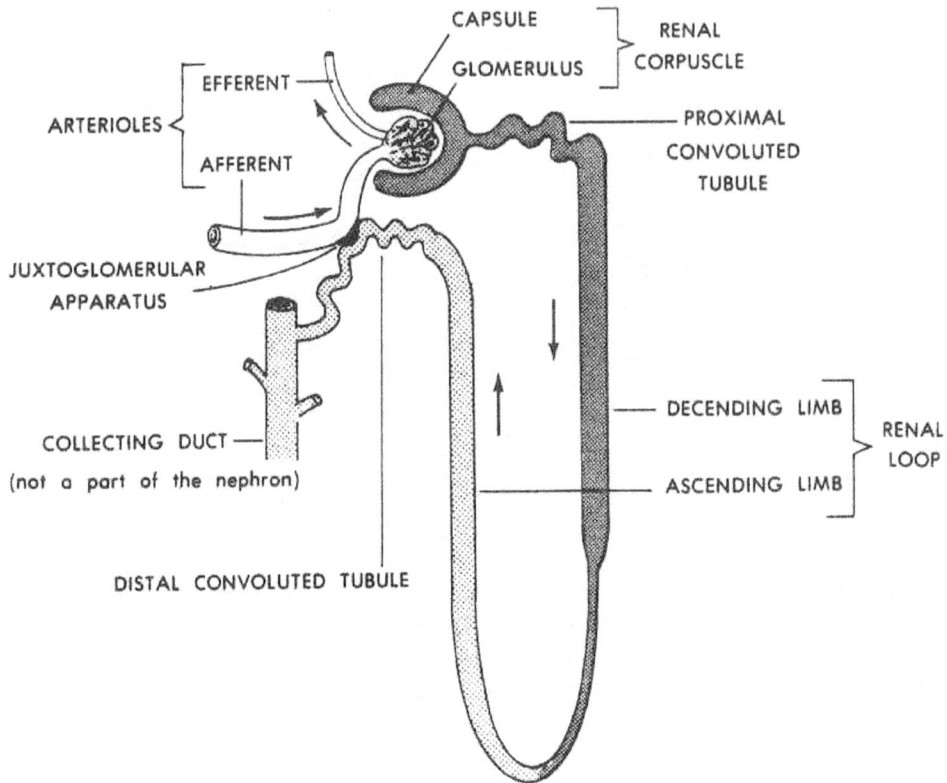

Figure 6-3. A "typical" nephron.

　　　d.　**The Collecting Tubule.** The distal convoluted tubules of several nephrons empty into a collecting tubule. The urine is then passed from the collecting tubule at the papilla of the medullary pyramid. Several collecting tubules are present in each pyramid.

　　　e.　**Renal Pelvis.** The renal pelvis is a hollow sac within the sinus of the kidney. Urine from the pyramids collects into the funnel-shaped renal pelvis. The ureter then drains the urine from the renal pelvis.

6-6.　HORMONES INVOLVED IN THE FORMATION OF URINE

　　　There are two main hormones involved in the formation of urine. These hormones are the antidiuretic hormone (ADH), and aldosterone.

　　　a.　**Antidiuretic Hormone.** The antidiuretic hormone is a hormone secreted by the pituitary gland. It acts on the distal and collecting tubules to increase water reabsorption. Since more water is reabsorbed, the urine becomes more concentrated.

b. **Aldosterone.** The aldosterone is secreted by adrenal cortex, that is situated above each kidney. Aldosterone increases sodium reabsorption in the distal tubules and collecting ducts. This leads to an increase in sodium reabsorption and of concentration of the urine.

6-7. URETERS

The ureters are tubes that connect the kidneys to the urinary bladder. The smooth muscle walls of the ureters produce a peristalsis (wave-like movement) that moves the urine along drop by drop.

6-8. URINARY BLADDER

a. The urinary bladder is a muscular organ for storing the urine. Near the inferior posterior corners of the urinary bladder are openings where the ureters empty into the bladder. Also at the inferior aspect of the urinary bladder is the exit, the beginning of the urethra. The triangular area, between the openings of the ureters and the urethra, is called the trigone, or base of the urinary bladder.

b. The urinary bladder wall is stretchable to accommodate varying volumes of urine.

c. Nerve endings called stretch receptors are found in the wall of the urinary bladder. Usually, the pressure within the urinary bladder is low. However, as the volume of the enclosed urine approaches the bladder's capacity, stretching of the wall stimulates the stretch receptors. The cycle of events controlling urination (voiding or emptying of the urinary bladder) is known as the voiding reflex.

6-9. URETHRA

The urethra is a tube that conducts the urine from the urinary bladder to the outside of the body. It begins at the anterior base of the urinary bladder.

a. **Urethral Sphincters**. The urethral sphincters are circular muscle masses that control the passage of the urine through the urethra. There are two urethral sphincters: an internal urethral sphincter and an external urethral sphincter.

(1) The internal urethral sphincter is located in the floor of the urinary bladder. It is made of smooth muscle tissue. Nerves of the autonomic nervous system control it.

(2) The external urethral sphincter is inferior around the urethra in the area of the pelvic floor. It is made up of striated muscle tissue. It is controlled by the peripheral nervous system.

b. **Male-Female Differences**. The female urethra is short and direct. The male urethra is much longer and has two curvatures. Whereas the female urethra serves only a urinary function, the male urethra serves both the urinary and reproductive functions.

6-10. URINARY TRACT DISORDERS

Several disorders can affect the urinary system. Some of these disorders can present serious problems.

a. **Uremia.** Uremia, or as it is frequently called, toxemia, is a condition in which there is a build-up of toxic substances in the blood. These accumulated waste products are in the blood because of kidney failure. This condition can occur during pregnancy, since many pregnant women have fluid retention.

b. **Glomerulonephritis**. Glomerulonephritis is an inflammation of the nephrons--mainly centered in the glomerulus. This condition is due to toxic material produced by bacteria.

c. **Pyelonephritis.** Pyelonephritis is another condition caused by bacteria. Pyelonephritis is an inflammation of the kidney and pelvis area of the kidney.

d. **Edema**. Edema is a build-up of fluids in the tissues. It is found in a variety of conditions (that is, pregnancy, congestive heart failure, and renal disease).

e. **Diabetes Insipidus**. Diabetes insipidus is an increased urine output due to a low production of the antidiuretic hormone. As previously mentioned, the antidiuretic hormone increases the reabsorption of water. A lack of the antidiuretic hormone thus prevents water from being reabsorbed and leads to increased urine output.

f. **Cystitis.** Cystitis is an inflammation of the urinary bladder, which may spread to the kidneys.

Section III. INTRODUCTION TO HUMAN GENITAL (REPRODUCTIVE) SYSTEMS

6-11. SEXUAL DIMORPHISM

The human male and human female each has a system of organs specifically designed for the production of new humans. These systems are known as <u>reproductive</u> or <u>genital</u> systems. Since there are different systems for males and females, the genital systems are an example of sexual dimorphism.

```
         MORPH   = form, shape
           D1    = two
         SEXUAL = according to sex (gender)
SEXUAL DIMORPHISM = having two different forms according to sex
```

6-12. ADVANTAGES OF DOUBLE PARENTING

The existence of two parents for each child means that genetic materials are recombined to produce a new type. This new type may be an improvement over previous generations.

6-13. MAJOR COMPONENT CATEGORIES OF THE GENTIAL SYSTEMS

Components of the genital systems may be considered in the following categories:

a. **Primary Sex Organs (Gonads)**. Primary sex organs produce sex cells (gametes). A male gamete and a female gamete may be united to form the one-cell beginning of an embryo (the process of fertilization). Primary sex organs also produce sex hormones.

b. **Secondary Sex Organs**. Secondary sex organs care for the product of the primary sex organ.

c. **Secondary Sexual Characteristics**. Secondary sexual characteristics are those traits that tend to make males and females more attractive to each other. Secondary sexual characteristics help to ensure mating. These characteristics first appear during puberty (10-15 years of age).

Section IV. THE HUMAN FEMALE GENITAL (REPRODUCTIVE) SYSTEM

6-14. PRIMARY SEX ORGANS (OVARIES)

The primary sex organ in the human female is the ovary. (See Figure 6-4 for an illustration of the female genital system.) The ovaries are located to the sides of the upper end of the uterus. They are anchored to the posterior surface of the broad ligaments. (The broad ligaments are sheets or folds of peritoneum inclosing the uterus and uterine tubes and extending to the sides of the pelvis.)

a. The ovary produces the egg cell or ovum (ova, plural).

b. The ovary produces female sex hormones (estrogens and progesterone).

c. The production of ova is cyclic. Usually, one ovum is released during each 28-day menstrual cycle.

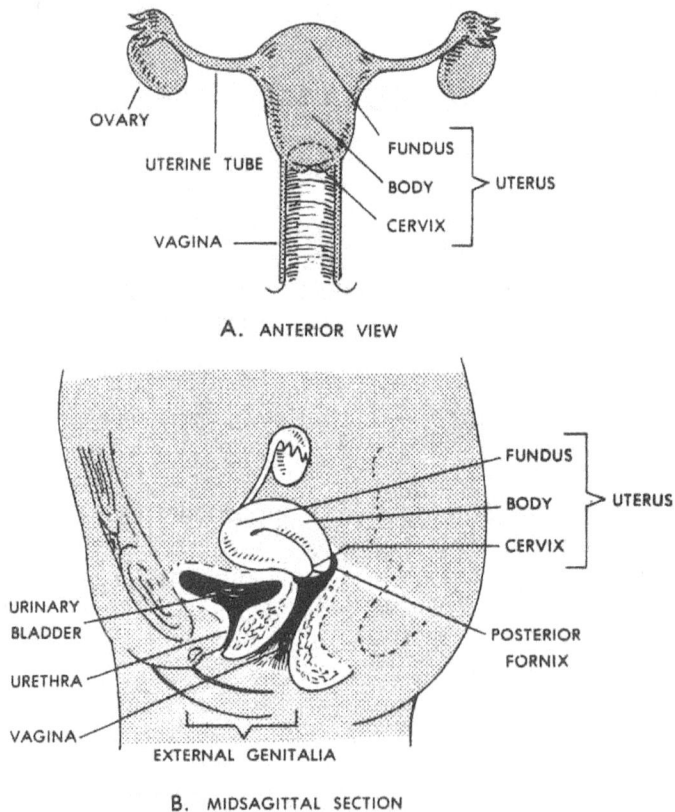

Figure 6-4. The human female genital system.

6-15. SECONDARY SEX ORGANS

a. **Uterine Tubes (Fallopian Tubes, Oviducts)**. Extending to either side of the uterus are two muscular tubes, which open at the outer ends like fringed trumpets. The fringe-like appendages encircle the ovaries. At their medial ends, the uterine tubes open into the uterus. The function of the uterine tubes is to pick up the ovum when released from the ovary and hold it UNTIL one of the following happens:

(1) Fertilization. Then it is fertilized. After fertilization, the initial stages of embryo development take place. The developing embryo is eventually moved into the uterus.

(2) Death of Ovum. The nutrient stored within the ovum is used up, and the ovum dies. This may take 3-5 days.

b. **Uterus**. The uterus is the site where all but the first few days of embryo development takes place. After 8 weeks of embryonic development, it is known as the fetus.

(1) Main subdivisions. The uterus is shaped like a pear, with the stem (cervix) facing downward and toward the rear. The fundus is the portion of the uterus above the openings of the uterine tubes. The main part, or body, is the portion between the cervix and the fundus. The uterus usually leans forward with the body slightly curved as it passes over the top of the urinary bladder. The cervix opens into the upper end of the vagina.

(2) Wall structure. The inner lining of the uterus is called the endometrium. Made up of epithelium, it is well supplied with blood vessels and glands. The muscular wall of the uterus is called the myometrium. In the body of the uterus, the muscular tissue is in a double spiral arrangement. In the cervix, it is in a circular arrangement.

(3) Age differences. The uterus of an infant female is undeveloped. During puberty the uterus develops. The uterus of an adult is fully developed. The uterus of an old woman is reduced in size and nonfunctional.

c. **Vagina**. The vagina is a tubular canal connecting the cervix of the uterus with the outside. It serves as a birth canal and as an organ of copulation. It is capable of stretching during childbirth. The low opening of the vagina may be partially closed by a thin membrane known as the hymen.

d. **External Genitalia**. Other terms for the external genitals of the human female are vulva and pudendum. Included are the:

(1) Mons pubis. The mons pubis is a mound of fat tissue covered with skin and hair in front of the symphysis pubis (the joint of the pubic bones).

(2) Labia majora. Extending back from the mons pubis and encircling the vestibule (discussed below) are two folds known as the labia majora. Their construction is similar to the mons pubis, including fatty tissue and skin. The outer surfaces are covered with hair. The inner surfaces are moist and smooth. The corresponding structure in the male is the scrotum.

LABIA = lips   LABIUM, singular

(3) Labia minora. The labia minora are two folds of skin lying within the labia majora and inclosing the vestibule. In front, each labium minus (minus = singular or minora) divides into two folds. The fold above the clitoris (discussed below) is called the prepuce of the clitoris. The fold below is the frenulum.

(4) Clitoris. The clitoris is a small projection of sensitive erectile tissue that corresponds to the male penis. However, the female urethra does not pass through the clitoris.

(5) Vestibule. The cleft between the labia minora and behind the clitoris is call the vestibule. It includes the urethral opening in front and the vaginal opening slightly to the rear.

e. **Pregnancy and Delivery.** When an embryo forms an attachment to the endometrium, a pregnancy exists. The attachment eventually forms a placenta, an organ joining mother and offspring for such purposes as nutrition of the offspring. The fetal membranes surround the developing individual (fetus), and are filled with the amniotic fluid.

(1) During the first 8 weeks, the developing organism is known as an embryo. During this time, the major systems and parts of the body develop.

(2) During the remainder of the pregnancy, the developing organism is known as the fetus. During this time, growth and refinement of the body parts occur.

(3) Parturition is the actual delivery of the fetus into a free-living state. The delivery of the fetus is followed by a second delivery--that of the placenta and fetal membranes.

f. **Menstruation and Menopause.** About 2 weeks after an ovum is released, if it is not fertilized, menstruation occurs. Menstruation involves the loss of all but the basal layer of the endometrium. This process includes bleeding. It first occurs at puberty and lasts until menopause (45-55 years of age). After menopause, pregnancy is no longer possible.

6-16. SECONDARY SEXUAL CHARACTERISTICS

The secondary sexual characteristics of females include growth of pubic hair, development of mammary glands, development of the pelvic girdle, and deposition of fat in the mons pubis and labia majora.

6-17. MAMMARY GLANDS

Secretion of milk begins after parturition. Stimulation from suckling helps to maintain the normal rate of milk secretion. At the time of menopause, breast tissue becomes less prominent.

Section V. THE HUMAN MALE GENITAL (REPRODUCTIVE) SYSTEM

6-18. PRIMARY SEX ORGANS (TESTES)

The primary sex organ of the human male is the testis. See Figure 6-5 for an illustration of the male genital system. The testes are egg-shaped.

a. **Location.** The paired testes lie within the scrotum. The scrotum is a sac of loose skin attached in the pubic area of the lower abdomen. The scrotum provides a site cooler than body temperature to maintain the viability of the spermatozoa (see below). However, when the air is too cold, muscles and muscular fibers draw the testes and scrotum closer to the body to maintain warmth. Otherwise, the scrotum hangs loosely. The tunica vaginalis is a serous cavity surrounding each testis.

b. **Functions.** The testis produces the male sex cells, called spermatozoa (spermatozoon, singular). The millions continuously produce the spermatozoa. One such cell may eventually fertilize an ovum of a human female. The testes also produce male sex hormones, called androgens.

6-19. SECONDARY SEX ORGANS

a. **Epididymis.** The epididymis is a coiled tube whose function is to aid in the maturation of spermatozoa. Its coiled length is only about 1 1/2 inches. Its uncoiled length is about 16 feet. When coiled, it extends downward along the posterior side of each testis. Its lining secretes a nutritive medium for spermatozoa. It receives spermatozoa from the testes in an immature state. As the spermatozoa pass through the nutrient, they mature.

b. **Ductus (Vas) Deferens.** The ductus deferens is a transporting tube that carries the mature sperm from the epididymis to the prostate. Each tube enters the abdomen through the inguinal canal. Each passes over a ureter to reach the back of the urinary bladder and then down to the prostate gland.

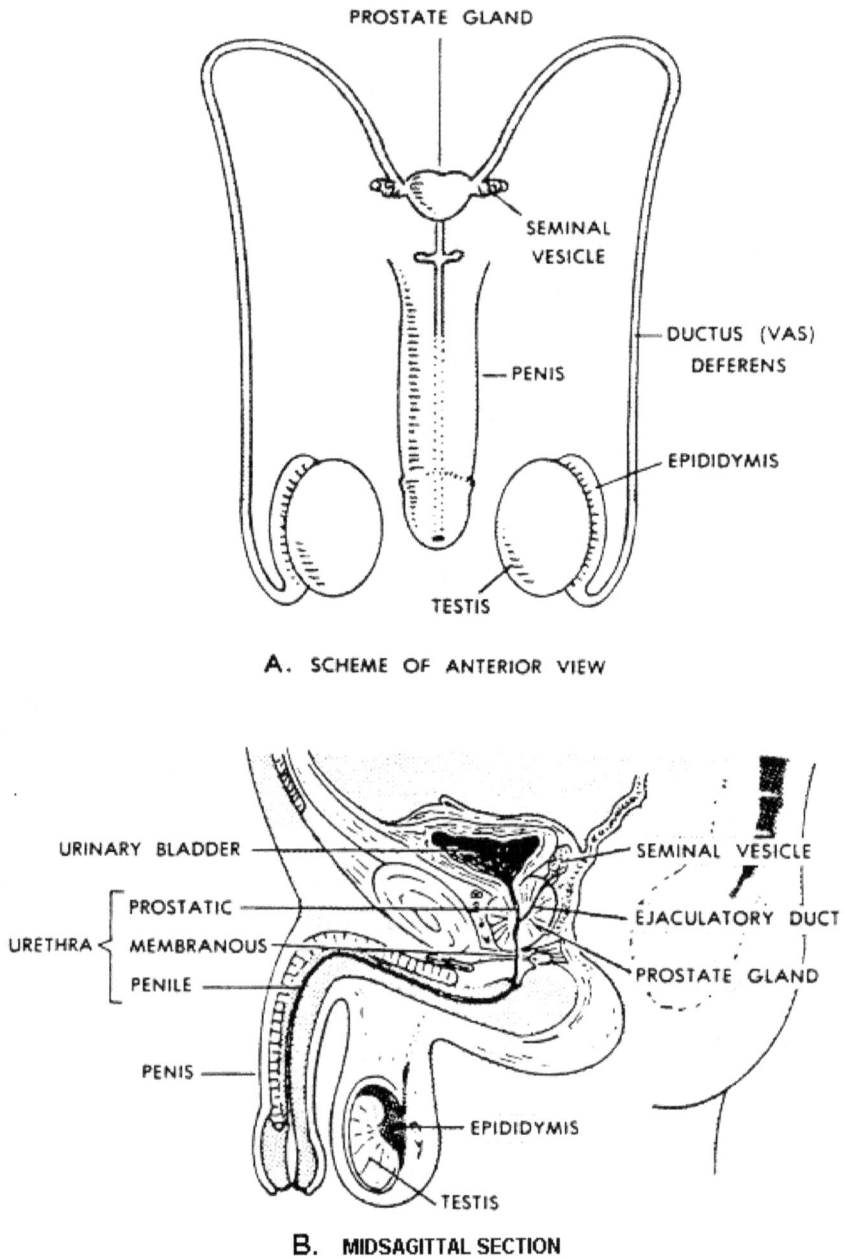

PROSTATE GLAND

SEMINAL
VESICLE

DUCTUS (VAS)
DEFERENS

PENIS

EPIDIDYMIS

TESTIS

A. SCHEME OF ANTERIOR VIEW

URINARY BLADDER

SEMINAL VESICLE

EJACULATORY DUCT

PROSTATIC

URETHRA { MEMBRANOUS

PENILE

PROSTATE GLAND

PENIS

EPIDIDYMIS

TESTIS

B. MIDSAGITTAL SECTION

Figure 6-5. The human male genital system.

c. **Seminal Vesicles**. Lying alongside each ductus deferense as it crosses the back of the bladder is a tubular structure called the seminal vesicle. The seminal vesicle produces a fluid that becomes part of the ejaculate (see below).

d. **Ejaculatory Duct**. Each ductus deferens and its corresponding seminal vesicle converge to form a short tube called the ejaculatory duct. The ejaculatory duct opens into the urethra within the prostate gland (see below). The ejaculatory duct carries both spermatozoa and seminal vesicle fluid.

e. **Prostate Gland**. As the urethra leaves the urinary bladder, a chestnut-size gland called the prostate gland surrounds its first inch. The prostate gland provides an additional fluid to be added to the spermatozoa and seminal vesicle fluid.

f. **Penis**. As the urethra leaves the abdomen, it passes through the penis, the male organ of copulation.

(1) Surrounding the urethra is a central cylinder of erectile tissue called the corpus spongiosum. This cylinder is bulb-shaped at each end. The posterior end is attached to the base of the pelvis. The sensitive anterior end is known as the glans.

CORPUS SPONGIOSUM = spongy body

(2) Overlying the corpus spongiosum is a pair of cylinders of erectile tissue called the corpora cavernosa. These two cylinders are separate in their proximal fourth and joined in their distal three-fourths. They are attached to the pubic bones. Together, the corpus spongiosum and the corpora cavernosa combine to form the shaft of the penis.

CORPUS CAVERNOSUM = cavernous body

(3) The prepuce, or foreskin, is a covering of skin for the glans. It may be removed in a surgical procedure called circumcision.

6-20. SECONDARY SEXUAL CHARACTERISTICS

The secondary sexual characteristics of male include growth of facial pubic, and chest hair, growth of the larynx to deepen the voice, and deposition of protein to increase muscularity and general body size.

Continue with Exercises

EXERCISES, LESSON 6

REQUIREMENT. The following exercises are to be answered by marking the lettered response that best answers the question; or by completing the incomplete statement; or by writing the answer in the space provided at the end of the question.

After you have completed all the exercises, turn to "Solutions to Exercises," at the end of the lesson, and check your answers with the solutions.

1. Which of the following are components of the human urogenital system?

   a. Urinary organs.

   b. Pleural space.

   c. Reproductive organs.

   d. Pituitary gland.

2. Select the major components of the human urinary system.

   a. Urethra.

   b. Urinary bladder.

   c. Ureters.

   d. Kidneys.

   e. All the above.

3. Referring to the drawing below, match the name of each component of the urinary system with its location on the drawing.

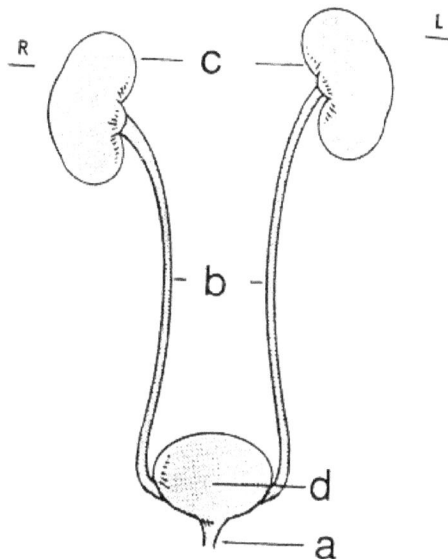

_____ Ureter

_____ Urethra

_____ Kidney

_____ Urinary bladder

4. From the list below, select the function(s) of the nephron.

    a. Remove the wastes of protein usage from the blood.

    b. Remove the secretions of endocrine glands from the blood.

    c. Conserve water and other materials for continued use by the body.

    d. All the above.

5. Which of the following statements is true concerning the role of the renal tubule?

    a. The renal tubule drains into the renal capsule.

    b. The renal tubule decreases sodium reabsorption when acted on by aldosterone.

    c. The renal tubule selectively removes the wastes of protein usage from the glomerular filtrate.

    d. The renal tubule selectively removes blood cells and large proteins from the glomerular filtrate.

6. The antidiuretic hormone is one of the two main hormones involved in the formation of urine. What is its role in the formation of urine?

    a. The antidiuretic hormone dilutes the concentration of urine by increasing the amount of water reabsorbed in the distal and collecting tubules.

    b. The antidiuretic hormone dilutes the concentration of the urine by increasing sodium reabsorption in the distal tubules and collecting ducts.

    c. The antidiuretic hormone concentrates the urine by decreasing sodium and water absorption in the distal tubules and collecting ducts.

    d. The antidiuretic hormone increases water absorption in order to concentrate the urine.

7. The ureter can be best described as a _____.

    a. Tube that conducts the urine from the urinary bladder to the outside of the body.

    b. Tube that allows for reabsorption of water from the glomerular filtrate in order to concentrate the urine.

    c. Tube that connects the kidneys to the urinary bladder.

    d. Tube that collects the urine after it has passed through the distal convoluted tubule.

8. Uremia is a condition-characterized by_____.

    a. An inflammation of the nephrons caused by toxic material produced by certain bacteria.

    b. A build-up of toxic substances in the blood because of kidney failure.

    c. Increased urine output due to a low production of the antidiuretic hormone.

    d. A burning and stinging sensation in the urinary bladder due to some type of chronic inflammation.

9. What is the primary sex organ in the human female?

    a.   The ovary.

    b.   The vagina.

    c.   The uterus.

    d.   The cervix.

10. The vagina is best described as _____.

    a. A mound of fat tissue covered with skin and hair in front of the symphysis pubis.

    b. A small projection of sensitive erectile tissue which corresponds to the male penis.

    c. A tubular canal that connects the cervix of the uterus with the outside.

    d. The cleft between the labia minora and behind the clitoris.

11. The primary sex organ in the human male is the _____.

    a. Epididymis.

    b. Penis.

    c. Seminal vesicle.

    d. Testis.

12. Select the function(s) of the testis.

    a. Production of androgens.

    b. Production of estrogens.

    c. Production of spermatozoa.

    d. Production of a fluid that retards the development of spermatozoa.

    e. All the above.

    f. b and d only.

    g. a and c only.

13. The prostate gland _____.

    a. Provides an additional fluid that is added to the spermatozoa and seminal vesicle fluid.

    b. Is the gland that produces spermatozoa.

    c. Is a coiled gland that secretes a nutritive medium for spermatozoa so they mature.

    d. Is the tissue responsible for the production of the male sex hormones called androgens.

Check Your Answers on Next Page

SOLUTIONS TO EXERCISES, LESSON 6

1. a Urinary organs. (para 6-1)

    c Reproductive organs. (para 6-1)

2. e All the above. (para 6-4b)

3.

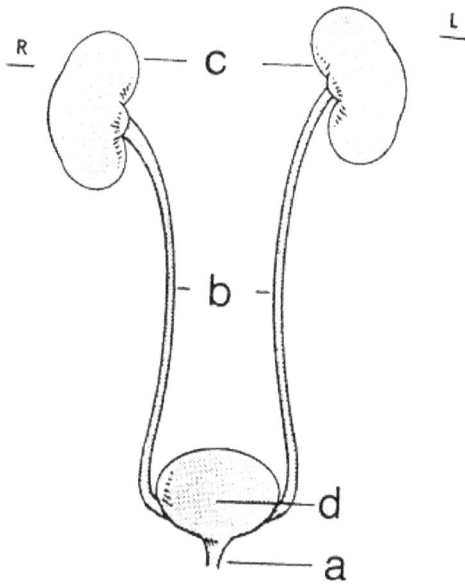

b Ureter

a Urethra

c Kidney

d Urinary bladder

(Figure 6-1)

4. a Remove the wastes of protein usage from the blood. (para 6-5c)

    c Conserve water and other materials for continued use by the body.
       (para 6-5c)

5. c The renal tubule selectively removes the wastes of protein usage
       from the glomerular filtrate. (para 6-5c)

6. d The antidiuretic hormone increases water absorption in order to
       concentrate the urine. (para 6-6a)

7. c Tubes that connect the kidneys to the urinary bladder. (para 6-7)

8. b A build-up of toxic substances in the blood because of kidney failure.
       (para 6-10a)

9. a   The ovary. (para 6-14)

10. c   A tubular canal that connects the cervix of the uterus with the outside. (para 6-15d)

11. d   Testis. (para 6-18)

12. g   a and c only. (para 6-18b)

13. a   Provides an additional fluid which is added to the spermatozoa and seminal vesicle fluid. (para 6-19e)

End of Lesson 6

LESSON ASSIGNMENT

LESSON 7	Antihypertensive Agents.
LESSON ASSIGNMENT	Paragraphs 7-1--7-12.
TASKS	081-824-0001, Perform Initial Screening of a Prescription.
	081-824-0026, Evaluate a Prescription.
	081-824-0002/3, Fill a Prescription for a Controlled/Non-Controlled Drug.
	081-824-0027, Evaluate a Completed Prescription.
	081-824-0028, Issue Outpatient Medications.
LESSON OBJECTIVES	After completing this lesson you will be able to:

7-1.   From a group of statements, select the statement which best defines the term <u>essential hypertension</u>.

7-2.   Given the name of a type of essential hypertension and a group of statements, select the statement that best describes that type.

7-3.   Given a group of statements, select the statement that best describes why diuretics are used to treat hypertension.

7-4.   Given a group of trade and/or generic names of antihypertensive agents match each trade name with its corresponding generic name.

7-5.   Given the trade and/or generic name of an antihypertensive agent and a group of indications, side effects, or patient warnings; select the indication(s), side effect(s), or patient warning(s) associated with that agent.

SUGGESTION   After completing the assignment, complete the exercises at the end of this lesson. These exercises will help you to achieve the lesson objectives.

LESSON 7

ANTIHYPERTENSIVE AGENTS

Section I. INTRODUCTION TO HYPERTENSION

7-1. INTRODUCTION

a. It is estimated that 23 million people in the United States suffer from hypertension. Of this number, it is thought that 11.5 million people have been diagnosed as having the condition and that 5.75 million of those people are being treated for it. Unfortunately, it is estimated that only 2.875 million of those persons treated for hypertension are being treated properly. Therefore, it is obvious that hypertension is a major medical problem which should be a concern of all medical personnel.

b. Hypertension (high blood pressure) is prevalent in both men and women. It frequently contributes to the death of many persons. The cause of most cases of hypertension is unknown. This type of hypertension is referred to as primary or essential hypertension. Hypertension that has a known cause (kidney disease, hyperthroidism) is called secondary hypertension. Blood pressure is the force that the blood exerts on the vessel wall while the heart is contracting and at rest. The force against the vessel wall during contraction or systole is the systolic pressure and the force during rest or diastole is the diastolic pressure. The blood pressure is expressed in terms of millimeters of mercury (Hg). Normal blood pressure is less than 135 mm Hg (systolic) and less than 85 mm Hg (diastolic) = 135/85 mm Hg.

7-2. TREATMENT OF HYPERTENSION

There is no cure for hypertension. Most patients who have a bacterial infection are accustomed to taking a 10-day treatment regimen of an antibiotic in order to rid themselves of the infection. The same is not true with hypertension. Once a person begins taking an antihypertensive agent, it is likely that he will continue taking some type of antihypertensive agent for the rest of his life.

7-3. DEFINITION OF ESSENTIAL (PRIMARY) HYPERTENSION

Essential (primary) hypertension can be defined as a disorder of unknown origin characterized mainly by an elevated systolic or diastolic blood pressure associated with generalized arteriolar vasoconstriction (see Lesson 2). Essential hypertension may be divided into three classes according to the severity of the condition. Labile hypertension is a condition of elevated blood pressure with intervening periods of normal blood pressure.

7-4. CLASSES OF ESSENTIAL HYPERTENSION

a. **Stage I Hypertension**. Stage I hypertension is characterized by sustained, documented systolic pressure 140 to 159 mm Hg and or diastolic pressure measurements 90-99 mm Hg. Signs of this type include increased heart rate (tachycardia) and increased cardiac output with normal total peripheral vascular resistance, however the majority of patients cannot tell that they have hypertension.

b. **Stage II Hypertension**. Stage II hypertension is characterized by sustained, systolic elevation (160 to 179 mm of Hg) and or diastolic pressure (100 to 109 mm Hg). Symptoms are the same as noted in Stage I. Patients with Stage I or II DO NOT show signs of target end organ damage. The organs of most concern are the heart, kidneys, and eyes. Stage I and II hypertension may be treated nonpharmacologically with diet and exercise or pharmacologically with antihypertensive medications.

c. **Stage III Hypertension**. Stage III hypertension is characterized by a persistent elevation (systolic >180mm Hg; diastolic >110mm Hg) with target end organ damage. Damage to the heart may include strain or enlargement of the left ventricle. Kidney damage may appear as abnormal laboratory values that indicate inefficiency. Damage to the eyes may appear as small hemorrhages due to the sustained blood pressure in these small vessels. This stage is often treated immediately with antihypertensive medications.

d. **Hypertensive urgency** is a condition of persistent elevation in blood pressure without target end organ damage. However, the pressure is high enough that the patient presents for treatment because of symptoms of dizziness, chest pain, or confusion. The goal in treatment of this condition is to normalize the blood pressure as quickly as possible (usually over 1-3 days). **Hypertensive crisis** is a similar condition, however the patient has symptoms of target end organ damage. This may be a life-threatening condition. The goal of therapy is to normalize the blood pressure in 12-24 hours. Both conditions are usually treated with intravenous (IV) antihypertensives.

7-5. REVIEW OF IMPORTANT FACTORS RELATING TO HYPERTENSION

Essential hypertension is a process of variable course and severity. Several options are open to the physician depending upon the severity of the drug therapy. Condition weight reduction and diet control may be adequate treatment; however, drug therapy is sometimes needed. When drug therapy is required, it usually begins with a diuretic followed by the addition of the other agents based on the patient's response. However, certain classes of drugs may be more advantageous (fewer side effects) when patients have other diseases. It is not unreasonable to see patients treated by the same provider on different drugs.

7-6. DIURETICS IN THE TREATMENT OF HYPERTENSION

The effectiveness of diuretics in the treatment of essential hypertension arises from the fact that diuretic agents decrease tubular reabsorption of sodium, which caused a reduction in blood pressure. Some of the common diuretics include hydrochlorothiazide, spironolactone (Aldactone®), furosemide (Lasix®), and triamterene (Dyrenium®). These agents will be discussed in detail in Lesson 8 of this subcourse.

7-7. COMBINATION THERAPY IN THE TREATMENT OF HYPERTENSION

When diuretics alone are ineffective in controlling hypertension, it is necessary to combine the diuretic therapy with one or more additional agents. The physician may use many combinations of agents in order to control the patient's high blood pressure. The patient should be encouraged to discuss any questions he might have concerning the side effects (for example, drowsiness), which might be caused by an agent or agents.

Section II. DRUGS USED IN THE TREATMENT OF HYPERTENSION

NOTE: For this discussion commonly used antihypertensive agents will be classified into the following categories.

7-8. DRUGS WHICH ACT ON THE SYMPATHETIC NERVOUS SYSTEM

NOTE: For a review of the sympathetic nervous system you should refer to Subcourse MD0805, Pharmacology II.

a. **Methyldopa (Aldomet®).** Methyldopa is one of the drugs of this type. It is believed to produce its effects by its being metabolized to a substance which is very similar to norepinephrine--but with considerably less vasoconstricting activity than is shown by epinephrine. Thus, methyldopa competes with norepinephrine and thereby depresses the activity of the sympathetic nervous system. This medication is rarely used but is still one of the drugs of choice for pregnancy-induced hypertension. Side effects associated with this agent include bradycardia, swelling of the feet and lower legs (because sodium and water retention), drowsiness, and mental depression.

b. **Clonidine (Catapres®, Catapres TTS®).** Clonidine is an agent that is believed to act by decreasing sympathetic outflow from the brain and consequently inhibit vasoconstriction. It is used in mild to moderate hypertension. Side effects associated with this agent include swelling of the feet and lower legs (due to sodium and water retention) and mental depression. The patient taking this drug should be cautioned to check with his physician before suddenly discontinuing the medication because abrupt withdrawal from the drug may cause serious hypertension problems. Clonidine is also used in the treatment of symptoms associated with alcohol withdrawal.

7-9. BETA ADRENERGIC BLOCKERS

As you remember, beta adrenergic blocking agents block the effect of the sympathetic neurotransmitters by competing for receptors.

a. **Propranolol (Inderal®).** Propranolol is a drug used in the treatment of hypertension, angina pectoris, and cardiac arrhythmias. Side effects associated with propranolol include dizziness, mental confusion, and mental depression. It may also exacerbate congestive heart failure and mask the symptoms of hypoglycemia.

b. **Metoprolol (Lopressor®, Toprol XL®).** Metoprolol is prescribed for the same conditions as propranolol and is also indicated used in the treatment of myocardial infarction and treatment of congestive heart failure. Normal doses for hypertension are 25 – 100 mg twice daily. The dose for heart failure is 6.25 – 12.5 mg twice daily and adjusted upward as tolerated by the patient. This agent is available as an oral and injectable preparation.

c. **Other Beta Adrenergic Blockers.** Other beta blockers used in the treatment of hypertension include betaxolol (Kerlone®), bisoprolol (Zebeta®), labetolol (Trandate®, Normodyne®), nadolol (Corgard®), and carvedilol (Coreg®). Carvedilol is also indicated for congestive heart failure.

7-10. SMOOTH MUSCLE RELAXANTS

Drugs in this category treat hypertension by acting directly on vascular smooth muscle by relaxing the blood vessels. Consequently, they cause vasodilation and a decrease in peripheral resistance results in a lower blood pressure.

a. **Hydralazine (Apresoline®).** Hydralazine is given orally or injected in the management of hypertension. Preferably, it is used in conjunction with other antihypertensive agents. Side effects associated with this agent include chest pain (angina pectoris), a general feeling of weakness, unexplained sore throat, joint pain, and headache. The patient should to be told to avoid getting up suddenly from a lying or a sitting position.

b. **Alpha adrenergic blockers.** Alpha adrenergic blockers block alpha receptors in peripheral vessels, therefore causing vasodilation. Agents in the class include prazosin (Minipress®), doxazosin (Cardura®), and terazosin (Hytrin®). Doxazosin and terazosin offer the advantage of once daily dosing and the added benefit of relieving the symptoms of benign prostatic hyperplasia (enlarged prostate gland). Dizziness, drowsiness, and headache are common side effects associated with these agents, especially with the first dose. Patients must be counseled on these side effects and instructed to take the first dose in the evening at home. Some patients who have taken this drug have also experienced syncope (unconsciousness due to decreased oxygen supply to the brain).

c. **Calcium Channel Blockers**. Calcium channel blockers are potent peripheral vasodilators used in the treatment of hypertension. Similar to beta blockers that can slow the heart rate, calcium channel blockers are also used in the treatment of atrial fibrillation to control the heart rate. Many of the products are available in oral and injectable form and may be administered once daily. Side effects include dizziness, headache, heartburn, edema, and constipation. Agents include diltiazem (Cardizem®, Tiazac®, Dilacor®), verapamil (Calan®, Isoptin®, Covera®, Verelan®), amlodipine (Norvasc®), felodipine (Plendil®), and nifedipine (Procardia XL®, Adalat CC®).

d. **Angiotensin Converting Enzyme Inhibitors (ACE Inhibitors)**. ACE inhibitors work by inhibiting the enzyme which converts angiotensin I to angiotensin II. Angiotensin II is one of the most potent vasoconstrictors known to man. By inhibiting the enzyme, these agents produce vasodilation and are used in the treatment of hypertension and heart failure. Most products are administered 1-2 times daily. The most common side effects are rash, dry cough, and hyperkalemia. These agents are contraindicated in pregnancy. Selected agents include benazepril (Lotensin®), captopril (Capoten®), enalapril (Vasotec®), lisinopril (Prinivil®, Zestril®), and ramipril (Altace®). Enalapril is available in an injectable form.

e. **Angiotensin II receptor blockers (ARBs)**. ARBs work by directly blocking the angiotensin II receptor to cause vasodilation and lower blood pressure. They appear to have less side effects than ACE inhibitors, especially the dry cough. Selected agents include irbesartan (Avapro®), losartan (Cozaar®), and valsartan (Diovan®).

7-11. COMBINATION PRODUCTS

It should be apparent that in order to control hypertension the patient may be required to take extremely large amounts of medication. In an attempt to develop a more convenient method of controlling hypertension, researchers have combined diuretic and antihypertensive agents in order to maximize the best attributes of each. These combination products are very convenient for the patient to use if the dosage of the product is exactly what the patient needs to control his hypertension. Since these combination products tend to be rather expensive, military pharmacies frequently have a limited selection of these items in stock. Two examples of combination products are listed below.

a. **Aldactazide® (Spironolactone and Hydrochlorothiazide)**. Spironolactone and hydrochlorothiazide are both diuretics. This particular drug is used in the treatment of hypertension, congestive heart failure and cirrhosis of the liver. The patient taking this medication should be told to take the preparation with or after meals to minimize stomach upset.

b. **Dyazide® (Triamterene and Hydrochlorothiazide)**. Triamterene and hydrochlorothiazide are both diuretics. This product is used as a diuretic and as an antihypertensive agent.

7-12. THE TREATMENT OF A HYPERTENSIVE CRISIS OR EMERGENCY

Patients presenting with extreme elevations of blood pressure and symptoms of impending stroke, pulmonary edema, kidney failure, or heart attack must be promptly. The following agents are used to treat hypertensive crisis:

a. **Diazoxide (Hyperstat® I.V.)** This agent is administered by rapid intravenous (I.V.) injection (150 to 300 milligrams immediately, repeated in 30 minutes and every four hours if needed). When administered, this agent produces a fall in blood pressure in from one to five minutes. Hyperglycemia and sodium retention are side effects associated with this agent.

b. **Nitroprusside (Nipride®).** Nitroprusside is administered by continuous intravenous infusion at a rate of 0.5 to 0.8. micrograms per kilogram of patient weight per minute. The patient must be closely observed, when he is receiving this drug since overdosage of nitroprusside results in cyanide poisoning. Nitroprusside is not intended for direct injection. Instead, the drug must be used as an infusion with sterile 5 percent dextrose in water. The intravenous infusion must be used within four hours once it is prepared. Furthermore, the prepared intravenous infusion must be protected from light (for example: the bottle must be wrapped with foil). Nausea, vomiting, and headache are side effects commonly associated with this agent.

Continue with Exercises

EXERCISES, LESSON 7

REQUIREMENT: The following exercises are to be answered by marking the lettered response that best answers the question; or by completing the incomplete statement; or by writing the answer in the space provided at the end of the question.

After you have completed all the exercises, turn to "Solutions to Exercises," at the end of the lesson, and check your answers with the solutions.

1.   Match the drug name in <u>Column A</u> with its corresponding name listed in <u>Column B.</u>

COLUMN A	COLUMN B
_____ Lisinopril.	a. Cardura®
_____ Spironolactone and hydrochlorothiazide combination.	b. Catapres®
	c. Adalat CC®
_____ Doxazosin.	d. Inderal®
_____ Diltiazem.	e. Calan®
_____ Metoprolol.	f. Cardizem®
_____ Propranolol.	g. Zestril®
_____ Clonidine.	h. Lopressor®
_____ Verapamil.	i. Aldactazide®
_____ Nifedipine.	

2. Which of the following statements best defines the term essential hypertension?

        a. A disorder of unknown origin characterized mainly by an elevated systolic or diastolic pressure associated with generalized arteriolar vasoconstriction.

        b. A disorder caused by too many fats in the diet and by an excess of sodium in the intracellular fluid.

        c. A disorder produced by unknown causes which results in a diastolic pressure which is higher than the systolic pressure.

        d. A disorder of unknown origin that can be cured by a 10-day treatment regimen of diuretics and antihypertensives.

3. Which of the following statements best describes Stage I primary hypertension?

        a. A type of essential hypertension characterized by documented pressure measurements greater than159 mm Hg (systolic) and/or greater than 99 mm Hg (diastolic).

        b. A type of essential hypertension characterized by a persistent elevation in diastolic pressure with minor target organ (heart and kidney damage).

        c. A type of essential hypertension characterized by marked elevated blood pressure with definite target organ (heart and kidney) damage.

        d. A type of essential hypertension characterized by a mild, but sustained, elevation in diastolic pressure without target organ (heart and kidney) damage.

4.   Stage III primary hypertension is best described as a type of essential hypertension characterized by _____.

   a. Persistent elevated diastolic pressure with minor damage to the heart and/or kidneys.

   b. Documented diastolic pressure associated with generalized arteriolar vasoconstriction.

   c. A mild, but sustained, elevation in diastolic pressure without damage to the heart and/or kidneys.

   d. Marked elevated blood pressure with definite damage to the heart and/or kidneys.

5.   The indication for nitroprusside (Nipride®) is _____.

   a. Treatment of essential hypertension.

   b. Treatment of a hypertensive crisis.

   c. Treatment of labile primary hypertension.

   d. Treatment of moderate primary hypertension.

6.   Select the side effect associated with beta blockers.

   a. Swelling of the feet and lower legs.

   b. Tachycardia.

   c. Restlessness.

   d. Mask symptoms of hypoglycemia.

7. What should the patient taking terazosin be told?

    a. To be aware that many patients taking the drug experience impotence or decreased sexual interest.

    b. To take the medication one hour before meals in order to increase the absorption of the drug.

    c. To arise slowly from a lying or sitting position because of the possibility of orthostatic hypotension and syncope.

    d. To avoid taking the medication with fats because absorption of the drug is affected.

8. The patient taking nitroprusside should be closely monitored because _____.

    a. Hyperglycemia and sodium retention occur so abruptly with this agent that death can result if the drug is not withdrawn after their onset.

    b. Overdosage of nitroprusside results in cyanide poisoning.

    c. Abrupt withdrawal of this agent can result in an extreme hypertensive crisis.

    d. Too rapid administration of this product can result in a cerebrovascular accident.

9. Which of the following is a side effect associated with the use of enalapril?

    a. Hypokalemia (low potassium).

    b. Dry cough.

    c. Syncope.

    d. Chest pain.

10. What is/are the indications for Coreg®?

    a. Antihypertensive.

    b. Congestive Heart Failure.

    c. Antianginal agent (treatment of angina pectoris).

    d. a and b only.

    e. a, b, and c.

Check Your Answers on Next Page

SOLUTIONS TO EXERCISES, LESSON 7

COLUMN A	COLUMN B
1. ___g___ Lisinopril (para 7-10d).	a. Cardura®
___i___ Spironolactone and hydrochlorothiazide combination. (para 7-11a)	b. Catapres®
	c. Adalat CC®
___a___ Doxazosin (para 7-10b).	d. Inderal®
___f___ Diltiazem (para 7-10c).	e. Calan®
___h___ Metoprolol (para 7-9b).	f. Cardizem®
___d___ Propranolol (para 7-9a).	g. Zestril^v
___b___ Clonidine (para 7-8b).	h. Lopressor®
___e___ Verapamil (para 7-10c).	i. Aldactazide®
___c___ Nifedipine (para 7-10c).	

2.   a   A disorder of unknown origin characterized mainly by an elevated systolic or diastolic pressure associated with generalized arteriolar vasoconstriction. (para 7-3)

3.   a.   A type of essential hypertension characterized by documented pressure measurements greater than159 mm Hg (systolic) and/or greater than 99 mm Hg (diastolic). (para 7-4a)

4.   d   Marked elevated blood pressure with definite damage to the heart and/or kidneys. (para 7-4c)

5.   b   Treatment of a hypertensive crisis. (para 7-12b)

6.   d.   Mask symptoms of hypoglycemia. (para 7-9a)

7.   c   To arise slowly from a lying or sitting position because of the possibility of orthostatic hypotension. (para 7-10b)

8.   b   Overdosage of nitroprusside results in cyanide poisoning. (para 7-12b)

9.   b   Syncope. (para 7-10d)

10.   d   a and b only. (para 7-9c)

End of Lesson 7

LESSON ASSIGNMENT

LESSON 8   Diuretic and Antidiuretic Agents.

LESSON ASSIGNMENT   Paragraphs 8-1--8-7.

TASKS   081-824-0001, Perform Initial Screening of a
                        Prescription.

                        081-824-0026, Evaluate a Prescription.

                        081-824--0002/3, Fill a Prescription For a
                        Controlled/Non-Controlled Drug.

                        081-824-0027, Evaluate a Completed Prescription.

                        081-824-0028, Issue Outpatient Medications.

LESSON OBJECTIVES   After you finish this lesson you should be able to:

                        8-1.   Given a group of statements, select the
                        statement that best defines the term diuretic.

                        8-2.   Given a list of conditions, select the
                        condition(s) that are treated with diuretic therapy.

                        8-3.   Given the name of a type of diuretic and a
                        group of statements describing the mechanisms of
                        action of different types of diuretics, select the
                        mechanism of action for that type of diuretic.

                        8-4.   Given the trade and/or generic name of a
                        diuretic agent or antidiuretic agent and a list of
                        indications, uses, side effects, or precautionary
                        statements, select the indication(s), use(s), side
                        effect(s), or precautionary statements(s) for that
                        particular agent.

                        8-5.   Given a group of trade and/or generic names
                        of various diuretic or antidiuretic agents match each
                        trade or generic name with its corresponding trade or
                        generic name.

8-6.   Given the trade or generic name of a diuretic agent and a list of types of diuretic agents select the type of diuretic to which that agent belongs.

SUGGESTION

After completing the assignment, complete the exercises at the end of this lesson. These exercises will help you to achieve the lesson objectives.

LESSON 8

DIURETIC AND ANTIDIURETIC AGENTS

Section I. DIURETIC AGENTS

8-1. INTRODUCTION

In Lesson 3 of this subcourse, congestive heart failure was described as a condition characterized by sodium retention that results in expanded extracellular fluid volume or edema. This same process of increased tubular reabsorption of sodium-resulting in an accumulation of fluid--may accompany cirrhosis of the liver, renal disease, toxemia of pregnancy, the side effects of drugs, and other states of fluid retention. In all of these conditions, treatment of sodium retention is what is desired. REMEMBER: WHERE SODIUM GOES, WATER GOES! Therefore, the treatment as sodium retention by sodium excretion--not just the increase in urine volume--is the desired goal. Diuretic agents increase the amount of sodium excreted from the body.

8-2. DEFINTION OF DIURETIC

A diuretic is any agent that produces diuresis (an increase in the volume of urine output that results in the mobilization of edema fluid). You have heard the term edema before. Edema is the presence of abnormally large amounts of fluid in the body. Many diuretics reduce edema by increasing the amount of sodium removed from the body. Remember, where sodium goes, water goes. Thus, when sodium is removed from the body, there is a corresponding increase in the volume of urine produced.

8-3. USES OF DIURETICS

The general uses of diuretics include the treatment of congestive heart failure, hypertension, glaucoma, ascites, toxemia of pregnancy, and diabetes insipidus. Congestive heart failure has been discussed in Lesson 3 of this subcourse, hypertension has been discussed in Lesson 7 of this subcourse, and glaucoma has been discussed in MD0805, Pharmacology II. Review these materials if you have a need. The other conditions will be explained in this paragraph. Ascites is the accumulation of fluid in the abdominal cavity. Toxemia of pregnancy is a group of pathologic conditions--essentially metabolic disturbances--which sometimes occurs in pregnant women. Toxemia of pregnancy is manifested by preeclampsia (a toxemia of late pregnancy characterized by hypertension, albuminuria, and edema) and fully developed eclampsia (this condition includes convulsions and coma, which might occur in a pregnant woman or in a woman who has just delivered). Hypertension, edema, and/or proteinuria characterize eclampsia. Diabetes insipidus is a metabolic disorder caused by a lack of production of antidiuretic hormone (ADH), which is marked by great thirst and the passage of a large amount of dilute urine with no excess of sugar.

8-4. TYPES OF DIURETICS

There are several types of diuretics. The categories are defined based upon their mechanism of action.

a. **Osmotic Diuretics**. Osmostic diuretics produce a diuresis of water rather than a diuresis of sodium. The body does not metabolize osmotic diuretics. Instead, the drug molecules are not reabsorbed in the kidney tubules. This greatly affects the tonicity of every part of the kidney tubules through which the glomerular filtrates pass. By the process of osmosis, the drug molecules draw an increased amount of water from the interstitial fluid compartment. The result is that a great volume of urine is produced (water diuresis). It just so happens that sodium is contained in that urine and is subsequently removed from the body. Thus, the osmotic diuretics indirectly produce a removal of sodium from the body. Following is one example of an osmotic diuretic:

Mannitol. Mannitol is used to prevent acute renal (kidney) failure, evaluate kidney functioning, treat glaucoma (by the reduction of intraocular pressure), promote the urinary excretion of toxic substances (diuresis in certain drug intoxications) and reduce intracranial pressure (pressure in the head). The usual dosage of mannitol is from 50 to 200 grams in a 24-hour period by intravenous infusion. Side effects associated with the use of mannitol include pulmonary congestion, fluid and electrolyte imbalance, acidosis, electrolyte loss, and dryness of mouth and dehydration. Since mannitol may crystallize on exposure to low temperatures, you should observe mannitol vials and premixed bags for such crystals. When you observe these crystals, you should warm the vials or bags in a 500° C water bath in order to dissolve the crystals. The product should be cooled to body temperature before the mannitol solution is administered. Mannitol is available in a 5, 10, 15, 20, and 25 percent injection.

b. **Thiazide Diuretics**. Thiazide diuretics work by the inhibition of sodium reabsorption in the first portion of the distal tubule. The passive diffusion of the accompanying water and chloride is correspondingly reduced. Thus, the result is an increased excretion of sodium, water, and chloride from the body. When the thiazide acts on the proximal tubule, the carbonic anhydrase activity in the distal tubule is also decreased. This causes increased secretion of potassium. Consequently, the water lost contains sodium, potassium, and chloride. This loss of potassium can present problems to the patient.

(1) Hydrochlorothiazide (Hydrodiuril®). Hydrochlorothiazide is used in the treatment of essential hypertension and edema found in congestive heart failure. The usual dose of this drug is from 12.5 to 100 milligrams per day. Side effects commonly associated with hydrochlorothiazide include hypokalemia, hyperglycemia, and hyperuricemia. This drug should be used in caution in patients suffering from diabetes or gout and in patients who take digitalis.

(2) Chlorothiazide (Diuril®). This drug is used as a diuretic and as an antihypertensive. It is available in both parenteral and oral dosage forms. For side effects, refer to hydrochlorothiazide.

(3) Chlorthalidone (Hygroton®). Although chlorthalidone is not the same chemically as the thiazide diuretics, it has the same effects as these agents. For indications and side effects, you should refer to hydrochlorothiazide.

c. **Potassium-Sparing Diuretics**. This type of diuretic is used when there is a need to maintain normal levels of potassium in the patient along with the diuresis. The specific mechanisms of actions of selected drugs in this category.

(1) Spironolactone (Aldactone®). Spironolactone causes sodium diuresis and potassium retention by acting as an aldosterone competitive antagonist. That is, this drug acts on the distal tubule to block the sodium-potassium exchange mechanism. The net result is sodium loss and potassium retention. Consequently, by antagonizing aldosterone, sodium as well as water diuresis and potassium retention are affected. Spironolactone is used for primary hyperaldosteronism, edema associated with congestive heart failure, cirrhosis of the liver or ascites, essential hypertension, and in hypokalemia when other means are considered inappropriate or inadequate. The usual dose of this drug is from 25 to 400 milligrams per day depending upon the condition of the patient. Although spironolactone is a mild diuretic, it can hasten major side effects such as gastrointestinal symptoms (for example: cramping and diarrhea), lethargy, hyperkalemia, and hyponatremia. Hyperkalemia is a major side effect that occurs in patients who have impaired renal function. Hyperkalemia can cause irregularities that may be fatal. Spirolactone also causes estrogen-like side effects because of its hormone-like structure.

(2) Triamterene (Dyrenium®). While triamterene produces effects similar to those of spironolactone, the effects produced by triamterene are not dependent on the presence of aldosterone. This agent acts directly on the distal tubule where it prevents the passage of sodium across the membrane of the tubule. Thus, by blocking sodium reabsorption, potassium loss is reduced. Triamterene is used for edema associated with congestive heart failure and cirrhosis of the liver. The usual dosage of this drug is from 25 to 200 milligrams per day. The daily dose should not exceed 300 milligrams. Side effects associated with this agent include electrolyte imbalances, hyperkalemia, weakness, and dry mouth. Like spironolactone, hyperkalemia is a major side effect which can occur in patients who have impaired renal function or when the drug is administered alone.

d. Carbonic Anhydrase Inhibitor Diuretics. Carbonic anhydrase inhibitors produce diuresis by inhibiting carbonic anhydrase in the renal tubules. Carbonic anhydrase is an enzyme that catalyzes the following reaction:

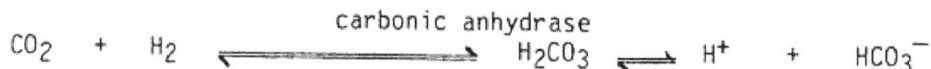

$$CO_2 \; + \; H_2 \; \underset{\xleftarrow{\hspace{2cm}}}{\overset{\text{carbonic anhydrase}}{\xrightarrow{\hspace{2cm}}}} \; H_2CO_3 \; \rightleftharpoons \; H^+ \; + \; HCO_3^-$$

From the reaction above, it can be deduced that removal of or blocking the enzyme carbonic anhydrase would result in a much slower reaction. Consequently, there would be a greatly reduced production of hydrogen ions and bicarbonate ions. This interferes with the ion exchange mechanism at the distal tubule, where the sodium ion that accompanies the bicarbonate ion is reabsorbed only by exchange for hydrogen or potassium ions secreted into the tubule. Normally the bicarbonate ion that accompanies the sodium ion (provided by the glomerular filtrate) is reabsorbed almost complete at the distal tubule. With reduced production of hydrogen ion due to inhibition of the carbonic anhydrase, the bicarbonate ion, together with the sodium ion will not be reabsorbed. Thus, the sodium will be excreted in an unusually large amount--with a corresponding loss of water (remember, where sodium goes, water goes).

Acetazolamide (Diamox®). Acetazolamide is one example of a carbonic anhydrase inhibitor. Although rarely used today, it may be used in the treatment of edema because of congestive heart failure; drug-induced edema; petit mal and unlocalized seizures; and open-angle and secondary glaucoma. The usual dosage of this drug ranges from 250 milligrams to 2 grams--depending on the type of condition being treated. Actually, the dosage recommendations for glaucoma and epilepsy differ considerably from those of congestive heart failure, since the first two conditions are not dependent on carbonic anhydrase inhibition in the kidney which requires intermittent dosage if it is to recover from the inhibitory effect of the therapeutic agent. The side effects of this agent include loss of appetite, transient myopia (nearsightedness), drowsiness, and acidosis. Acetazolamide is available in the injectable form.

e. **Inhibition of Sodium Transport in the Ascending Limb of the Loop of Henle, the Distal Tubule, and the Proximal Sites Diuretics**. Diuretics of this type are extremely potent and rapidly acting. In fact, they are used only after less potent--but safer--diuretics have failed. As the category type states, this type of diuretic acts by inhibiting sodium transport in the ascending limb of the loop of Henle, the distal tubule, and in the proximal sites. Thus, a greater fraction of filtered sodium can escape reabsorption. Thereby, increased sodium and water excretions occur. Diuretics of this type are called "loop diuretics".

(1) Furosemide (Lasix®). Furosemide is used in the treatment of edema associated with congestive heart failure, cirrhosis of the liver and renal disease, pulmonary edema, and hypertension. It is particularly useful when an agent with a greater diuretic potential than that of those commonly used is desired. This agent is also a rapidly acting diuretic. When administered orally it acts within one hour. When administered by injection it acts within 5-10 minutes. However, the agent does produce massive changes in electrolyte and water balance in the body. The usual dosage of furosemide is 20 to 80 milligrams given in a single dose--preferably in the morning. Depending on the patient's response, this dose can be repeated, maintained, or reduced. There are numerous adverse effects associated with the use of furosemide. These adverse effects include hypokalemia, hyponatremia, hyperglycemia, electrolyte depletion, and hypovolemia. Reservsible and irreversible hearing impairment and loss may occur with any of the loop diuretics. It is often associated with rapid infusion and

the use of extremely high doses. The injectable form of the drug must be stored at controlled room temperature and should not be used if the solution is yellow. The oral solution and tablet preparations should be dispensed in light--resistant containers.

(2)   Other loop diuretics include bumetanide (Bumex®), ethacrynic acid (Edecrin®), and torsemide (Demadex®).

f.   **Inhibition of Sodium and Chloride Reabsorption Diuretics**. The mechanism of action of this type is very similar to the thiazide diuretics. That is, drugs of this category inhibit sodium and chloride reabsorption that results in the increased excretion of sodium, chloride, and water.

Chlorthalidone (Hygroton®). This agent differs from the thiazide diuretics only in chemical structure. Chlorthalidone's pharmacological action is indistinguishable from the thiazide diuretics. Chlorthalidone is used in the management of hypertension--either as the sole therapeutic agent or to enhance the effect of other antihypertensive drugs in patients who have the more severe forms of hypertension. It is also used as adjunctive therapy in the treatment of edema associated with congestive heart failure, hepatic cirrhosis, and various forms of renal dysfunctions. Refer to the information on hydrochlorothiazide for side effect information.

g. **Combination Diuretics (Potassium-Sparing and Thiazide Diuretic Combination).** The potassium-sparing and thiazide diuretics have different but complementary mechanisms and sites of action. Therefore, when given together they produce additive diuretic and antihypertensive effects. The thiazide component blocks the reabsorption of sodium and chloride ions and thus increases the quantity of sodium traversing the distal tubule and the volume of water excreted in the urine. This characteristically induces potassium loss. The potassium-sparing component inhibits the reabsorption of sodium in exchange for potassium and hydrogen ions at the distal tubule, so that sodium excretion is greatly favored and the excess loss of potassium, as well as hydrogen and chloride ions induced by the thiazide, is reduced.

(1) Aldactazide® (combination of spironolactone and hydrochlorothiazide). This drug is used for the treatment of edema associated with congestive heart failure, cirrhosis of the liver and ascites and for essential hypertension.

(2) Dyazide® (combination of triamterene and hydrochlorothiazide). This agent is used in the treatment of edema associated with congestive heart failure, cirrhosis of the liver, and hypertension. The usual dosage of this product from 1 to 2 capsules taken twice daily after meals. The patient should take no more than four capsules per day. The side effects associated with this agent include hyperglycemia, hyperuricemia, and gastrointestinal disturbances. Each Dyazide® capsule contains 37.5 milligrams of triamterene and 25 milligrams of hydrochlorothiazide. There are other combinations of these diuretics available as generics or as Maxide® (75/50; 50/25). One must be very careful and doublecheck the active ingredients to ensure that the correct product is dispensed.

Section II. ANTIDIURETIC AGENTS

8-5. INTRODUCTION

The antidiuretic hormone has been discussed in Lesson 6 of this subcourse. As you will remember, it is a hormone secreted by the pituitary gland. The antidiuretic hormone (ADH) acts on the distal tubule and collecting ducts to increase water reabsorption (and thus to <u>decrease urine output</u>). The agents discussed below are those that work in a manner opposite the diuretics. This process is called <u>antidiuresis</u>. Antidiuresis is the suppression of urinary secretion. Consequently, an antidiuretic is an agent that suppresses urine formation as well as the rate of urine formation.

8-6. MECHANISM OF ACTION OF ANTIDIURETICS

Antidiuretics work by increasing the reabsorption of water at the distal tubule and collecting ducts without significantly modifying the rate of glomerular filtration.

8-7. EXAMPLES OF ANTIDIURETIC AGENTS

Two examples of antidiuretic agents are presented below.

a. **Vasopressin (Pitressin®).** This agent is used for the control or prevention of the symptoms and complications of diabetes insipidus. For vasopressin injection, the dose is 5 to 10 units (0.25 to 0.5 milliliters) by intramuscular or subcutaneous injection as required (usually every 2 to 3 hours as needed). The side effects associated with this product include abdominal cramps, fluid retention, and increased blood pressure. It is dispensed for hospital use only and should never be administered intravenously. This drug is available as a solution containing 20 pressor units per milliliter.

b. **Lypressin (Diapid®).** This agent is also used for the control or prevention of the symptoms and complications of diabetes insipidus. The usual dosage of this drug is 1 to 2 sprays applied to each nostril four times daily. The side effects associated with lypressin are abdominal cramps, nasal congestion, fluid retention, and increased bowel movements. Lypressin is useful in patients suffering from diabetes insipidus who have become unresponsive to other therapy or who experience allergic or other undesirable reactions to antidiuretic hormone of animal origin. The product has to be kept refrigerated. This product has an expiration date of 36 months. It is available as a nasal spray, 0.185 milligrams of lypressin per milliliter of solution (equivalent to 50 units per milliliter).

Continue with Exercises

EXERCISES, LESSON 8

REQUIREMENTS: The following exercises are to be answered by marking the lettered response that best answers the question; or by completing the incomplete statement; or by writing the answer in the space provided at the end of the question.

After you have completed all the exercises, turn to "Solutions to Exercises," at the end of the lesson, and check your answers with the solutions.

1. Which of these conditions is/are treated with diuretics?

    a. Asthma.

    b. Congestive heart failure.

    c. Diabetes mellitus.

    d. Gallstones.

2. Select the statement that best describes the mechanism of action for the thiazide diuretics.

    a. Thiazide diuretics cause sodium diuresis and potassium retention by acting as an aldosterone competitive antagonist.

    b. Thiazide diuretics produce a diuresis of water by drawing water from the cells in the body and thus by increasing the glomerular filtrate.

    c. Thiazide diuretics work by the inhibition of sodium reabsorption in the first portion of the distal tubule.

    d. Thiazide diuretics inhibit sodium transport--and thus sodium excretion--in the ascending limb of the Loop of Henle, the distal tubule, and in the proximal tubule.

3. Mannitol is used to _____.

    a. Prevent or treat acute liver failure.

    b. Treat dehydration and electrolyte imbalance.

    c. Promote the excretion of toxic substances in the urine.

    d. Treat epilepsy.

4. Hydrochiorothiazide is used to treat _____.

    a. Essential hypertension.

    b. Diabetes mellitus.

    c. Hyperglycemia.

    d. Cramping and diarrhea.

5. Vasopressin is used _____.

    a. For the control or prevention of the symptoms and complications of diabetes insipidus.

    b. To treat hypovolemia.

    c. To treat nasal congestion.

    d. To prevent hyperkalemia.

6. Which of the following is/are side effect(s) associated with Dyazide®?

    a. Hypouricemia.

    b. Hyperglycemia.

    c. Hypernatremia.

    d. Fluid retention.

7. Select the use(s) of Diamox®.

    a. The treatment of edema because of congestive heart failure.

    b. The treatment of drug-induced edema.

    c. The treatments of open--angle glaucoma and secondary edema.

    d. All the above.

8.   Match the drug name in <u>Column A</u> with its corresponding trade or generic name listed in <u>Column B.</u>

<u>Column A</u>

_____Aldactazide®.

_____Spironolactone.

_____Furosemide.

_____Diapid®

_____Diuril®.

_____Dyrenium®.

<u>Column B</u>

a. Chlorothiazide.

b. Aldactone.

c. Combination of spironolactone and hydrochlorothiazide.

d. Lypressin.

e. Lasix®.

f. Triamterene.

Check Your Answers on Next Page

SOLUTIONS TO EXERCISES, LESSON 8

1. b Congestive heart failure. (para 8-3)

2. c Thiazide diuretics work by the inhibition of sodium reabsorption in the first portion of the distal tubule. (para 8-4b)

3. c Promote the excretion of toxic substances in the urine. (para 8-4a)

4. a Essential hypertension. (para 8-4b(1))

5. a For the control or prevention of the symptoms and complications of diabetes insipidus. (para 8-7a)

6. b Hyperglycemia. (para 8-4g(2))

7. d All the above. (para 8-4d)

8.

Column A	Column B
c Aldactazide®. (para 8-4g(1))	a. Chlorothiazide.
b Spironolactone. (para 8-4c(1))	b. Aldactone.
e Furosemide. (para 8-4e(1))	c. Combination of spironolactone and hydrochlorothiazide.
d Diapid®. (para 8-7b)	d. Lypressin.
a Diuril®. (para 8-4b(2))	e. Lasix®.
f Dyrenium®. (para 8-4c(2))	f. Triamterene

End of Lesson 8

LESSON ASSIGNMENT

LESSON 9	Toxicology and Poison Control.
LESSON ASSIGNMENT	Paragraphs 9-1--9-13.
TASKS	081-824-0001, Perform Initial Screening of a Prescription.
	081-824-0026, Evaluate a Prescription.
	081-824-0002/3, Fill a Prescription For a Controlled/Non-Controlled Drug.
	081-824-0027, Evaluate a Completed Prescription.
	081-824-0028, Issue Outpatient Medications.
LESSON OBJECTIVES	After completing this lesson you will be able to:

9-1.   Given a list of numbers, select the number of deaths per year which are caused by accidental poisonings.

9-2.   Given a list of statements and one of the following terms: poison and toxicology, select the definition of the given term.

9-3.   Given a group of statements, select the purpose of the Poison Prevention Packaging Act of 1970.

9-4.   From a group of statements, select the requirement(s) of the Poison Prevention Packaging Act of 1970.

9-5.   Given a prescription and a list of types of prescription containers, select the type of container that should be used to contain the medication when it is dispensed to the patient.

9-6.   Given a group of statements, select the statement(s) that best explain(s) the exceptions to the Poison Prevention Packaging Act of 1970.

9-7.   Given a statement pertaining to the treatment of a poisoning victim, select the statement that best describes the best treatment.

9-8.   Given a situation involving an accidental poisoning and a list of references, select the reference that would provide the information required by the description of the situation.

SUGGESTION

After completing the assignment, complete the exercises at the end of this lesson. These exercises will help you to achieve the lesson objectives.

LESSON 9

TOXICOLOGY AND POISON CONTROL

Section I. INTRODUCTION

9-1. GENERAL

It is estimated that accidental poisonings result in about 4,000 deaths per year, while suicides by chemical agents result in about 6,000 deaths per year in the United States. Each year there are some 500,000 children involved in accidental poisonings. Approximately 90 percent of these poisonings occur in children who are too young to attend school. You have probably read and heard about many cases of accidental poisonings. As a pharmacy technician you may be asked to provide information to professional personnel or to the public in an emergency situation. It is therefore imperative that you be familiar with some general treatment procedures and information sources pertinent to poisoning. Just as important, you can provide guidance which can help persons avoid the tragedy associated with an accidental poisoning.

9-2. DEFINITIONS

a. **Poison**. A poison is any substance which when ingested, inhaled, absorbed, applied, injected, or even manufactured by the organism itself may cause damage to the structure of that organism or destruction to the normal functioning of that organism.

b. **Toxicology**. Toxicology is the scientific study of poisons--their actions, detection, and the treatment of the conditions they produce.

9-3. CAUSES OF POISONING

a. **Intentional**. Individuals for a variety of reasons can intentionally ingest poisons. Some of these reasons are:

    (1)   To commit suicide.

    (2)   To gain personal attention.

    (3)   To commit child abuse.

b. **Accidental**. Accidental poisonings usually affect children. In the years from 1972 through 1976, there were from one to two million cases of accidental poisoning per year in the United States. Since 1976, this number of accidental poisonings has dropped to approximately 500,000 cases per year. This decrease is attributed to the Poison Prevention Packaging Act and to poison prevention publicity. The most common sources of accidental poisoning were plants, various types of cleaners (soaps, detergents, and cleaners), vitamins and minerals, and aspirin. It is interesting to note that aspirin is no longer the most common cause of accidental poisoning (this is probably due to child resistant packaging).

Section II. THE PHARMACY AND POISON PREVENTION

9-4. THE POISON PREVENTION PACKAGING ACT OF 1970

The purpose of the Poison Prevention Packaging Act of 1970 is to reduce poisonings among small children. The Act provides that certain household products (such as aspirin and certain other drugs, including oral prescription drugs; furniture polish; oil of wintergreen, antifreeze; some cleaners for drains and ovens; turpentine; and cigarette lighter fluid), which are found to be hazardous or potentially hazardous must be sold in safety packaging. This safety packaging must be designed so that most children under five years of age cannot open the packages.

9-5. THE REQUIREMENTS OF THE POISON PREVENTION PACKAGING ACT OF 1970

a.   The Act requires the previously mentioned products to be packaged in containers which are sufficiently difficult to open in order to prevent 80 percent of children under five years of age from opening them. However, the containers must allow access to at least 90 percent of adults who will be able to open and properly close the packaging conveniently.

b.   The Act requires that the prescription filled in the pharmacy--with the exceptions noted in paragraph 9-6 below--be dispensed in child-resistant containers. The requirements below are especially important:

(1)   <u>Prescriptions which are not to be refilled.</u> For a prescription that is not to be refilled, the medication must be dispensed in either a glass or a plastic container with a child-resistant top.

(2)   <u>Prescriptions which are to be refilled.</u> For a prescription that is to be refilled, the medication must be dispensed in either a glass or a plastic container which has a child-resistant top. If the medication is dispensed in a glass container, a new child-resistant top <u>must</u> be placed on the container whenever the prescription is refilled. If the medication is dispensed in a plastic container, upon refilling, the medication must be placed in a new plastic container with a new child-resistant top. That means that a new label must be prepared for the refill when the medication is placed in a plastic container.

9-6. EXCEPTIONS TO THE ACT

Some patients (that is, those who have arthritis) may find child-resistant packaging too difficult to open. Furthermore, some patients (for example: those with certain types of heart conditions) may wish to obtain their medications from the container in a short period of time when they need them. For these types of patients, alternatives to child--resistant packaging are available.

a. **Nitroglycerin Must NOT be Dispensed in Child--Resistant Packaging.** This drug is for patients who have certain types of heart conditions. These patients must be able to obtain their nitroglycerin quickly in the event they need it.

b. **Alternative Packaging.** The manufacturer can market one size of a product in conventional (not child-resistant) packaging--if the same product is also available in child-resistant packaging. However, the conventional packaging must have a label which clearly states:

This packaging for household without young children or if the package is small:

Package not child-resistant

c. **Patient or Physician Request.** The patient or prescribing physician may request that prescription medicines be put into ordinary packaging without safety features. Although some pharmacists may ask for a written statement from a patient before providing a conventional closure, this is not a requirement of the Federal law.

9-7. CONSIDERATIONS FOR THE OUTPATIENT PHARMACY

Child--resistant packaging has been in use for quite some time. It has, without a doubt, decreased the number of cases of accidental poisonings. If you have purchased items or received prescriptions packaged in child-resistant containers, you are aware of the advantages and disadvantages of this means of preventing accidental poisonings. In your position in the pharmacy, you may hear comments about the packaging. Some patients are quick to complain about the packaging. Here are some considerations about the act that are pertinent to you:

a. You should be very familiar with your pharmacy's policies regarding child-resistant packaging. For example, if a patient requests conventional packaging for a prescription item, does your pharmacy require the patient to sign or initial the prescription or a special form? You should carefully read and study your local Standing Operating Procedures (SOP) to insure you do what is required.

b. Some patients may request conventional packaging. Suppose a retired individual asks you to package his prescription in a conventional container. Does this person have grandchildren who frequently come to the home? Remember, many poisonings occur when a small child visits grandparents and goes through the medicine cabinet or grandmother's purse.

c. Some pharmacies sponsor poison prevention campaigns. These campaigns focus on the basics of poison prevention. Frequently overlooked basics include keeping materials (cleaners, drugs, insecticides, and so forth) in their original containers and disposing of unused medications. Many persons repackage substances (like insecticides in soft drink bottles) only to tragically discover that a young child has ingested the poison thinking it was something else. Above all, these publicity campaigns seek to make people aware of dangerous practices which could result in tragedy.

Section III. THE TREATMENT OF POISONING

9-8. INTRODUCTION

Suppose a poisoning has occurred. What should be done to treat the patient? Because of your position in the pharmacy you probably will not be called upon to treat persons who are victims of intended or accidental poisoning. You should know the essentials of first aid and you should know to immediately take the victim to medical professionals who have been trained to treat poisoning victims. The information given below is not intended to serve as a strict procedure for the treatment of poisonings. Instead, it is intended to give general guidelines. Remember, the treatment given depends, to a great extent, on the poison ingested, absorbed, or inhaled.

9-9. TREATMENT GUIDELINES FOR POISONING VICTIMS

a. **Screen the Patient**. In the screening process it is important to identify the specific poison affecting the person and how the person was exposed to it. That is, if a child is suffering from poisoning from a particular insecticide (for example, malathion) was the insecticide swallowed or was it absorbed through the skin?

b. **Minimize Absorption**. There are two ways in which the amount of poison absorbed into the patient's system may be decreased.

(1) Remove the poison. The poison, if swallowed, can sometimes be removed by emesis (having the patient to vomit). Depending upon the type of poison ingested, the physician may or may not have the patient to vomit. Syrup of Ipecac and apomorphine are recognized as effective emetics. Emetic agents should not be administered to all patients. Specifically, emetic agents should not be administered to patients who are unconscious or convulsing, to persons who have ingested caustic or corrosive agents, or to patients who have ingested volatile petroleum products. One should not administer sodium bicarbonate ($NaHCO_3$) to a patient who has ingested a substance containing a corrosive agent such as hydrochloric acid (HCl), because the

two chemicals might react to form carbon dioxide gas ($HCl + NaHCO_3 \rightarrow NaCl + CO_2(\uparrow) + H_2O$) that could distend or even perforate the stomach.

     (2)   Administer gastric lavage.

     (3)   Administer cathartics.

    c. **Retard Absorption**. There are two methods by which the absorption of toxins can be retarded.

     (1)   Dilute the poison. Water, milk, flour or cornstarch suspension can be used to dilute (lower the concentration of) the poison. When the concentration of the poison is lowered, the amount of poison absorbed in a given period of time is usually lower.

     (2)   Administer activated charcoal. The activated charcoal adsorbs the poison and thereby reduces the amount of the poison which is available for adsorption. It should be noted that if both syrups of ipecac and activated charcoal are to be used, the activated charcoal must not be given until after the ipecac-induced emesis has occurred since the charcoal will render the ipecac ineffective.

    c. **Administer Systemic Antidotes (when possible)**. As you know, antidotes are substances which counteract the effects of other substances. Unfortunately, not every substance which is a toxin has an antidote which will serve to render its effects harmless. When the physician sees the poisoning victim, he must know what the identity of the ingested poison is before he considers giving an antidote. Furthermore, even after the identify of the poison is known, there must be an antidote in existence for that particular poison. Some examples of antidotes are naloxone (Narcan®), for narcotic poisonings--atropine, for the treatment of certain insecticide poisonings--BAL in Oil, for arsenic, gold, and mercury poisoning--Edetate Calcium Disodium, for lead poisoning-- and flumazenil (Romazicon®) for benzodiazepine overdose.

    d. **Speed the Elimination of the Poison**. As you might expect the effects of a toxin can be reduced in many instances if that substance is quickly eliminated from the body. Methods such as forced diuresis, through the administration of hypertonic solutions and through adjustment of urine pH; peritoneal dialysis, and hemodialysis (hematodialysis) can be used to speed the elimination of certain poisons from the body.

    e. **Support the Patient**. In all poisonings the patient must be supported. That is, the physician must carefully monitor the patient--through observation and by laboratory tests. When required, the physician may administer drugs for pain, replace fluids and electrolytes, regulate body temperature, maintain respiration, and maintain the nutrition of the patient.

Section IV. POISON CONTROL AND INFORMATION

9-10. INTRODUCTION

As with many types of emergencies, the poisoning emergency happens without notice. It is important that information sources pertaining to poisoning be maintained in the pharmacy and at certain other locations (that is, hospital emergency rooms and poison control centers). These sources of information must be up to date. Furthermore, the personnel who work in the area must be trained in the rapid use of these references.

9-11. POISON INFORMATION/CONTROL CENTERS

Poison control/information centers provide ready sources of information concerning poisons and chemical substances. These centers are usually staffed on a 24-hour basis. The Physicians' Desk Reference contains a section entitled "Directory of Poison Control Centers" which states the location and telephone number of poison control centers located in the United States. Regardless of the size of the medical treatment facility or the pharmacy, the number of the closest Poison Control Center should be posted on the wall or telephone where everyone can see the number.

9-12. SUGGESTED REFERENCES TO BE MAINTAINED IN THE PHARMACY IN RELATION TO POISONING INFORMATION

Lesson 1 of MD0804, Pharmacology I, discussed journals and texts pertinent to the practice of pharmacy. In addition to the references listed in that lesson, the pharmacy should maintain, at a minimum, the following references.

a. **Physician's Desk Reference.** This reference contains product information (that is, the ingredients in a particular product). It is indexed so that the information can be found if the manufacturer, trade name, or chemical composition of the product is known. The Product Identification Section of the Physicians' Desk Reference is very helpful in that if a tablet or capsule of the medication is on hand, this section can be used to rapidly identify it in most instances. Also helpful is the "Guide to Management of Drug Overdose" found on the back inside cover.

b. **American Drug Index.** In this text the trade and generic names of the medications are cross-indexed. No specific information on toxicity's is included in this text.

c. **Merck Index.** In this text the trade and generic names of the products are cross--indexed. Foreign as well as American products are included in this text.

d. **Handbook of Poisoning.** This text is organized according to the type of setting in which poisoning might occur (that is, agricultural, industrial, household, plant, insect, and so forth.). The text also presents an excellent discussion of such pertinent topics as poison prevention, emergency treatment, and poisoning diagnosis.

e. **Handbook of Nonprescription Drugs**. This reference identifies the ingredients of over-the-counter products.

f. **Clinical Toxicology of Commercial Products**. This comprehensive text contains information on over 17,000 products and ingredients. It discusses the signs, symptoms, and treatment of various types of poisonings. One caution: It is rather a complex book to use. Therefore, you should acquaint yourself with this text before you have to use it in an emergency situation.

g. **Poisindex**®. Poisindex®, as part of the subscription to Micromedex is available as a quick, thorough reference. Most drug information centers and emergency departments will have Poisindex® set up as an icon on their desktop computers for quick reference.

9-13. CONCLUDING COMMENTS

The references just described contain essential information on topics related to poisoning. The quick use of these references to learn of poisoning signs, symptoms, and treatment have saved many a patient's life. Just think, <u>many accidental poisonings can be prevented.</u> The best therapy is that of prevention. You are in a unique position to help the patient realize that they should safeguard their medications in order to prevent any type of accidental poisoning. It is much easier to prevent most poisonings than it is to treat those poisonings. Some pharmacies emphasize poisoning prevention through such programs as the collection of unused medication. You can have your own poisoning prevention program in your own home.

Continue with Exercises

EXERCISES, LESSON 9

REQUIREMENT. The following exercises are to be answered by marking the lettered response that best answers the question; or by completing the incomplete statement; or by writing the answer in the space provided at the end of the question.

After you have completed all the exercises, turn to "Solutions to Exercises," at the end of the lesson, and check your answers with the solutions.

1.   Select the number of deaths per year caused by accidental poisonings.

    a.   2,000.

    b.   4,000.

    c.   6,000.

    d.   500,000.

2.   The term poison is best defined as _____.

    a.   A chemical which will cause death if it is ingested.

    b.   Any substance which will cause destruction of living cells.

    c.   Any substance which when ingested, inhaled, absorbed, applied, injected, or even manufactured by the organism itself will cause damage to the organism or will interfere with its normal functioning.

    d.   Any substance or chemical which when ingested, inhaled, or in any other way taken into the body, will cause death to the cells of the organism.

3.   What is the purpose of the Poison Prevention Packaging Act of 1970?

    a.   To reduce poisonings among small children.

    b.   To reduce the number of intentional poisonings among children and adults.

    c.   To reduce the number of accidental deaths caused by aspirin.

    d.   To require packaging which could be opened only by children over the age of 13.

4.   You are to fill the prescription below. Select the type of container which must be used to dispense the drug to the patient.

```
                  DD , FORM , 1289
                       NOV 71
                  DOD PRESCRIPTION
───────────────────────────────────────────────
FOR (Full name, address & phone number.) (If under 12 years, give age.)

    William Paxton      11 years old
    614 Arbor Lane      Dep/LTC Paxton
    San Antonio, TX
───────────────────────────────────────────────
MEDICAL FACILITY              DATE
   Alamo Army Hosp            12 Feb 83
───────────────────────────────────────────────
Rx                                    Gm. or ml.

      Methylphenidate HCl        5mg
           #20

   Sig: ī tab before breakfast
         and lunch


   No Refills      FOR INSTRUCTIONAL USE ONLY
───────────────────────────────────────────────
MFGR:                  EXP DATE:
LOT NO:                FILLED BY:
                         James Anderson M.D. USAF
                         Col, MC    246-90-1011
   Rx NUMBER           SIGNATURE, RANK AND DEGREE
        EDITION OF 1 JAN 60 MAY BE USED.
```

a.   A glass container without a child-resistant top.

b.   A plastic container without a child-resistant top.

c.   A plastic or glass container without a child-resistant top.

d.   A glass or plastic container with a child-resistant top.

5.   Which of the following statements best explains an exception to the Poison Prevention Packaging Act of 1970?

   a.   Aspirin (ASA) must not be dispensed in child-resistant packaging for the convenience of those patients who have arthritis.

   b.   Nitroglycerin must not be dispensed in child-resistant packaging.

   c.   Federal law requires that patients who desire their medications be dispensed in conventional packaging must sign a disclaimer statement on the back of the prescription form.

   d.   Only persons who suffer from heart disease or arthritis may request their medications be dispensed in conventional packaging.

6.   You suspect that your two-year-old child has just ingested some poisonous substance. Select the first thing you should do.

   a.   Make the child ingest some syrup of ipecac.

   b.   Identify the substance to which the child was exposed and how he was exposed to it.

   c.   Make the child drink a 5 percent solution of sodium bicarbonate (NaHCO3).

   d.   Administer a hypertonic solution intravenously to the child.

7.   The Chief, Pharmacy Service, has asked you to prepare a brief report on poison prevention. Which of the following references would you use to prepare the report?

   a.   Handbook of Nonprescription Drugs.

   b.   Physicians' Desk Reference.

   c.   Merck Index.

   d.   Handbook of Poisoning.

8.   You are asked to find some information on an insecticide not used in the United States. Which of the references below would you use to locate some information on this product?

        a.   Clinical Toxicology of Commercial Products.

        b.   Handbook of Nonprescription Drugs.

        c.   Handbook of Poisoning.

        d.   Merck Index.

Check Your Answers on Next Page

SOLUTIONS TO EXERCISES, LESSON 9

1. b 4,000. (para 9-1)

2. c Any substance which when ingested, inhaled, absorbed, applied, injected, or even manufactured by the organism itself will cause damage to the organism or will interfere with its normal functioning. (para 9-2b)

3. a To reduce poisonings among small children. (para 9-4)

4. d A glass or plastic container with a child-resistant top. (para 9-5b(1))

5. b Nitroglycerin must not be dispensed in child-resistant packaging. (para 9-6a)

6. b Identify the substance to which the child was exposed and how he was exposed to it. (para 9-9a)

7. d Handbook of Poisoning. (para 9-12d)

8. d Merck Index. (para 9-12c)

End of Lesson 9

ANNEX

DRUG PRONUNCIATION GUIDE

This Drug Pronunciation Guide was developed to help you to learn how the trade and generic names of commonly prescribed medications are frequently pronounced. Not all the drugs in the guide are discussed in this subcourse. Remember, it is not enough to be able to know the uses, indications, cautions and warnings, and contraindications for a drug--you must also know how to pronounce that drug's name.

Trade Name	*Generic Name*
Actifed (Ak'-ti-fed)	Triprolidine (Tri-pro'-li-deen) and Pseudoephedrine (Soo-do-e-fed'-rin)
Adapin (Ad'-a-pin)	Doxepin (Dok'-se-pin)
Sinequan (Sin'-a-kwan)	" "
Afrin (Af'-rin)	Oxymetazoline (Ok-see-met-az'-o-leen)
Aldactazide (Al-dak'-ta-zide)	Spironolactone (Spi-ro-no-lak'-tone) and Hydrochlorothiazide (Hy-dro-klor-thi'-a-zide)
Aldactone (Al-dak'-tone)	Spironolactone (Spi-ro-no-lak'-tone)
Aldomet (Al'-do-met)	Methyldopa (Meth-il-do'-pah)
Alupent (Al'-u-pent)	Metaproterenol (Met-a-pro-ter'-eh-nol)
Amoxil (Am-ok'-sil)	Amoxicillin (Ah-moks'-i-sil-in)
Amphojel (Am'-fo-jel)	Aluminum (Al-loo'-mi-num) Hydroxide (Hy-drok'-side)
Ampicillin (Amp'-I-sil-in)	Same
Antepar (Ab'-te-par)	Piperazine (Pi-per'-ah-zeen)
Anturane (An'-tu-rain)	Sulfinpyrazone (Sul-fin-pie'-ra-zone)
Anusol (An'-u-sol)	Pramoxine (Pram-ok'-seen)
Apresoline (A-press'-o-leen)	Hydralazine (Hy-dral'-ah-zeen)
Aralen (Ar'-a-len)	Chloroquine (Klor'-o-kwin)
Aristocort (A-ris'-to-cort)	Triamcinolone (Tri-am-sin'-o-lone)
Artane (Ar'-tane)	Trihexyphenidyl(Tri-hek-see-fen'-i-dil)
A.S.A.	Aspirin (As'-per-in)
Atromid S (A'-tro-mid)	Clofibrate (Klo-fi'-brate)
Avlosulfon (Av-lo-sul'-fon)	Dapsone (Dap'-sone)
Azolid (Az'-o-lid)	Phenylbutazone (Fen-il-bute'-a-zone)
Bactrim (Bak'-trim)	Sulfamethoxazole (Sul-fah-meth-oks'-ah-zole) and Trimethoprim (Tri-meth'-o-prim)
Bellergal (Bel'-er-gal)	Ergotamine (Er-got'-a-meen), Phenobarbital (Feen-o-bar'-bi-tal) and Belladonna (Bel-la-don'-na) Alkaloids
Benadryl (Ben'-a-dril)	Diphenhydramine (Di-fen-hy'-dra-meen)

Trade Name	Generic Name
Bendectin (Ben-dek'-tin)	Doxylamine (Dok-sil'-a-meen)
Benemid (Ben'-eh-mid)	Probenecid (Pro-ben'-eh-sid)
Bonine (Bo'-neen)	Meclizine (Mek'-li-zeen)
Cafergot (Kaf'-er-got)	Ergotamine (Er-got'-a-meen) and Caffeine (Kaf'-feen)
Calamine (Kal'-a-mine)	Same
Catapres (Kat'-a-press)	Clonidine (Klo'-ni-deen)
CeeNu (See'-new)	Lomustine (Lo-mus'-teen)
Chlor-Trimeton (Klo-tri '-meh-ton)	Chlorpheniramine (Klor-fen-it'-a-meen)
Clomid (Klo'-mid)	Clomiphene (Klo'-mi-feen)
Clonopin (Klo-o-pin)	Clonazepam (Klo-na'-ze-pam)
Codeine (Ko'-deen)	Same
Cogentin (Ko-jen'-tin)	Benztropine (Benz'-tro-peen)
Colace (Ko'-lace)	Dioctyl(Di-ok'-til) Sodium (So'-dee-um) Sulfosuccinate (Sul-fo-suk'-si-nate)
Colchicine (Kol'-chi-seen)	Same
Compazine (Kom'-pa-zeen)	Prochlorperazine (Pro-klor-per'-a-zeen)
Cordran (Kor'-dran)	Flurandrenolide (Floor-an-dren'-o-lide)
Coumadin (Koo'-mah-din)	Warfarin (War'-fah-rin)
CP	Cloroquine (Klor'-o-kwin) and Primaquine (Prim'-a-kwin)
Cyclogyl (Si'-klo-jel)	Cyclopentolate (Si-klo-pen'-to-late)
Cytomel (Si'-to-mel)	Liothyronine (Li-o-thy-ro-neen)
Cytoxan (Si-tok'-san)	Cyclophosphamide (Si-klo-fos'-fa-mide)
Dalmane (Dal '-mane)	Flurazepam (Floor-az'-e-pam)
Darvocet (Dar'-vo-set)	Propoxyphene (Pro-pok'-se-feen) and Acetaminopen (As-et-am'-ino-fen)
Darvon (Dar'-von)	Propoxyphene (Pro-pok-se-feen)
Decadron (Dek'-a-dron)	Dexamethasone (Dek-sa-meth'-ah-sone)
Deltasone (Del '-ta-sone)	Prednisone (Pred'-ni-sone)
Demerol (Dem'-er-ol)	Meperidine (Meh-pair'-i-deen)
Dexedrine (Deks '-eh-dreen)	Dextroamphetamine (Deks-tro-am-fet'-a-meen)
Diabinese (Di-ab'-i-nees)	Chlorpropamide (Klor-prop'-a-mide)
Diethylstilbestrol (Di-eth-il-stil-bes'-trol)	Same
Dilantin (Di-lan'-tin)	Phenytoin (Fen'-i-toin)
Dilaudid (Di-law'-did)	Hydromorphone (Hy-dro-more' -fon)
Dimetane (Di'-meh-tane)	Brompheniramine (Brom-fen-ir'-a-meen)

Trade Name	Generic Name
Dimetapp (Di'-meh-tap)	Brompheniramine (Brom-fen-ir'-a-meen) Phenylephrine (Fen-il-ef'-rin) and Phenylpropanolamine (Fen-il-pro-pan-ol'-a-meen)
Disophrol (Dice'-o-frol)	Dexbrompheniramine (Deks-brom-fen-ir'-a-meen) and Pseudoephedrine (Soo-do-e-fed'-rin)
Dolophine (Dol'-o-feen)	Methadone (Meth'-a-done)
Domeboro (Dome-bor'-o)	Aluminum (Ah-loo'-mi-num) Acetate (As'-e-tate)
Donnatal (Don'-na-tal)	Belladonna (Bel-la-don'-na) Alkaloids (Al'-ka-loids) and Phenobarbital (Feen-o-barb'-i-tal)
Doxidan (Dok'-si-dan)	Danthron (Dan'-thron) and Dicctyl (Di-ok'-til) Calcium (Kal'-see-um) Sulfosuccinate (Sul-fo-suk'-si-nate)
Drixoral (Driks'-or-al)	Dexbrompheniramine (Deks-brom-fen-ir'-a-meen) and Pseudoephedrine (Soo-do-e-fed'-rin)
Dulcolax (Dul'-ko-laks)	Bisacodyl (Bis-a'-ko-dil)
Dyazine (Di'-a-zide)	Triamterene (Tri-am'-ter-een) and Hydrochlorothiazide (Hy-dro-klor-o-thi'-a-zide)
Dymelor (Die'-meh-lor)	Acetohexamide (As-e-to-heks'-a-mide)
Dyrenium (Die-ren'-i-um)	Triamterene (Tri-am'-ter-een)
Efudex (Ef'-u-deks)	Fluorouracil (Floo-ro-ur'-ah-sil)
Elavil (El'-ah-vil)	Amitriptyline (Am-i-trip'-til-een)
Elixir Terpin (Ter'-pin) Hydrate	Same
Empirin (Em'-per-in)	Codeine (Ko'-deen) and Aspirin (As'-per-in)
E-Mycin (E-mie'-sin)	Erythromycin (E-rith-ro-mie'-sin)
Equanil (Ek'-wa-nil)	Meprobamate (Me-pro-bam'-ate)
Ergomar (Er'-go-mar)	Ergotamine (Er-got'-a-meen)
Ergotrate (Er'-go-trate)	Ergonovine (Er-go-no'-veen)
Erythrocin (Er-eeth'-ro-sin)	Erythromycin (Er-eeth-ro-my'-sin) Stearate (Stare'-rate)
Esidrix (Es'-i-driks)	Hyrochlorothiazide (Hy-dro-klor-o-thi'-a-zide)
Feosol (Fe'-o-sol)	Ferrous (Fer'-rus) Sulfate (Sul'-fate)
Fergon (Fer'-gon)	Ferrous (Fer'-rus) Gluconate (Glu'-con-ate)

Trade Name	Generic Name
Fiorinal (Fee-or'-i-nal)	Butalbi tal (Bu-tal'-bi-tal), Apririn, Phenacetin (Fen-ass'-eh-tin), and Caffeine (Kaf'-feen)
Flagyl (Fla'-jil)	Metronidazole (Me-tro-ni'-dah-zole)
Flexeril (Flek'-sa-ril)	Cyclobenzaprine (Si-klo-benz'-a-preen)
Fulvicin (Ful'-vi-sin)	Griseofulvin (Griz-e-o-ful'-vin)
Guantanol (Gan'-ta-nol)	Suiphamethoxazole (Sul-fah-meth-oks'-ah-zole)
Gantrisin (Gan'-tri-sin)	Sulfisoxazole (Sul-fi-sok'-sah-zole)
Gelusil (Jel'-u-sil)	Aluminum (Ah-loo'-mi-num) Hydroxide (Hy-drok'-side) and Magnesium (Mag-nee'-zee-um) Hydroxide
Grifulvin (Gri-ful'-vin)	Griseofulvin (Griz-e-o-ful'-vin)
Gynergen (Jin'-er-jen)	Ergotamine (Er-got'-a-meen)
Haldol (Hal'-dol)	Haloperidol (Hal-o-pair'-i-dol)
Halotestin (Hal-o-tes'-tin)	Fluoxymesterone (Floo-ok-see-mes-teh-rone)
Hexadrol (Hek'-sa-drol)	Dexamethasone (Dek-sa-meth'-a-sone)
Hydrodiuril (Hy-dro-di'-ur-il)	Hydroclorothiazide (Hy-dro-kior-thi'-a-zide)
Hygroton (Hy-grow'-ton)	Chiorthalidone (Kior-thal'-i-done)
Ilosone (I'-low-sone)	Erythromycin (Er-ith-ro-mi'-sin) Estolate (Es'-to-late)
Inderal (In'-der-al)	Propranolol (Pro-pran'-o-lol)
Indocin (In'-do-sin)	Indomethacin (In-do-meth'-a-sin)
INH	Isoniazid (I-so-ni'-a-zid)
Insulin (In'-sul-in)	Same
Intal	Cromolyn (Kro'-mo-lin)
Ismelin (Is'-meh-lin)	Guanethidine (Gwan-eth'-i-dine)
Isopto-Atropine (I-sop-to-at'-ro-peen)	Atropine (At'-ro-peen)
Isopto-Carpine (I-sop-to-car'-peen)	Pilocarpine (Pile-o-car'-peen)
Isordil (I'-sor-dil)	Isosorbide (I-so-sor'-bide)
Keflex (Kef'-lex)	Cephalexin (Sef-ah-lek'-sin)
Lanoxin (Lan-ok'-sin)	Digoxin (Di-jok'-sin)
Larodopa (Lar-o-do'-pa)	Levodopa (Le-o-do'-pa)
Larotid (Lar'-o-tid)	Amoxicillin (Ah-moks'-i-sil-in)
Lasix (La'-siks)	Furosemide (Fu-ro'-se-mide)
Leukeran (Lu'-ker-an)	Chlorambucil (Klor-ram'-bu-sil)
Librium (Lib'-ree-um)	Chlordiazepoxide (Klor-die-az-eh-pok'-side)

Trade Name	Generic Name
Lidex (Lie'-deks)	Fluocinoide (Floo-o-sin'-o-nide)
Lomotil (Lo'-mo-til)	Diphenoxylate (Die-fen-ok'-si-late)
Lopressor (Lo'-pres-sor)	Metoprolol (Met-o-pro'-lol)
Lotrimin (Lo'-tri-min)	Chlotrimazole (Klo-trim'-ah-zole)
Maalox (May'-loks)	Aluminum (Ah-loo'-mi-num) and Magnesium (Mag-nee'-zee-um) Hydroxides
Macrodanton (Ma-kro-dan'-tin)	Nitrofurantoin (Ni-tro-fur-an'-toin)
Mandelamine (Man-del'-a-meen)	Methenamine (Meth-en'-a-meen) Mandelate (Man'-deh-late)
Medihaler-Iso (Med-i-hail-er-I'-so)	Isoproterenol (I-so-pro-ter'-en-ol)
Mellaril (Mel'-la-ril)	Thioridazine (Thi-o-rid'-a-zeen)
Metamucil (Met-a-mu'-sil)	Psyllium (Sil'-e-um)
Metaprel (Meh'-ta-prel)	Metaproterenol (Meh'-ta-pro-ter'-eh-nol)
Methotrexate (Meth-o-treks'-ate)	Amethopterin (Ah-meth-op'-ter-in)
Milk of Magnesia	Same
Minipress (Min'-i-press)	Prazosin (Pra'-zo-sin)
Minocin (Min'-o-sin)	Minocycline (Mi-no-si'-kleen)
Monistat (Mon'-i-stat)	Miconazole (Mi-kon'-ah-zole)
Motrin (Mo'-trin)	Ibuprofen (I-bu'-pro-fen)
Myambutol (My-am'-bu-tol)	Ethambutol (Eth-am'-bu-tol)
Mycostatin (My-co-stat'-in)	Nystatin (Ny-stat'-in)
Mylanta (My-lan'-ta)	Aluminum (Ah-loo'-mi-num) and Magnesium (Mag-nee'-zee-um) Hydroxides and Simethicone (Si-meth'-i-kone)
Myleran (My-ler-an)	Busulfan (Bu-sul'-fan)
Mylicon (My'-li-kon)	Simethicone (Si-meth'-i-kone)
Mysoline (My'-so-leen)	Primidone (Pri'-mi-done)
Nalfon (Nal'-fon)	Fenoprofen (Fen-o-pro'-fen)
Naprosyn (Na'-pro-sin)	Naproxen (Na-prok'-sen)
Nembutal (Nem'-bu-tal)	Pentobarbital (Pen-to-barb'-i-tal)
Neosynephrine (Nee-o-sin-eh'-frin)	Phenylephrine (Fen-il-eh'-frin)
Nitrobid (Ni'-tro-bid)	Nitroglycerin (Ni-tro-gli'-ser-in)
Nitrol (Ni'-trol)	" "
Nitrostat (Ni-tro-stat)	" "
Noctec (Nok'-tek)	Chloral Hydrate (Klor'-al- Hy'-drate)
Norfiex (Nor'-fleks)	Orphenadrine Citrate (Or-fen'-a-dreen)
Norpace (Nor'-pace)	Disopyramide (Di-so-peer'-a-mide)

Trade Name	Generic Name
Novahistine (No-va-his'-teen) Expectorant	Guaifenesin (Gwi-fen'-eh-sin), Phenylpropanolamine (Fen-il-pro-pan-ol'-a-meen), and Codeine (Ko'-deen)
NTG	Nitroclycerin (Ni-tro-gli'-ser-in)
Nupercainal (New-per-kain'-al)	Dibucaine (Die'-bu-kain)
Oretic (O-ret'-ik)	Hydrochiorothiazide (Hy-dro-kior-thi'-a-zide)
Orinase (Or'-in-ase)	Tolbutamide (Tol-bu'-tah-mide)
Ornade (Or'-nade)	Chlorpheniramine (Klor-fen-ir'-a-meen), Triprolidine (Tri-pro-li-deen) and Pseudoephedrine (Su-do-eh-fed'-rin)
Parafon Forte (Pair'-a-fon For'-tay)	Chlorzoxazone (Klor-zok'-sa-zone)
Percodan (Per'-ko-dan)	Oxycodone (Ok-si-ko'-done)
Periactin (Per-ee-ak'-tin)	Cyproheptadine (Si-pro-hep'-tah-deen)
Persantine (Per-san'-teen)	Dipyridamole (Di-pi-rid'-ah-mole)
Phenobarbital (Feen-o-barb'-it-al)	Same
Phenylpropanolamine (Fen-il-pro-pan-ol'-a-meen)	Same
Pitocin (Pi-tow'-sin)	Oxytocin (Ok-see-tow'-sin)
Pontocaine (Pon'-to-kain)	Tetracaine (Teh'-tra-kain)
Povan (Po'-van)	Pyrvinium (Pire-vin'-ee-um)
Premarin (Prem'-ar-in)	Conjugated (Kon'-joo-gay-ted) Estrogens (Es-tro-jens)
Presamine (Press'-a-meen)	Imipramine (Im-ip'-rah-meen)
Primaquine (Pri'-mah-kwin)	Same
Probanthine (Pro-ban'-theen)	Propantheline (Pro-pan'-the-leen)
Pronestyl (Pro-nes'-til)	Procainamide (Pro-kain'-a-mide)
Prophylthiouracil (Pro-pil-thi-o-u'-rah-sil)	Same
Prostaphlin (Pro-staff'-lin)	Oxacillin (Oks'-ah-sil-in)
Provera (Pro-ver'-ah)	Medroxyprogesterone (Med-rok-see-pro-jes'-ter-one)
Pyridium (Pie-rid'-ee-um)	Phenazopyridine (Fen-ahs-o-per'-i-deen)
Quinidine (Kwin'-i-deen)	Same
Quinine (Kwie'-nine)	Same
Reserpine (Ree-ser'-peen)	Same
Retin A (Reh'-tin A)	Tretinoin (Tret'-i-noin)
Rifadin (Rie-fad'-in)	Rifampin (Rie-fam'-pin)
Riopan (Rie'-o-pan)	Magaidrate (Mag'-al-drate)

Trade Name	Generic Name
Rimactane (Rim-act'-ane)	Rifampin (Rie-fam'-pin)
Ritalin (Rit'-a-lin)	Methylphenidate (Meth-il-fen'-i-date)
Robaxin (Ro-bak'-sin)	Methocarbamol (Meth-o-kar'-ba-mol)
Robitussin (Row-i-tus'-sin)	Guaifenesin (Gwie-fen'-eh-sin)
Robitussin DM	Guiafenesin and Dextromethorphan (Dek-tro-meh-or'-fan)
Sansert (San'-sert)	Methysergide (Meth-ee-ser'-jide)
Seconal (Sek'-o-nal)	Secobarbital (Sek-o-bar'-bi-tal)
Selsun (Sel'-sun)	Selenium (Se-leh'-nee-um)
Septra (Sep'-tra)	Sulfamethoxazole (Sul-fah-meth-oks'-a-zole) and Trimethroprim (Tri-meth'-o-prim)
Serax (See'-raks)	Oxazepam (Oks-az'-eh-pam)
Silvadene (Sil'-va-deen)	Silver Sulfadiazine (Sul-fa-die'-a-zeen)
Sinemet (Si'-ne-met)	Levodopa (Le-vo-do'-pa)
Sinequan (Sin'-a-kwan)	Doxepin (Dok'-seh-pin)
Sorbitrate (Sor'-bi-trate)	Isosorbide (I-so-sor'-bide)
Stelazine (Stel'-a-zeen)	Trifluoperazine(Tri-floo-o-per'-a-zeen)
Sudafed (Soo'-da-fed)	Pseudophedrine (Soo-do-eh-feh'-drin)
Sulamyd (Sul'-a-mid)	Sulfacetamide (Sul-fah-set'-a-mide)
Sulfamylon (Sul-fa-mie'-lon)	Mafenide (Maf'-eh-nide)
Sultrin (Sul'-trin)	Sulfathiazole (Sul-fah-thi'-ah-zole) Sulfacetamide (Sul-fah-set'-ah-mide) and Sulfabenzamide (Sul-fah-benz'-ah-mide)
Surfak (Sur'-fak)	Dioctyl (Di-ok'-til) Calcium (Kal'-see-um) Sulfosuccinate (Sul-fo-suk'-si-nate)
Synalar (Sine'-a-lar)	Fluocinolone (Floo-o-sin'-o-lone)
Synthroid (Sin'-throid)	Levothyroxine (Lee-vo-thi-rok'-sin)
Tace (Tace)	Chlorotrianisene (Klor-o-tri-an'-I-seen)
Tagamet (Tag'-a-met)	Cimetidine (Si-met'-i-deen)
Talwin (Tal'-win)	Pentazocine (Pen-taz'-o-seen)
Tandearil (Tan'-da-ril)	Oxyphenbutazone (Ok-see-fen-bute'-a-zone)
Tegretol (Teg'-reh-tol)	Carbamazepine (Kar-ba-maz'-eh-peen)
Tessalon (Tess'-a-lon)	Benzonatate (Benz-on'-a-tate)
Tetracycline (Tet-ra-si'-kleen)	
Thorazine (Thor'-a-zeen)	Chlorpromazine (Klor-pro'-ma-zeen)
Thyroid (Thy'-roid)	Same
Tigan (Tie'-gan)	Trimethobenzamide (Tri-meth-o-benz'-a-mide)
Timoptic (Tim-op'-tic)	Timilol (Tim'-o-lol)

Trade Name	Generic Name
Tinactin (Tin-act'-in)	Tolnaftate (Tol-naf'-tate)
Titralac (Ti'-tra-lak)	Calcium (Kal-see-um) Carbonate (Kar'-bon-ate) and Glycine (Gly'-seen)
Tofranil (Toe'-fra-nil)	Imipramine (I-mip'-rah-meen)
Tolectin (Tow-lek'-tin)	Tolmetin (Tol-met'-in)
Triavil (Tri'-a-vil)	Perphenazine (Per-fen'-a-zeen) and Amitriptlyline (Am-i-trip'-ti-leen)
Trilafon (Try'-la-fon)	Perphenazine (Per-fen-a-zeen)
Tylenol (Tie'-leh-nol)	Acetaminophen (As-et-am'-ino-fen)
Tylenol #3	Acetaminophen and Codeine (Ko'-deen)
Unipen (U'-ni-pen)	Nafcillin (Naf-sil-lin)
Urecholine (Ur-eh-ko'-leen)	Bethanecol (Beth-an'-eh-kol)
Valisone (Val'-i-sone)	Betamethasone (Beh-tah-meth'-a-sone)
Valium (Val'-ee-um)	Diazepam (Die-aze-eh-pam)
Vermox (Ver'-moks)	Mebendazole (Meh-ben'-dah-zole)
Vibramycin (Vie-bra-my'-sin)	Doxycycline (Doks-see-si'-kleen)
Xylocaine (Zie'-low-kain)	Lidocaine (Lie-do-kain)
Zarontin (Zar-on'-tin)	Ethosuximide (Eh-tho-suks'-a-mide)
Zyloprim (Zie'-low-prim)	Allopurinol (Al-lo-pure'-in-ol)

COMMENT SHEET

SUBCOURSE MD0806 Pharmacology III   **EDITION 100**

Your comments about this subcourse are valuable and aid the writers in refining the subcourse and making it more usable. Please enter your comments in the space provided. ENCLOSE THIS FORM (OR A COPY) WITH YOUR ANSWER SHEET **ONLY** IF YOU HAVE COMMENTS ABOUT THIS SUBCOURSE..

FOR A WRITTEN REPLY, WRITE A SEPARATE LETTER AND INCLUDE SOCIAL SECURITY NUMBER, RETURN ADDRESS (and e-mail address, if possible), SUBCOURSE NUMBER AND EDITION, AND PARAGRAPH/EXERCISE/EXAMINATION ITEM NUMBER.

PLEASE COMPLETE THE FOLLOWING ITEMS:
(Use the reverse side of this sheet, if necessary.)

1.   List any terms that were not defined properly.

_____
_____
_____
_____

2.   List any errors.

   <u>paragraph</u>   <u>error</u>   <u>correction</u>

_____
_____
_____
_____
_____
_____
_____
_____

3.   List any suggestions you have to improve this subcourse.

_____
_____
_____
_____

4.   Student Information (optional)

Name/Rank _____
SSN _____
Address _____
        _____
E-mail Address _____
Telephone number (DSN) _____
MOS/AOC _____

PRIVACY ACT STATEMENT (AUTHORITY: 10USC3012(B) AND (G))

PURPOSE: To provide Army Correspondence Course Program students a means to submit inquiries and comments.

USES: To locate and make necessary change to student records.

DISCLOSURE: VOLUNTARY. Failure to submit SSN will prevent subcourse authors at service school from accessing student records and responding to inquiries requiring such follow-ups.

U.S. ARMY MEDICAL DEPARTMENT CENTER AND SCHOOL   Fort Sam Houston, Texas 78234-6130

This page intentionally left blank.

Pharmacology IV

Subcourse MD0807

This page intentionally left blank.

U.S. ARMY MEDICAL DEPARTMENT CENTER AND SCHOOL
FORT SAM HOUSTON, TEXAS 78234-6100

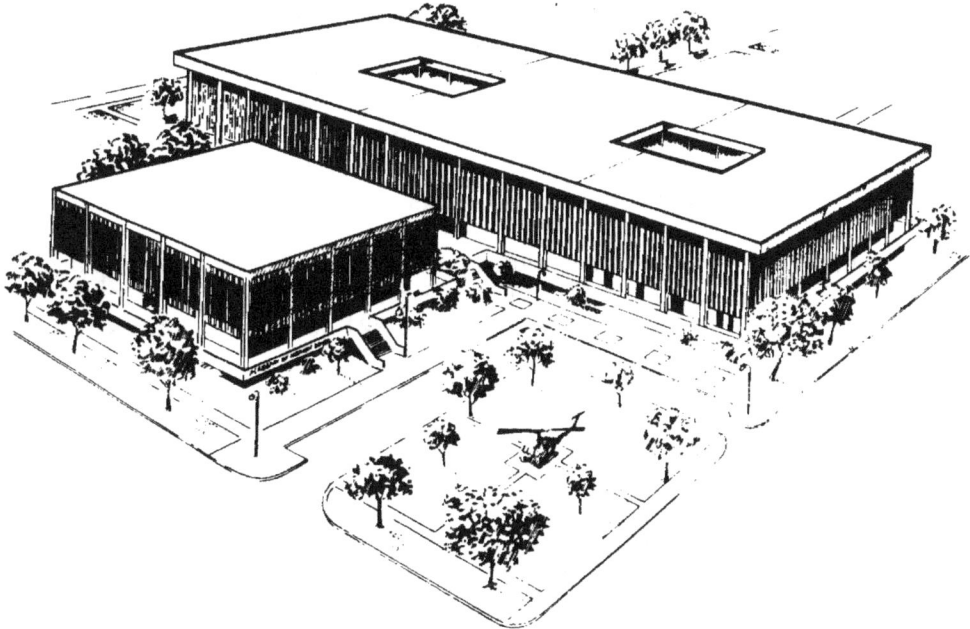

PHARMACOLOGY IV

SUBCOURSE MD0807   EDITION 100

DEVELOPMENT

This subcourse is approved for resident and correspondence course instruction. It reflects the current thought of the Academy of Health Sciences and conforms to printed Department of the Army doctrine as closely as currently possible. Development and progress render such doctrine continuously subject to change.

ADMINISTRATION

Students who desire credit hours for this correspondence subcourse must enroll in the subcourse. Application for enrollment should be made at the Internet website: http://www.atrrs.army.mil. You can access the course catalog in the upper right corner. Enter School Code 555 for medical correspondence courses. Copy down the course number and title. To apply for enrollment, return to the main ATRRS screen and scroll down the right side for ATRRS Channels. Click on SELF DEVELOPMENT to open the application; then follow the on-screen instructions.

For comments or questions regarding enrollment, student records, or examination shipments, contact the Nonresident Instruction Branch at DSN 471-5877, commercial (210) 221-5877, toll-free 1-800-344-2380; fax: 210-221-4012 or DSN 471-4012, e-mail accp@amedd.army.mil, or write to:

> NONRESIDENT INSTRUCTION BRANCH
> AMEDDC&S
> ATTN: MCCS-HSN
> 2105 11TH STREET SUITE 4191
> FORT SAM HOUSTON TX 78234-5064

Be sure your social security number is on all correspondence sent to the Academy of Health Sciences.

CLARIFICATION OF TERMINOLOGY

When used in this publication, words such as "he," "him," "his," and "men" 'are intended to include both the masculine and feminine genders, unless specifically stated otherwise or when obvious in context.

USE OF PROPRIETARY NAMES

The initial letters of the names of some products may be capitalized in this subcourse. Such names are proprietary names, that is, brand names or trademarks. Proprietary names have been used in this subcourse only to make it a more effective learning aid. The use of any name, proprietary or otherwise, should not be interpreted as endorsement, deprecation, or criticism of a product; nor should such use be considered to interpret the validity of proprietary rights in a name, whether it is registered or not.

TABLE OF CONTENTS

CORRESPONDENCE COURSE OF THE
U.S. ARMY MEDICAL DEPARTMENT CENTER AND SCHOOL

SUBCOURSE MD0807

PHARMACOLOGY IV

INTRODUCTION

In Subcourses MD0804, MD0805, and MD0806, various topics pertaining to anatomy, physiology, pathology, and pharmacology were presented. Specifically, topics like drug references, the physiology of the nervous system, nervous system drugs, and dermatological agents were introduced.

In this subcourse, MD0807, other systems of the body (for example, the digestive system) and the drugs used to treat conditions of those systems will be discussed. As in the other pharmacology subcourses, you will be provided background material in anatomy, physiology, and pathology in order to help you learn about the specific drugs discussed in the subcourse.

Remember, this subcourse is not intended to be used as an authoritative source of drug information. As you know, new drugs are being discovered and new uses for existing drugs are being found through research. Therefore, this subcourse can serve as a means for your review or initial learning of pharmacological concepts. You are strongly encouraged to use other references (see MD0804, Pharmacology I) to gain additional information which will help you to do your job in a better way. Knowing more about pharmacology can help you to better serve your patients.

Subcourse Components:

This subcourse consists of eleven lessons as follows:

➢ Lesson 1 The Human Digestive System.

➢ Lesson 2, Antacids and Digestants.

➢ Lesson 3, Emetics, Antiemetics, and Antidiarrheals.

➢ Lesson 4, Cathartics.

➢ Lesson 5, Fluid and Electrolyte Therapy.

➢ Lesson 6, Review of the Endocrine System.

➢ Lesson 7, Thyroid, Antithyroid, and Parathyroid Preparations.

➢ Lesson 8, Reproductive Hormones and Oral Contraceptives.

➢ Lesson 9, Adrenocortical Hormones.

➢ Lesson 10, Insulin and the Oral Hypoglycemic Agents.

➢ Lesson 11, Oxytocics and Ergot Alkaloids.

Here are some suggestions that may be helpful to you in completing this subcourse:

--Read and study each lesson carefully.

--Complete the subcourse lesson by lesson. After completing each lesson, work the exercises at the end of the lesson, marking your answers in this booklet.

--After completing each set of lesson exercises, compare your answers with those on the solution sheet that follows the exercises. If you have answered an exercise incorrectly, check the reference cited after the answer on the solution sheet to determine why your response was not the correct one.

Credit Awarded:

Upon successful completion of the examination for this subcourse, you will be awarded 14 credit hours.

To receive credit hours, you must be officially enrolled and complete an examination furnished by the Nonresident Instruction Branch at Fort Sam Houston, Texas.

You can enroll by going to the web site http://atrrs.army.mil and enrolling under "Self Development" (School Code 555).

A listing of correspondence courses and subcourses available through the Nonresident Instruction Section is found in Chapter 4 of DA Pamphlet 350-59, Army Correspondence Course Program Catalog. The DA PAM is available at the following website: http://www.usapa.army.mil/pdffiles/p350-59.pdf.

LESSON ASSIGNMENT

LESSON 1   The Human Digestive System.

TEXT ASSIGNMENT   Paragraph 1-1 through 1-24.

LESSON OBJECTIVES   After completing this lesson, you should be able to:

1-1.   Given a group of statements, select the statement that best defines the human digestive system.

1-2.   From a list of names of organs, select the organ(s) which are part of the human digestive system.

1-3.   Given a group of statements, select the statement that best describes the function of a digestive enzyme.

1-4.   Given a diagram of the human digestive system and a list of names of organs of the human digestive system, match the name of an organ with its location on the diagram.

1-5.   Given the name of a part of the human digestive system and a group of statements, select the statement that best describes that part of the human digestive system.

1-6.   Given the name of a part of the human digestive system and a group of statements, select the statement(s) that best describe the function(s) of that part of the digestive system.

1-7.   From a group of statements, select the statement that best describes the digestion of fats, carbohydrates, or proteins.

1-8.   Given the name of a disease or disorder of the human digestive system and a group of statements, select the statement that best describes that disease or disorder.

SUGGESTION   After completing the assignment, complete the exercises at the end of this lesson. These exercises will help you to achieve the lesson objectives.

LESSON 1

THE HUMAN DIGESTIVE SYSTEM

Section I. INTRODUCTION

1-1. GENERAL

a. **Definition.** The <u>human digestive system</u> is a group of organs designed to take in foods, initially process foods, digest the foods, and eliminate unused materials of food items. It is a <u>hollow tubular</u> system from one end of the body to the other end. See figure 1-1.

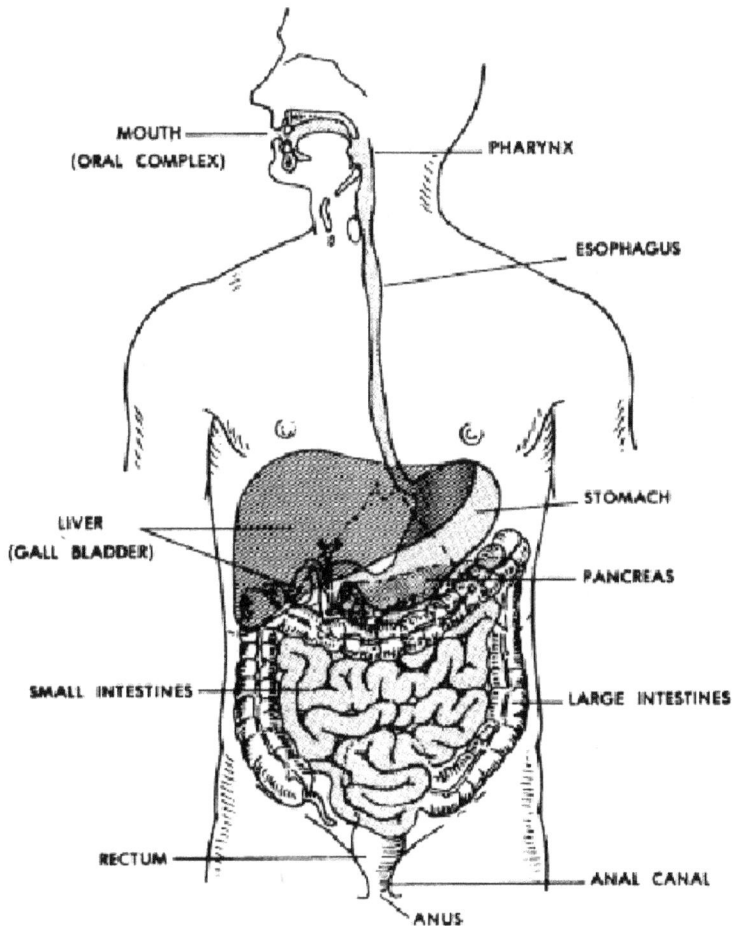

Figure 1-1. The human digestive system.

b. **Major Organs.** The major organs involved in the human digestive system are listed below. They are each discussed later in this lesson.

    (1)   Mouth or oral complex.

    (2)   Pharynx.

    (3)   Esophagus.

    (4)   Stomach.

    (5)   Small intestines and associated glands.

    (6)   Large intestines.

    (7)   Rectum.

    (8)   Anal canal and anus.

c. **Digestive Enzymes.** A catalyst is a substance that accelerates (speeds up) a chemical reaction without being permanently changed or consumed itself. A digestive enzyme serves as a catalyst, aiding in digestion. Digestion is a chemical process by which food is converted into simpler substances that can be absorbed or assimilated by the body. Enzymes are manufactured in the salivary glands of the mouth, in the lining of the stomach, in the pancreas, and in the walls of the small intestine.

1-2. FOODS AND FOODSTUFFS

Examples of food items are a piece of bread, a pork chop, and a tomato. Food items contain varying proportions of foodstuffs. Foodstuffs are the classes of chemical compounds that make up food items. The three major types of foodstuffs are carbohydrates, lipids (fats and oils), and proteins. Food items also contain water, minerals, and vitamins.

Section II. THE SUPRAGASTRIC STRUCTURES

1-3. ORAL COMPLEX

The oral complex consists of the structures commonly known together as the mouth. It takes in and initially processes food items. See figure 1-2.

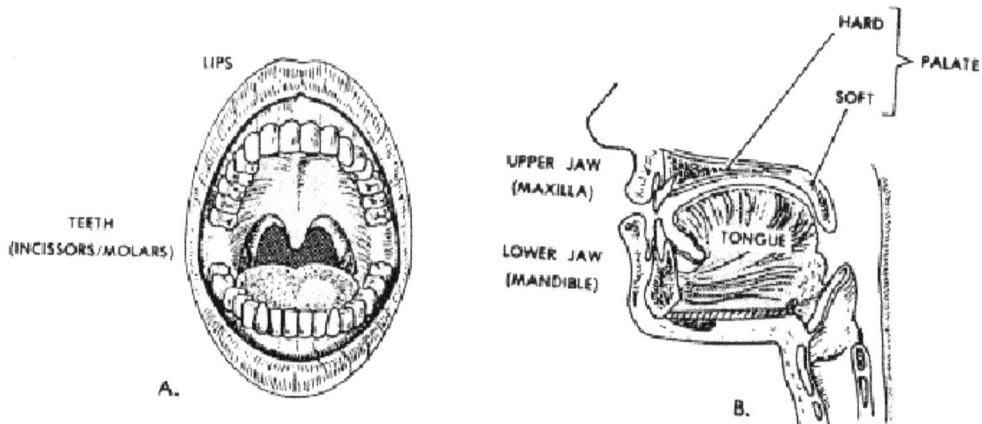

Figure 1-2. Anatomy of the oral complex.

a. **Teeth.**

(1) A tooth (figure 1-3) has two main parts, the crown and the root. The root canal passes up through the central part of the tooth. The root is suspended within a socket (called the alveolus) of one of the jaws of the mouth. The crown extends up above the surface of the jaw. The root and inner part of the crown are made of a substance called dentin. The outer portion of the crown is covered with a substance known as enamel. Enamel is the hardest substance of the human body. The nerves and blood vessels of the tooth pass up into the root canal from the jaw substance.

(2) There are two kinds of teeth, anterior and posterior. The anterior teeth are also known as incisors and canine teeth. The anterior teeth serve as choppers. They chop off mouth-size bites of food items. The posterior teeth are called molars. They are grinders. They increase the surface area of food materials by breaking them into smaller and smaller particles.

(3) Humans have two sets of teeth, deciduous and permanent. Initially, the deciduous set includes 20 baby teeth. These are eventually replaced by a permanent set of 32.

> **DECIDUOUS** = to be shed

TEETH:

1. STRUCTURE:

    A.   CROWN / ROOT / ROOT CANAL

    B.   ENAMEL / DENTIN

2. ALVEOLI OF JAWS

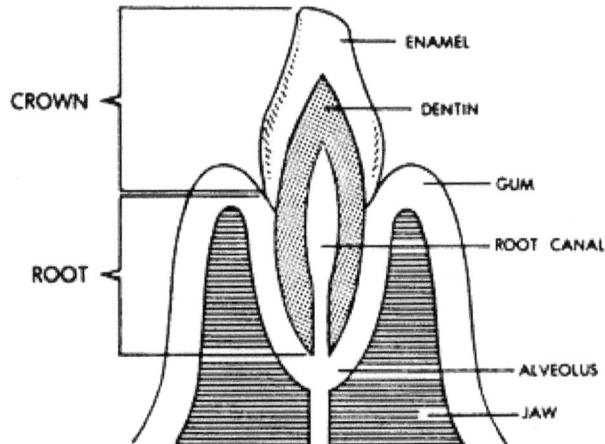

Figure 1-3. Section of a tooth and jaw.

b. **Jaws.** There are two jaws, the upper and the lower. The upper is called the maxilla. The lower is called the mandible.

(1) In each jaw, there are sockets for the teeth. These sockets are known as alveoli. The bony parts of the jaws holding the teeth are known as alveolar ridges.

(2) The upper jaw is fixed to the base of the cranium. The lower jaw is movable. There is a special articulation, (T-MJ, temporo-mandibular joint), with muscles to bring the upper and lower teeth together to perform their functions.

c. **Palate.** The palate serves as the roof of the mouth and the floor of the nasal chamber above. Since the anterior two-thirds is bony, it is called the hard palate. The posterior one-third is musculo-membranous, and is called the soft palate. The soft palate serves as a trap door to close off the upper respiratory passageway during swallowing.

d. **Lips and Cheeks.** The oral cavity is closed by a fleshy structure around the opening. Forming the opening are the lips. On the sides are the cheeks.

e. **Tongue.** The tongue is a muscular organ. The tongue is capable of <u>internal</u> movement to shape its body. It is moved as a whole by muscles outside the tongue. Interaction between the tongue and cheeks keeps the food between the molar teeth during the chewing process. When the food is properly processed, the tongue also initiates the swallowing process.

f. **Salivary Glands.** Digestion is a chemical process that takes place at the wet surfaces of food materials. The chewing process has greatly increased the surface area available. The surfaces are wetted by saliva produced by glands in the oral cavity. Of these glands, three pairs are known as the <u>salivary glands proper</u>.

g. **Taste Buds.** Associated with the tongue and the back of the mouth are special clumps of cells known as <u>taste buds</u>. These taste buds literally taste the food. That is, they check its quality and acceptability.

1-4. PHARYNX

The pharynx (pronounced "FAIR-inks") is a continuation of the rear of the mouth region, just anterior to the vertebral column (spine). It is a common passageway for both the respiratory and digestive systems.

1-5. ESOPHAGUS

The esophagus is a muscular, tubular structure extending from the pharynx, down through the neck and the thorax (chest), and to the stomach. During swallowing, the esophagus serves as a passageway for the food from the pharynx to the stomach.

Section III. THE STOMACH

1-6. STORAGE FUNCTION

The stomach is a sac-like enlargement of the digestive tract specialized for the storage of food. Since food is stored, a person does not have to eat continuously all day. One is freed to do other things. The presence of <u>valves</u> at each end prevents the stored food from leaving the stomach before it is ready. The <u>pyloric valve</u> prevents the food from going further. The inner lining of the stomach is in folds to allow expansion.

1-7. DIGESTIVE FUNCTION

a. While the food is in the stomach, the digestive processes are initiated by juices from the wall of the stomach. The musculature of the walls thoroughly mixes the food and juices while the food is being held in the stomach. In fact, the stomach has an extra layer of muscle fibers for this purpose.

b. When the pyloric valve of the stomach opens, a portion of the stomach contents moves into the small intestine.

Section IV. THE SMALL INTESTINES AND ASSOCIATED GLANDS

1-8. GENERAL

a. Digestion is a chemical process. This process is facilitated by special chemicals called digestive enzymes. The end products of digestion are absorbed through the wall of the gut into the blood vessels. These end products are then distributed to body parts that need them for growth, repair, or energy.

b. There are associated glands, the liver and the pancreas, which produce additional enzymes to further the process.

c. Most digestion and absorption takes place in the small intestines.

1-9. ANATOMY OF THE SMALL INTESTINES

a. The small intestines are classically divided into three areas, the duodenum, the jejunum, and the ileum. The duodenum is C-shaped, about 10 inches long in the adult. The duodenum is looped around the pancreas. The jejunum is approximately eight feet long and connects the duodenum and ileum. The ileum is about 12 feet long. The jejunum and ileum are attached to the rear wall of the abdomen with a membrane called a mesentery. This membrane allows mobility and serves as a passageway for nerves and vessels (NAVL) to the small intestines.

DUODENUM = Length equal to width of 12 fingers

JEJUNUM = empty

ILEUM = lying next to the illume (bone of the pelvic girdle)

PELVIS = basin

b. The small intestine is tubular. It has muscular walls that produce a wave-like motion called peristalsis moving the contents along. The small intestine is just the right length to allow the processes of digestion and absorption to take place completely.

c. The inner surface of the small intestine is NOT smooth like the inside of new plumbing pipes. Rather, the inner surface has folds (plicae). On the surface of these plicae are fingerlike projections called villi (villus, singular). This folding and the presence of villi increase the surface area available for absorption.

Section V. THE LARGE INTESTINES

1-10. GENERAL FUNCTION

The primary function of the large intestines is the salvaging of water and electrolytes (salts). Most of the end products of digestion have already been absorbed in the small intestines. Within the large intestines, the contents are first a watery fluid. Thus, the large intestines are important in the conservation of water for use by the body. The large intestines remove water until a nearly solid mass is formed before defecation, the evacuation of feces.

1-11. MAJOR SUBDIVISIONS

The major subdivisions of the large intestines are the cecum (with vermiform or "worm-shaped" appendix), the ascending colon, the transverse colon, the descending colon, and the sigmoid colon. The fecal mass is stored in the sigmoid colon until passed into the rectum.

1-12. RECTUM, ANAL CANAL, AND ANUS

Rectum means "straight". However, this six inch tubular structure would actually look a bit wave-like from the front. From the side, one would see that it was curved to conform the sacrum (at the lower end of the spinal column). The final storage of feces is in the rectum. The rectum terminates in the narrow anal canal, which is about 1 1/2 inches long in the adult. At the end of the anal canal is the opening called the anus. Muscles called the anal sphincters aid in the retention of feces until defecation.

Section VI. ASSOCIATED PROTECTIVE STRUCTURES

1-13. GENERAL

Within the body, there are many structures that aid in protection from bacteria, viruses, and other foreign substances. These structures include cells that can phagocytize (engulf) foreign particles or manufacture antibodies (which help to inactivate foreign substances). Collectively, such cells make up the reticuloendothelial system (RES). Such cells are found in bone marrow, the spleen, the liver, and lymph nodes.

1-14. STRUCTURES WITHIN THE DIGESTIVE SYSTEM

Lymphoid structures make up the largest part of the RES. Lymphoid structures are collections of cells associated with circulatory systems.

a. Tonsils are associated with the posterior portions of the respiratory and digestive areas in the head, primarily in the region of the pharynx. The tonsils are masses of lymphoid tissue.

b. Other lymphoid aggregations are found in the walls of the small intestines.

c. The <u>vermiform appendix</u>, attached to the cecum of the large intestine, is also a mass of lymphoid tissue. It is the "tonsil" of the intestines.

Section VII. ACCESSORY STRUCTURES OF THE DIGESTIVE SYSTEM

1-15. THE LIVER

The liver is a massive glandular organ. In fact, the liver is the largest gland in the body. The major function of the liver, as far as digestion is concerned, is the production of bile, a substance that aids in the digestion of lipids (fats). There are salts contained in the bile (bile salts) that help to emulsify fat globules so that they can be digested by intestinal lipases. Bile also aids in making the end products of fat digestion more soluble so that they are absorbed through the intestinal mucosa. Bile is continuously being made and excreted by the liver. Bile is stored in the gallbladder until it is needed. The function of the gallbladder is to store bile and release it when it is needed in the small intestine. The liver also has functions that are not related to the digestive system.

a. **Glycogen Storage.** When carbohydrates are digested and the end product sugars are not immediately utilized by the body, they are made into a substance called glycogen and stored in the liver in that form until needed.

b. **Hematopoiesis.** The liver is an important organ in the hematopoietic system. It functions as a blood reservoir during venous pooling and it polices up iron from destroyed red cells so that it can be used for synthesis of new red cells by the bone marrow.

c. **Phagocytosis.** The liver has phagocytic cells called Kupffer's cells that can remove bacteria and foreign particles from the blood.

d. **Detoxification.** This is not the most accurate word to describe this function, but the liver is responsible for metabolizing many drugs and other substances in the blood from an active to an inactive form. For example, alcohol is active and is metabolized by the liver to an inactive substance and the drink wears off.

e. **Vitamin Storage and Synthesis.** The liver can store large quantities of Vitamins A and B_{12}. It also functions in the synthesis of Vitamin D from precursors in the body, a very important vitamin affecting bone structure and function, and blood Ca++ levels.

f. **Blood Coagulation.** The liver is the organ responsible for the production of fibrinogen, prothrombin, and other factors important in the blood clotting mechanism. Impairment could result in inhibition of the clotting process.

g. **Antibody (Ab) Production.** Antibodies are an important defense mechanism against infection and invasion of body tissues by bacteria. They are formed in the plasma cells found in lymphoid tissue. The liver contains a very large amount of lymphoid tissue, lymph nodes, and lymph. Damage may severely impair the immune process of the body.

1-16. THE PANCREAS

The other accessory organ important to the gastrointestinal tract is the pancreas. The pancreas functions as both an endocrine and exocrine gland and it is the exocrine portion that is concerned with digestion. The pancreas secretes lipases and proteases that are responsible for the digestion of fats and proteins in the small intestine. The endocrine portion of the pancreas is composed of groups of cells scattered throughout the pancreas called the Islets of Langerhans. There are alpha and beta cells in the pancreas. These alpha and beta cells have specific functions. The alpha cells secrete glucagon, a hormone which promotes the breakdown of glycogen and sugar stores and causes their release into the bloodstream. The beta cells secrete insulin, a hormone which promotes the movement of glucose from the bloodstream into the cells and the subsequent oxidation of the glucose. The release of insulin promotes a lowering of blood sugar. Diabetics have insulin deficiency and hence have unusually high blood sugar levels that "spill over" into the urine.

Section VIII. ABSORPTION AND METABOLISM IN THE DIGESTIVE SYSTEM

1-17. INTRODUCTION

Once foodstuffs are taken into the body and have passed through the gastrointestinal tract, their end products are either stored or used by our cells for energy. The only substance that can be used by our body cells for the purpose of obtaining energy is glucose. Our bodies can obtain glucose directly from the absorption and digestion of carbohydrates or from the production of glucose from other substances (if necessary).

1-18. THE DIGESTION OF CARBOHYDRATES

a. The digestion of carbohydrates begins in the mouth by the enzyme alpha-amylase or ptyalin, which is found in saliva. The process of turning complex carbohydrates (starches) into simple disaccharide units thus begins in the mouth. The mouth is very important in the digestion of carbohydrates--food is chewed, mixed with saliva, and swallowed. This occurs within a very short period of time, which allows for only about five percent of the starch to split. As the bolus moves on to the stomach, the low pH of the stomach prevents further action by salivary amylase. Hence, very little further digestion of carbohydrates occurs in the stomach.

b. After the carbohydrates pass into the small intestine, their digestion is completed. In the small intestine, pancreatic amylase acts on the remaining starch and completely breaks it down to disaccharide (maltose and isomaltose). Sucrose, maltase, isomaltase, and lactase finally break down this disaccharide, along with other disaccharides ingested in foods (sucrose, lactose) to the monosaccharides glucose, fructose, and galactose. These simple sugars are the end products of carbohydrate digestion and are absorbed through the intestinal mucosa into the bloodstream via a carrier-mediated transport system. They can be either oxidized immediately by the cells to do work or they can be stored until they are needed by the body. They can be stored in two ways:

(1) Synthesized to glycogen in the liver, or

(2) Synthesized to fat and stored in fat cells.

1-19. THE DIGESTION OF FAT

a. There is virtually no fat digestion in the mouth or stomach. The first step in the digestion of fats is emulsification, the physical break up of fat globules into small droplets. This occurs in the small Intestine by the action of bile and bile salts. Emulsification permits the digestive enzymes (lipases) to act upon the fat molecules and break them down into monoglycerides, fatty acids, and glycerol, the end products of fat digestion and the form in which they are absorbed through the intestinal mucosa.

b. The absorption occurs through a rather complex and poorly understood mechanism. The end products of lipid digestion can be either oxidized by the cells or transformed into glucose that, in turn, is then oxidized by the cells to do work. They may also be stored as fat.

1-20. THE DIGESTION OF PROTEINS

The digestive process of proteins begins in the stomach. In the stomach, pepsin, an enzyme activated by the low pH of the stomach, breaks apart long chain polypeptides and proteins into simpler short-chain peptides referred to as proteoses and peptones. Further hydrolysis of these fragments to dipeptides and amino acids is accomplished in the small intestine by the enzymes chymotrypsin and trypsin. Ultimately, all peptide fragments are broken down to their constituent amino acids, the end products of protein digestion, by various carboxypeptidases and aminopeptidases present all along the walls of the small intestine. The mechanism by which the amino acids are absorbed across the small intestine walls is poorly understood.

Section IX. DISORDERS AND DISEASES OF THE DIGESTIVE TRACT

1-21. INTRODUCTION

There are several common disorders of the digestive system. Many of these disorders can be treated by drugs that you will dispense in the pharmacy.

1-22. DISORDERS OF THE MOUTH CAVITY

a. **Dental Caries (Tooth Decay).** Dental caries is a weakening or decay of the enamel coating of teeth. If allowed to progress unchecked, eventual destruction of the entire tooth (including the root and pulp) can result. Destruction of the root necessitates extraction.

b. **Mumps.** Mumps are a typical childhood disease in which the salivary glands (principally the parotid) become swollen and inflamed. Mumps are caused by a virus and the condition is highly infectious. There is a vaccine available that can protect persons from mumps.

c. **Trench Mouth (Vincent's Disease).** Trench mouth is an acute inflammation of the gums. Bleeding and pain are usually present. Probably the disease is not communicable and may be due to poor oral hygiene, mononucleosis, or nonspecific viral infection. This disorder is treated with antibiotics and oxygenating mouthwashes such as hydrogen peroxide.

d. **Thrush.** Thrush is due to an overgrowth of a normally occurring oral fungus, Candida albicans. Thrush is characterized by creamy-white, curd-like patches that may occur anywhere in the mouth. Pain and fever are usually present and treatment must include the removal of the causative factor. The patient should have a nutritious diet with adequate intake of vitamins and rest. Saline rinses help promote healing. If thrush is not treated, it can lead to ulcers and stomach problems.

1-23. DISORDERS OF THE STOMACH

a. **Peptic Ulcer.** Probably the best known stomach disease is peptic ulcer. Peptic ulcers are presumed to be caused by the action of pepsin upon the stomach lining until it becomes eroded, exposing the layers of the cells underneath. Continual secretion of stomach acid irritates the exposed layers of the stomach lining resulting in pain and bleeding. There is no specific cure or treatment for ulcers and the cause or initiating factor in the disease process is not known. People who have peptic ulcers usually are told to avoid stress and are maintained on strict diets. Ulcers may eventually erode completely through a region of the stomach (called a perforation) and cause excessive bleeding.

b. **Duodenal Ulcer.** Duodenal ulcers are ulcers that occur in the duodenum, usually along the initial two inch segment just distal to the stomach. The symptoms for a duodenal ulcer are virtually the same as for a stomach ulcer, but duodenal ulcers are much more common and death due to perforation and hemorrhage is a major problem. Duodenal ulcers also appear to penetrate other organs (migration of the ulcerative crater). Treatment usually consists of preventing or controlling stress in the patient and maintaining the patient on a strictly controlled diet and administering certain drugs (like sucralfate or cimetidine). Although the ulcer will "heal" in three to four weeks, periodic recurrence has never successfully been prevented. The origin of the condition is not understood.

c. **Cancer.** The stomach is susceptible to cancer or neoplasms of the mucosal lining. A cancer is an uncontrollable growth of cells. Neither the cause nor the cure for cancer of the stomach is known. If discovered early, surgery can prove beneficial.

1-24. DISORDERS OF THE INTESTINES

a. **Sprue.** Sprue, or malabsorption of nutrients from the small intestine, can be very serious. It usually involves impaired absorption of fats and vitamins that leads to vitamin deficiency and anemia (inadequate red blood cell count). Treatment of sprue usually consist s of a high carbohydrate, low protein, low fat diet with vitamin supplements. Emergency replenishment of vital nutrients, if necessary, can be accomplished by intravenous injection.

b. **Diarrhea.** Diarrhea is the frequent excretion of excessive, soft, or watery stools. In some cases, the excretion may be totally liquid. Nausea and vomiting may be present. Although the condition is obviously unpleasant for the patient, mild diarrhea is usually not serious. However, if a patient has severe diarrhea, loss of nutrients and electrolytes may occur which requires replacement therapy and medical care. Cholera, a very serious condition, is characterized by a large loss of fluids and nutrients in watery stools.

c. **Colitis.** Colitis is simply an inflammation of the colon that sometimes results in diarrhea. If the condition is ulcerative colitis, then changes in the colon wall and scar tissue formation may result. Anemia, malaise, and weakness may be present. Treatment of colitis usually consists of rest, careful administration of anti-infectives, and restricted diet. Symptoms usually go away after a period of two to three weeks, but there is no cure for the condition.

d. **Appendicitis.** Appendicitis is simply an inflammation of the veriform appendix, usually due to an obstruction. Treatment consists of surgical removal. If left untreated, perforation into the peritoneal cavity with generalized peritonitis usually results.

e. **Hemorrhoids (Piles).** Hemorrhoids (or piles) are ulcerations of the hemorrhoidal vein (a vein which lies in close proximity to the external mucosa of the anus). Pain, itching, and general discomfort are the usual symptoms associated with hemorrhoids. However, complications such as infection or obstruction may arise. It is surgically possible to remove hemorrhoids.

f. **Hepatitis.** There are two types of hepatitis, serum (or long-term incubation) and infectious (or short-term incubation). Infectious hepatitis is spread via the oral route and the danger of an epidemic exists in close environments such as military bases and hospitals. Serum hepatitis is transmitted by blood transfusion or by the use of an unsterilized syringe or "dirty" needle. The incubation period for hepatitis ranges from six weeks to six months. The type of hepatitis a patient has can be identified in some patients. There can be a wide variety of clinical symptoms and signs of hepatitis ranging from mild infection to death. The disease is usually centered in the liver and jaundice (yellow coloration of skin) is usually present along with hepatomegaly (enlarged liver). Liver damage may result in hepatitis. Most patients recover from hepatitis. Bed rest is usually required during the first phase of the disease. Hepatitis is viral in nature. Therefore, there is no specific treatment or cure other than to let the disease run its course. The physician treating a person who has hepatitis must carefully observe the patient and treat symptoms and complications when they arise.

g. **Cirrhosis.** Cirrhosis is a disease of the liver characterized by degeneration and necrosis of liver cells with fatty deposits. Although the specific cause is unknown, malnutrition, vitamin deficiency, and alcoholism definitely are causative factors and contribute to progression of the disease process. The liver has a number of vital functions in the body and, hence, cirrhosis is a serious condition. A wide variety of symptoms may be present, but treatment almost always consists of adequate rest, abstinence from alcohol, and a carefully selected diet. Vitamin supplements may be necessary for the patient. There is no "cure" for cirrhosis and the outlook for the improvement of the patient is not good. Only 50 percent of the patients who have cirrhosis survive beyond two years and only 35 percent survive beyond five years.

h. **Cholecystitis.** Cholecystitis is an inflammation of the gallbladder. An infection may be the source of the inflammation. If an infection is present, the patient may be prescribed antibiotics. Cholecystitis is usually treated by placing the patient on a low-fat diet. The gallbladder may be surgically removed if the inflammation becomes too severe.

i. **Cholelithiasis.** Cholelithiasis is the presence of gallstones, calcified deposits of cholesterol, bilirubin, and bile salts. Cholecystitis usually must be treated with the surgical removal of the gallstones.

j. **Diabetes Mellitus.** Diabetes mellitus is insulin deficiency. This insulin deficiency results in the inability of body cells to take up and use glucose. Therefore, the glucose (sugar) remains in the blood and the blood levels eventually rise to extremely high levels and eventually "spill over" into the urine. This is one of the classic signs of diabetes mellitus. There is no cure for diabetes mellitus--treatment consists of insulin replacement therapy with commercially available insulin and a very strictly controlled diet.

k. **Ascites.** Ascites is edema or the presence of fluid in the peritoneal cavity. Ascites can be caused by a variety of factors, with cardiac or renal insufficiency or disease being the most common.

Continue with Exercises

EXERCISES, LESSON 1

INSTRUCTIONS: The following exercises are to be answered by marking the lettered response that best answers the question or best completes the incomplete statement or by writing the answer in the space provided.

After you have completed all the exercises, turn to "Solutions to Exercises" at the end of the lesson and check your answers.

1. The human digestive system is best defined as:

   a. A group of organs intended to provide energy to the body.

   b. A group of organs designed to take in, process, and digest foods and eliminate unused materials of food items.

   c. A group of organs involved in the absorption of foods.

   d. A group of organs which convert food into simpler substances which can be used by the body.

2. Which of the organs below is/are in the human digestive system?

   a. Esophagus.

   b. Spleen.

   c. Large intestines.

3. Select the function(s) of the stomach.

   a. The digestion of food.

   b. The initiation of food digestion.

   c. The salvaging of water and electrolytes from the food.

4. The esophagus is best described as:

   a. A continuation of the rear of the mouth region which is just anterior to the vertebral column.

   b. A structure with tubular muscular walls that has villi on the inner surfaces which moves the food through an action called peristalsis.

   c. A mass of lymphoid tissue that is located just anterior to the stomach.

   d. A muscular, tubular structure that serves as a passageway for the food from the pharynx to the stomach.

5. Which of the statements below best describes the digestion of fats?

   a. Fats are emulsified by bile and bile salts in the small intestine and absorbed as fatty acids in the large intestine.

   b. Fats are emulsified in the stomach and then broken down to fatty acids, monoglycerides, and glycerol which are absorbed in the small intestine.

   c. Fats are emulsified by bile and bile salts in the large intestine and are then absorbed as fatty acids and glucose through the intestinal mucosa.

   d. Fats are emulsified in the stomach and are absorbed as fatty acids, monoglycerides, and glycerol through the intestinal mucosa.

6. What is the major function of the liver (as far as digestion is concerned)?

   a. The production of insulin.

   b. The production of bile.

   c. The production of fatty acids and monoglycerides.

   d. The production of Vitamins A and B_{12}.

7. Mumps is best described as a viral infection of the:

   a. Salivary glands.

   b. Liver.

   c. Esophagus.

   d. Ileum.

8. Appendicitis is best described as:

   a. An inflammation of the veriform appendix typically caused by an obstruction.

   b. An inflammation of the liver characterized by degeneration and necrosis of the cells with fatty deposits.

   c. An inflammation of the colon which sometimes results In diarrhea.

   d. An inflammation of the small intestines due to an Infection usually caused by a gallstone.

9. Ascites is:

   a. An inflammation of the gallbladder due to infection that is usually precipitated by a gallstone.

   b. An inflammation of the colon that usually results in diarrhea.

   c. A condition in which there is malabsorption of nutrients from the small intestine.

   d. Edema or the presence of fluid in the peritoneal cavity.

SPECIAL INSTRUCTIONS FOR EXERCISES 10 THROUGH 12. The drawing below is used in questions 10, 11, and 12. Match the question in Column A to its correct location in Column B.

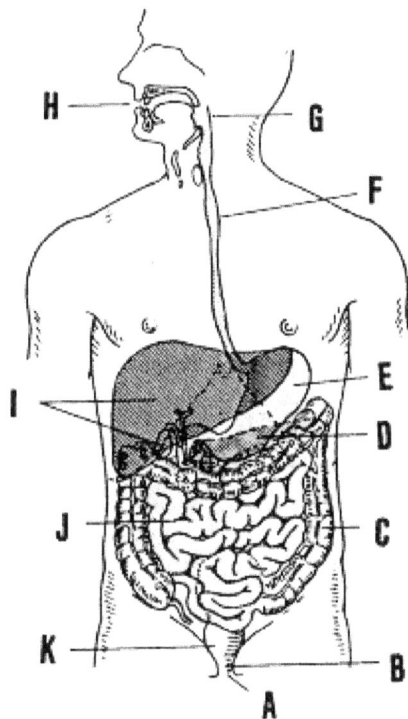

10. Which letter is pointing to the pancreas? _____

11. Which letter is pointing to the small intestines? _____

12. Which letter is pointing to the rectum? _____

Check Your Answers on Next Page

SOLUTIONS TO EXERCISES, LESSON 1

1. b   (para 1-1a)

2. a and c   (para 1-1b (3), (6))

3. a and b   (para 1-6, 1-7)

4. d   (para 1-5)

5. b   (para 1-19)

6. b   (para 1-15)

7. a   (para 1-22b)

8. a   (para 1-24d)

9. d   (para 1-24k)

10. D   (Figure 1-1)

11. J   (Figure 1-1)

12. K   (Figure 1-1)

End of Lesson 1

LESSON 2   Antacids and Digestants.

LESSON ASSIGNMENT   Paragraphs 2-1 through 2-6.

LESSON OBJECTIVES   After completing this lesson, you should be able to:

2-1.   Given a group of statements and one of the following terms: antacid or digestant, select the statement that best defines the given term.

2-2.   Given a group of indications, select the indication(s) for the use of antacids or digestants.

2-3.   From a group of statements, select the statement that describes a consideration involved in the selection of an antacid for use.

2-4.   Given the trade and/or generic name of an antacid or digestant product and a group of uses, actions, indications, side effects, or cautions and warnings, select the use(s), indication(s), side effect(s), or caution(s) and warning(s) associated with that product.

2-5.   Given the trade or generic name of an antacid or digestant product and a list of trade and/or generic names, select the trade or generic name which corresponds to the given trade or generic name.

SUGGESTION   After completing the assignment, complete the exercises at the end of this lesson. These exercises will help you to achieve the lesson objectives.

LESSON 2

ANTACIDS AND DIGESTANTS

Section I. ANTACIDS

2-1. INTRODUCTION

Many of the patients you will see at the outpatient pharmacy window will be there to receive antacid preparations. You will usually see these patients every several months because they will return to obtain more antacids. Thus, one can see that many of the patients who take antacid preparations will be taking them for many years. You must be familiar with the antacid preparations so that you can adequately serve these patients.

2-2. GENERAL CONSIDERATIONS FOR ANTACIDS

a. **Definition.** Antacids are drugs which neutralize part of the hydrochloric acid in the stomach.

b. **Indications for the Use of Antacids.** Antacids are indicated in ulcer therapy, minor stomach irritations, and other conditions depending on the type of antacid prescribed.

c. **Factors Considered When an Antacid is Prescribed.** Before a patient is prescribed a particular antacid preparation, the prescriber must consider the patient's condition as well as a group of other factors. Some of these factors are listed below:

(1) Gastric acid neutralization. The chief reason for prescribing an antacid preparation is the neutralization of the hydrochloric acid in the stomach. Antacid preparations contain one or more drugs which chemically neutralize this hydrochloric acid. Not all chemicals neutralize the same amount of stomach acid on a weight-by-weight basis. Therefore, the prescriber must be aware of the active ingredient(s) present in an antacid preparation and how effectively that preparation is able to neutralize stomach acid in relation to other antacid preparations.

(2) Effect on systemic pH. Most antacid agents remain in the gastrointestinal system when they are taken to neutralize stomach acid. However, some agents (e.g., sodium bicarbonate ($NaHCO_3$)), because of their ability to ionize, are capable of going into systemic circulation in the bloodstream once they are ingested. For example, if enough sodium bicarbonate is ingested, the bicarbonate ion (HCO_3) can be systemically absorbed and affect the pH of the blood. This effect is highly undesirable.

(3)   Speed of action. It is desirable that an antacid product act quickly once it has been ingested.

(4)   Acid rebound.

(5)   Drug interactions.

(6)   Other side effects specific to individual agents.

2-3.   ANTACID PREPARATIONS

a. **Sodium Bicarbonate (NaHCO₃).** Sodium bicarbonate is used as a gastric antacid, urinary alkalizing agent, and an agent used to counteract the lowering of the pH of the blood in heart failure (raising the pH of the blood during heart failure increases the pharmacological effectiveness of epinephrine). The usual dosage of sodium bicarbonate is 0.3 to 2 grams as needed. Side effects associated with this agent include systemic alkalization (raising the pH of the blood) and acid rebound. The patient receiving sodium bicarbonate for antacid purposes should be told that it should not be used frequently and that it should not be used for prolonged periods. Sodium bicarbonate is available in tablets of various strengths and in powder form.

b. **Calcium Carbonate and Glycine (Titralac®).** Titralac® is used as a gastric antacid. The usual dosage of this product is from one to four tablets or from one to four teaspoonsful four times daily. Side effects associated with this product include acid rebound and systemic alkalization. The patient receiving this product should be cautioned not to use it for prolonged periods. Persons receiving the tablets should be told to chew them thoroughly before swallowing them. Patients receiving the suspension should be told to shake the preparation well before taking the medication. Titralac® is available in both suspension form (1 gram calcium carbonate and 300 milligrams of glycine per 5 milliliters) and tablet form (300 milligram tablets and 600 milligram tablets).

c. **Magnesium Hydroxide (Milk of Magnesia).** Magnesium hydroxide is used both as an antacid and as a cathartic (laxative). The antacid dose of milk of magnesia (MOM) is one to two teaspoonsful as needed. The cathartic dose of MOM for adults is one to two tablespoonsful taken with one or more glasses of water. Patients taking this product should be cautioned that they can obtain the laxative effect if they take too large a dose or if they take the antacid dose too often. A side effect associated with MOM is diarrhea. Patients who receive MOM in suspension form should be told to shake the suspension thoroughly, while patients taking the tablet form of the product should be cautioned to chew the tablets thoroughly.

d. **Aluminum Hydroxide (Amphojel®).** Aluminum hydroxide is used as a gastric antacid and as an agent in ulcer therapy. The usual dose of aluminum hydroxide is one teaspoonful to two tablespoonsful of the suspension four or more times daily or one to four tablets four or more times daily. Constipation is a side effect associated with the use of aluminum hydroxide. When you dispense the tablets, you should tell the patient to chew them thoroughly before swallowing them. When you dispense the suspension, you should tell the patient to shake the container well before taking the dose. Aluminum hydroxide is available in both suspension form (320 milligrams per teaspoonful) and in tablet form (300 and 600 milligram tablets).

e. **Magaldrate (Riopan®).** Magaldrate is used as a gastric antacid and as an agent in the treatment of ulcers. It acts as a buffer/antacid. Side effects associated with magaldrate include constipation and diarrhea. This preparation is available in three forms: suspension, chew tablets, and swallow tablets. The information you provide the patient when dispensing the product depends on the particular dosage form being dispensed:

(1) Suspension. Tell the patient to shake the container well. The usual dosage of this form is one or two teaspoonsful between meals and at bedtime.

(2) Chew tablet. Tell the patient to chew the tablet(s) thoroughly before swallowing. The usual dosage of the chew tablets is one to two tablets between meals and at bedtime.

(3) Swallow tablet. Tell the patient to take the tablet(s) with enough water to swallow them properly. The usual dosage of the swallow tablet is one or two tablets between meals and at bedtime.

CAUTION: Magaldrate should not be taken by persons who are taking a prescription antibiotic drug containing any form of tetracycline.

f. **Aluminum Hydroxide and Magnesium Hydroxide (Maalox®).** Maalox® is used as a gastric antacid and as an agent in ulcer therapy. This product is available in both a suspension form (225 milligrams of aluminum hydroxide and 200 milligrams of magnesium hydroxide per teaspoonful) and in tablet form (200 milligrams of aluminum hydroxide and 200 milligrams of magnesium hydroxide per tablet). Depending on the amount of the preparation taken, diarrhea and constipation are side effects associated with the product.

g. **Aluminum Hydroxide and Magnesium Trisilicate Tablets (Gaviscon®).** This tablet product is used as a gastric antacid and as a protectant for the lower esophagus. Gaviscon® produces a foam when ingested. This foam floats on the stomach contents. Thus, the foam protects the delicate mucosa of the esophagus from irritation when stomach contents are forced into the esophagus. Gaviscon® produces a local effect--the entire stomach contents are not neutralized. The usual dose is two to four tablets four times daily, after meals and at bedtime. Side effects of this product, depending on the dose, are either diarrhea or constipation. When you dispense these tablets to the patient, you should tell him to chew them thoroughly before swallowing. Each tablet has 80 milligrams of aluminum hydroxide and 20 milligrams of magnesium trisilicate.

h. **Aluminum Hydroxide and Magnesium Carbonate Liquid (Gaviscon® liquid antacid).** Like the product in paragraph g above, this liquid antacid preparation is used as a gastric antacid and as a protectant for the lower esophagus. The usual dose of this product is one to two tablespoonsful four times daily. The product contains 95 milligrams of aluminum hydroxide and 412 milligrams of magnesium carbonate in each 15 milliliters (one tablespoonful). When you dispense this product to a patient, tell him that the container should be shaken well before the dose is taken.

i. **Simethicone (Mylicon®).** Simethicone is used as an antiflatulent. An antiflatulent is a product which relieves the painful symptoms of excess gas in the gastrointestinal system by breaking apart mucous surrounded gas pockets or preventing their formation. The usual dose of this product is 40 to 80 milligrams four times daily after meals and at bedtime. When you dispense this product in tablet form, you should tell the patient to chew the tablet(s) thoroughly before swallowing. Mylicon® is supplied in two forms--tablets (40 or 80 milligrams per tablet) and drops (40 milligrams per 0.6 milliliters).

j. **Aluminum Hydroxide, Magnesium Hydroxide, and Simethicone (Mylanta®, Gelusil®).** This product is used as a gastric antacid, antiflatulant, and as an agent useful in ulcer therapy. The side effects associated with this preparation (depending on the dose) are diarrhea and constipation. This product is available in both suspension and tablet form. The formulation of the product by form basis is below:

	Aluminum Hydroxide	Magnesium Hydroxide	Simethicone
Tablets	200 milligrams	200 milligrams	25 milligrams (Gelusil®)
Suspension (per 5 milliliters)	200 milligrams	200 milligrams	20 milligrams (Mylanta®)

CAUTION: When you dispense the tablets, you should tell the patient to chew them thoroughly before swallowing. When you dispense the suspension, you should tell the patient to shake the container well before taking the dose.

k. **Other**. Many other antacid preparations are stocked in military and civilian pharmacies. You should use available references (Physicians' Desk Reference, United States Pharmacopeia Dispensing Information, etc.) to discover any specific information you want to learn about a particular product. Some of these products are:

(1) Aluminum carbonate (Basojel®).

(2) Dihydroxyaluminum sodium carbonate (Rolaids®).

(3) Dihydroxyaluminum amino acetate.

(4) Aluminum phosphate (Phosphajel®).

(5) Magnesium oxide.

(6) Magnesium carbonate.

Section II. DIGESTANTS

2-4. DEFINITION

Digestants are a group of drugs used to promote the process of digestion in the gastrointestinal tract.

2-5. INDICATION OF DIGESTANT THERAPY

A digestant is indicated when there is evidence of insufficient functioning of some part of the digestive system responsible for producing a substance necessary for the digestion of food. Viewed from this area, the digestants are substances used in deficiency states. Digestants commonly employed are the choleretics (e.g., bile salts), pancreatic enzymes, and hydrochloric acid.

2-6. EXAMPLES OF DIGESTANTS

a. **Glutamic Acid Hydrochloride.** Glutamic acid hydrochloride is used in the treatment of patients who are either secreting no stomach acid (achlorhydria) or are secreting little stomach acid (hypochlorhydria). Once prepared, the acid solution is sipped through a glass straw in order to minimize damage to the teeth.

b. **Dehydrocholic Acid, NF.** Dehydrocholic acid is used to increase the volume of bile produced and secreted in the digestive system. It is used to relieve excessive constipation as well as to remove fragments of gallstones from the body. The usual dose of this drug is 3 to 5 milliliters of a 20 percent solution administered intravenously.

c. **Pancrelipase (Cotazyme®).** This product is used as a pancreatic enzyme supplement. The usual dosage of pancrelipase is one to three capsules or one to two packets of the powder before or with meals. The preparation is available in both capsule or powder (regular and cherry flavor). When you dispense the granules, tell the patient to mix the granules with food or with water.

d. **Pancreatin (Panteric®).** Pancreatin is used as a pancreatic enzyme supplement. The usual dosage of the product is one to three tablets with meals.

e. **Other**. Other digestants are commonly stocked in military and civilian pharmacies. To learn of the specific uses and side effects of these agents, you should read a reference such as Physicians' Desk Reference. Examples of these digestants are:

(1) Glutamic acid hydrochloride (Acidulin®).

(2) Ox bile extract.

(3) Ox bile extract, pancreatin, pepsin, glutamic acid, hydrochloride, and cellulose (Kanulase®).

Continue with Exercises

EXERCISES, LESSON 2

INSTRUCTIONS: The following exercises are to be answered by marking the lettered response that best answers the question or best completes the incomplete statement or by writing the answer in the space provided.

After you have completed all the exercises, turn to "Solutions to Exercises" at the end of the lesson and check your answers.

1. A digestant is defined as:

    a. A drug used to promote the process of digestion in the gastrointestinal tract.

    b. A product used to reduce the amount of hydrochloric acid in the stomach.

    c. A drug used to break apart mucous--surrounded gas pockets in order to relieve painful symptoms of excess gas.

    d. A drug used as an antiflatulent.

2. Antacids are indicated in the treatment of:

    a. Minor stomach irritations.

    b. Flatulence.

    c. Ulcers.

    d. Both a and b above.

    e. Both a and c above.

3. Which of the following is a consideration involved in the selection of an antacid?

    a. The speed at which the antacid neutralizes stomach acid.

    b. The amount of the antacid required to neutralize the stomach acid.

    c. The tendency of the antacid to be absorbed systemically and affect the blood pH.

    d. All of the above.

4. From the statements below, select the one which describes a consideration involved in the selection of an antacid.

  a. Whether or not the antacid has a tendency to produce acid rebound.

  b. The degree to which the antacid acts as an antiflatulent.

  c. The inability of the antacid product to ionize in the intestines.

  d. The ability of the product to produce catharsis.

5. Titralac® is used as a(n):

  a. Pancreatic enzyme replacement.

  b. Gastric antacid.

  c. Laxative/antacid.

  d. Antiflatulent.

6. Magnesium hydroxide (milk of magnesia) is used as a(n)

  a. Laxative and an antiflatulent.

  b. Laxative and an antacid.

  c. Antacid and an antiflatulent.

  d. Digestant and an antiflatulent.

7. Calcium carbonate and glycine has what side effect(s)?

  a. Acid rebound.

  b. Systemic alkalization.

  c. Both a and b above.

8. A patient is about to receive Gaviscon® tablets. What caution and warning should be told to the patient?

    a. Swallow the tablets without chewing them.

    b. Chew the tablets thoroughly before you swallow.

    c. The tablets should not be taken by a person who has hypotension.

    d. The tablets should be quickly swallowed in order to avoid damage to the tissues of the mouth.

9. You have just dispensed some pancrelipase granules to a patient. Which of the statements below should you tell the patient?

    a. Chew the tablets before swallowing.

    b. Do not take the granules within two hours after taking a prescription antibiotic.

    c. Mix the granules with food or with water.

    d. Mix the granules in orange juice and swallow the solution quickly to avoid damage to the tissues of the mouth.

10. Dehydrocholic acid, NF, is used to:

    a. Provide hydrochloric acid to patients whose stomachs make little or no stomach acid.

    b. Stimulate the production of insulin in patients who have diabetes mellitus.

    c. Reduce flatulence.

    d. Increase the volume of bile produced and secreted in the digestive system.

SPECIAL INSTRUCTIONS FOR EXERCISES 11 THROUGH 14. In exercises 11 through 14, match the trade name in Column B with its corresponding generic name in Column A.

	Column A		**Column B**
11. _____	Aluminum hydroxide, magnesium hydroxide, and simethicome	a.	Cotazyme®
		b.	Mylanta®
12. _____	Pancrelipase	c.	Mylicon®
13. _____	Calcium carbonate and glycine	d.	Titralac®
14. _____	Simethicone		

Check Your Answers on Next Page

SOLUTIONS TO EXERCISES, LESSON 2

1. a   (para 2-4)

2. e   (para 2-2b)

3. d   (para 2-2c)

4. a   (para 2-3c(4))

5. b   (para 2-3b)

6. b   (para 2-3c)

7. c   (para 2-3b)

8. b   (para 2-3g)

9. c   (para 2-6c)

10. d   (para 2-6b)

11. b   (para 2-3j)

12. a   (para 2-6c)

13. d   (para 2-3b)

14. c   (para 2-3i)

End of Lesson 2

LESSON ASSIGNMENT

LESSON 3   Emetics, Antiemetics, and Antidiarrheals.

LESSON ASSIGNMENT   Paragraphs 3-1 through 3-8.

LESSON OBJECTIVES   After completing this lesson, you should be able to:

3-1.   Given one of the following terms: emetic, antiemetic, or antidiarrheal and a group of statements, select the statement that best defines the given term.

3-2.   Given a group of situational statements and one of the following terms: emetic, antiemetic, or antidiarrheal, select the statement that best describes an indication for the use of that type of agent.

3-3.   Given the trade and/or generic name of an emetic, antiemetic, or antidiarrheal and a group of indications, uses, side effects, cautions or warnings, or patient instructions, select the indication(s), use(s), side effect(s), caution(s) or warning(s), or patient instruction(s) for the given agent.

3-4.   Given the trade or generic name of an emetic, antiemetic, or antidiarrheal and a list of trade and/or generic names, select the corresponding trade or generic name for the given drug name.

SUGGESTION   After completing the assignment, complete the exercises at the end of this lesson. These exercises will help you to achieve the lesson objectives.

LESSON 3

EMETICS, ANTIEMETICS, AND ANTIDIARRHEALS

Section I. OVERVIEW

3-1. INTRODUCTION

Emetics, antiemetics, and antidiarrheals are three categories of drugs that affect the gastrointestinal system. Each category of agents has its own distinct use for the relief of patient discomfort. You must be familiar with these agents in order to provide the patient with information which will enhance the medication's therapeutic effect and/or provide greater patient safety and comfort.

3-2. DEFINITIONS

Before any discussion is made of individual categories and specific agents, it is necessary for you to learn/review the definition of each of these categories.

a. **Emetic.** An emetic is a chemical agent which will cause the patient to vomit (i.e., produce emesis). Emesis is <u>sometimes</u> indicated when a patient ingests certain chemical substances.

b. **Antiemetic.** An antiemetic is an agent which prevents or alleviates nausea and vomiting. Antiemetics are sometimes used to treat the nausea and vomiting associated with motion sickness, pregnancy, or an illness.

c. **Antidiarrheal.** An antidiarrheal is an agent used to control diarrhea. Antidiarrheals are sometimes prescribed to patients who have severe diarrhea.

Section II. EMETICS

3-3. INTRODUCTION

An emetic is a chemical agent that will cause the patient to vomit (i.e., to produce emesis). A physician may administer an emetic to a patient who has ingested a certain type of chemical substance. <u>Emetics are not indicated for all poisonings</u>. Prior to administering an emetic to a poisoning victim, the local poison control center should be consulted to determine if this is the best procedure to follow.

3-4. EXAMPLES OF EMETIC AGENTS

a. **Ipecac Syrup, USP.** Ipecac syrup is a clear, amber, hydroalcoholic preparation used in the treatment of poisoning and/or drug overdoses. This product acts by stimulating the chemoreceptor trigger zone and by irritating the gastric mucosa. Emesis usually occurs within 15 minutes after ingestion. The recommended dose of ipecac syrup is one or two <u>teaspoonsful</u> in children who are less than one year old and three <u>teaspoonsful</u> in persons over one year old. To aid emesis, one or two glasses of water or fruit juice can be ingested after the ipecac syrup is taken. Carbonated beverages, milk, or activated charcoal should not be taken with this product. In particular, milk and activated charcoal are thought to decrease the effectiveness of ipecac syrup. If it is thought necessary to administer activated charcoal, the activated charcoal should be given <u>after</u> emesis has occurred.

b. **Ipecac Tincture and Ipecac Fluidextract.** Ipecac syrup, USP, has replaced ipecac tincture and ipecac fluidextract as the preferred form of ipecac. Ipecac fluidextract is 14 times more concentrated than ipecac syrup. Hence, giving the patient three teaspoonsful of ipecac fluidextract can be potentially dangerous to the patient.

Section III. ANTIEMETICS

3-5. INTRODUCTION/INDICATIONS FOR ANTIEMETIC THERAPY

Antiemetics are agents which prevent or alleviate nausea and vomiting. These agents are indicated when the physician wishes to prevent or alleviate nausea and vomiting, especially when it is associated with motion sickness, pregnancy, or an illness. For example, a child with the flu, with serious vomiting, can lose large volumes of fluid. An antiemetic can help to reduce that vomiting with a resultant reduction in fluid loss.

3-6. EXAMPLES OF ANTIEMETICS

a. **Prochlorperazine (Compazine®).** Prochlorperazine is an agent that is widely used to control severe nausea and vomiting. As an antiemetic, the usual oral dose is five to 10 milligrams three or four times a day. When given rectally in suppository form, the dose is 25 milligrams two times a day. Intramuscular injection in a dosage of 5 to 10 milligrams a day is sometimes ordered, the patient may repeat the dosage every three to four hours, but the total dosage should not exceed 40 milligrams per day. Compazine is supplied as 5, 10, and 25 milligram tablets; 2.5, 5, and 25 milligram suppositories; and 5 milligrams per milliliter injection. When you dispense this product, tell the patient that prochlorperazine may cause drowsiness and warn him to avoid taking the product with alcohol.

b. **Trimethobenzamide (Tigan®).** Trimethobenzamide is indicated for use as an antiemetic in the treatment of nausea and vomiting. The usual side effect associated with this drug is drowsiness. Patients taking this product should be warned not to take it with alcohol. The usual oral dose of trimethobenzamide is 250 milligrams three to four times daily, while the rectal and injection routes of administration have the usual dosage of 200 milligrams given three to four times daily. This product is supplied as 100 to 250 milligram capsules, 200 milligram suppositories, and 100 milligrams per milliliter intramuscular injection.

c. **Dimenhydrinate (Dramamine®).** Dimenhydrinate has been used for many years in the treatment of motion sickness. The usual side effect associated with the administration of this agent is drowsiness. The patient taking this medication should be informed about the drowsiness and that alcohol should not be consumed while taking this drug. Dimenhydrinate has as its usual dose one tablet two hours before travel, then one tablet every four hours as needed for nausea and vomiting. Dramamine® is supplied as a 50 milligram tablet.

d. **Meclizine (Bonine®).** Meclizine is an antiemetic normally used in the treatment of motion sickness. It is frequently prescribed for vertigo; hence, one company's trade name for meclizine is Antivert®. Drowsiness is the most prominent side effect associated with this product. You should inform the patient of this side effect when you dispense it. Likewise, you should tell the patient that meclizine should not be taken with alcohol. The usual dose for motion sickness is 25 to 50 milligrams one hour before travel. This dose may be taken every 24 hours if necessary. In the treatment of vertigo (dizziness), the recommended dose is 25 to 100 milligrams per day in divided doses. Bonine® is supplied as 25 milligram chewable tablets, while Antivert® is available in 12.5 and 25 milligram tablets.

Section IV. ANTIDIARRHEALS

3-7. INTRODUCTION

Antidiarrheals are agents used to control diarrhea. Antidiarrheals are indicated in patients who have severe diarrhea. Antidiarrheals not only can make life more pleasant for persons so afflicted, they can really prevent the body from losing a great volume of fluid.

3-8. EXAMPLES OF ANTIDIARRHEAL AGENTS

a. **Attapulgite (Kaopectate®).** It is used for its adsorbent and protectant action. This product is effective for minor diarrhea. The usual dose of Kaopectate® is two to four tablespoonsful after each loose bowel movement.

b. **Paregoric.** The active ingredient in paregoric is its morphine component. This morphine component is helpful in treating diarrhea because it reduces the intestinal motility and digestive secretions. The result is that the movement of the stool through the small and large intestines is slowed. This effect allows more water to be absorbed out of the stool. This helps produce a stool of a more solid mass. Furthermore, paregoric causes the tone of the anal sphincter to be increased and this, combined with the dulling of the sensation to defecate aids in the constipating effect of the drug. The patient taking paregoric should be cautioned against taking the drug with alcohol or any other central nervous system (CNS) depressant. Furthermore, the patient should be informed that the product can cause drowsiness. The usual dosage of paregoric is 5 to 10 milliliters (one to two teaspoon(s)full four times a day. Paregoric is supplied as a liquid. It is a Note Q item.

c. **Diphenoxylate with Atropine (Lomotil®).** Lomotil® is an antidiarrheal that acts by slowing intestinal motility. Since this drug may cause drowsiness, patients taking it should be cautioned about this. Theoretically, at high doses Lomotil® can be addicting. Therefore, Lomotil® is a Note Q item. A subtherapeutic dose of atropine is added to the product to discourage deliberate overdosage. The usual dose of Lomotil® is one or two tables four times a day. It is supplied in tablet form, each tablet contains 2.5 milligrams of diphenoxylate and 0.025 milligram of atropine sulfate and in liquid form containing the same amount of each drug in 5 milliliters (one teaspoonful) of solution.

d. **Loperamide (Imodium®).** Loperamide is another drug which acts by slowing intestinal motility. Since this agent may cause drowsiness, the patient should be cautioned against doing anything requiring mental alertness while taking the drug. Imodium® is supplied in the form of 2 milligram capsules. The usual dose is 4 milligrams (two capsules) immediately, then 2 milligrams (one capsule) after each loose bowel movement.

e. **Attapulgite (Parepectolin®).** Attapulgite is used in the treatment of diarrhea. A side effect associated with this agent is stool may temporarily appear gray-black. Also if diarrhea is accompanied by high fever or continues for more then 2 days, consult physician. The patient should be informed of this side effect.

Continue with Exercises

EXERCISES, LESSON 3

INSTRUCTIONS: The following exercises are to be answered by marking the lettered response that best answers the question or best completes the incomplete statement or by writing the answer in the space provided.

After you have completed all the exercises, turn to "Solutions to Exercises" at the end of the lesson and check your answers.

1.   An emetic is best defined as:

    a.   A chemical agent that will prevent or alleviate nausea and vomiting.

    b.   A chemical agent that will produce diuresis.

    c.   A chemical agent that will control fluid bowel movements.

    d.   A chemical agent that will cause a person to vomit.

2.   An antidiarrheal is indicated in some instances in which the patient:

    a.   Has severe diarrhea with resultant fluid loss.

    b   Has soft stool.

    c.   Has nausea and vomiting.

    d.   Has intestinal cramps and stomach pain.

3.   Lomotil® is used as a(n):

    a.   Antiemetic.

    b.   Laxative.

    c.   Antidiarrheal.

    d.   Emetic.

4. The patient taking paregoric should be cautioned:

   a. That the product can produce central nervous system (CNS) stimulation.

   b. Not to take the product with alcohol or any other central nervous system depressant.

   c. To take the product only on a full stomach.

   d. That the product can produce excess intestinal gas.

5. Meclizine is a product normally used in the treatment of:

   a. Motion sickness.

   b. Diarrhea.

   c. Stomach cramps.

   d. Flatulence.

6. The side effect usually associated with trimethobenzamide is:

   a. Nausea.

   b. Drowsiness.

   c. Vomiting.

   d. Diarrhea.

7. Dramamine is used in the treatment of:

   a. Drug overdoses.

   b. Vertigo.

   c. Motion sickness.

   d. Diarrhea.

8. Patients taking Compazine® should be warned:

   a. Not to take the drug with carbonated beverages, milk, or activated charcoal.

   b. That the drug can cause severe constipation.

   c. Not to take the drug with alcohol.

   d. That the drug can produce nausea and vomiting.

9. Kaopectate® is used in the treatment of:

   a. Stomach cramps.

   b. Drug overdoses.

   c. Excess gas in the gastrointestinal tract.

   d. Minor diarrhea.

SPECIAL INSTRUCTIONS FOR EXERCISES 10 THROUGH 13. In exercises 10 through 13, match the trade name in Column B with its corresponding generic name in Column A.

Column A	Column B
10. ___ Meclizine	a. Lomotil®
11. ___ Diphenoxylate with Atropine	b. Imodium®
12. ___ Prochlorperazine	c. Compazine®
13. ___ Loperamide	d. Bonine®

Check Your Answers on Next Page

SOLUTIONS TO EXERCISES, LESSON 3

1. d   (para 3-3)

2. a   (para 3-7)

3. c   (para 3-8c)

4. b   (para 3-8b)

5. a   (para 3-6d)

6. b   (para 3-6b)

7. c   (para 3-6c)

8. c   (para 3-6a)

9. d   (para 3-8a)

10. d   (para 3-6e)

11. a   (para 3-6a)

12. c   (para 3-6a)

13. b   (para 3-8d)

End of Lesson 3

LESSON ASSIGNMENT

LESSON 4   Cathartics.

LESSON ASSIGNMENT   Paragraphs 4-1 through 4-10.

LESSON OBJECTIVES   After completing this lesson, you should be able to:

4-1. Given a group of statements, select the statement that best defines the term cathartic.

4-2. From a group of statements, select the statement that best describes the cathartic (laxative) habit.

4-3. Given a list of factors, select those factors that can help most people maintain normal bowel   habits.

4-4. Given a group of statements, select the statement(s) which best describe(s) precautions associated with the use of cathartics.

4-5. Given a group of statements, select the information statement that should be told to persons taking cathartics.

4-6. Given the name of one of the categories of cathartics (by mechanism of action) and a group of statements, select the statement that best describes the mechanism of action for that cathartic category.

4-7. Given the trade and/or generic name of a cathartic and a list of categories of cathartics (by mechanism of action), select the category for which that particular agent belongs.

4-8. Given the name of one of the five categories of cathartics (by mechanism of action) and a group of statements, select the statement that describes an important dosage consideration, precaution, or patient information associated with that category

4-9. Given the trade and/or generic name of a cathartic and a group of uses, side effects, cautions and warnings, or patient information statements, select the use(s), side effect(s), caution(s), and warnings or patient information statement(s) associated with the given agent.

4-10. Given the trade or generic name of a cathartic agent and a list of trade and/or generic names, select the corresponding trade or generic name of the given agent.

SUGGESTION

After completing the assignment, complete the exercises at the end of this lesson. These exercises will help you to achieve the lesson objectives.

LESSON 4

CATHARTICS

Section I. INTRODUCTION

4-1. OVERVIEW

Cathartics are a group of drugs which cause an evacuation of the bowel (i.e., bowel movement). This group is one of the most abused categories of drugs. Why? The answer is simple, most people believe that something is wrong with them if they don't have at least one bowel movement a day.

4-2. DEFINITION OF A CATHARTIC

A cathartic is any agent which causes an evacuation of the bowel (i.e., causes a bowel movement). You may have heard the term laxative used instead of cathartic. Not all cathartics have to be purchased in a drug store. Remember, food such as prunes and bran may be categorized as cathartics because of their ability to cause evacuation of the bowels.

4-3. THE CATHARTIC (LAXATIVE) HABIT

The physician seldom has the opportunity to prescribe cathartics, except in the hospital setting, since valid indications for the use of laxatives are limited. More commonly, the physician is faced with the problem of chronic misuse of these agents by his patients. The task the physician faces is a difficult one; the patient must be helped to break the cathartic habit. The cathartic habit is the extensive, chronic misuse of self-prescribed cathartics by a bowel-conscious person. Cathartics are taken by many people because they believe they must have a bowel movement at least once each day.

4-4. THE NORMAL FUNCTIONING OF THE BOWELS

The digestive process, from the intake of food to the elimination of the waste products from that ingestion, may take from one to three days depending on the composition of the food. The number of times a healthy person defecates can vary from once or twice a day to one bowel movement every one or two days. Many persons who don't know a great deal about bowel habits often take cathartics so they can have daily bowel movements. After a while, this results in an inability of the bowel to be stimulated by normal body function. The person then begins to rely entirely on the ingestion of cathartics for bowel movements. This is known as the cathartic habit. Time and education are required before the person can remove this dependence upon cathartics.

4-5. FACTORS WHICH HELP TO MAINTAIN NORMAL BOWEL HABITS

The following factors, if followed, can help most people maintain normal (whatever that means for each person) bowel habits without the use of cathartics.

a. **Exercise.** Exercise helps to maintain muscle tone.

b. **Proper Diet.** Ingesting foods containing high fiber content provides the bulk needed by the digestive system for normal bowel functioning.

c. **Fluids.** Each person should drink several glasses of water a day (unless this is not allowed by the physician) in order to give the body the water it needs for the proper functioning of <u>all</u> its systems.

d. **Routine.** Slow down and relax. Establish a time and a place (i.e., a routine) where you can relax and have bowel movements.

4-6. PRECAUTIONS ASSOCIATED WITH THE USE OF CATHARTICS

It is important that persons not believe that they should take a cathartic every time they fail to have a daily bowel movement. The precautions below are important in that they provide some basic guidelines dealing with the ingestion of cathartics.

a. Do not take a cathartic within two hours after having taken another drug. Taking a drug with a cathartic will have an effect upon the absorption of that drug, it may result in either more or less of the drug being absorbed.

b. Do not take a cathartic if you do not have a bowel movement for several days.

c. Do not take a cathartic just to take one. Some persons believe it is therapeutic to periodically take a cathartic. This is not true. In fact, too frequently taking a cathartic can result in a patient's having the "laxative habit."

d. Do not take a cathartic if you developed a skin rash after having taken it the last time.

e. Do not take a cathartic for more than one week unless your physician has told you otherwise.

f. Do not take a cathartic if you have the following signs --tenderness in the stomach or lower abdominal area, soreness in the abdomen, bloating, vomiting, or nausea.

Section II. CATHARTIC AGENTS

4-7. INTRODUCTION

Not all cathartics have the same mechanism of action. In fact, there are several categories of cathartics, each has a particular mechanism of action. These categories are bulk-forming cathartics, lubricant cathartics, stimulant cathartics, emollient cathartics (also known as stool softeners), and hyperosmotic cathartics.

4-8. IMPORTANT INFORMATION FOR PERSONS TAKING CATHARTICS

Persons who take cathartics should be told of the importance of drinking extra fluids. In fact, a person who is taking a laxative should drink at least six to eight full glasses of fluid (each glass should be equal to 8 fluid ounces, 240 milliliters). This extra fluid helps the cathartic to produce its effects faster. Certain cathartics (e.g., those in the bulk-forming category) require fluid in addition to the six to eight glasses of fluid they should be drinking. This additional fluid should be taken when ingesting the cathartic.

4-9. MECHANISMS OF ACTION OF CATHARTICS

Each category of cathartics has its own particular mechanism of action. The mechanisms of action are important because the physician may select a particular agent because of the specific favorable results obtained as a direct effect of a mechanism of action.

a. **Bulk-Forming Cathartics.** These cathartics absorb water and provide bulk for the gastrointestinal tract. The increased bulk provides stimulation to the bowels (peristalsis).

b. **Lubricant Cathartics.** Lubricant cathartics increase the fluid level in the small intestines. They do this by coating the surfaces of the stool and the intestines. This coating results in decreased absorption of water and increase in the volume of water in the intestines. This effect also eases the flow of stool through the intestines by lubrication.

c. **Stimulant Cathartics.** Stimulant cathartics increase the rate of peristalsis in the intestine by directly acting on the smooth muscle of the intestine.

d. **Emollient Cathartics.** Emollient cathartics reduce the surface film tension of the stool. This allows for fluids to penetrate the stool and thus to make the stool softer.

e. **Hyperosmotic Cathartics.** Hyperosmotic cathartics are concentrated solutions of substances which draw water into the intestine. Increased water content of the stool further stimulates peristalsis.

4-10. CATEGORIES AND SPECIFIC EXAMPLES OF CATHARTICS

Many cathartics are on the shelves of military and civilian pharmacies. You can help yourself (and your patients) if you are able to categorize a specific agent into a particular category of agents. Why? Because each category of cathartics has certain general information that pertain to drug interactions, side effects, and patient precautionary statements. Therefore, if you are able to correctly categorize an agent, you should be able to predict side effects and precautionary statements related to that product. The information below provides you with general information pertaining to each category of drugs. Invest some time learning this material. Specific statements pertaining to side effects and precautionary statements will not be repeated when the individual agents are discussed.

    a. **Bulk-Forming Cathartics.** The person taking a bulk-forming cathartics should be told to drink a full glass of fluid (one glass = 8 fluid ounces = 240 milliliters) when ingesting the cathartic. Persons taking bulk-forming cathartics should not expect immediate results. Instead, they should be told that the bulk-forming cathartics take from one to three days to produce their effects. Furthermore, it is generally recommended that the patient taking antibiotics, anticoagulants, digitalis preparations, or salicylates wait at least two hours after they take a dose of these drugs before they ingest the cathartics. This is recommended because the interaction between the drug and the cathartic could result in less of the drug being absorbed. Side effects are rare with the bulk-forming cathartics. However, intestinal impaction has occurred in patients who did not drink enough water while taking the products. The cathartic habit does not occur with bulk-forming laxatives. Consequently, they are sometimes prescribed for extended use.

    (1) <u>Malt soup extract (Maltsupex®)</u>. This product is available in tablet, liquid, and powder form. Label these products "Take with a full glass of water."

    (2) <u>Methylcellulose (Cellothyl®)</u>. Methylcellulose is available in tablet, capsule, solution, and powder form. Label these products "Take with a full glass of water."

    (3) <u>Polycarbophil calcium (Mitrolan®)</u>. This product is available in tablet form. The patient should be told to chew or crush the tablets before swallowing them.

NOTE: This product is sometimes given at 1/2 hour intervals in the treatment of diarrhea.

    (4) <u>Psyllium (Effersyllium®, Serutan®)</u>. This product is available in powder form. The powder should be placed in 1/2 glass of water (one full teaspoonful in 1/2 glass of water). When the product is dispensed, tell the patient to keep the container in a dry place and keep it tightly capped.

b. **Lubricant Cathartics.** Lubricant cathartics are usually ingested at bedtime. The patient should not take a lubricant cathartic with meals, since this could interfere with the absorption of food, vitamins, and minerals in the gastrointestinal tract. Furthermore, patients should be warned not to take lubricant cathartics for long periods because of the absorption problems (e.g., reduced absorption of vitamins) associated with their use. Lubricant laxatives usually provide results within 12 hours after ingestion. Lastly, patients taking lubricant cathartics should be cautioned to protect their clothing, since some leakage might occur from the rectum.

Product: Mineral Oil (Nujol®). The oral dosage of this product, one to three tablespoonsful, is usually given at bedtime. Several strengths of this product are available (emulsion-50%; jell-55%; and plain-100%).

---

c. **Stimulant Cathartics.** Side effects associated with stimulant cathartics include belching, diarrhea, and cramping. Stimulant cathartics should be taken on an empty stomach in order to produce faster effects. Potassium loss, cramping, the laxative habit, and pinkish urine or stool are effects associated with stimulant cathartics.

(1) Bisacodyl (Dulcolax®). Bisacodyl is available in tablet form (five milligrams per tablet). The usual dose is two to three tablets. Only one dose of the medication is taken. The tablets should be swallowed whole with a full glass of water (8 fluid ounces = 240 milliliters). The patient taking this product should be warned not to chew or crush the tablet (the contents have a bitter taste). Furthermore, the patient should be cautioned not to take this product within one hour after taking antacids or milk, since these products may cause the enteric coating of the tablet to be prematurely removed in the stomach and result in gastric irritation.

(2) Cascara (Cas-Evac®). Cascara is available as the aromatic cascara fluid extract and as cascara tablets. Persons receiving the fluid extract should be told to thoroughly shake the container before taking the dose. Persons taking either product should be told that cascara can discolor the urine.

(3) Castor oil (Alphamul®, Neoloid®). Castor oil is available in an emulsified form as well as in an aromatic form. The usual adult dose of this product is from one to four tablespoonsful.

(4) Danthron (Dorbane®). This product is available in both tablet and solution form. The solution dosage form contains five percent ethyl alcohol. Persons taking this drug should be warned that their urine may become discolored because of the preparation.

(5) Dehydrocholic acid (Decholin®). This product is available in 250 milligram tablets. The usual adult dose of dehydrocholic acid is one tablet three or four times a day. This product is not recommended for patients under 12 years of age.

(6) Phenolphthalein (Alophen®, Evac-U-Gen®, Ex-Lax®, Feen-A-Mint®). Phenolphthalein is available in the form of chewing gum, tablets, and chewable tablets. Patients taking the gum should be told to chew the gum well and not to swallow it. Patients receiving this product should be told that phenolphthalein may discolor their urine.

(7) Senna (Black Draught®, Fletcher's Castoria®). Senna is available in a variety of forms. Patients taking this product should be told that it may discolor their urine.

d. **Emollient Cathartics.** Skin rashes, gastric cramping, and irritated throats (with liquid preparations) are sometimes associated with emollient agents. In general, emollients are used to soften hard, dry stools in order to ease defecation. Results are not immediately obtained with emollient cathartics. Instead, it takes approximately one to three days for this type of cathartic to produce results after the first dose is taken. Patients taking emollient cathartics should be cautioned not to take mineral oil or other laxatives since they might be absorbed to a greater degree. Since some emollient products have a rather bitter taste, the patient can take the preparations with milk or fruit juice to mask the unpleasant taste. Emollient cathartics will not produce the cathartic habit, but they will increase absorption through the lipid membrane. Consequently, they are not prescribed for extended periods.

(1) Docusate calcium (Surfak®). Docusate calcium is available in 50 and 240 milligram tablets. The usual adult dose of the product is one (240 milligram) tablet a day taken with a full glass of water. Ensure that you tell the patient to drink adequate fluids while taking the medication, since this will enhance the stool softening effect of the medication. Docusate is available in several salts (calcium, potassium, and sodium) and in several dosage forms. Docusate sodium is a product available under the trade name of Colace®.

(2) Poloxamer 188 (Alxin®, Magcyl®). This product is available in 240 and 250 milligram capsules. The usual adult dose of Poloxamer 188 is one capsule one to three times a day with a glass of water.

e. **Hyperosmotic Cathartics.** Hyperosmotic cathartics are divided into two categories, lactulose and saline cathartics. Because saline cathartics tend to produce nonabsorbable complexes with tetracyclines, patients taking saline cathartics should be cautioned not to take them within one to three hours after taking tetracycline. Saline cathartics produce rapid results--defecation is achieved within two to eight hours after taking the product. Therefore, the person should not take a saline cathartic late at night or immediately before going to bed. Since some saline cathartics contain sugar and/or sodium, diabetics and persons who must reduce their intake of sodium should check each product for its composition. Saline cathartics should not be given to children six years of age and under.

(1) Lactulose (Chronulac®). Lactulose is available in syrup form with 10 grams of lactulose per tablespoonful. The usual adult dose of this product is from one to two tablespoonful a day. This product should be protected from freezing. The prolonged exposure of this product to high temperatures may produce a darkening of the product; however, the darkening does not decrease the therapeutic effectiveness of the active ingredient. When you dispense this product, you should tell the patient that the dose may be combined with water, milk, or fruit juice to improve the taste. Lactulose produces results in one to two days.

(2) Magnesium citrate (citrate of magnesia). This product is available in the form of an effervescent solution. The usual oral dose of this product is 200 milliliters of the solution. The solution may lose some of its effervescence upon standing, but this does not reduce its therapeutic effectiveness (although it does affect the taste of the product).

(3) Magnesium sulfate crystals (epsom salts). This product is supplied in crystal form which is to be dissolved in water before taking. The usual adult dose of the product is 15 grams in a glass of water (8 fluid ounces = 240 milliliters) as one dose. The crystals may be placed in a lemon-lime carbonated beverage in order to improve the taste.

(4) Sodium phosphate (Fleets Phospho-Soda®). Sodium phosphate is available in the form of effervescent sodium phosphate powder and sodium phosphate oral solution. The powder should be dissolved in one full glass of water and then ingested (adult dose--10 to 20 grams per glass of water).   The usual adult dose of the oral solution is 10 to 40 milliliters (as one dose) mixed in a glass of water (240 milliliters).   You should note that sodium phosphate contains large amounts of sodium. This information is important for persons who must restrict their intake of sodium.

Continue with Exercises

EXERCISES, LESSON 4

INSTRUCTIONS: The following exercises are to be answered by marking the lettered response that best answers the question or best completes the incomplete statement or by writing the answer in the space provided.

After you have completed all the exercises, turn to "Solutions to Exercises" at the end of the lesson and check your answers.

1. The term cathartic is best defined as an agent that:

    a. Causes an evacuation of the bowel.

    b. Produces emesis.

    c. Causes the bowels to move on a daily basis.

    d. Softens the stool in order to produce a bowel movement with less effort.

2. Which of the following can help people maintain normal bowel habits?

    a. Establishing a time of day when they can relax and have a bowel movement.

    b. Eating foods high in protein and carbohydrates.

    c. Eating food which is soft and not bulky.

    d. All of the above.

3. What precaution(s) is/are associated with the use of cathartics?

    a. Do not take a cathartic if there is tenderness in the stomach or lower abdominal area.

    b. Do not take a cathartic if a skin rash developed immediately after the last dose of the drug was taken.

    c. Do not take a cathartic just for the sake of taking one.

    d. All of the above.

4. Select the statement that best describes the mechanism of action of emollient cathartics.

    a. These agents increase the fluid level In the small intestines which helps move the ingested material through the bowels.

    b. These agents increase the rate of peristalsis in the intestine by directly acting on the smooth muscle of the intestine.

    c. These agents reduce the surface film tension of the stool allowing fluids to penetrate the stool and make the stool softer.

    d. These agents absorb water and provide bulk for the gastrointestinal tract.

5. Phenolphthalein (Alophen®) is classified as a(n) _____ cathartic.

    a. Lubricant.

    b. Emollient.

    c. Bulk-forming.

    d. Stimulant.

6. Mineral oil (Nujol®) is classified as a(n) _____ cathartic.

    a. Emollient.

    b. Lubricant.

    c. Stimulant.

    d. Bulk-forming.

7. A patient taking a lubricant cathartic should be told:

    a. To take the product on an empty stomach in order to obtain faster results.

    b. Not to take this type of cathartic for a long period because this cathartic can decrease the absorption of vitamins from the gastrointestinal tract.

    c. That this type of agent usually requires two to three days to produce a bowel movement.

    d. Take the product with an emollient cathartic in order to produce faster results.

8. Patients taking senna (Black Draught®) should be told:

    a. The drug may discolor their urine.

    b. They should not take the product for a long period because it can interfere with vitamin absorption in the gastrointestinal tract.

    c. They should protect their clothing since some leakage of the product may occur from the rectum.

    d. They should not expect the product to produce bowel movements until three to four days after they initially take the product.

9. Select the special labeling information which should be included on the label when you dispense methylcellulose (Cellothyl®) tablets.

    a. "Chew tablets thoroughly before swallowing."

    b. "Warning: This product may cause your urine to become pinkish."

    c. "Protect this product from light since light may cause discoloration."

    d. "Take with a full glass of water."

10. Patients taking polycarbophil calcium tablets should be told to:

    a. Avoid chewing or crushing the tablets because of their bitter taste.

    b. Chew or crush the tablets before taking them.

    c. Expect their urine to be pinkish or red in color because of the medication.

    d. They should take the medication with milk or fruit juice to mask the medication's unpleasant taste.

SPECIAL INSTRUCTIONS FOR EXERCISES 11 THROUGH 14. In exercises 11 through 14, match the trade name in Column B with its corresponding generic name in Column A.

Column A	Column B
11. __ Bisacodyl	a. Dulcolax®
12. __ Lactulose	b. Chronulac®
13. __ Psyllium	c. Ex-Lax®
14. __ Phenolphthalein	d. Serutan®

Check Your Answers on Next Page

SOLUTIONS TO EXERCISES, LESSON 4

1. a   (para 4-2)

2. a   (para 4-5)

3. d   (para 4-6)

4. c   (para 4-9d)

5. d   (para 4-10c(6))

6. b   (para 4-10b)

7. b   (para 4-10b)

8. a   (para 4-10c(7))

9. d   (para 4-10a(2))

10. a   (para 4-10a(3))

11. a   (para 4-10c(1))

12. b   (para 4-10e(1))

13. d   (para 4-10a(4))

14. c   (para 4-10c(6))

End of Lesson 4

LESSON ASSIGNMENT

LESSON 5	Fluid and Electrolyte Therapy
LESSON ASSIGNMENT	Frames 1 through 81 (programmed text) and Paragraphs 5-1 through 5-10.
LESSON OBJECTIVES	After completing this lesson, you should be able to

5-1.   Given one of the categories of body fluid and a group of statements, select the statement that best describes that type of body fluid.

5-2.   From a group of statements, select the definition of an electrolyte.

5-3.   Given a list of the names of electrolytes, select the electrolyte which is the primary positive electrolyte in either intracellular fluid or extracellular fluid.

5-4.   Given the name of an electrolyte and a group of functions, select the function performed by that electrolyte.

5-5.   From a list of means by which fluids and electrolytes are lost from the body, select those which are either normal or abnormal means of fluid and electrolyte loss.

5-6.   Given a group of statements, select the statement that describes the effect an intravenously administered hypertonic solution might have on the cells near the administration site.

5-7.   Given a group of statements, select the statement that describes the effect an intravenously administered hypotonic solution might have on the cells near the administration site.

5-8.   Given a group of statements, select the statement that describes the effect an intravenously administered acidic or alkaline solution might have on the cells near the administration site.

5-9. Given a list of volumes, select the maximum recommended volume of intravenous fluid that should be administered to an adult during a 24-hour period.

5-10. From a group of statements, select the statement that defines fluid and electrolyte maintenance therapy.

5-11. From a group of statements, select the statement that defines fluid and electrolyte replacement therapy.

5-12. Given one of the two basic categories of intravenous preparations (intravenous solutions or intravenous admixtures) and a group of statements, select the statement that best describes the given type of preparation.

5-13. From a list of characteristics, select the requirements of intravenous preparations.

5-14. Given a group of statements, select the statement that best describes a precaution pertaining to intravenous fluid therapy.

5-15. From a list of possible complications, select the possible complication(s) of intravenous fluid therapy.

5-16. Given the name of one of the types of intravenous fluid and a group of statements, select the statement that best describes the use of that type of fluid.

5-17. Given the name of an intravenous fluid and a list of the categories of intravenous fluids, select the category to which the given intravenous fluid belongs.

SUGGESTION

After completing the assignment, complete the exercises at the end of this lesson. These exercises will help you to achieve the lesson objectives.

INSTRUCTIONS   This text is set up differently from most subcourse lessons. The first section of this lesson uses a programmed instruction format. The numbered "frames" present information and/or a question about presented information. You should work through the frames in the order presented. Answer each question that is presented. To check your answers, go to the shaded box of the NEXT frame. For example. the solution to the question presented in Frame 7 is found in the shaded box of Frame 8.

DISCLAIMER   The language used in this subcourse was chosen to make the lesson easier to understand and may not be as precise as definitions and terminology you will learn in the future.

FRAME 1

Section I. INTRODUCTION TO FLUID AND ELECTROLYTE PHYSIOLOGY

SPECIAL NOTE: The material in Section I, Fluid and Electrolyte Therapy, is presented to you in the form of a programmed text. The content of this section is designed to review the basic concepts of fluid and electrolyte therapy. An understanding of the principles set forth in this section is essential for a thorough understanding of the use of intravenous solutions. The questions and answers dispersed throughout the programmed text will take the place of the practice exercises usually seen at the end of the lesson. The remaining sections of this lesson will be presented in their usual format.

GO TO FRAME 2.

FRAME 2

The average size person (154 pounds or 70 kilograms) has water amounting to 60 to 70 percent of his total body weight. Electrolytes are found in body fluids. Electrolytes are chemical compounds which are ionized in the aqueous solutions of the body. These electrolytes perform essential physiological functions in the body. Fluctuations in the levels of body fluids and/or electrolytes can result in illness and even death.

FRAME 3

As a person who prepares sterile products, you will have the responsibility of preparing sterile solutions which are meant to be intravenously administered to patients. These solutions will always consist of sterile water. Many times these solutions will also have electrolytes (like sodium chloride) added.

FRAME 4

In this module, the topic of fluid and electrolyte therapy will be discussed. Parts of this module will be a review for many of you, while others will be learning these concepts for the first time. In either event, the knowledge you gain during this time will give you a broader background in fluid and electrolyte therapy.

FRAME 5

The first portion of this module discusses fluid and electrolyte distribution in the body. These principles form a foundation for the remainder of the module.

FRAME 6

As previously mentioned, the average 70 kilogram adult's body weight is approximately 60 to 70 percent water. This water is divided into two primary types. These two types are the intracellular fluid and the extracellular fluid. These two types can be represented as below:

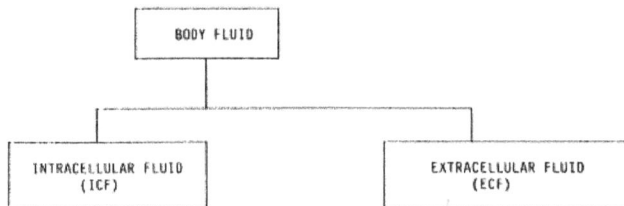

FRAME 7

QUESTION: What are the two primary types of body fluids.

a. _____.

b. _____.

FRAME 8

The first type of fluid we shall discuss is the intracellular fluid (ICF), that fluid which is contained <u>inside</u> the body cells. Intracellular fluid composes approximately two-thirds of a person's total body water and approximately 50 percent of the person's body weight.

Solution to Frame 7

ANSWER:

<u>Intracellular fluid (ICF)</u>

<u>Extracellular fluid (ECF)</u>

FRAME 9

The intracellular fluid serves several functions. One, it serves as a transporting medium in that it carries food and oxygen into the cells and wastes and carbon dioxide from the cells. The intracellular fluid also maintains the shape and size of each cell in the body.

FRAME 10

QUESTION: The intracellular fluid composes approximately _____ percent of a person's body weight.

FRAME 11

The second type of body fluid is the extracellular fluid. The extracellular fluid is located <u>outside</u> the body cells. The extracellular fluid (ECF) composes approximately one-third of the water contained in the body and it accounts for approximately 20 percent of a person's body weight. The extracellular fluid also has several functions. One, it carries nutrients and oxygen to the cells and waste materials from the cells. Also, it serves to bathe the cells in order to keep the cells moist.

Solution to Frame 10

ANSWER:
The intracellular fluid composes approximately <u>50%</u> of a person's body weight.

FRAME 12

QUESTION: State the body's two major types of fluids and the approximate percentage of total body water each contains.

BODY FLUID	APPROXIMATE % OF TOTAL BODY WATER
a. _____	_____
b. _____	_____

FRAME 13

The body's extracellular fluid can be further divided into two types, <u>interstitial fluid and intravascular fluid</u>. The interstitial fluid surrounds cells and it serves as a transporting medium to carry materials to and from cells. Approximately three-fourths of the extracellular fluid is contained in the interstitial fluid. Interstitial fluid accounts for approximately 15 percent of a person's body weight. The second division of the extracellular fluid is the intravascular fluid (plasma). The intravascular fluid is found in the body's circulatory system. It accounts for approximately five percent of a person's body weight.

Solution to Frame 12

Answer:

BODY FLUID	APPROXIMATE % OF TOTAL BODY WATER
Intracellular Fluid	2/3 (or 66.6%)
Extracellular Fluid	1/3 (or 33.3%)

FRAME 14

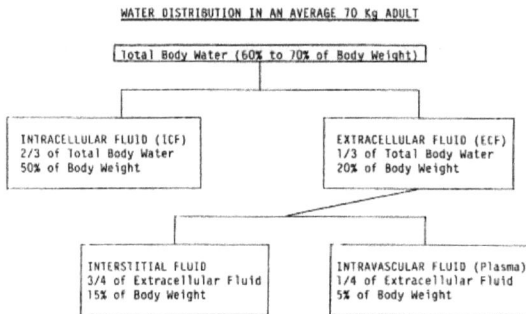

WATER DISTRIBUTION IN AN AVERAGE 70 Kg ADULT

Total Body Water (60% to 70% of Body Weight)

INTRACELLULAR FLUID (ICF)
2/3 of Total Body Water
50% of Body Weight

EXTRACELLULAR FLUID (ECF)
1/3 of Total Body Water
20% of Body Weight

INTERSTITIAL FLUID
3/4 of Extracellular Fluid
15% of Body Weight

INTRAVASCULAR FLUID (Plasma)
1/4 of Extracellular Fluid
5% of Body Weight

FRAME 15

QUESTION: State the two main types of fluid found in the body.

a. _____.

b. _____.

FRAME 16

QUESTION: The extracellular fluid composes

approximately _____ percent of total body

water and _____ percent of body weight.

Solution to Frame 15

ANSWER:
Intracellular fluid (ICF)

Extracellular fluid (ECF)

FRAME 17

QUESTION: The intracellular fluid composes

approximately _____ percent of total body

water and _____ percent of body weight.

Solution to Frame 16

ANSWER: The extracellular fluid composes approximately 33% of total body water and 20% of body weight.

FRAME 18

The amount of intracellular and extracellular fluid contained in a person s body is extremely important to his proper physiological functioning. Losses of body fluids by vomiting, diarrhea, and perspiration can produce illness. Whenever body fluids are lost, certain substances are also lost. For example, diuretics produce increased urine flow. Electrolytes like potassium are lost in this urine. Electrolytes, ions like potassium and chloride, are inorganic substances which are found in solution in body fluids. Therefore, a loss of body fluids usually means a corresponding loss of electrolytes. The particular ion(s) and the number of each ion lost will depend upon whether the fluid lost arises from the interstitial fluid or the intravascular fluid. The situation is complicated by the fact that fluid can move from one type of fluid compartment to another.

Solution to Frame 17

ANSWER: The intracellular fluid composes approximately 66% of total body water and 50% of body weight.

FRAME 19

Below are the major electrolytes and the amount of each contained in a liter of extracellular fluid.

Sodium (Na^+)	140 mEq
Chloride (Cl^-)	100 mEq
Bicarbonate (HCO_3)	27 mEq
Potassium (K^+)	4 mEq
Magnesium (Mg^{+2})	3 mEq

FRAME 20

QUESTION: What is the most abundant positive

ion found in extracellular fluid? _____.

FRAME 21

Electrolytes are also found in intracellular fluid. Below is a listing of the major electrolytes found in intracellular fluid. The concentrations are listed in terms of milliequivalents of the electrolytes per liter of the fluid.

ELECTROLYTE	NO. OF MILLIEQUIVALENTS PER LITER
Potassium (K^+)	160
Phosphate (PO_4^{-3})	110
Magnesium (Mg^{-2})	25
Sodium (Na^+)	5
Chloride (Cl^-)	3

Solution to Frame 20

ANSWER: Sodium (Na^+) is the most abundant positive ion in extracellular fluid.

FRAME 22

QUESTION: What is the primary positive

electrolyte present in intracellular fluid? _____

FRAME 23

In the earlier sections of this module, the distribution of body fluids and electrolytes was discussed. It has been previously stated that electrolytes are essential in the proper physiological functioning of the body. In this section, the primary physiological function(s) of the major body electrolytes will be discussed.

First, sodium (Na^+) is the most abundant positive electrolyte in extracellular fluid. Sodium is essential in maintaining the osmotic pressure of extracellular fluid.

Solution to Frame 22

ANSWER: Potassium is the primary positive electrolyte in intracellular fluid.

FRAME 24

Chloride is the most abundant negative electrolyte present in extracellular fluid. The chloride ion is essential in maintaining the normal osmotic pressure of extracellular fluid. The chloride ion is also found in the stomach as a result of the ionization of hydrochloric acid (HCl).

FRAME 25

Potassium is the most abundant positive electrolyte present in intracellular fluid. Postassium is required for the conversion of dextrose into energy in the body. Potassium also helps to maintain the osmotic pressure of intracellular fluid, as well as aid in the transmission of nervous impulses within the heart.

FRAME 26

The bicarbonate radical helps maintain the acid-base balance in the body.

FRAME 27

The phosphate radical is essential in the formation of bones and teeth and in the formation of body enzymes.

FRAME 28

Magnesium is essential in the formation of enzymes in the body.

FRAME 29

Finally, calcium is essential in the formation of bones and teeth. It also plays key roles in the clotting of blood and in maintaining the rhythm of the heart beat.

FRAME 30

As you have seen, concentrations of body electrolytes are expressed in units called milliequivalents (mEq). The concentration of these electrolytes are expressed in the number of milliequivalents present in a liter of solution (mEq/L).

FRAME 31

Whenever fluid is lost from the body, certain electrolytes tend to be lost with the fluid. A liter of extracellular fluid contains approximately 140 mEq of sodium. Therefore, if a liter of extracellular fluid were lost from the body, the sodium lost in that fluid would have to be replaced along with the liter of fluid. To further complicate matters, extracellular fluid in the stomach has a different electrolyte composition than extracellular fluid in the intestine. Therefore, a liter of fluid lost during severe vomiting would not contain the same electrolytes (in regard to type and number) as a liter of fluid lost during a severe case of diarrhea. Therefore, in replacing lost fluid, the type of fluid lost and the volume of lost fluid must be closely monitored.

FRAME 32

Up to now, body fluids and electrolytes have been discussed. Normally, people are unaware of the loss or gain of body fluids or electrolytes, it is only when one begins to lose a large volume of fluid through diarrhea and vomiting that this loss becomes acutely apparent. Just think of a time when you experienced acute fluid loss. You will have to agree that the body usually does a superb job of maintaining fluid and electrolyte balance.

FRAME 33

Each and every day the body loses fluids and electrolytes. These fluid and electrolyte losses are normal. These fluid losses normally occur through four main routes, perspiration, digestion, respiration, and urination.

FRAME 34

First, perspiration is that fluid which is lost through the skin. Normally, a person is unaware of perspiration unless the temperature is extremely hot or strenuous exercise has just taken place. Perspiration contains approximately 45 mEq of sodium, 4.5 mEq of potassium, and 57.5 mEq of chloride in each liter.

FRAME 35

NOTE: Most people have difficulty grasping the significance of the volume of perspiration lost during a 24-hour period of time. In order to illustrate this point, the next question will ask you to estimate the volume of fluid lost during a 24-hour period of time in the form of perspiration. Do not attempt to find this figure in the above paragraph. Sufficient data has not been provided for an accurate estimate. Do not be surprised if your estimate is off by 25 or 50 milliliters.

FRAME 36

QUESTION: About _____ ml of fluid lost in the form of perspiration over a 24-hour period of time.

FRAME 37

A small volume of fluid is lost every day in the feces. Usually only 100 milliliters of fluid is lost in normal stools. This demonstrates the efficiency of the large intestine in absorbing the water passing through it. A third means of fluid loss is by respiration. Respiration occurs around-the-clock; however, most people are unaware that they are exhaling fluid (water vapor) every time they breathe. This fluid loss through the lungs only becomes apparent during cold weather. During cold weather, the water vapor can be seen when it is exposed to low temperatures.

Solution to Frame 36

ANSWER: Approximately 650 milliliters of perspiration is lost during a normal day by a normal individual.

FRAME 38

NOTE: Most people have difficulty grasping the significance of the volume of fluid lost during a 24-hour period of time during respiration. In order to illustrate this point, the next question will ask you to estimate the volume of fluid lost during a day in respiration. <u>Do not</u> attempt to find this figure in the above paragraph.

FRAME 39

QUESTION: Estimate the volume of fluid lost in a 24-hour period of time in respiration.

_____ milliliters

FRAME 40

The fourth major route of normal fluid loss is through urination. The volume of urine excreted during a 24-hour period of time will vary; however, the normal person will excrete approximately 1,300 milliliters of urine in 24-hours. One liter of urine will contain approximately 75 mEq of sodium, 40 mEq of potassium, and 80 mEq of chloride.

Solution to Frame 39

ANSWER: Approximately <u>450</u> milliliters of fluid are lost during a 24-hour period of time in respiration.

FRAME 41

Adding these normal fluid losses:

PERSPIRATION	650 ml/day
FECES	100 ml/day
RESPIRATION	450 ml/day
URINATION	1,300 ml/day
	2,500 ml/day

Approximately 2,500 milliliters of fluid are normally lost during a 24-hour period of time by the average individual.

FRAME 42

QUESTION: In order to maintain body fluid balance, approximately _____ milliliters of fluid must be taken into the body during each 24 hour period of time.

FRAME 43

A person normally loses approximately 2,500 milliliters of fluid each day. Most people are unaware that these fluid losses are occurring because the losses are replaced as they occur. For example, a person drinks a 240 ml soft drink; then he might go directly to the restroom (latrine) and urinate 240 milliliters. How often have you had a spot of tea only to find yourself needing to go to the restroom several minutes later?

Solution to Frame 42

ANSWER: In order to maintain body fluid balance, approximately 2,500 milliliters of fluid must be taken into the body during each 24-hour period of time.

FRAME 44

Abnormal losses of fluid are not subtle. Everyone is aware when abnormal fluid losses occur. Obviously, the most obvious fluid losses occur when a person suffers from severe vomiting and diarrhea. However, more subtle abnormal fluid losses can occur.

FRAME 45

Vomiting, a very noticeable way of losing fluids, accounts for more fluid loss than one would expect. That is, a person who experiences severe vomiting not only loses those fluids he has taken orally, he also loses fluids (like gastric juices) which are secreted into the stomach. Gastric juices are rich in electrolytes. For example, a liter of gastric juice contains approximately 50 mEq of bicarbonate.

FRAME 46

A second way fluids are abnormally lost is by diarrhea. Most people have had "bugs" that cause diarrhea, loose, watery stools. Not only is diarrhea unpleasant, it also accounts for a large loss of body fluids. Diarrhea causes a loss of fluids and electrolytes (to include sodium, potassium, and chloride). In addition, the digested nutrients present in the diarrhea are not absorbed by the body. Thus, after a bout with severe diarrhea, weakness promptly ensues.

FRAME 47

QUESTION: List two of the most obvious abnormal ways fluids and electrolytes are lost from the body.

a. _____.

b. _____.

FRAME 48

A third means of abnormal fluid loss is by severe perspiration. Strenuous exercise in a hot environment can lead to this excessive perspiration. Sodium, potassium, and chloride are examples of electrolytes lost in perspiration.

Solution to Frame 47

ANSWER:

Vomiting.

Diaherra.

FRAME 49

Fourth, severe burns can cause an abnormal loss of body fluids. In certain types of burns, blisters containing fluid are made, imagine the water loss of a patient who has such blisters over 60 percent of his body. In more severe burns where the skin is actually burned, the loss of body fluids is more noticeable. In cases of very severe burns, fluids actually seep out of the burned skin directly onto the patient's bedding. Along with these fluids, electrolytes are also lost. Thus, this severely injured person must face both fluid and electrolyte losses.

FRAME 50

Several other abnormal means of losing fluids and electrolytes also exist. These abnormal ways are the subtle ways of losing large volumes of fluids and large numbers of electrolytes. One subtle means of abnormal fluid loss is by gastric suction. The Gomco® Pump can be used to remove gastric juices from a patient's stomach. Often, a nurse will give the patient small amounts of water to relieve thirst. When this occurs, the gastric fluid, the water, and large numbers of electrolytes are withdrawn from the stomach. Before long, the patient has lost a tremendous number of electrolytes. Bleeding also produces a loss of fluid (plasma), blood cells, and other important substances. Lastly, a person who is being treated with a thiazide diuretic also loses fluids and electrolytes (primarily potassium). In such cases, potassium must be given to the patient in order to prevent potassium deficiencies.

FRAME 51

QUESTION: List five abnormal ways fluid can be lost from the body.

a. _____.

b. _____.

c. _____.

d. _____.

e. _____.

FRAME 52

In the earlier sections of this module, the concepts of body fluid distribution, electrolyte distribution, and fluid and electrolyte loss by both normal and abnormal means were discussed. A certain volume of fluid will be lost from the body each day and this fluid will contain electrolytes. The fluids and electrolytes lost each day must be replaced in order to maintain proper physiological functioning. If abnormal losses of fluids and electrolytes occur, these losses must be corrected. Two main ways of maintaining fluid and electrolyte balance and replacing abnormal fluid and electrolyte losses are available to the physician. These two methods of maintenance and replacement are through the oral (by mouth) route and by the intravenous route.

Solution to Frame 51

ANSWER: (Any 5 of the following)

Diarreha.
Vomiting.
Excessive perspiration.
Gastric suction.
Bleeding.
Burns.
Diueretics.

FRAME 53

The oral route of administration offers the safest and easiest method of replacing fluids and electrolytes. For example, a patient being treated with a thiazide diuretic can be given orange juice to replace the potassium that is being lost in the urine. Orange juice contains approximately 15 milliequivalents of potassium in each eight fluid ounces. Also available are effervescent tablets containing potassium. These tablets are supplied in several palatable flavors. When the oral route is used, the patient is able to move about freely and the psychological impact of intravenous administration is not present.

FRAME 54

The second major route used to administer fluids and electrolytes is by the intravenous route. The intravenous route makes it possible to control the volume of fluid and the numbers of each electrolyte to be given. One problem inherent in the intravenous administration of fluids is that frequently the patient is immobilized, it is very difficult to maneuver with all the intravenous apparatus hanging from one's arm.

FRAME 55

There are several other considerations concerning intravenous therapy. First, and extremely important, is the topic of infection. If microorganisms enter the patient through a contaminated intravenous solution, administration set, or administration site, potential problems could result. Remember, the patient who is receiving intravenous solution frequently is the patient least able to ward off an infection.

FRAME 56

Another consideration of intravenous therapy is the total volume of fluid to be administered to the patient over a given period of time. As a general rule, an adult patient should be administered a maximum of four liters (4,000 milliliters) of intravenous fluid per 24 hours. Of course, the volume of fluid to be administered would depend upon such factors as body weight, age, etc. Pediatric patients would be administered proportionally lower volumes of fluid. At first though, only the major fluids being administered to the patient would seem to apply. However, every milliliter of solution (to include "piggy-back", hyperalimentation, and "to-keep-open" solutions) must be taken into account when calculating the volume of fluid that is being administered to the patient.

FRAME 57

The renal condition of the patient also influences the volume of intravenous solution to be administered. In circumstances where the patient is suffering from insufficient kidney function, the volume of administered fluid would have to be decreased to preclude fluid overload.

FRAME 58

Infection, volume of intravenous fluid to be administered, and the renal condition of the patient are all considerations involved in the intravenous administration of drugs. Bearing these considerations in mind, answer the following questions.

FRAME 59

QUESTION: A patient who has undergone three days of intravenous therapy has shown the signs of an infection. You believe the infection has resulted from the intravenous therapy. State three possible sources of the responsible microorganisms based upon your suspicions.

a. _____ .

b. _____ .

c. _____ .

FRAME 60

QUESTION: A patient has been administered 2,500 ml of a hyperalimentation solution, one gram of an antibiotic administered piggyback in 300 ml of intravenous solution, and 800 ml of Lactated Ringer's solution during a 24-hour period of time. Was this patient administered too much intravenous fluid during this 24-hour period?

a. Yes.

b. It depends.

c. No.

Solution to Frame 59

ANSWER:

The intravenous solutions.

The adminisration sets.

The administration site.

FRAME 61

A fourth consideration of intravenous therapy is the tonicity of the intravenous solution being administered. In your previous pharmacy related courses, you were exposed to the concept of osmotic pressure and tonicity. In brief, solutions are classified into three broad categories based upon tonicity, isotonic, hypotonic, and hypertonic.

Solution to Frame 60

ANSWER: It depends. The age, size, and renal condition of the patient have been omitted on purpose. Without these bits of information, a definite answer cannot be given.

FRAME 62

To begin, an isotonic solution has the same concentration as that of body fluids. Below is a diagrammatic representation of the response a cell exhibits when placed in an isotonic solution:

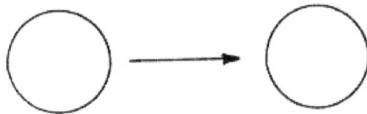

FRAME 63

Observe that when a cell is placed in an isotonic solution no noticeable change in size occurs. Therefore, no cell irritation (related to the tonicity of the solution) would occur. Examples of isotonic solutions are 0.9% Sodium Chloride Solution and Lactated Ringer's Injection.

FRAME 64

A hypertonic solution is more concentrated than that of body fluids. Saying it another way, the hypertonic solution has more solute present per volume than does cell fluid. Therefore:

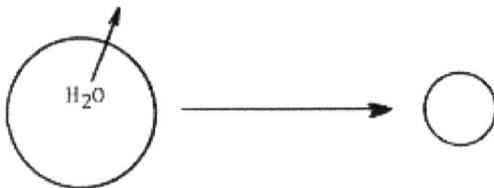

FRAME 65

Observe that fluid was "drawn" from the cell in order to achieve equilibrium. Therefore, the cell was reduced in size. Such an experience is traumatic for the cell unfortunate enough to be placed in such a situation. In relation to intravenous fluids, a hypertonic solution would cause cell irritation to blood cells and the cells lining the circulatory system. The patient who is being administered a hypertonic solution would experience localized pain in the area of the administration site. Examples of hypertonic solutions are most hyperalimentation solutions and 10% dextrose solution.

FRAME 66

A hypotonic solution is less concentrated than that of body fluids. That is, the hypotonic solution has less solute per volume than that of body fluid. When placed in a hypotonic solution, a cell will increase in size because water will enter the cell in an attempt to equalize the concentrations of the cell and the hypotonic solution:

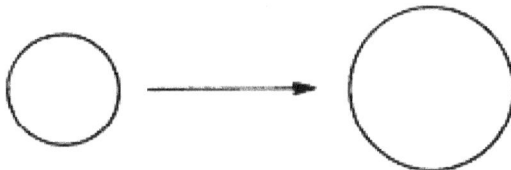

FRAME 67

As you can see, unfortunate cells exposed to hypotonic solutions could become irritated and damage to them could result. Examples of hypotonic solutions are 0.45% sodium chloride solution and sterile water for injection.

FRAME 68

A final consideration in intravenous therapy is the pH of the solution to be administered to the patient. Solutions with an alkaline (pH greater than 7.0) or an acidic (pH less than 7.0) pH value have been associated with irritation of the veins (thrombophlebitis). In order to reduce the incidence of thrombophlebitis, buffering agents can be added to solutions with highly acidic or alkaline pH values in order to bring the pH of these solutions closer to pH 7.4, the approximate pH of blood. However, the alteration of some intravenous solutions' pH values can affect their stability as well as the stability of drugs added to those solutions. Consequently, appropriate pharmaceutical references must be consulted prior to adding buffering solutions.

FRAME 69

Below are the pH ranges for various intravenous solutions:

0.9 Sodium Chloride Solution	5.7 (Abbott) 5.5 (Baxter) 5.0 (Travenol)
Lactated Ringer's Injection	6.7 (Abbott) 6.5 (Baxter) 6.6 (Cutter)
Dextrose 5% in Water	pH range of solutions are from 4.0 to 5.0.

FRAME 70

Two considerations of intravenous therapy have just been discussed. These two considerations, the tonicity and the pH of infused fluids, are pertinent topics when discussing the preparation and the administration of intravenous fluids.

FRAME 71

QUESTION: Briefly state the effect of the intravenous administration of isotonic, hypertonic, and hypotonic solutions on a patient's veins.

a. Isotonic solution-_____.

b. Hypertonic solution-_____.

c. Hypotonic solution-_____.

FRAME 72

QUESTION: The administration of an acidic or an alkaline intravenous solution can irritate the patient's veins. What is this occurrence called?

_____

Solution to Frame 71

ANSWER:
a. Isotonic solution-no significant effect.
b. Hypertonic solution-can cause irritation to vein.
c. Hypotonic solution- can cause irritation to vein.

FRAME 73

QUESTION: Is the addition of a buffering agent to

an intravenous solution always desirable? _____

Explain. _____

_____

Solution to Frame 72

ANSWER: Thrombophlebitis.

FRAME 74

The pros and cons of intravenous therapy have been discussed. Many formulations of intravenous solutions can be obtained. These formulations can be categorized into two main areas in regard to intended therapeutic use. These two broad therapeutic categories are <u>maintenance</u> and <u>replacement</u>.

Solution to Frame 73

ANSWER: No. Alteration of a solution's pH can affect its stability and the stability of drugs that are added to it.

FRAME 75

Maintenance therapy is designed to meet the ordinary fluid and electrolyte requirements of patients who have a restricted oral intake, but who are without extra losses caused by vomiting, diarrhea, or other stress. In short, maintenance therapy is designed to replace the fluids and electrolytes lost during a normal day.

FRAME 76

Few solutions can be used alone as maintenance solutions because the body requires a specified number of certain electrolytes each day. Most solutions contain only a limited number of electrolytes. For example, 0.9% Sodium Chloride Solution contains 154 mEq of sodium and 154 mEq of chloride in each 1,000 milliliters. 5% Dextrose Solution contains approximately 170 calories per liter of solution. Observe that the sodium chloride solution contains only sodium and chloride ions, while the dextrose solution contains absolutely no electrolytes. Lactated Ringer's injection contains 130 mEq of sodium, 109 mEq of chloride, 3 mEq of calcium, *28* mEq of lactate, and 4 mEq of potassium in each liter of the solution. Although more electrolytes are contained in the Lactated Ringer's injection, the amount of each electrolyte supplied is usually below that amount the patient needs each day.

FRAME 77

The second broad therapeutic category of intravenous therapy involving fluids and electrolytes is referred to as replacement. Replacement therapy is designed to help patients with pre-existing or continuing fluid and electrolyte losses requiring replacement of extracellular fluid. Solutions used for replacement therapy should be tailored to fill the needs of the patient. For example, a patient who has had severe diarrhea for three days would have different fluid and electrolyte requirements than a patient who has suffered from severe vomiting for three days. Laboratory tests can be used to gain an idea of the electrolytes and the numbers of each electrolyte that need to be replaced. Once laboratory results are obtained, a solution can be prepared to replace depleted fluids and electrolytes. A solution such as 5% dextrose solution can be used as a parent solution for such a preparation.

FRAME 78

Remember, in cases where deficiencies in fluids and electrolytes exist, fluid and electrolyte maintenance and replacement therapy must be instituted in most cases.

FRAME 79

Two broad therapeutic uses of intravenous solutions in regard to fluid and electrolyte therapy are referred to as maintenance and replacement.

FRAME 80

QUESTION: What is the difference between maintenance and replacement therapy in reference to fluid and electrolyte therapy?

_____

_____

_____

_____

_____

_____

_____

FRAME 81

This completes Section I. Go on to Section II.

Solution to Frame 80

ANSWER: Maintenance therapy is used to replace fluids and electrolytes that are lost during the course of a normal day. Replacement therapy seeks to replace those fluids and electrolytes that are lost due to extraordinary losses of these essential substances.

Section II. PRECAUTIONS AND COMPLICATIONS ASSOCIATED WITH INTRAVENOUS THERAPY

5-1. INTRODUCTION

Normally, a person obtains the fluids and electrolytes needed to live by the oral route. This route has certain built-in safeguards against bacterial invasion. When the intravenous route of administration must be used, the material being given is injected directly into the circulatory system through the veins. Although this route of administration is certainly effective in terms of getting the fluid into the patient, the intravenous route is not completely safe. Complications (e.g., infection) can arise. In the case of infection, the fluid being administered, the intravenous administration set (the equipment between the bottle or the bag and the patient), or the technique used to start the fluid administration are potential sources of bacterial contamination. In short, the intravenous administration of fluids is to be taken seriously.

5-2. TWO BASIC CATEGORIES OF INTRAVENOUS PREPARATIONS

We have all seen intravenous solutions being administered to a patient. We have known that the bottle or bag connected to the patient by a plastic tube means life to many patients. For the purpose of discussion, this subcourse divided intravenous preparations into two major categories: intravenous solutions and intravenous admixtures. The purpose of this division is to help you understand that the pharmacy does not prepare every intravenous product which is administered to a patient.

   a. **Intravenous Solutions.** Intravenous solutions are products which meet certain rigid requirements and are supplied ready for use by manufacturers. Examples of such intravenous solutions are 5% Dextrose Injection, 0.9% Sodium Chloride Injection, and Lactated Ringer's Injection. These solutions are ready for use as soon as they arrive from the manufacturer. You will see the 5% Dextrose Injection and the 0.9% Sodium Chloride Injection used as "to keep open" (TKO) solutions. That is, they are slowly administered to a patient in order to provide fluid. In addition, they serve as a ready and rapid way by which drugs could be given to the patient should the patient go into shock. These solutions serve as a "base" for the category below.

   b. **Intravenous Admixtures.** Intravenous admixtures are intravenous solutions to which have been added one or more drugs. For example, it is common for a patient to be administered a liter of 5% Dextrose Injection which has 20 mEq of potassium chloride added to it. Thus, the patient received fluid, nutrients (dextrose), and electrolytes (potassium and chloride). Typically, patients receive much more complicated intravenous admixtures. These intravenous admixtures are prepared in the Pharmacy Sterile Products Section by specially trained persons who use aseptic techniques.

5-3. REQUIREMENTS FOR INTRAVENOUS SOLUTIONS/INTRAVENOUS ADMIXTURES

Any solution administered through a patient's veins must be:

a. **Sterile.** Sterile means that no living microorganisms are present in the solution.

b. **Pyrogen-Free.** Pyrogens are substances which produce fever when injected into the circulatory system.

c. **Free from Visible Particulate Matter.** Visible particles in an intravenous preparation mean that the product should be discarded. These particles could have been present in the solution when it arrived in the pharmacy or they may have been accidentally added to the solution when other substances were added. Regardless of origin, these visible particles, if intravenously administered, could cause a blockage in the patient's circulatory system. Filters with very small pores are available which can remove these visible particles as the product is being administered. But remember, the origin of the particles is unknown--it is possible that some particles could be undissolved drug. Removing the drug particles would be good, but the patient should receive the prescribed amount of medication to achieve the desired therapeutic effect.

5-4. PRECAUTIONS PERTAINING TO FLUID THERAPY

You could be in the position of seeing that an intravenous solution prepared for a patient does not do more harm than good. If you have received special training in the preparation of intravenous solutions in the Pharmacy Sterile Products Section, you are well familiar with the tasks you must perform In order to insure the patient receives what is intended in an intravenous product. Below are some of the precautions which are of primary importance in protecting the welfare of a patient who is on intravenous therapy.

a. **Contamination.** A solution intravenously administered to a patient must be free from living microorganisms. Microorganisms are capable of entering the admixture when it is prepared. Therefore, the person who prepares the admixture in the Pharmacy Sterile Products Section has the great responsibility of using aseptic technique. When there is doubt about the sterility of the admixture (or intravenous solution), the product should be discarded. Microorganisms are also present in the environment of the hospital room. They are on the hands of the person who will start (i.e., begin the administration) the intravenous product. Therefore, this person is responsible for using care and aseptic technique to make the venipuncture.

b. **Incompatibilities.**

(1)   Certain drugs or chemicals react when they are placed in a solution. The result is changed drugs or chemicals. This same type of chemical change can occur when a drug is added to an intravenous solution. Remember the chemical reaction below?

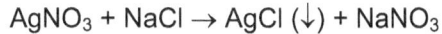

$$AgNO_3 + NaCl \rightarrow AgCl (\downarrow) + NaNO_3$$

(2)   In the laboratory, silver nitrate ($AgNO_3$) is added to sodium chloride (NaCl) and white precipitate (silver chloride, AgCl) is formed.   You can actually see the silver chloride formed. Unfortunately, one cannot see all the chemical reactions which could happen when a drug is added to an intravenous solution. But remember, when this type of reaction occurs, the patient is not receiving the drug(s) the physician ordered. How can such incompatibilities be prevented? The answer is simple, the person who prepares the admixture in the Pharmacy Sterile Products Section must use the references available there to determine if a drug (or combination of drugs) may be safely added to an intravenous solution. Furthermore, nursing personnel should be cautioned never to add a drug to the contents of the intravenous product without checking with the person in the Pharmacy Sterile Products Section.

c. **Irritating Drugs.** The veins are very sensitive. Therefore, any intravenous product which has an extreme pH or which is very concentrated can irritate the veins. In some cases, the physician can decide to place the drug in another intravenous solution with a resultant pH which will not irritate the veins to a great degree. In other cases, the site through which the irritating solution is being administered can be changed on a frequent basis in order to allow that part of the vein to recover.

d. **Particulate Matter.** Hold a bottle or bag of intravenous solution up in front of a light. See how it is sparkling clear. Actually, small particles called particulate matter are present in the solution. Standards allow for extremely small particles to be present in the solution in certain concentrations. Intravenous solutions or admixtures should never be administered to a patient when the products contain visible particulate matter. A product which is cloudy in nature might actually be cloudy because of suspended particulate matter. Remember, filters are available which can filter most particulate matter from intravenous products, but in some cases the particulate matter is actually drug particles.

5-5.   COMPLICATIONS OF INTRAVENOUS FLUID THERAPY

Various complications are associated with the administration of intravenous fluid therapy. Some of these complications are:

a. **Infection.** When microorganisms enter the circulatory system through the venipuncture site, an infection can result. The microorganisms--primarily bacteria--can be present in the intravenous solution or admixture, in the intravenous administration set, or around the administration site when the product is administered. The infection can be localized or systemic.

b. **Infiltration.** Infiltration occurs when the needle or catheter through which the product is entering the veins is removed from the vein. In this case the fluid enters the tissue surrounding the vein. Although this condition is not usually serious, it can be very uncomfortable for the patient. To remedy this problem, the product is started in another administration site.

c. **Phlebitis.** Phlebitis is the inflammation of vein tissue. Phlebitis is caused by mechanical, chemical, or bacterial irritation. This condition is characterized by pain and redness at the administration site. When phlebitis occurs, the solution is usually administered at a different site.

d. **Pyrogenic Reaction.** A pyrogenic reaction is one in which the patient's body temperature increases after certain types of substances enter the circulatory system. Bacteria (or their parts), various chemicals, and certain types of particles are capable of causing a pyrogenic reaction. A pyrogenic reaction is characterized by chills followed by a fever.

e. **Circulatory Overload.** The "average" person has a blood volume of approximately five liters. Blood is approximately 93 percent fluid. The body has intricate mechanisms for compensating with changes in blood volume. For example, when you give blood, some fluid from the inside of the cells as well as fluid surrounding the cells enters the circulating blood volume. Likewise, there is a reverse flow when the blood volume is normal and intravenous fluids are administered. Unfortunately, when too much fluid is administered too rapidly circulatory overload can result. When circulatory overload occurs, the heart cannot efficiently pump the blood. Circulatory overload is a potentially dangerous condition which must be treated by the physician.

f. **Air Embolism.** An air embolism occurs when a sizeable volume of air enters the circulatory system. An air embolism can be caused by the movement of air through the intravenous administration set into the circulatory system. This can occur when the intravenous administration set has not been properly "bled" (i.e., had all the air replaced by intravenous solution) or by an intravenous solution or admixture bottle which has been allowed to empty completely resulting in air flow down the administration set. An air embolism is potentially dangerous because an air bubble can occlude cardiac, cerebral, or pulmonary circulation.

g. **Thrombus.** A thrombus is a clot which is formed in the blood vessels. A thrombus is usually a further complication of phlebitis. A clot formed in the vessels can produce damage to tissue below the stoppage.

Section III. CATEGORIES OF INTRAVENOUS FLUIDS AND THEIR USES

5-6. INTRODUCTION

Many patients in hospitals receive intravenous fluid therapy. The reasons for their receiving intravenous fluid therapy are not the same. Likewise, the solutions they receive are not all alike. Some patients have intravenous solutions tailored to meet their specific fluid, nutritional, and electrolyte needs. This section of the subcourse will focus on those solutions commonly used and/or prepared in the hospital setting.

5-7. HYDRATING SOLUTIONS

a. **Use.** Hydrating solutions are used to provide the patient with required fluid (i.e., water). The volume of preparation administered depends on the fluid needs of the patient.

b. **Examples of Hydrating Solutions.** Below are some examples of preparations commonly used as hydrating solutions.

(1) 5% Dextrose Injection (D5W). This solution consists of dextrose and water. One liter of the 5% Dextrose Injection contains approximately 170 calories. This solution contains no appreciable electrolytes. Therefore, electrolytes are sometimes added to the 5% Dextrose Injection (e.g., 15 mEq KCl in one liter of D5W). The 5% Dextrose Injection is used to provide fluid replacement and energy.

NOTE: Dextrose solution is available in several concentrations. For example, you will see 10% Dextrose Injection and 50% Dextrose Injection in the pharmacy. Because of its high concentration, 50% Dextrose Injection should never be injected before it is diluted.

(2) 0.9% Sodium Chloride Injection (Normal Saline). This product is a solution of sodium chloride and water. Each 100 milliliters of solution contains 0.9 gram of sodium chloride. 0.9% Sodium Chloride Injection contains 154 milliequivalents of sodium and 154 milliequivalents of chloride in each 1,000 milliliters of solution. This product is used to provide fluid replacement and to replace moderate losses of the sodium ion (Na^+).

NOTE: Sodium chloride solutions are also available in other concentrations. For example, 0.45% Sodium Chloride Injection is commonly seen.

(3) 5% Dextrose Injection in 0.9% Sodium Chloride Injection. This product has in each 100 milliliters five grams of dextrose and 0.9 grams of sodium chloride. As you might think, it is a combination of products "a" and "b" above. Not only does this product provide a source of fluid, it also serves as a source of both energy (170 calories/liter) and sodium. This product is used in fluid replacement, in the replacement of moderate losses of sodium, and as a source of energy.

NOTE: Various combinations of dextrose and sodium chloride are available. For example, 5% Dextrose in 0.45% Sodium Chloride Injection, and 2.5% Dextrose in 0.9% Sodium Chloride Injection.

5-8. ELECTROLYTE REPLACEMENT SOLUTIONS

a. **Use.** Electrolyte replacement solutions provide both electrolytes (like sodium, potassium, etc.) and fluid to the patient. Special electrolyte replacement solutions can be prepared in order to meet the needs of particular patients.

b. **Examples of Electrolyte Replacement Solutions.** Below are only two of the solutions commonly used to replace electrolytes.

(1) Lactated Ringer's Injection (LR. Ringer's Lactate, RL, Hartmann's Solution). This product is a solution of electrolytes in water. This product contains sodium, potassium, calcium, chloride, and lactate ions. The lactate ion in the product has an alkalizing effect and is metabolized in the liver to glycogen and ends up as carbon dioxide and water. Lactated Ringer's Injection is used as a fluid replacement and as an electrolyte replacement.

(2) Lactated Ringer's Injection with 5% Dextrose (D5RL). This product is a combination of Lactated Ringer's Injection and 5% Dextrose Injection. The dextrose supplies 170 calories per 1,000 milliliters of solution. D5RL is used as a fluid replacement, electrolyte replacement, and as a source of energy.

NOTE: Other combination products are available.

5-9. PLASMA EXPANDERS

a. **Use.** Plasma expanders are used to treat or prevent acute and severe fluid loss due to trauma or surgery. These products are usually used instead of whole blood in emergency situations in which whole blood is not available.

b. **Examples of Plasma Expanders.**

(1) Normal human serum albumin. Normal human serum albumin is a fraction of whole blood. It is a clear, moderately viscous, brownish fluid which contains 25 grams of serum albumin in 100 milliliters of product. Because each gram of albumin holds approximately 18 milliliters of water, it is used as blood volume expander in the treatment of hemorrhage or shock. In this use, the albumin draws fluid into the circulatory system from the surrounding tissues. This product has also been used as a protein replacement in cases where the level of protein in the serum is very low (e.g., in nephrosis). Normal human serum albumin should not be given to dehydrated patients since it draws fluid from the body tissues. If necessary, the product may be administered to dehydrated patients if 0.9% Sodium Chloride Injection or 5% Dextrose

Injection is administered at the same time. Fortunately, this product is very stable. Therefore, it is not necessary to keep it refrigerated in its liquid state.

(2) <u>Plasma protein fraction (Plasmanate)</u>. Plasma protein fraction is a sterile solution of stabilized human plasma proteins in 0.9% Sodium Chloride Injection. Each 100 milliliters of this product contains approximately five grams of protein. This product is nearly colorless (slightly brown). Plasma protein fraction is used in the treatment of nonhemorrhagic shock (i.e., shock not associated with loss of whole blood). Side effects associated with this product are uncommon, but they include increased salivation, nausea, and vomiting.

5-10. NUTRIENT SOLUTIONS (HYPERALIMENTATION PRODUCTS)

These products provide total parenteral nutrition for those patients who cannot, should not, or will not ingest the nutrients they need to live. It should be noted that a hyperalimentation can supply all the patient's nutritional needs by administration through the circulatory system. However, these solutions are quite expensive and, because of their nutrient content, are highly susceptible to bacterial growth. Most of the solutions contain high concentrations of carbohydrates (e.g., dextrose). Because of this high concentration, the solutions must be administered through a large-bore vein. Just placing the needle or catheter into such a large-bore vein is a surgical procedure in itself. The hyperalimentation solution is prepared in the Pharmacy Sterile Products Section by a specially trained person. Extreme care must be taken to prevent microbial contamination. The preparation of the product itself is quite a task because the preparer must add ingredients in a certain sequence since many of the components of a hyperalimentation solution are incompatible in certain concentrations. The components of most hyperalimentation solutions are water, dextrose, amino acids, electrolytes, and vitamins. One product, Intralipid®, is an oil in water emulsion. Intralipid® is one hyperalimentation product which can be administered through a small-bore vein such as those found in the arm.

Continue with Exercises

EXERCISES, LESSON 5

INSTRUCTIONS: The following exercises are to be answered by marking the lettered response that best answers the question or best completes the incomplete statement or by writing the answer in the space provided.

After you have completed all the exercises, turn to "Solutions to Exercises" at the end of the lesson and check your answers.

1. An intravenous admixture is best described as an intravenous:

    a. Product which is at least 1,000 milliliters in volume.

    b. Solution which has one or more drugs added to it.

    c. Solution which contains only water and a high concentration of glucose.

    d. Product which is not prepared in the pharmacy.

2. Which of the following statements best describes a precaution pertaining to intravenous fluid therapy?

    a. All intravenous solutions must be visually checked for the presence of bacteria before the solution is administered.

    b. An intravenous product with visible particulate matter can be administered to a patient if the product is filtered immediately prior to administration.

    c. Two chemicals which are known to be incompatible can be mixed in an intravenous solution as long as no visible particulate matter is observed.

    d. Some intravenous solutions, because of their pH or concentration, may cause irritation to the vein in which they are administered.

3. Select the possible complication associated with intravenous fluid therapy.

    a. Dehydration.

    b. Phlebitis.

    c. Nausea and vomiting.

    d. Cardiac arrest.

4. Hyperalimentation products can be best described as products that:

   a. Provide the patient with only protein and fluid needs.

   b. Provide total parenteral nutrition for those patients who cannot, should not, or will not ingest the nutrients they need to live.

   c. Are designed to provide severely burned patients with the substances required for life for a short period.

   d. Contain fluids and trace amounts of proteins and fat.

5. Normal human serum albumin is classified as a(n):

   a. Plasma expander solution.

   b. Electrolyte replacement solution.

   c. Hydrating solution.

   d. Hyperalimentation solution.

6. Five percent Dextrose Injection in 0.9% Sodium Chloride Injection is classified as a(n):

   a. Plasma expander solution.

   b. Electrolyte replacement solution.

   c. Hydrating solution.

   d. Hyperalimentation solution.

Check Your Answers on Next Page

SOLUTIONS TO EXERCISES, LESSON 5

1. b (para 5-2b)

2. d (para 5-4c)

3. b (para 5-5a)

4. b. (para 5-10)

5. a (para 5-9b(1))

6. c (para 5-7b(3))

End of Lesson 5

LESSON ASSIGNMENT

LESSON 6   Review of the Endocrine System.

LESSON ASSIGNMENT   Paragraphs 6-1 through 6-18.

LESSON OBJECTIVES   After completing this lesson, you should be able to:

6-1.   Given one of the following terms: gland, hormone, exocrine glands, endocrine glands, or negative feedback and a group of statements, select the statement that best defines the given term.

6-2.   Given a list of the names of various glands or organs, select those that are endocrine glands.

6-3.   Given a diagram of the body with the endocrine glands present and a list of the names of the endocrine gland, match each name with its appropriate location.

6-4.   Given the name of an endocrine gland and a group of statements, select the statement that best describes the location or the function of that gland.

6-5.   Given the name of an endocrine gland and a list of hormones, select the hormone(s) produced by that gland.

6-6.   From a list of statements, select the statement(s) that best describe the physiological effects produced by a given endocrine hormone.

6-7.   Given the name of an endocrine hormone and a group of statements, select the statement that best describes the effects of too much or too little of that particular hormone in the body.

6-8. From a group of statements, select the statement that best describes the changes that occur during a female's menstrual cycle.

6-9. From a group of statements, select the statement that best describes the changes that occur in a female after fertilization of an ovum occurs.

6-10. From a group of statements, select the statement that best describes the changes that occur at menopause.

6-11. Given the name of a disorder that affects the human reproductive system and a group of statements, select the statement that best describes that disorder.

SUGGESTION   After completing the assignment, complete the exercises at the end of this lesson. These exercises will help you to achieve the lesson objectives.

LESSON 6

REVIEW OF THE ENDOCRINE SYSTEM

Section I. INTRODUCTION

6-1. OVERVIEW

a. Many of the drugs you will dispense will directly affect one or more of the endocrine glands or will perform some function intended to be performed by one of the endocrine glands. As you review the endocrine system, be aware of the importance of this system to your daily life.

b. The endocrine system is an interconnected system of glands that produces substances known as hormones. These glands are not connected directly, but are nonetheless connected by the circulatory system. The hormones these glands produce have wide-ranging effects on the body. The production of the proper hormone in the proper amount at the proper time is absolutely essential for the maintenance of good health. An imbalance of one of these hormones causes widely varying effects upon the body.

6-2. BASIC DEFINITIONS

a. **Gland.** A gland is a secreting organ. The process of secretion includes the production of a chemical substance and the release of that substance into the blood or a body cavity.

b. **Hormone.** A hormone is a specific chemical substance that is produced in one organ (that is, endocrine gland) and transported by the blood to distant parts of the body. The hormones stimulate these various parts of the body to perform a function.

c. **Exocrine Glands.** The exocrine glands are duct glands. That is, exocrine glands secrete a chemical substance through a system of ducts into a body cavity or onto the body surface. Examples of exocrine glands are the liver, salivary glands, and sweat glands.

d. **Endocrine Glands.** Endocrine glands are ductless glands. That is, endocrine glands secrete hormones directly into the bloodstream instead of through a duct or duct system. Examples of endocrine glands include the pituitary body and the thyroid gland.

e. **Negative Feedback.** Negative feedback enables the endocrine glands to regulate themselves. Negative feedback means that once the normal physiological function of the hormones has been achieved, information is transmitted back to the glands in some way and the producing glands stops or slows the production of that particular hormone. The presence of increased amounts of a hormone will depress the endocrine gland responsible for the production of this hormone and cause less of this hormone to be produced. Conversely, a decrease in the blood levels of a hormone will cause the endocrine gland to produce more of this hormone.

6-3. GENERAL COMMENTS

a. **Control "Systems" of the Human Body.** The structure and function of the human body is controlled and organized by several different "systems."

(1) Heredity/environment. The interaction of heredity and environment is the fundamental control "system." Genes determine the range of potentiality and environment develops it. For example, good nutrition will allow a person to attain his full body height and weight within the limits of his genetic determination. Genetics is the study of heredity.

(2) Hormones. The hormones of the endocrine system serve to control the tissues and organs In general. (Vitamins have a similar role.) Both the hormones and vitamins are chemical substances required only in small amounts.

(3) Nervous system. More precise and immediate control of the structures of the body is carried out by the nervous system.

b. **The Endocrine System.** In the human body, the endocrine system consists of a number of ductless glands that produce their specific hormones. Because these hormones are carried to their target organs by the bloodstream, the endocrine glands are richly supplied with blood vessels.

c. **Better Known Endocrine Organs of Humans.** The better known endocrine glands are the:

(1) Pituitary body.

(2) Thyroid gland.

(3) Parathyroid glands.

(4) Pancreatic islets (Islets of Langerhans).

(5) Suprarenal (adrenal) glands.

(6)   Gonads (ovaries in the female, testes in the male).

(7)   In addition, there are several other endocrine glands whose function is less well understood and there are other organs that are suspected to be of the endocrine type. Figure 6-1 shows some of the better known endocrine glands and their locations.

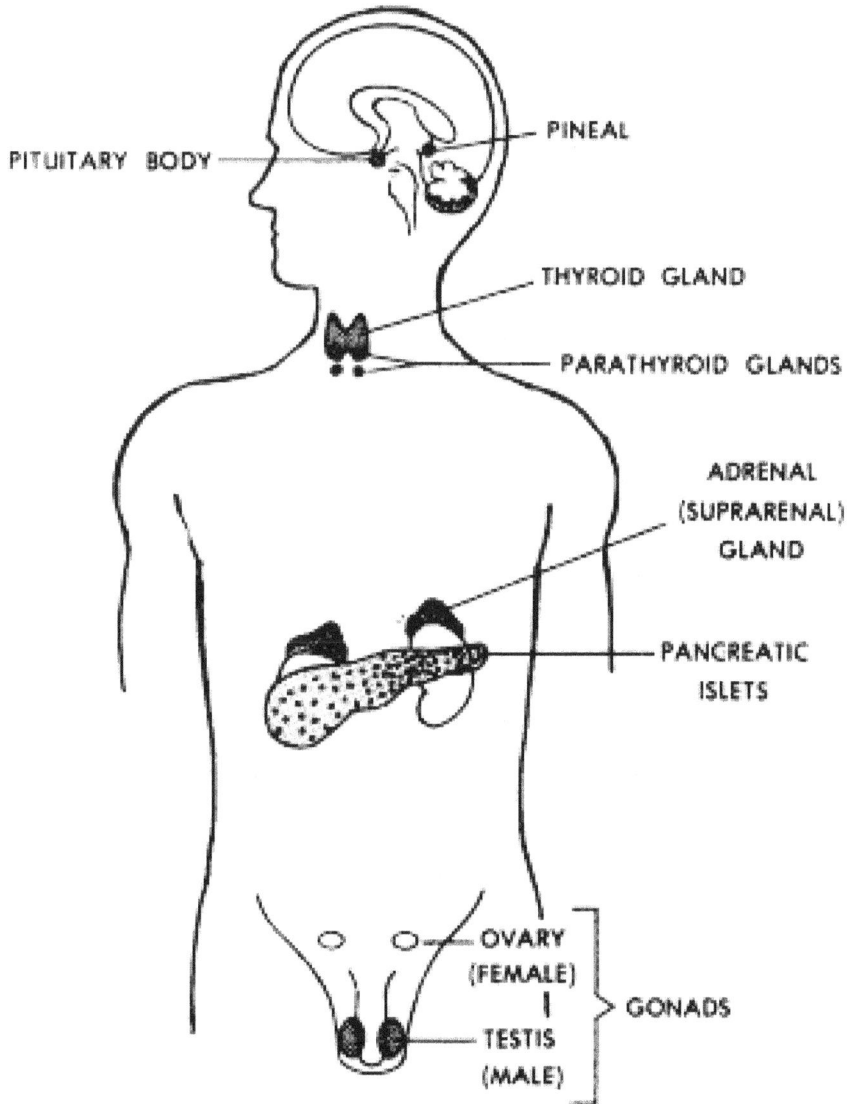

Figure 6-1. The endocrine glands of the human body and their locations.

Section II. ENDOCRINE GLANDS

6-4. INTRODUCTION

In order to gain an understanding of some of the drugs that will be presented later in the subcourse, you must become familiar with the endocrine glands and the functions they perform. As you read the paragraphs below, associate the gland with the substance(s) it produces and with the function(s) performed by the/those substance(s).

6-5. THE PITUITARY BODY

a. **Location.** The pituitary body is a small pea-sized and pea-shaped structure. It is attached to the base of the brain in the region of the hypothalamus. In addition, it is housed within a hollow of the bony floor of the cranial cavity. The hollow is called the sella trucica ("Turk's saddle"). This gland is sometimes referred to as the "master gland" of the body because of the many effects it produces.

b. **Major Subdivisions of the Pituitary Body.** The pituitary body is actually two glands, the posterior pituitary gland and the anterior pituitary gland. Initially separate, these glands join together during development of the embryo.

6-6. THE POSTERIOR PITUITARY GLAND

The posterior pituitary gland is the portion that comes from and retains a direct connection with the base of the brain. The hormones of the posterior pituitary gland are actually produced in the hypothalamus of the brain. From the hypothalamus, the hormones are delivered to the posterior pituitary gland where they are released into the bloodstream. At present, we recognize two hormones of the posterior pituitary gland.

a. **The Antidiuretic Hormone.** The Antidiuretic Hormone (ADH, Vasopressin) is involved with the resorption or salvaging of water within the kidneys. Therefore, this hormone produces its main effects in the kidneys. In the kidney, ADH increases the permeability of the distal tubules collecting tubules, thus causing the antidiuretic effect by osmosis. In large doses, vasopressin increases blood pressure by direct stimulation of the smooth muscles in the vessels. This effect is seen only with injections of vasopressin. Diabetes insipidus is a disorder that may be caused by hyposecretion of vasopressin. Diabetes insipidus is characterized by polyuria (excessive urine production). As much as 20 to 40 liters of urine may be excreted in one day by a patient who has diabetes insipidus. Polydipsia (excessive thirst) is another characteristic of diabetes insipidus.

b. **Oxytocin.** Oxytocin is a hormone concerned with contractions of smooth muscle in the uterus and with milk secretion. The contractions occur in the pregnant female. Milk secretion is an effect of oxytocin that occurs after the female has delivered the baby.

6-7. THE ANTERIOR PITUITARY GLAND

The anterior pituitary gland originates from the roof of the embryo's mouth. It then attaches itself to the posterior pituitary gland. The anterior pituitary gland is indirectly connected to the hypothalamus by means of a venous portal system. By "portal," we mean that the veins carry substances from the capillaries at one point to the capillaries at another point (hypothalamus to the anterior pituitary gland). In the hypothalamus, certain chemicals known as releasing factors are produced. These are carried by the portal system to the anterior pituitary gland. Here, they stimulate the cells of the anterior pituitary gland to secrete their specific hormones. The anterior pituitary gland produces many hormones. In general, these hormones stimulate the target organs to develop or produce their own products. This stimulating effect is referred to as tropic. Of the many hormones produced by the anterior pituitary gland, we will examine these:

a. **Somatotropic Hormone (Growth Hormone).**

(1)   The target organs of this hormone are the growing structures of the body. This hormone influences such structures to grow. Growth is produced because cell division is increased--stimulating increased growth of all tissues capable of growing. This hormone produces an increased utilization of amino acids to produce proteins. It also causes a renal depression followed by accumulation of sodium chloride and water. Inhibition of carbohydrate utilization also occurs, producing hyperglycemia.

(2)   Unfortunately, the anterior pituitary gland does not always function properly. For instance, the anterior pituitary gland may produce too much or too little somatotropin. The hyposecretion of somatotropin in childhood produces a condition known as pituitary dwarfism that results in a lack of physical development. A 20-year old person with this disease may have the same physical appearance as a 5-year old child. Conversely, the hypersecretion of somatotropin in childhood may cause giantism. This is distinguished by accelerated, undiminished growth. An extreme example of the results of this condition is a man who has grown to a height of eight feet, 6-1/2 inches and weighs 375 pounds. This same hypersecretion sometimes occurs in adulthood. This condition is called acromegaly. In acromegaly, there is no increase in the height of the person since the epiphyses of the long bones have been fused. However, the membraneous bones such as the facial bones become enlarged and the person gains coarse facial features. Other symptoms of acromegaly include enlarged hands, feet, and internal organs. Hyposecretion of somatotropin in the adult causes a condition known as Simmond's disease. This disease produces what appears to be advanced physical senility, although the patient may be quite young.

b. **Thyroid-Stimulating Hormone.** The thyroid-stimulating hormone (Thyrotropic Hormone, TSH). stimulates the growth of the thyroid gland. It thus promotes the growth of the thyroid gland as well as the production and secretion of the hormones made by the thyroid gland. The secretion of the thyroid-stimulating hormone as well as the thyroid hormones is controlled by a negative feedback mechanism. That is, a high level of TSH causes an increase in the amount of thyroid hormones produced. Once the levels of the thyroid hormones reach a certain level in the bloodstream, the amount of TSH secreted is reduced and the secretion of the thyroid hormones is decreased.

      c. **Pituitary Gonadotropic Hormones.** The pituitary gonadotropic hormones are three in number. These hormones control the development and function of the sex glands (gonads). However, these hormones have differing effects in the different sexes. Each of these hormones will be discussed below.

      (1)   Follicle-stimulating hormone. In the female, the follicle-stimulating hormone (FSH)acts in the ovary to stimulate the growth and maturation of the ovarian follicles that contain the ovum (egg). The FSH also stimulates the secretion of estrogen, a female hormone, by the ovaries. In the male, the FSH acts on structures called the seminiferous tubules in the testes to cause spermatogenesis (the production of sperm).

      (2)   Luteinizing hormone. In the female, luteinizing hormone (LH) acts to cause ovulation, the release of a mature egg from the ovary. In the male, LH is known as the interstitial cell-stimulating hormone (ICSH). The ICSH controls the production of testosterone, a male hormone, in the testes.

      (3)   Prolactin (luteotropic hormone). In the female, prolactin causes the secretion of milk from the fully developed mammary gland (breast) after the breast has been stimulated by progesterone and estrogen.

6-8.   THE THYROID GLAND

      The thyroid gland is located in the neck just below the larynx (voice box). The thyroid gland secretes the hormone thyroxin.

      a. **Background.** Thyroxin is synthesized within the thyroid gland by the combination of several amino acids with four atoms of iodine. Once made, the hormone is stored in the thyroid gland in combination with a protein. This protein-hormone complex is called thyroglobulin. The hormone is released into the blood by breaking the bonds between thyroxin and the protein. The thyroxin is then released into the bloodstream. The release of the hormone is stimulated by the thyroid-stimulating hormone from the anterior pituitary gland.

      b. **Effects of Thyroxin.** When thyroxin reaches the cells of the body, it stimulates them to use more oxygen. This increases the metabolic rate, or basal metabolism, of the body. Basal metabolism is defined as the amount of oxygen the body uses per unit of weight when the body is at rest. Thyroxin also functions to regulate the growth of organs; aid in mental development; aid in sexual development; and aid in the metabolism of water, electrolytes, proteins, glucose, and lipids. The Basal Metabolic Rate test may be used to measure the effect of thyroxin on the body.

The Protein Bound Iodine test may be used to measure the amount of thyroxin present in the blood.

c. **Diseases Involving the Thyroid Gland.** There are several diseases involving the thyroid gland.

(1) Goiter. Goiter is an abnormal enlargement of the thyroid gland producing a distinct swelling at the base of the neck just below the larynx ("Adam's Apple"). Simple goiters result from a dietary lack of iodine. This occurs most commonly in areas in which the soil is relatively free of iodine and where no seafood, material high in iodine content-is eaten. The thyroid gland, because of the lack of iodine, does not produce enough active thyroxin. Because of this lack of thyroxin, increased amounts of thyroid-stimulating hormone are produced, stimulating the thyroid and causing it to increase in size. Hence, a goiter (abnormal enlargement) is formed.

(2) Graves' disease. Another form of goiter is called Graves' Disease. Graves' Disease is the result of an overactivity of the thyroid (or hyperthyroidism). It is also called exophthalmic goiter because of the protruding eyeballs that are characteristic of the disease. Other symptoms associated with Graves' Disease include nervous tension, fatigue, fast and irregular heart beat, and eventually, congestive heart failure. The cause of Graves' disease is unknown. The result of Graves' disease is an enlarged and hyperactive thyroid gland. Graves' disease is treated by the use of antithyroid drugs and/or surgical removal of part of the thyroid gland. Many of the clinical signs and symptoms typical of Graves' Disease may also be seen in patients who take an overdose of a thyroid drug.

(3) Cretinism. Diseases involving thyroid underactivity may be seen in children and adults. Hyposecretion of thyroxin in the fetus or newborn produces a disease called cretinism. This lack of thyroxin causes retardation of skeletal and nervous system growth. Untreated, this hyposecretion of thyroxin in a newborn can result in a mentally retarded dwarf. If the disease is detected very early, the child can be given thyroxin replacement therapy so development can be normal. Lack of thyroxin in adults may produce myxedema. Characteristics of myxedema include edema, fatigue, lethargy, sensitivity to cold, and other degenerative changes. The disease reaches its peak of severity in a hypothermic coma, in which the patient goes into a coma and the body temperature decreases to between 80 to 90 degrees Fahrenheit.

6-9. THE PARATHYROID GLANDS

The parathyroid glands are usually four in number. They are embedded in the posterior portion of the thyroid. Their principal action is the production of parathormone.

a. **Parathormone.** Parathormone is a hormone that works in conjunction with another hormone, calcitonin, to regulate the calcium and phosphate in the body. The storehouse of calcium in the body is bone. That is, bone is being formed and reabsorbed at the same time. Parathormone acts on bone by increasing bone reabsorption and increasing serum calcium. Parathormone also acts on the kidneys to increase calcium reabsorption and on the intestinal tract to increase the absorption of calcium. The net effect is an increase in serum calcium level.

b. **Diseases Involving the Parathyroid Glands.**

(1) Hypoparathyroidism. Hypoparathyroidism is a disease usually caused by inadvertent surgical removal of the parathyroid glands. This removal results in a lack of parathromone that decreases the serum calcium. Lowering the serum calcium level causes increased neuromuscular irritability that results in tetany. Tetany is characterized by intermittent muscular contractions, tremor, and muscular pain.

(2) Hyperparathyroidism. Occasionally, the parathyroid glands produce too much parathormone. This condition is called hyperparathyroidism. Hyperparathyroidism causes erosion of the skeletal muscle system. Such an erosion results in weak, painful, and brittle bones.

c. **Calcitonin.** Calcitonin apparently performs as a sort of fine control of the blood's calcium level. Its action is essentially the reverse of parathormone. Calcitonin causes the body to build more bone-thus decreasing the serum calcium level. Calcitonin is produced by both parathyroid and thyroid glands.

6-10. THE ADRENAL GLANDS

The adrenal glands (also known as suprarenal glands) are embedded in the fat above each kidney. Both adrenal glands have an internal medulla and an external cortex.

a. **Hormones of the Adrenal Medulla.** The medullary (inside the gland) portion of each adrenal gland produces a pair of hormones, epinephrine (adrenalin) and norepinephrine (noradrenalin). These hormones are both involved in the mobilization of energy during the stress reaction ("fight or flight" response). These hormones are also produced in the autonomic nervous system. Therefore, production of these hormones in the adrenal medulla is not necessary for life. After production, these hormones are stored in the adrenal medulla and are released in large quantities during the stress reaction.

(1) Epinephrine (adrenalin). Epinephrine has the following effects on the body, constriction of arterioles which produces a rise in blood pressure, increased heart rate and force of contraction, inhibition of intestinal activity, contraction of the gallbladder, dilation of the pupils, stimulation of glycogenolysis, stimulation of adrenocorticotropic hormone (ACTH) production, and bronchodilation.

(2) Norepinephrine (noradrenalin). Norepinephrine has less an effect on the gastrointestinal tract and a greater effect on blood pressure than does epinephrine. Norepinephrine has no effect on the bronchioles. Tumors of the adrenal medulla are

called pheochromocytomas. These tumors produce hypertension (either chronic or acute), elevation of basal metabolism, and glucosuria.

   b. **Hormones of the Suprarenal Cortex (Outside Area).** Approximately 28 hormones are produced by the suprarenal cortex. These hormones are produced only in the suprarenal cortex and are essential to life. The hormones of the suprarenal cortex are of most importance during times of stress (like trauma and disease). The hormones produced here tend to keep body metabolism stable during such periods of stress. The hormones reduce fluid loss, stabilize blood glucose, reduce inflammation, and prevent shock. Animals that have had their adrenal glands removed die under much less stress than do animals that have their adrenal glands. Occasionally, the suprarenal cortex malfunctions. When its function is reduced, a condition called Addison's disease results. Fatigue, muscle weakness, weight loss, low blood pressure, gastronintestinal upset, and collapse are clinical signs of Addison's disease. When the suprarenal cortex too actively secretes its hormones, a condition called Cushing's disease results. Cushing's disease is characterized by the abnormal disposition of fat in the face (called moon face) and back of the neck (called buffalo hump), obesity, edema, hypertension, acne, abnormalities in carbohydrate metabolism (in 90 percent of patients), and diabetes mellitus (in 20 percent of patients). The hormones produced here can be grouped into two major categories according to their action. These two categories are the mineralocorticoids and the glucocorticoids.

   (1) <u>Mineralocorticoids.</u> The mineralocorticoids affect the electrolytes and water in the body. These hormones cause a conservation of sodium (Na+) and chloride (Cl-) by increasing the renal reabsorption of these ions. Conversely, they increase the excretion of potassium (K+). This retention of sodium and chloride also causes a retention of water. The principle mineralocorticoid is aldosterone. Other hormones in this group also exhibit, to some degree, some glucocorticoid activity.

   (2) <u>Glucocorticoids.</u> Glucocorticoids have several different metabolic effects. They cause deposition of glycogen in the liver, gluconeogenesis (conversion of amino acids to glucose), liberation of amino acids from proteins, mobilization of fats, decreased utilization of glucose, and an increase in blood glucose levels. Hydrocortisone is the principal example of a glucocorticoid. Hydrocortisone and cortisone both have sodium-retention effects. Both hydrocortisone and cortisone have anti-inflammatory actions and cause dissolution of lymphoid tissue. Synthetic steriods have more effect on inflammation than do naturally occurring steroids.

6-11. THE PANCREAS

   The pancreas is located behind the stomach in the curve of the duodenum. The pancreas may be considered both an endocrine and an exocrine gland since pancreatic juices are secreted through the common pancreatic duct. Two types of tissue make up the pancreas. The acini secrete digestive juices into the duodenum. The Islets of Langerhans is the endocrine tissue. The Islets of Langerhans contains two types of cells, each type produces a particular hormone. Alpha cells produce glucagon. Beta cells produce insulin, a hormone essential to the body's metabolism.

a. **Glucagon.** Glucagon is frequently called the hyperglycemic factor. Glucagon causes glycogenolysis (the conversion of glycogen into glucose) and tends to prevent hypoglycemia. Glucagon is released when blood glucose levels drop, thus, glucagon tends to raise the level of sugar in the blood.

b. **Insulin.** Insulin's principal effect is to increase the cells' permeability to glucose. When the glucose enters the cells, it is metabolized to produce energy. Insulin also increases glycogenesis in the liver, thus, it increases glycogen stored there. A hyposecretion of insulin is known as diabetes mellitus. There are essentially two types of diabetes, juvenile diabetes and maturity-onset diabetes. Juvenile diabetes develops early in life, usually about the time of puberty, and is frequently associated with ketoacidosis. This form of diabetes is treated with insulin therapy. Maturity-onset diabetes frequently does not appear until middle age. Maturity-onset diabetes is usually milder than juvenile diabetes. Furthermore, maturity-onset diabetes is sometimes managed by the administrating of oral hypoglycemics and by controlling the patient's weight and diet. The lack of insulin decreases the amount of glucose that enters the cells of the body and increases the amount of glucose present in the person's blood (hyperglycemia). Hyperglycemia causes sugar to spill over into the urine. This results in glycosuria and polyuria (due to the osmotic effect of the glucose). The lack of glucose entering the cells causes gluconeogenesis and fat catabolism. This result in wasting of the cells and ketoacidosis. Ketoacidosis leads to coma and death. Uncontrolled diabetes mellitus may be accompanied by hyperglycemia, glycosuria, polyuria, polydipsia (excessive thirst leading to increased water intake), ketoacidosis, wasting coma, and death. A person who has diabetes mellitus may be required to take insulin to treat the lack of insulin present in the body. If a person must take insulin, it is likely that this individual must take insulin for the remainder of his or her life. Remember, insulin taken by the diabetic does not cure diabetes. In the opposite fashion, an overdose of insulin may cause hypoglycemia, depression of the central nervous system, and death. One possible treatment of this condition is an injection of glucagon. Remember, when injected, glucagon causes glycogenesis that results in an elevated level of blood sugar.

6-12. THE GONADS

Both the male and female sexes have gonads. The female and male cells, or gametes, are produced by the reproductive glands or gonads. In the male, the gonads are the two testes. In the female, the gonads are the two ovaries. In addition to these primary sex glands, there are a number of accessory organs. In the male, these accessory organs are the vas deferens, seminal vesicles, prostate gland, and the penis. In the female, the accessory organs are the fallopian tubes (oviducts), uterus, vagina, and mammary glands. For a review of the human reproductive system, review Lesson 6 in MD0806, Pharmacology III.

a. **Male.** In the male, the actual reproductive cells are the spermatozoa (sperm). The spermatozoa are produced in the seminiferous tubules of the testes. In the testes, germinal cells produce spermatozoa by a process called spermatogenesis. Once formed, the spermatozoa travel into another portion of the testes called the epididymis. The spermatozoa are stored in the epididymis until they mature. From the epididymis, the spermatozoa travel in two ducts called the vas deferens. The vas deferens unite with the urethra. In the vas deferens, the spermatozoa are joined by a fluid produced by the seminal vesicle. This fluid, together with the secretions of the prostate gland and the bulbo-urethral gland which flow into the urethra, compose the semen that nourishes the spermatozoa and provides the electrolytes and proper pH In the proper concentration range. The vas deferens is separated from the urethra by the ejaculatory duct (a muscular sphincter). During the process of ejaculation, the sphincter relaxes and the spermatozoa are propelled by powerful peristaltic waves. At the onset of puberty in the male, the pituitary gland produces follicle-stimulating hormones (FSH) which stimulate the seminiferous tubules to undergo spermatogenesis and produce spermatozoa. At the same time, the pituitary gland releases interstitial cell-stimulating hormones (ISCH or LH), that stimulate the interstitial cells in the testes to produce androgens. Androgens are masculinizing hormones. The principal androgen is testosterone. Testosterone, in turn, stimulates the secondary sexual characteristics of the male. These androgens are produced throughout the male's life.

b. **Female.** In the female reproductive system, the ovaries produce the egg cell or ovum. The ovum then passes the short distance between the ovary and the fallopian tube (in the abdominal cavity) and enters the fallopian tube (oviduct). The ovum then travels down the oviduct by peristalsis and ciliary movement of the cells lining the oviduct. The fallopian tubes connect the ovaries with the uterus. The uterus is a pear-shaped organ in the center of the female reproductive system. It is lined with a tissue called the endometrium. The base of the uterus is a diaphragm-like structure called the cervix. Below the cervix is a muscular tube called the vagina.

(1) Hormone production. The production of hormones in the female is considerably more complex than in the male. The hormones of the female reproductive system do not remain at a constant level, as in the male, but are in a cyclic balance. Each cycle takes, on the average, 28 days. To understand this cycle properly, one should first consider the production of the ovum in more detail. The ovaries are composed of several hundred thousand ova. These are surrounded by granulosa cells. This combination is called a primary follicle. Under the influence of hormones, the follicle enlarges and begins to secrete a fluid that fills the cavity inside the follicle, creating an antrum (cavity) in the follicle. Numerous follicles enlarge at the same time until one follicle ruptures. The remaining follicles then return to their normal state. The ova, which is released then migrates through the abdominal cavity until it reaches the fallopian tube. The ovum then takes from three to seven days to reach the uterus. However, the ova must be fertilized within 24 hours after it is released. Thus, the ova must be fertilized while it is in the oviduct. Occasionally, more than one follicle ruptures at the same time and more than one ova are released. This is the chief cause of multiple births. Pituitary gonadotropins function in the process of releasing ova.

(2) <u>Follicle growth.</u> Growth of the primary follicle is initiated by the folliclestimulating hormone (FSH). The FSH causes a proliferation of the granulosa cells and the production of the fluid filling the antrum. The luteinizing hormone (LH) causes a further production of fluid that continues until the follicle bursts. The ovum is then expelled and the remainder of the follicle undergoes a transformation into a mass of yellow cells known as the corpus luteum.

(3) <u>Release of FSH.</u> The release of FSH by the adenohypohysis, in addition to causing the growth of the follicle, also causes the follicles to secrete one of the two female hormones--estrogen. Estrogen is the principal female hormone. Estrogen is a composite of several hormones called estradiol, estriol, and estrone. These three substances have slightly different molecular structures, but they produce the same activity in the body. Estrogens are responsible for the secondary sexual characteristics of the female. Estrogens also cause the lining of the uterus, the endometrium, to increase in thickness by about threefold. The corpus luteum, under the stimulation of the luteotropic hormone secreted by the pituitary gland, begins to secrete large amounts of estrogen and progesterone. Unless fertilization of the ova occurs, the corpus luteum persists for about two weeks, after which time it begins to degenerate. Progesterone is the other female hormone. Its principal effect is on the endometrium. Progesterone causes the endometrium to secrete a nutrient fluid to nourish the ovum under its implantation, to deposit fats and glycogen in the endometrium, and to increase the blood supply to the endometrium. Progesterone also prepares the breasts for the secretion of milk and inhibits contractions of the uterus, since contractions might expel the ovum. Thus, if fertilized, the ovum would be able to stay in the uterus.

6-13. THE FEMALE'S MENSTRUAL CYCLE

The rhythmical cycle of events in the female's reproductive system is known as the menstrual cycle. The menstrual cycle depends on the interplay of the hypophyseal gonadotropins and the estrogens. At the beginning of the cycle, estrogen levels are low. Because estrogens act to inhibit the pituitary's production of the follicle-stimulating hormone (FSH), the FSH level is allowed to increase. The increase in the FSH acts on the ovaries to stimulate the production of estrogens. The level of estrogens as produced by the follicles then increases, causing a drop in the FSH level. At midcycle, the luteinizing hormone (LH) is secreted by the pituitary gland. The luteinizing hormone stimulates ovulation, followed by the conversion of the follicle to a corpus luteum and the secretion of estrogen and progesterone by the corpus luteum. The high levels of progesterone cause a decrease in secretion of the luteinizing hormone. If the egg is not fertilized by a sperm cell, the corpus luteum degenerates, causing a drop in levels of both estrogen and progesterone that completes the cycle. This drop in estrogen and progesterone levels causes the endometrium to degenerate and slough off and also causes small hemorrhages in the uterus. This is the cause of the periodic menstrual flow in women.

6-14. CHANGES DUE TO FERTILIZATION OF THE OVUM

If the ovum is fertilized by a sperm cell, the menstrual cycle ceases. After the fertilized ovum passes through the fallopian tube, it implants into the already prepared endometrium. The embryo (fertilized egg) grows rapidly and soon develops a placenta. The placenta is a tissue that eventually covers about one-fourth of the uterus. The placenta is located between the endometrium and the fetus. The placenta is supplied with blood vessels from the mother and blood vessels from the embryo through the umbilical cord. There is no direct exchange of blood between the mother and the embryo; however, the embryo is able to receive nutrients, electrolytes, and oxygen from the mother's blood by the processes of diffusion and active transport. Likewise, waste products from the embryo's system are diffused from the embryo's blood to the mother's blood. The fetus is surrounded by its own membranes and is supported by the amniotic fluid in the amniotic sac filling the uterus. The endometrium and placenta are maintained by high levels of progesterone, which acts to cause an increase in the concentration of nutrients in the endometrium, reduce uterine contraction, and prepare the breasts for lactation. For about the first trimester of pregnancy, the progesterones are supplied by the corpus luteum. The corpus luteum, which normally degenerates after two weeks, is itself maintained by another hormone, chorionic gonadotropin, which is produced by the cells of the fetus (embryo) very soon after implantation. After the first trimester of pregnancy, the corpus luteum degenerates and the progesterone becomes produced by the placenta. If, at any time during this "change over" the progesterone level falls too low, the endometrium will degenerate causing a spontaneous abortion. The estrogens produced during pregnancy come from the same sources as do the progesterones. The estrogens function to enlarge the uterus and the breast.

6-15. MENOPAUSE

Women usually stop menstruating at about the age of 45. This is known as the menopause. At this time, nearly all the primary follicles in the ovaries have been released or have become involuted (returned to normal size). Since the primary follicles supply most of the body's estrogen, the cyclic increase and decrease of estrogens cannot occur. Thus, the menstrual cycle is ended. Some women experience various effects (for example, hot flashes, fatigue, anxiety, and irritability) because of the metabolic changes the body is undergoing because of the decreased production of estrogen. The physician may prescribe estrogen therapy to the woman during this time.

Section III. DISORDERS OF THE HUMAN REPRODUCTIVE SYSTEM

6-16. INTRODUCTION

There are numerous disorders of the human reproductive system that can occur. This section of the lesson will consider some of these disorders.

6-17. ECTOPIC PREGNANCY

An ectopic pregnancy occurs when a fertilized ovum implants in a location other than the uterus. The usual site of such an implantation in an ectopic pregnancy is the fallopian tube. When the fertilized egg becomes attached to a site other than the uterus, it invades the tissues to which it is implanted and it forms a placenta, amniotic sac, etc. The weakness of the placenta may allow bleeding, fetus necrosis (death), or the fetus may develop normally. If the fertilized ovum implants somewhere in the abdominal cavity severe damage may result to the organ against which it implants.

6-18. TOXEMIA OF PREGNANCY

Toxemia of pregnancy is a condition characterized by hypertension, edema, proteinuria, and other variable symptoms. In its more severe form, it is called eclampsia. In severe cases, lesions of the liver, kidney, and brain of the mother can result. These lesions may be caused by an anti-immune process in which antibodies attack these organs. Eclampsia may be severe enough to require termination of the pregnancy in order to save the mother.

Continue with Exercises

EXERCISES, LESSON 6

INSTRUCTIONS: The following exercises are to be answered by marking the lettered response that best answers the question or best completes the incomplete statement or by writing the answer in the space provided.

After you have completed all the exercises, turn to "Solutions to Exercises" at the end of the lesson and check your answers.

1.   Endocrine glands are best described as:

    a.   Duct glands that secrete a chemical substance through a system of ducts into a body cavity or onto the surface of the body.

    b.   Glands that secrete chemical substances through the lymphatic system of the body.

    c.   Ductless glands which secrete their hormones directly into the bloodstream instead of through a duct or duct system.

    d.   Glands that have no ducts, but are actively involved in the production of perspiration and stomach acid.

2.   Which of the following are endocrine glands?

    a.   Pituitary gland, parathyroid gland, and the gonads.

    b.   Suprarenal (adrenal) glands, thyroid gland, and salivary glands.

    c.   Thyroid gland, Islets of Langerhans, and sweat glands.

    d.   Pancreas, pituitary gland, and gallbladder.

3.   The principle function of the parathyroid glands is the production of :

    a.   Calcitonin.

    b.   Parathormone.

    c.   Thyroxin.

    d.   Prolactin.

4. Select the hormone(s) produced by the suprarenal cortex.

    a. Glucagon and noradrenalin.

    b. Hydrocortisone and cortisone.

    c. Interstitial cell-stimulating hormone and estrogen.

    d. Testosterone and calcitonin.

5. Select the hormone(s) produced by the alpha cells of the Islets of Langerhans.

    a. Insulin.

    b. Hydrocortisone.

    c. Parathormone.

    d. Glucagon.

6. From the statements below, select the statement that best describes the physiological effect produced by testosterone.

    a. Testosterone stimulates the secondary sexual characteristics of the male.

    b. Testosterone stimulates the seminal vesicle to undergo spermatogenesis and to produce spermatozoa.

    c. Testosterone stimulates the pineal gland to produce the folliclestimulating hormone (FSH).

    d. Testosterone stimulates the process of glycogenolysis.

7. Addison's disease, a condition caused by reduced functioning of the suprarenal cortex, is characterized by:

    a. Moon face and buffalo hump.

    b. Hyperglycemia and ketoacidosis.

    c. Fatigue, muscle weakness, and weight loss.

    d. The early onset of secondary male sexual characteristics.

8. Which of the statements below best describes the changes that occur during a female's menstrual cycle?

   a. The secretion of estrogen directly influences the production of progesterone that causes the endometrium to degenerate and slough off.

   b. A deficiency of estrogen caused by the overproduction of the follicle stimulating hormone (FSH) causes the endometrium to degenerate and slough off.

   c. When the corpus luteum degenerates, progesterone and estrogen levels decrease causing the endometrium to slough off.

   d. The luteinizing hormone directly influences the level of the follicle-stimulating hormone that, in turn, affects the level of estrogen in the woman's body.

9. Which of the statements below best describes the changes that occur at menopause?

   a. Due to changes in the primary follicles, the increases in the estrogen and progesterone do not occur.

   b. The primary follicles secrete more progesterone than estrogen.

   c. The endometrium degenerates and sloughs off producing hot flashes and anxiety.

   d. The ovaries become degenerated because of lack of estrogen and the follicle stimulating hormone.

10. An ectopic pregnancy occurs when a fertilized ovum:

    a. Implants in the uterus.

    b. Implants in the placenta.

    c. Implants in an amniotic sac.

    d. Implants in a location other than the uterus.

SPECIAL INSTRUCTIONS FOR EXERCISES 11 THROUGH 13. For each question in Column A, select the appropriate answer in Column B based upon the following figure.

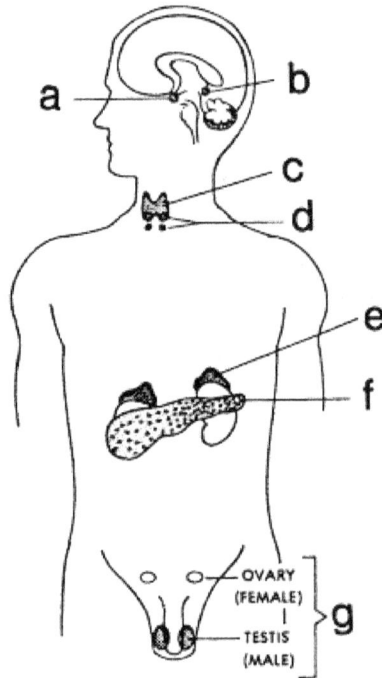

Column A	Column B
11. The arrow labeled "d" is pointing to:	a. Pituitary body.
12. The arrow labeled "f" is pointing to:	b. Parathyroid glands.
13. The arrow labeled "a" is pointing to:	c. Pineal gland.
	d. Adrenal (suprarenal) gland.
	e. Thyroid gland.
	f. Pancreatic islets.

Check Your Answers on Next Page

SOLUTIONS TO EXERCISES, LESSON 6

1. c   (para 6-2d)

2. a   (para 6-3c)

3. b   (para 6-9)

4. b   para 6-10b(2))

5. d   (para 6-10b)

6. a   (para 6-12a)

7. c   (para 6-10b)

8. c   (para 6-13)

9. a   (para 6-15)

10. d   (para 6-17)

11. b   (Figure 6-1)

12. d   (Figure 6-1)

13. a   (Figure 6-1)

End of Lesson 6

LESSON ASSIGNMENT

LESSON 7   Thyroid, Antithyroid, and Parathyroid Preparations.

LESSON ASSIGNMENT   Paragraphs 7-1 through 7-12.

LESSON OBJECTIVES   After completing this lesson, you should be able to:

7-1.   From a list of functions, select the function performed by the thyroid hormones.

7-2.   Given the name of a condition caused by either hyposecretion or hypersecretion of thyroxin and a group of statements, select the statement that best describes that condition.

7-3.   Given a group of statements, select the statement(s) that best describe precautions for persons who take thyroid preparations.

7-4.   Given the trade and/or generic name of a thyroid preparation and a group of uses and side effects, select the use(s) or side effect(s) associated with the given agent.

7-5.   Given a group of indications, select the indication(s) of antithyroid preparations.

7-6.   Given the trade and/or generic name of an antithyroid preparation and a group of uses, side effects, or cautions and warnings, select the use(s), side effect(s), and caution(s) and warning(s) associated with the given agent.

7-7.   From a group of statements, select the statement that best describes the indication for parathyroid preparations.

7-8.   From a group of statements, select the statement that best describes hypoparathyroidism.

7-9. Given the trade or generic name of a thyroid, antithyroid, or parathyroid preparation and a group of trade and generic names, select the trade or generic name that corresponds to the given name.

SUGGESTION

After completing the assignment, complete the exercises at the end of this lesson. These exercises will help you to achieve the lesson objectives.

LESSON 7

THYROID, ANTITHYROID, AND PARATHYROID PREPARATIONS

Section I. OVERVIEW

7-1. INTRODUCTION

The thyroid gland is a very important endocrine gland. This gland is located in the neck just below the larynx. This gland secretes the hormone thyroxin. Proper functioning of the thyroid gland is essential to normal functioning of the body. Either increased or decreased thyroid activity can present real problems to the patient. This lesson will focus attention on the thyroid gland and present some of the drugs available to treat both hypoactivity and hyperactivity of this important endocrine gland.

7-2. THE NATURAL THYROID HORMONES

Two hormones are responsible for the major functions of the thyroid. These hormones are thyroxine (T_4) and triiodothyronine (T_3). The notation T_4 reflects that the thyroxine nucleus has four iodine atoms attached to it. The notation T_3 means that three iodine atoms are attached to the thyroxine nucleus. Approximately, 10 times as much T_4 is secreted from the thyroid than T_3. As the T_4 circulates, some of it has iodine removed from the molecule. Hence, in terms of availability to body tissues, only about three times as much T_4 is available than T_3. Basically, because of differences in serum concentration and activity, the effects produced by these two hormones are identical for practical purposes. In order for these hormones to be synthesized in the body, sources of iodine must be present. When sufficient iodine is lacking in the diet, underlined endemic goiters (enlarged thyroid) result. Such enlargement is due to hypersecretion of thyroid stimulating hormone (TSH) in an attempt by the body to obtain the required level of thyroid hormone secretion.

7-3. FUNCTION OF THE THYROID HORMONES

The hormones produced by the thyroid gland exert effects on most of the tissues of the body. Basically, the thyroid hormones maintain normal metabolic rate, allow the body to more rapidly use carbohydrates for energy, and promote the growth of tissues in the body.

7-4. HYPOTHYROIDISM

Hypothyroidism occurs when there is not enough thyroxin being secreted into the bloodstream. Depending on the age of the individual affected, various problems can result because of hypothyroidism.

a. **Cretinism.** Cretinism is the hyposecretlon of thyroxin in the newborn. This lack of thyroxin causes retardation of skeletal and nervous system growth. Untreated, this hyposecretion of thyroxin in a newborn can result in a mentally retarded dwarf. Early diagnosis and treatment of hypothyroidism is critical. Once detected, the newborn or infant can be given thyroxin so that development can be normal.

b. **Myxedema.** Myxedema is the hyposecretion of thyroxin in an adult (person after puberty). Myxedema is characterized by edema, fatigue, lethargy, sensitivity to cold, and other degenerative changes. In general, individuals suffering from myxedema feel tired and want to sleep a great deal (perhaps from 14 to 16 hours per day).

7-5. HYPERTHYROIDISM

Because the Irish physician, Robert Graves, first described hyper-thyroidism around 1835, this condition is usually referred to as Graves disease. Hyperthyroidism is increased secretion of thyroxine. Graves disease is characterized by anxious behavior, rapid pulse rate, increased appetite, weight loss, elevated metabolic rate, tremor of the hands, and exophthalmos (a condition in which the eyeballs slightly protrude from the sockets giving the patient a startled appearance). Graves's disease can be treated by the administration of Iodine 131 (I^{131}) or by surgery. Surgery is the first choice of treatment in patients whose age is between 25 and 40 and the second choice of treatment in patients 0 to 25 years.

Section II. THYROID PREPARATIONS

7-6. PRECAUTIONS FOR PATIENTS WHO ARE TAKING THYROID PREPARATIONS

From the preceding discussion, it is obvious that thyroid preparations affect the entire body. Therefore, persons who take these medications should be told of the following precautions.

a. **Regular Checkups.** An individual taking a thyroid preparation should schedule regular visits with the prescribing physician. These regular visits give the physician the opportunity to monitor the patient's progress. Changes in the dosage of the medication may be required, the dosage of each of the agents below must be tailored to meet the individual needs of the patient. These regular checkups also give the patient an opportunity to tell the physician of any side effects the patient might be experiencing (e.g., changes in appetite, changes in menstrual periods, etc.).

b. **Exercise or Physical Work.** If the patient has certain types of heart disease, thyroid medication may cause shortness of breath or chest pain when the patient exerts himself when exercising or performing physical work. Hence, they should be cautioned against overdoing exercise or physical work. Specified questions the patient has concerning this precaution should be directed to the physician.

c. **Emergency Medical Treatment, Surgery, or Dental Surgery.** If the patient requires any emergency medical treatment, surgery, or dental surgery, the physician or dentist in charge should be told that the patient is taking thyroid medication.

d. **Over-The-Counter Medications.** Patients who take thyroid medications should be told not to take any other drug(s) unless the prescribing physician knows about the drug(s). The category of drugs includes over-the-counter medications. This is especially true of over-the-counter cold, cough, and appetite suppressant medications.

7-7. THYROID PREPARATIONS

You will see a variety of thyroid preparations in the pharmacy. Some of the medications you may dispense are discussed below.

a. **Thyroid, USP.** Thyroid, USP, is prepared from the thyroid glands of domesticated animals. Once the thyroid gland is obtained from the slaughtered animal, the gland is cleaned, dried, and powdered. Thyroid, USP, contains both the T_3 and T_4 hormone. This preparation is used in the treatment of hypo-thyroidism. The dosage of this product must be tailored to meet the needs of the individual patient. Side effects associated with this agent include changes in appetite, chest pain, diarrhea, and hand tremors.

b. **Levothyroxine (Synthroid®).** Levothyroxine is a synthetic source of the T_4 hormone. Once taken, approximately 30 percent of the levothyroxine is converted to the T_3 hormone. Levothyroxine is used in the treatment of hypothyroidism. Like Thyroid, USP, the dosage of levothyroxine must be individualized to meet the patient's needs. The usual dosage prescribed is from 0.1 milligram to 0.2 milligram taken daily in a single dose. Side effects associated with this agent include changes in appetite, chest pain, diarrhea, and hand tremors.

c. **Sodium Liothyronine (Cytomel®).** Liothyronine is a synthetic source of the T_3 hormone. This product is used in the treatment of hypothyroidism and male sterility due to hypothyroidism. As with the other thyroid preparations, the dosage of this product must be tailored to meet the needs of the individual patient. The dose usually prescribed is 25 to 50 micrograms daily in a single dose. Changes in appetite, chest pain, diarrhea, and hand tremors are side effects usually associated with this agent.

d. **Liotrix (Euthroid®).** Liotrix is a synthetic source of both T_3 and T_4 hormones. Liotrix is used in the treatment of hypothyroidism. The dosage of this product must be tailored to meet the needs of the individual patient. Side effects associated with this product include changes in appetite, chest pain, diarrhea, and hand tremors.

e. **Thyroglobulin (Proloid®).** Thyroglobulin is obtained from a purified extract of hog thyroid glands. This product provides both T_3 and T_4 hormones. Thyroglobulin is used in the treatment of hypothyroidism. The dosage of this preparation must be tailored to meet the needs of the individual patient. Adverse reactions associated with the use of this product include nervousness, sweating, and tachycardia.

7-8. MISCELLANEOUS PREPARATION

Strong Iodine Solution, USP (Lugol's solution). This preparation is used to provide the patient with a source of iodine. As noted in paragraph 7-2, a sufficient amount of iodine must be available to synthesize thyroid hormones. If iodine in the required amounts is lacking in the diet, the thyroid gland can become enlarged. The usual dosage of this product is 0.1 milliliters to 0.3 milliliters three times a day. The patient can take this medication in orange juice to mask the iodine taste.

Section III. ANTITHYROID PREPARATIONS

7-9. INTRODUCTION AND INDICATIONS

An anti-thyroid preparation inhibits the synthesis of thyroid hormones by interfering with the binding of iodine into an organic form. The administration of such a product is indicated in the treatment of hyperthyroidism and is sometimes given to a patient before thyroid surgery.

7-10. ANTITHYROID PREPARATIONS

a. **Methimazole (Tapazole®).** Methimazole is an antithyroid preparation used in the treatment of hyperthyroidism. It is also sometimes given to patients who are to undergo thyroid surgery or radiotherapy. Side effects associated with this agent include unexplained sore throat, fever, or chills; loss of hearing; swollen lymph nodes; increase in urination; and unusual bleeding or bruising. The dosage of this drug must be tailored to meet the individual needs of the patient. This medication should not be taken by pregnant women. Further, a woman should not take this preparation if she is breast-feeding an infant. You should also inform the patient that the medication should be taken each day in regularly spaced doses in order to achieve its desired effect. The medication should be taken at about the same time and the same way. This is, if the patient takes the medication with food, it should always be taken with food; if the medication is taken on an empty stomach, it should always be taken on an empty stomach. Two last precautions that should be communicated to the patient taking this drug are: (a) inform the physician or dentist before you have any type of surgery and (b) inform the physician immediately if you get an injury, infection, or illness of any type.

b. **Propylthiouracil (Propacil®).** Propylthiouracil is an antithyroid preparation used in the treatment of hyperthyroidism and it is sometimes given to patients who are to undergo thyroid surgery or radiotherapy. Side effects and precautions associated with the use of this agent are the same as those discussed under methimazole (Tapazole®) (para 7-10a). You should know that some prescribers will occasionally write PTU meaning propylthiouracil. Some patients go into remission after therapy with Tapazole® or Propacil®.

Section IV. PARATHYROID PREPARATIONS

7-11. INTRODUCTION AND INDICATION FOR USE

The parathyroid glands secrete the hormone parathormone (Lesson 6, para 6-9). This hormone regulates the amount of calcium in the intracellular fluid. The parathyroid preparations are used in the treatment of hypoparathyroidism. Hypoparathyroidism can occur spontaneously or with injury to the parathyroid glands. Hypoparathyroidism is characterized by a decrease in the concentration of calcium in the serum and an increase in the concentration of phosphorus in the serum. Overdosage of parathyroid preparations can be potentially dangerous because serum levels of calcium can reach very high levels. If the serum concentration of calcium reaches too high a level, calcification of kidneys and blood vessels can occur.

7-12. PARATHYROID PREPARATIONS

a. **Parathyroid Injection, USP.** This product is obtained from the parathyroid glands of freshly slaughtered domesticated animals like cattle. The preparation is used in the treatment of hypoparathyroidism.

b. **Dihydrotachysterol (Hytakerol®).** This product increases the level of calcium in the serum by mobilizing calcium from bones and by increasing calcium absorption from the intestines. Hence, it is used in the treatment of hypocalcemia.

Continue with Exercises

EXERCISES, LESSON 7

INSTRUCTIONS: The following exercises are to be answered by marking the lettered response that best answers the question or best completes the incomplete statement or by writing the answer in the space provided.

After you have completed all the exercises, turn to "Solutions to Exercises" at the end of the lesson and check your answers.

1. Select the function below that is performed by the thyroid hormones.

    a. Prevents the growth of tissues in the body.

    b. Maintains the normal metabolic rate of the body.

    c. Prevents the body from using carbohydrates for energy.

    d. Produces endemic goiters.

2. Cretinism is described as:

    a. A condition in which there is a hyposecretion of thyroxin in the newborn that can be treated with the administration of propythiouracil.

    b. A hyposecretion of thyroxin in the newborn that can result in retardation of the skeletal and nervous systems if left untreated.

    c. The hypersecretion of thyroxin in an adult that can result in mental retardation.

    d. A hyposecretion of thyroxin in an adult that is characterized by edema, fatigue, lethargy, and sensitivity to cold.

3. Which of the following statements best describes a precaution for persons who take thyroid preparations?

    a. Patients taking thyroid preparations should tell the dentist or physician they are taking these medications.

    b. Patients taking thyroid preparations should not exercise.

    c. Patients taking thyroid preparations should avoid any type of vitamin preparation.

    d. Patients taking thyroid preparations should avoid eating iodized salt.

4. One of the side effects associated with levothyroxine is:

    a. Hypotension.

    b. Hypothermia.

    c. Constipation.

    d. Changes in appetite.

5. Sodium liothyronine is a synthetic source of the _____ hormone.

    a. T_1.

    b. T_2.

    c. T_3.

    d. T_4.

6. An antithyroid preparation is sometimes indicated when the patient is:

    a. Diagnosed as having a diet lacking in iodine.

    b. Having difficulty with an infection.

    c. About to undergo thyroid surgery.

    d. Being treated for swollen lymph nodes.

7. All patients taking Tapazole® should be told:

    a. "Do not take any other medications while you are taking this drug."

    b. "Do not take this medication if you are breast feeding an infant."

    c. "Your lymph nodes may become sore and swollen after you take this medication for a while."

    d. "Take the medication at about the same time each day and take it the same way each time (that is, with food)."

8. While working in the outpatient pharmacy, you receive a prescription written for PTU. What is the name of this medication and what is it used?

    a. Propythlouracil, used in the treatment of hyperthyroidism.

    b. Parathroid, used in the treatment of hyperthyroidism.

    c. Para-amino-benzoic acid, used in the treatment of sunburn.

    d. Phenolated triethane urea, used in the treatment of kidney disease.

9. Hypoparathyroidism is described as:

    a. A condition characterized by a decrease in the concentration of calcium in the serum and an increase in the concentration of phosphorus in the serum.

    b. A condition that can result in the calcification of the blood vessels in the abdominal area.

    c. A condition caused by excessive intake of calcium and potassium.

    d. A condition caused by undersecretion of thyroxin.

SPECIAL INSTRUCTIONS FOR EXERCISES 10 THROUGH 13. In exercises 10 through 13, match the trade name in Column B with its corresponding generic name in Column A.

Column A	Column B
10. ___ Levothyroxine	a. Synthroid®
11. ___ Propythiouracil	b. Propacil®
11. ___ Dihydrotachysterol	c. Hytaberol®
13. ___ Thyroglobulin	d. Proloid®

Check Your Answers on Next Page

SOLUTIONS TO EXERCISES, LESSON 7

1. b   (para 7-3)

2. b   (para 7-4a)

3. a   (para 7-6c)

4. d   (para 7-11)

5. c   (para 7-7c)

6. c   (para 7-9)

7. d   (para 7-10a)

8. a   (para 7-10b)

9. a   (para 7-11)

10. a   (para 7-7b)

11. b   (para 7-10b)

12. c   (para 7-12b)

13. d   (para 7-7e)

End of Lesson 7

LESSON ASSIGNMENT

LESSON 8   Reproductive Hormones and Oral Contraceptives.

LESSON ASSIGNMENT   Paragraphs 8-1 through 8-22.

LESSON OBJECTIVES   After completing this lesson, you will be able to:

8-1.   Given the name of one of the three main categories of reproductive hormones and a group of statements, select the statement that best describes that hormone.

8-2.   Given the name of one of the three main categories of reproductive hormones and a group of statements, select the statement that describes the use of that hormone or the side effects associated with that hormone.

8-3.   Given the trade or generic name of a specific estrogen, progestin, or androgen agent and a list of uses, patient warning statements, and side effects, select the use(s), patient warning statement(s), and side effect(s) associated with the given agent.

8-4.   Given the trade or generic name of a specific estrogen, progestin, androgen agent, or oral contraceptive and a group of trade and/or generic names, select the trade or generic name that corresponds to the given name.

8-5.   Given the name of one of the methods of contraception and a group of statements, select the statement that best describes that method of contraception.

8-6.   Given a group of statements, select the statement that describes a mechanism of action of oral contraceptives.

8-7.   Given a group of statements, select the statement that best describes one of the three types of oral contraceptives.

8-8.   Given a group of effects, select the side effect associated with the use of oral contraceptives.

8-9.   Given a group of statements, select the statement that describes what a patient who is beginning to take oral contraceptives should be told.

8-10. Given the name of an oral contraceptive, classify that agent into one of three given categories of oral contraceptives (for example, estrogen product alone).

8-11. Given the trade or generic name of an ovulation-inducing agent and a group of statements, select the statement that describes the property, use, dispensing information, or side effects associated with that agent.

8-12. Given the trade or generic name of an ovulation-inducing agent and a group of trade and/or generic names of drugs, select the trade or generic name corresponding to the given name.

SUGGESTION

After completing the assignment, complete the exercises at the end of this lesson. These exercises will help you to achieve the lesson objectives.

LESSON 8

REPRODUCTIVE HORMONES AND ORAL CONTRACEPTIVES

Section I. INTRODUCTION

8-1. GENERAL COMMENTS

For many years people have attempted to better understand the reproductive process. The reasons why people have desired to learn more about reproduction are many. Some wish to identify and alleviate problems that prevent them from having children. Others want to identify and use ways to prevent pregnancy. You will dispense drugs that affect the reproductive process. Hence, you should be familiar with these agents and how they affect the reproductive system as well as the entire body.

8-2. REPRODUCTIVE HORMONES

There are three main categories of reproductive hormones, estrogens, progestins, and androgens.

    a. **Estrogens.** In females, estrogens are secreted by the developing ovarian follicle and by the corpus luteum (see Lesson 6, para 6-11b). During pregnancy, the placenta secretes estrogens. Estrogens are responsible for the development of the uterus, vagina, fallopian tubes, and breasts. Estrogen also produces such physiological effects as accelerating growth at puberty (causes epiphyses of long bones to close), increasing clotting factors in circulation, and decreasing bone reabsorption. Estrogen produces female secondary sex characteristics (like distribution of fat, development of pubic hair, high-pitch voice, and increased skin pigmentation). In males, there is limited estrogen secretion by the adrenal glands.

    b. **Progesterone.** Progesterone is the hormone that prepares the female's body for pregnancy and helps maintain pregnancy. That is, this hormone decreases the motility of the uterus, allowing the fertilized egg to implant and remain implanted in the uterus. Progesterone also develops the milk-secreting cells of the breasts. Decreased levels of progesterone cause irregularity of the menstrual cycle.

    c. **Androgens.** In males, the androgens are produced in the testes. Testosterone is the principal and most powerful androgen. Physiologically, the androgens affect the following:

        (1) Development of the testes, vas deferens, the prostate, seminal vessicles, penis, and scrotum.

        (2) Growth at puberty and the length of long bones (closes epiphyses of long bones).

(3) Anabolism increases the synthesis and decreases the breakdown of protein. Androgens also act to produce secondary sex characteristics associated with the male (like development of pubic hair and facial hair, development of a deeper pitched voice, and development of increased sebaceous secretions). In females, there is limited androgen production by the adrenal glands.

Section II. USES OF REPRODUCTIVE HORMONES

8-3. INTRODUCTION

In the previous section, the reproductive hormones were discussed in terms of their site of production and the effects produced on the body. As you have probably realized by now, these substances affect the body in many ways. Therapeutically, physicians take advantage of the different ways these substances affect the body in order to use them to treat certain disease conditions. This section will focus on the uses associated with the reproductive hormones discussed in Section I.

8-4. USES OF ESTROGEN

Estrogen has a variety of uses in medical practice. Following are some of those uses:

a. **Hormonal Replacement.** In cases where there is insufficient estrogen present, the woman can suffer various conditions (like dryness of the vagina). The lack of sufficient estrogen in the woman's body could be attributed to surgery (removal of the ovaries), to menopause, or to other conditions. In such cases, the physician might elect to prescribe estrogen therapy to provide the needed estrogen.

b. **Palliative Treatment of Breast Cancer and Prostatic Cancer.** Palliative refers to lessening the severity of symptoms or pain, such treatment does not necessarily mean cure. Estrogen is sometimes administered to relieve "bone pain," a condition experienced by some men who have cancer of the prostate that has metastasized to bone causing severe pain. In females, some breast tumors are sensitive to estrogens if there is an "estrogen receptor" present. The presence of such an estrogen receptor can be determined by laboratory tests. If such a receptor is present, estrogen therapy can lead to a decrease in the size of the tumor. At the present time, it is not known if an estrogen receptor is present in cases involving cancer of the prostrate. It is recommended that other treatment (for example, chemotherapy) be used in conjunction with estrogen therapy.

c. **Oral Contraceptive.** Estrogen alone, or in conjunction with progesterone, can be used to prevent pregnancy.

d. **Treatment of Postpartum Breast Engorgement and Bleeding.** Within 24 to 48 hours after delivery, the mother's breasts will become swollen and tender. If the mother intends to breast feed the infant, the nursing staff will provide care to help alleviate the pain. After a while, the pain will subside. If the mother does not wish to breast feed the infant, estrogen can be administered. A large dose of estrogen will feed back to the pituitary gland through the hypothalamus. Prolactin release will be inhibited and the breast engorgement will not occur. You should know that the use of estrogen to treat postpartum breast engorgement is not recommended because of the risk of clot formation. Such administration of estrogen is soon after delivery. Estrogen can also be given to decrease uterine bleeding, since estrogen stimulates the repair of the uterus and vagina (increases the lining of these structures).

e. **Treatment of Acne.** At one time physicians frequently prescribed estrogens in the treatment of severe acne. The estrogens caused the sebaceous secretions to be more fluid. Hence, the pores did not tend to clog so easily. You should know that this treatment is not as popular as it once was. Today other products are sometimes given in conjunction with antibiotics (for example, tetracyclines) in the treatment of acne.

8-5. SIDE EFFECTS ASSOCIATED WITH ESTROGEN THERAPY

As you might expect, there are some side effects associated with the use of estrogens. Some of these side effects are listed and discussed below:

a. **Bleeding.** Women on estrogen therapy sometimes experience vaginal bleeding. Such bleeding can be prolonged. When bleeding occurs with estrogen therapy, the patient should contact the physician.

b. **Headaches.** Headaches associated with estrogen therapy may be sudden in onset and/or severe in nature.

c. **Edema and Breast Tenderness.** The breast may enlarge because of fluid buildup, which cause the breasts to be very tender.

d. **Nausea and Vomiting.**

e. **Thrombo Embolic Disease.** Administration of estrogen can cause an increase in the likelihood of clot formation.

f. **Increased Incidence of Cancer.** There appears to be a higher incidence (five to 15 times) of endometrial cancer in postmenopausal patients that use estrogens, especially, patients who have taken estrogens for a long period of time (five years or longer).

g. **"In Utero" Effects on the Fetus.** In the 1950s and 1960s, females who were habitual aborters were given an estrogen product called diethylstilbestrol (DES). This drug was given in order for the habitual aborters to have children. The children they gave birth to have been found to have been affected by this drug. Some female offspring have been found to have an increased incidence of vaginal cancer. Some male offspring have decreased semen volume, sperm density, and mobility and hypertrophic testes.

h. **Increased Dietary Requirements for Vitamin B6 and Folic Acid.** Estrogens interfere with the absorption of these substances from the gastrointestinal tract. Hence, the patient may have to increase intake of these substances in order to absorb body requirements.

8-6. USES OF PROGESTINS

Progestins are used as listed and discussed below:

a. **Oral Contraceptive.** Progestins are used either alone or in combination with estrogens as oral contraceptives.

b. **Cancer Treatment.** Some progestins (for example, megestrol acetate) can be used in the treatment of certain types of cancer. Specifically, these agents are used in the treatment of breast cancer and cancer of the endometrium. The mechanism by which these products produce this anticancer effect is unknown. In the treatment of these cancers, the progestins are used in conjunction with other agents.

c. **Progestinic Supplement.** Progestins are prescribed in instances in which insufficient amounts of progestins are produced by the body.

8-7. SIDE EFFECTS ASSOCIATED WITH PROGESTIN THERAPY

Progestins may be estrogenic or androgenic in terms of the effects they produce. The various actions of progestins seem to be responsible for the side effects observed with their use. Immediately below are some of the side effects associated with progestins.

a. Changes in vaginal bleeding patterns (breakthrough bleeding or complete lack of bleeding can occur with these agents).

b. Severe or sudden headaches may occur with these agents.

c. Sudden loss of coordination.

d. Changes in appetite.

e. Changes in weight (can be caused by edema).

8-8. PRECAUTIONS ASSOCIATED WITH THE USE OF PROGESTINS

Progestins should not be taken during the first four months of pregnancy because of the potential harm they can cause the fetus. Progestins, because of the effects they produce, may delay the spontaneous abortion of a defective fertilized egg.

8-9. USES OF ANDROGEN THERAPY

a. **Androgen Replacement Therapy.** In some instances, there is a lack or insufficient amount of androgen produced by the testes. For example, the testes may have been surgically removed or damaged in some way. In these cases, androgens may be given to the man.

NOTE: Testicular cancer is most common in the young male from age 18 to 30. This type of cancer can be fatal if not diagnosed and treated early. Therefore, any lump on the testes should be cause for an immediate medical check. The loss of the testes will cause sterility. However, loss of the testes will not affect the ability to have an erection, ejaculation, or orgasm.

b. **Treatment of Osteoporosis.** Androgens are administered in osteoporosis in order to cause a rebuilding of bone.

c. **Treatment of Endometriosis.** Endometriosis is the uncontrolled growth of uterine endometrium. Androgens are given to treat endometriosis.

d. **Reduction of Protein Loss.** Androgens can be especially useful in the debilitated or geriatric patient to reduce the amount of protein lost from muscle tissue. In the use of androgens for this purpose, additional protein should be added to the diet in order for the body to synthesize the required proteins.

8-10. SIDE EFFECTS ASSOCIATED WITH ANDROGEN THERAPY

Because of the actions of androgens, they produce characteristic side effects. Some of the most widely observed side effects are:

a. **Edema.** To a slight extent androgens increase sodium and water retention in the kidney.

b. **Masculinizing Effects.** The androgens are responsible for producing the secondary male characteristics. Some of these characteristics include deepening the voice and increased hair on the body.

Section III. SPECIFIC REPRODUCTIVE HORMONES

8-11. INTRODUCTION

In the previous sections, general concepts related to reproductive hormones were presented. You were told of the effects, uses, and side effects associated with these agents. In this section, specific reproductive hormones will be discussed.

8-12. SPECIFIC ESTROGEN AGENTS

a. **Conjugated Estrogens (Premarin®).** Premarin® is used in estrogen replacement therapy. Side effects associated with Premarin® are listed in paragraph 8-5. Provide the patient with a patient package insert (PPI) when dispensing this product. Premarin® is available in tablet, topical cream, vaginal cream, and injectable forms.

b. **Chlorotrianisene (Tace®).** This estrogen is used to prevent postpartum breast engorgement. The usual dosage of this product is 12 milligrams four times daily for seven days or 50 milligrams every six hours for six doses. Because of the short duration of therapy associated with this product, nausea and vomiting are often associated with its use. Tace® also produces side effects such as those listed in paragraph 5-8 in some patients. When you dispense this product you should inform the patient that the medication should be taken until it is gone. Furthermore, a PPI should be provided to the patient when this product is dispensed. Tace® is supplied in capsule form.

c. **Ethinyl Estradiol (Estinyl®).** This estrogen product is used for estrogen replacement therapy, in the palliative treatment of cancer, and as a contraceptive. For the side effects associated with this agent, read paragraph 8-5. Provide the patient with a patient package insert when this product is dispensed. Estinyl® is available in tablet form.

d. **Dienestrol.** This estrogen product is used in estrogen replacement therapy and in the treatment of atrophic vaginitis. (Atrophic vaginitis is a condition sometimes observed in postmenopausal women. Dryness and itchiness of the vagina characterize it.) This preparation is supplied in the form of a cream. The usual dose of this product is one applicator full applied vaginally. Since this product is absorbed locally, the side effects associated with this agent are the same as for the other estrogens. Provide the patient with a PPI when you dispense this product.

e. **Diethylstilbestrol (Stilphostrol®).** This estrogen is used in estrogen replacement therapy, in the palliative treatment of breast and prostate cancer, and as a contraceptive (given as a single high dose following rape). Diethylstilbestrol (DES) is not routinely used as an oral contraceptive. The dosage of the product varies with the use. For the side effects associated with this agent, you should read paragraph 8-5. When you dispense the product, you must provide the patient with a PPI. If the product is being dispensed as a contraceptive, you should tell the patient to take the medication until it is gone. Since this preparation may affect the clotting of the blood, the patient should be told to inform the doctor or dentist the drug is being taken before any surgery is attempted. Furthermore, a female of childbearing age that is taking this product should be told that the drug can cause birth defects if it is taken during pregnancy. Diethylstilbestrol is available in tablet and suppository form.

8-13. SPECIFIC PROGESTIN AGENTS

> **IMPORTANT NOTE**: You must give the patient the PPI when you dispense these products.

a. **Medroxyprogesterone (Provera®).** This product is used in the treatment of amenorrhea and dysmenorrhea and in progestin replacement therapy. Side effects associated with this agent are few when it is taken in cycles. This product is available in tablet and injectable forms.

b. **Hydroxyprogesterone (Delalutin®).** This product is used in the treatment of amenorrhea and in the palliative treatment of uterine cancer. For the side effects associated with this agent, read paragraph 8-7. Delalutin® is available in an injectable form.

c. **Dydrogesterone (Duphaston®).** Dydrogesterone is used in the treatment of amenorrhea and in the palliative treatment of uterine cancer. For a description of the side effects associated with this product, you should read paragraph 8-7. This product is available in an injectable dosage form.

d. **Megestrol (Megace®).** Megestrol is only used in the treatment of cancer of the breast and endometrium. For product side effects, see paragraph 8-7.

e. **Norethindrone (Micronor®).** Norethindrone is used in the treatment of amenorrhea and endometriosis and as an oral contraceptive. For the side effects associated with norethindrone, read paragraph 8-7.

f. **Norgestrel (Ovrette®).** Norgestrel is only indicated for use as an oral contraceptive. See paragraph 8-7 for a description of the side effects associated with this agent.

g. **Progesterone (Luteogan®).** Progesterone is used in the treatment of amenorrhea and functional uterine bleeding. For the side effects associated with this agent, you should read paragraph 8-7.

8-14. SPECIFIC ANDROGEN AGENTS

a. **Danazol (Danocrine®).** Danazol is used in the treatment of endometriosis. (Endometriosis is a condition in which there is uncontrolled growth of uterine endometrium.) Side effects associated with danazol include increased oiliness of the hair or skin, acne, decreased breast size, and unnatural hair growth. This product is available in capsule form.

b. **Fluoxymesterone (Halotestin®).** Fluoxymesterone is used as an androgen hormonal supplement. Side effects associated with this agent include closing of the epiphyseal closures, hypercalcemia, and edema. This product should not be given to boys who are in puberty because of its effect on the epiphyseal closures. Fluoxymesterone is available in tablet form.

c. **Methyltestosterone.** Methyltestosterone is used as an androgen replacement. Side effects associated with this product include hypercalcemia, edema, and development of male secondary sexual characteristics (if used in women). Methyltestosterone is supplied in oral, buccal, or sublingual tablets.

Section IV. CONTRACEPTION

8-15. INTRODUCTION

For years people have been searching for a truly safe and effective contraceptive. Both physical and chemical means have been tried to prevent the process of fertilization. Some chemical means have been found which prevent contraception; however, this means also highly undesirable side effects. The topic of contraception will be presented and discussed in this section. Specifically, the methods of contraception will be examined in relation to their advantages and disadvantages.

8-16. METHODS OF CONTRACEPTION

Immediately below, some methods of contraception are discussed. You are probably familiar with most of these methods.

a. **Abstinence.** Abstinence, in this sense, means that one refrains from engaging in sexual intercourse. Theoretically, this means that abstinence is 100 percent effective in preventing pregnancy. However, intercourse does not have to occur in order for fertilization of the egg to occur. If sperm are deposited in one way or another in or around the vagina, it is possible that sperm could move themselves up the vaginal canal and eventually fertilize the egg.

b. **Coitus Interruptus/Withdrawal.** In this method, the penis is withdrawn from the vagina before ejaculation of sperm occurs. The advantages of this method are two: (1) no chemicals are involved and (2) no devices are used. The disadvantage of this method is that the method sounds better than it actually is. Realistically, some movement of sperm from the penis takes place before ejaculation. Actually, about one-fourth of the couples who practice this method end up with the female pregnant.

c. **Rhythm Method.** In an earlier lesson (see para 6-13), the topic of the female's monthly period (cycle) was discussed. Knowing what is involved in this cycle allows one to predict quite accurately (for many women) when intercourse could result in pregnancy. Many women have 28-day cycles, but other women deviate from this 28-day pattern. Various methods (for example, use of the basal body thermometer (BBT)) have been used to increase the accuracy of the method. As you might think, this method can be used to prevent pregnancy as well as to plan pregnancy. An advantage of this method is that no chemicals are used. A disadvantage is that miscalculation can result in pregnancy. Approximately one-fourth of the couples who used this method found that the female became pregnant.

d. **Spermicide Method.** The spermicide method involves the use of foams, creams, jellies, and suppositories to kill sperm after ejaculation has occurred. Individuals using this method should carefully follow the directions supplied with the spermicidal product. In terms of effectiveness, about 22 percent of the couples using this method find that the female becomes pregnant. One advantage of this product is that no hormones are involved. There are two primary disadvantages associated with this method. First, some products can cause irritation. Second, most products require that they be applied inside the vagina approximately 15 minutes before intercourse is to occur. This takes planning and is somewhat inconvenient.

e. **Prophylactic (Condom) Method.** In this method, a condom is used to cover the penis in order that ejaculated sperm cannot enter the vagina. Hence, this method is a mechanical block against pregnancy. This method also serves to reduce the chances of contracting of venereal disease from the sexual partner. In terms of effectiveness of pregnancy prevention, approximately 10 of 100 couples who use this method find the female becomes pregnant. The advantage of this method is that no chemicals are used and the method is convenient. The disadvantage of this method is that it affects the spontaneity of the sexual act. In addition, the condom may be defective. If defective, sperm can escape from the condom and enter the vagina. You should remember to use only a surgical lubricant (like K-Y® Jelly) on the condom since petroleum can dissolve the vulcanized rubber that is used to make most condoms.

f. **Diaphragm.** This method involves the use of a mechanical block in conjunction with spermicide. Specifically, a mechanical device is inserted in the vagina. A spermicidal product is applied around the diaphragm. Theoretically, this mechanical/chemical block should prevent pregnancy. Actually, approximately five of 100 couples who use this method find the female pregnant. The advantage of this method is that no hormone is used. The disadvantages of this method are that the diaphragm must be fitted (requires a prescription) and there is some difficulty in inserting the diaphragm.

g. **Intrauterine Device (IUD).** This method involves the use of a mechanical device (like a coil or loop) placed within the uterus. The IUD is believed to prevent the implantation of the fertilized ovum. There are various types of these intrauterine devices available. Some intrauterine devices contain chemicals (like copper or progesterone). Approximately five of 100 couples who use this method find the female becomes pregnant. The advantage of this method is that no chemicals are used (except in the two types that contain chemicals). Disadvantages associated with intrauterine devices are that they are not always inserted properly by the females and they can move and irritate tissue. Further, the intrauterine device can present problems to the female and fetus if the female becomes pregnant while the IUD is in place, if the IUD is removed there is a high likelihood of a miscarriage.

h. **Surgical Techniques.** A vasectomy is a surgical procedure that blocks the flow of sperm from the epididymis. This procedure is very effective. A tubal ligation is a surgical procedure that blocks the movement of ovum in the female. Both methods are extremely effective in making the individual sterile. The advantage of these surgical methods is that they are both effective and permanent. A disadvantage is that they are permanent, although some success has been achieved in surgically reversing the procedure.

i. **Oral Contraceptives.**

(1) Mechanism of action. Oral contraceptives act by three methods:

(a) Increase an estrogen level that inhibits ovulation by feedback action on the hypothalamus and subsequent suppression of the follicle-stimulating hormone (FSH) and lutinizing hormone (LH).

(b) Increases progesterone levels prior to ovulation, which inhibit the implantation of the ovum within the uterus.

(c) Affect the quality of the mucous in the vagina (the mucous becomes thick, scanty, and cellular) in order to hamper the movement of sperm.

(2) Types of oral contraceptives.

(a) Estrogen and progestin combination products. These preparations are supplied in a package containing 21 or 28 tablets. In that package, 21 of the tablets contain a combination of estrogen and progestin and seven tablets contain inert ingredients or iron (25 milligrams of elemental iron per tablet).

(b) Low dose progesterone products. These products contain progesterone. A tablet is to be taken each day of the cycle.

(c) High dose estrogen (DES). This tablet is taken within 72 hours of intercourse. High dose estrogen is not a routinely used oral contraceptive. It is only used in cases of rape and incest.

(3) Side effects. Some significant side effects are associated with the use of oral contraceptive agents. Some of these are:

(a) Breakthrough bleeding. This side effect is seen in patients taking low-dose estrogen.

(b) Thromboembolic disease. Symptoms associated with this particular side effect include severe headache, blurring or loss of vision, flashing lights, leg pains, chest pains, and shortness of breath.

(c) Candida vaginitis. This is a yeast infection of the vagina. This side effect is sometimes seen in patients taking high progestin products.

(d) Edema and breast enlargement. This side effect is seen most often in patients taking high estrogen and/or progestin products.

(e) Nausea and vomiting. This side effect is most often observed in patients taking high estrogen products.

(f) Skin reactions. Increased pigmentation can be aggravated by sunlight. This side effect is more common in individuals who have darker skin. This type of side effect is observed most often in patients who are taking high estrogen products.

(g) Libido changes. Oral contraceptives sometimes affect the individual's sex drive.

(h) Rebound fertility. Rebound fertility involves the increased likelihood of pregnancy. The cause of this side effect is unknown.

8-17. GENERAL DIRECTIONS FOR TAKING ORAL CONTRACEPTIVES

The patient should begin taking the medication on the fifth day after menstrual flow begins. Then, one tablet should be taken daily until all the tablets are gone. The patient should stop for seven days (if taking the 21-day packet) and then repeat the 21-day cycle. For patients who have 28-day packets, they should not stop taking tablets between cycles. If the menstrual period does not occur, check with the physician to rule out pregnancy.

NOTE: It is advisable to use alternative methods of contraception when using "the pill" for the first cycle. That is, use a combination of condom/spermicidal foam. Always provide the patient with a PPI each time you dispense an oral contraceptive.

8-18. GOAL OF CONTRACEPTIVE THERAPY

a. The goal of contraceptive therapy is to use as low a dose as possible. If a tablet is missed, it should be taken when remembered. If the patient vomits within two hours after taking the tablet, a second tablet should be taken. When in doubt, the patient should use a second method of contraception.

b. Not all estrogens and progestins are equipotent. For example, norethindrone acetate is twice as potent as norethindrone. Therefore, the lowest weight combination is not necessarily the least potent.

8-19. EXAMPLES OF ORAL CONTRACEPTIVES BY TYPE

a. **Progestin Product Alone.**

   (1)   Norethindrone (NOR-QD®, MICRONOR®).

   (2)   Norgestrol (Ovrette®).

b. **Combination Products (Estrogen and Progesterone).**

   (1)   Norethindrone/mestranol (Ortho-Novum®).

   (2)   Nogestrel/ethinyl estradiol (Ovral®).

   (3)   Ethynodiol acetate/ethinyl estradiol or mestranol (Demulen®).

   (4)   Norethindrone/ethinyl estradiol (Brevicon®).

8-20. PRECAUTIONARY STATEMENT

Oral contraceptives (just like any other type of legend drug) should not be given to friends. A physician must individually select the agent and tailor the dosage based on the history and needs of the patient. A physical examination should be performed every six months to one year. One part of this examination should be the PAP smear. Remember that oral contraceptives are potentially dangerous. A person should never be unless they have been prescribed for the person.

Section V. OVULATION INDUCING AGENT

8-21. INTRODUCTION

In some instances the physician may desire to stimulate ovulation in order that the patient can become pregnant. This section will focus on an agent that will stimulate ovulation.

8-22. CLOMIPHENE CITRATE (CLOMID®), AN OVULATION INDUCING AGENT

a. **Properties.** Clomiphene is a nonsteroidal compound. This agent has properties that are estrogenic and antiestrogenic properties. It has been used to stimulate ovulation in order that the female can become pregnant (if the male partner has adequate sperm production).

b. **Dispensing Information.** Frequently, a two or three month supply of Clomid® is dispensed to the patient since a month of therapy is usually not successful.

c. **Side Effects.** Side effects associated with this agent include enlarged ovaries (this can be painful), hot flashes, and multiple pregnancies.

Continue with Exercises

EXERCISES, LESSON 8

INSTRUCTIONS: The following exercises are to be answered by marking the lettered response that best answers the question or best completes the incomplete statement or by writing the answer in the space provided.

After you have completed all the exercises, turn to "Solutions to Exercises" at the end of the lesson and check your answers.

1. Progesterone is best described as:

   a. The hormone responsible for female secondary sexual characteristics.

   b. The hormone that prepares the female's body for pregnancy and helps maintain pregnancy.

   c. The hormone that affects the growth of bone during puberty (closes epiphyses of long bones).

   d. The hormone responsible for the development of the uterus, vagina, and fallopian tubes.

2. Estrogen is used in the palliative treatment of breast cancer and prostatic cancer. This means that:

   a. Estrogen lessens the severity of symptoms or pain, but it does not cure the patient.

   b. Estrogen causes a complete remission of the cancer in the patient.

   c. Estrogen is used in combination with other agents in order to slow the spread of the cancer throughout the body.

   d. Estrogen can be used to treat cancers that have not spread throughout the body.

3. When you dispense diethylstilbestrol to a patient you must:

   a. Inform the patient that the drug is used in estrogen replacement therapy and in the palliative treatment of breast and prostate cancer.

   b. Tell the patient to take the medication until it is gone.

   c. Tell the patient that the drug has been known to cause atrophic vaginitis in women who are of childbearing age.

   d. Provide the patient with a patient package insert (PPI).

4. The diaphragm method of birth control involves the use of:

   a. A mechanical device placed within the uterus.

   b. A spermicide in conjunction with a mechanical block inserted in the vagina.

   c. A condom used to cover the penis In order that ejaculated sperm cannot enter the vagina.

   d. A dome-shaped rubber device that is placed over the opening of the vagina.

5. Which of the following statements best describes a mechanism of action associated with some oral contraceptive agents?

   a. Some oral contraceptives make vaginal secretions (mucous) watery and noncellular in order to hamper the movement of the sperm.

   b. Some oral contraceptives increase progesterone levels that inhibit ovulation by feedback action on the hypothalamus and subsequent suppression of the follicle-stimulating hormone and lutinizing hormone.

   c. Some oral contraceptives increase progesterone levels prior to ovulation, which inhibit the implantation of the ovum within the uterus.

   d. Some oral contraceptives block the action of the follicle-stimulating hormone by depressing the action of the cilia of the fallopian tube.

6. Which of the following describes the category of oral contraceptives commonly referred to as "combination products"?

   a. Progesterone and estrogen products are together in the same product.

   b. Progesterone and androgen drugs are combined in order to affect ovulation and ovum implantation in the uterus.

   c. Estrogen and clomiphene citrate is combined in order to prevent pregnancy.

   d. Estrogen and androgens are administered in separate dosage forms in order to simulate pregnancy and interfere with progesterone levels in the blood.

7. Select the side effect associated with the use of oral contraceptives.

   a. Breakthrough bleeding.

   b. Hypertension.

   c. Hypotension.

   d. Hypoglycemia.

8. Which of the following statements should be told to the patient who has just started to take an oral contraceptive?

   a. The patient can miss as many as two consecutive days of taking the oral contraceptive, if the monthly menstrual cycle is regular.

   b. Use alternative methods of contraception when using "the pill" for the first cycle.

   c. If the patient vomits within two hours after taking the tablet, the patient should wait until the next day to take the next tablet.

   d. If the patient is on a trip and forgets to bring the oral contraceptive with her, she can take as many as three oral contraceptive tablets from a friend.

9. Diethylstilbesterol (DES) is used:

    a. Routinely as an oral contraceptive by many women.

    b. To prevent pregnancy in cases of rape and incest.

    c. To stimulate the production of milk.

10. Select the side effect associated with the use of clomiphene citrate.

    a. Increased likelihood of becoming pregnant.

    b. Changes in sex drive.

    c. Candida vaginitis.

    d. Multiple pregnancies.

SPECIAL INSTRUCTIONS FOR EXERCISES 11 THROUGH 14. In exercises 11 through 14, match the trade name listed in Column B with its corresponding generic name listed in Column A.

Column A	Column B
11. ___ Clomiphene citrate	a. Clomid®
12. ___ Norgestrel	b. Halotestin®
13. ___ Norethindrone/mestranol	c. Ortho-Novum®
14. ___ Fluoxymesterone	d. Ovrette®

Check Your Answers on Next Page

SOLUTIONS TO EXERCISES, LESSON 8

1. b   (para 8-2b)

2. a   (para 8-4b)

3. d   (para 8-12e)

4. b   (para 8-16f)

5. c   (para 8-16i(1)(b))

6. a   (para 8-19)

7. a   (para 8-16i(3)(a))

8. b   (para 8-17, Note 1)

9. b   (para 8-12e)

10. d   (para 8-22c)

11. a   (para 8-22)

12. d   (para 8-13f)

13. c   (para 8-19b(1))

14. b   (para 8-14b)

End of Lesson 8

LESSON ASSIGNMENT

LESSON 9   Adrenocortical Hormones.

LESSON ASSIGNMENT   Paragraphs 9-1 through 9-14.

LESSON OBJECTIVES   After completing this lesson, you should be able to:

9-1.   From a list of names of hormones, select the three general types of hormones produced by the cortex of the adrenal gland.

9-2.   From a list of names of hormones, select the primary mineralocorticoid or glucocorticoid.

9-3.   Given the name of the primary mineralocorticoid or glucocorticoid and a group of statements, select the statement that describes the physiological function of that hormone.

9-4.   Given a group of statements, select the statement that best describes the effects of either a hyposecretion or hypersecretion of either mineralocorticoids or glucocorticoids.

9-5.   From a group of statements, select the statement that describes Addison's disease or Cushing's disease.

9-6.   From a list of medical conditions, select the condition associated with the long-term administration of therapeutic amounts of glucocorticoids.

9-7.   Given the trade and/or generic name of a specific adreno-cortical hormone or synthetic agent and a group of uses, side effects, patient precautionary statements, or cautions and warnings, select the use(s), side effect(s), patient precautionary statement(s), or caution(s) and warning(s) associated with the given agent.

9-8. Given the trade or generic name of a specific adrenocortical hormone or synthetic agent and a group of trade and/or generic names of medications, select the trade or generic name corresponding to the given name.

SUGGESTION

After completing the assignment, complete the exercises at the end of this lesson. These exercises will help you to achieve the lesson objectives.

LESSON 9

ADRENOCORTICAL HORMONES

Section I. OVERVIEW

9-1. INTRODUCTION

The adrenocortical hormones are a group of chemical substances produced by the adrenal glands (suprarenal glands). These hormones are of particular importance to the body because they perform a variety of essential physiological functions. This lesson will review the physiology of these hormones and discuss some medications you have probably dispensed from your pharmacy.

9-2. THE ADRENAL GLANDS (SUPRARENAL GLANDS) AND THEIR PRODUCTS

Embedded in the fat above each kidney is an adrenal (suprarenal) gland. Both adrenal glands have an external portion and an internal portion. The external portion of the adrenal gland is called the cortex, while the internal portion of the gland is called the medulla. Both the cortex and the medulla produce specific hormones that are essential to the proper functioning of the body. As you will recall (Lesson 6, para 6-10a), the medulla produces epinephrine and norepinephrine. Epinephrine and norepinephrine are involved in the mobilization of energy during the stress reaction ("fight or flight" response). The cortex also produces hormones that are essential to the body. These hormones are introduced below.

9-3. HORMONES PRODUCED BY THE CORTEX OF THE ADRENAL GLANDS

The cortex of the adrenal gland produces hormones that can be grouped into three major groups of substances based on what they do in the body:

a. **Mineralocorticoids.** These hormones serve to control the electrolytes' potassium, sodium, and chloride in the body.

b. **Glucocorticoids.** These hormones serve to affect the metabolism of fat, glucose, and protein in the body.

c. **Androgens.** These hormones produce masculinizing effects in the body.

NOTE: This lesson will focus on the mineralocorticoids and glucocorticoids.

9-4. THE MINERALOCORTICOIDS

As stated above, the mineralocorticoids control the balance of potassium, sodium, and chloride in the body. The cortex secretes several different types of mineralocorticoids. The principal mineralocorticoid is <u>aldosterone</u>, since aldosterone is responsible for over 90 percent of the total mineralocorticoid activity.

a. **Physiological Actions of Aldosterone.** Aldosterone acts to increase the amount of sodium reabsorbed by the renal tubular epithelium. That is, the more aldosterone secreted by the cortex, the more sodium that is reabsorbed into the blood. Conversely, when extremely small amounts of aldosterone are secreted, very small amounts of sodium are reabsorbed into the blood and passed out of the body in the urine. Such control of sodium is crucial to the physiological balance in the body. Remember that sodium is the primary electrolyte in extracellular fluid. If there is too little sodium reabsorbed into the blood, the volume of extracellular fluid (and circulating blood volume) in the body could decrease to levels that could injure the body. Therefore, aldosterone helps to control the level of sodium in the body. In addition, aldosterone helps to decrease the amount of potassium reabsorbed (and thus increases the amount of potassium removed from the body in the urine) and increase the amount of chloride reabsorbed into the blood. To summarize, aldosterone helps to increase the amount of sodium and chloride present in the extracellular fluid and to decrease the amount of potassium present in the extracellular fluid.

b. **Hyposecretion of Mineralocorticoids.** As stated, hyposecretion of aldosterone can result in a lack of water in extracellular fluid (due to decreased amounts of sodium in the extracellular fluid). This can lead to decreased blood volume that can result in decreased cardiac output and hypotension.

c. **Hypersecretion of Mineralocorticoids.** Hypersecretion of mineralocorticoids (aldosterone) can lead to increased sodium reabsorption. This can also lead to decreased reabsorption of potassium into the blood. Ultimately, hypersecretion of aldosterone can result in an increased volume of extracellular fluid, which leads to increased volume of blood. This can increase cardiac output, ultimately resulting in hypertension.

9-5. THE GLUCOCORTICOIDS (HYDROCORTISONE (CORTISOL) AND OTHERS)

As stated previously, the glucocorticoids affect the metabolism of fat, glucose, and protein in the body. The principal glucocorticoid is hydrocortisone (cortisol).

a. **Physiological, Actions of the Glucocorticoids.** The glucocorticoids regulate blood/brain glucose levels. They also inhibit the inflammatory process. The glucocorticoids also decrease the immunological responses of the body by decreasing antibody formation. About 90 percent of the glucocorticoids produced is hydrocortisone (cortisol). One of the most significant metabolic actions of glucocorticoids is gluconeogenesis. Gluconeogenesis involves the formation of glycogen or glucose from noncarbohydrates such as fat or protein. This, of course, can act to raise the concentration of glucose in the blood. Glucocorticoids can also raise the concentration of glucose in the blood by decreasing the use of glucose by skeletal muscle. Glucocorticoids play an important role in the body's reaction to stress, although the specific mechanism for this role is not understood. Glucocorticoids also pay an important role as anti-inflammatory agents. As anti-inflammatory agents, they decrease the ability of histamine to dilate blood vessels, decrease the permeability of capillaries, impair the movement of phagocytes, and cause atrophy of lymphoid tissue (which causes a decrease in circulating antibodies).

b. **Hyposecretion of Glucocorticoids.** A decrease in circulating glucocorticoids often results in anemia, since the glucocorticoids have some effect on the production of red blood cells.

c. **Hypersecretion of Glucocorticoids.** An increase in the production of glucocorticoids can produce a number of serious effects. One such effect is osteoporosis, a thinning and weakening of bone. A second effect is the moon face and the buffalo hump, a condition characterized by atypical disposition of fat in the shoulder areas (buffalo hump) and in the face (moon face). A third effect is increased susceptibility to infection due to the anti-inflammatory action of the glucocorticoids.

9-6. ABNORMALITIES OF ADRENAL FUNCTIONING

In most individuals, the adrenal glands function as they should. That is, they produce the hormones needed in the body in the required amounts. However, for one reason or another, some persons find their adrenal glands not functioning as they should. Two such conditions are presented below:

a. **Addison's Disease.** Addison's disease results when the adrenal glands secrete too little of its hormones into the individual's system. Addison's disease is characterized by fatigue, muscle weakness, weight loss, low blood pressure, and gastrointestinal upset.

b. **Cushing's Disease.** Cushing's disease results when the adrenal glands secrete too great a quantity of its hormones into the patient's system. Cushing's disease is characterized by atypical disposition of fat in the face (referred to as moon face), in the shoulder areas (referred to as buffalo hump), edema, hypertension, acne, and diabetes mellitus.

Section II. GLUCOCORTICOIDS AND SYNTHETIC AGENTS

9-7. INTRODUCTION

In this section, you will be provided with information related to agents that can be classified as either mineralocorticoids or glucocorticoids.

9-8. ADRENOCORTICAL SUPPRESSION WITH GLUCOCORTICOID AGENTS

The long-term administration of therapeutic amounts of glucocorticoids may result in adrenocortical suppression. This adrenocortical suppression occurs because the therapeutic levels of the synthetic glucocorticoids tend to suppress the release of adrenocorticotropic hormone (ACTH) from the pituitary gland via a negative feedback mechanism. This negative feedback mechanism results in the suppression of secretion and synthesis of the naturally occurring glucocorticoids of the adrenal cortex. Prolonged suppression may cause the adrenal cortex to atrophy, thus resulting in adrenocortical insufficiency upon discontinuation of glucocorticoid therapy.

9-9. CLINICAL INDICATIONS FOR GLUCOCORTICOIDS

The glucocorticoids have specific indications for use in the treatment of certain conditions. These indications are discussed below:

a. **Replacement Therapy.** The glucocorticoids are used in replacement therapy for several conditions. These include:

(1) Chronic adrenal insufficiency (Addison's Disease). Addison's disease may develop as a result of adrenal surgery or due to destructive lesions of the adrenal cortex. The replacement therapy associated with this condition requires approximately 20 to 30 milligrams of hydrocortisone (cortisol) or its equivalent daily, with increased amounts of medication during periods of stress. (NOTE: Doses as high as 100 milligrams of hydrocortisone per day may be necessary during periods of stress.) Furthermore, mineralocorticoid therapy will also be necessary with monthly injections of deoxycorticosterone (Doca®, Percorten®).

(2) Acute adrenal insufficiency. Acute adrenal insufficiency is usually associated with disorders of the adrenal cortex. Acute adrenal insufficiency frequently follows abrupt withdrawal of high doses of corticosteroids (adrenocortical steroids). Patients who present with acute adrenal insufficiency are usually administered large doses of hydrocortisone (Solu-Cortef®).

(3) <u>Congenital adrenal hyperplasia syndrome (CAH)</u>. In CAH, the production of hydrocortisone (cortisol) and, at times, aldosterone is interfered with or prevented due to an inherited enzyme deficiency. The treatment of CAH requires the administration of hydrocortisone. The dosage of this agent must be adjusted over a long course of therapy to permit linear growth in children.

b. **Therapeutic Uses of Glucocorticoids in Nonendocrine Diseases.** The glucocorticoids are commonly used in the treatment of a variety of nonendocrine disorders. These products are useful because they produce anti-inflammatory and anti-immunologic actions in the body. The effects produced by these agents are seen with pharmacologic doses. Thus, patients who receive systemic glucocorticoid therapy for nonendocrine disorders risk developing adverse effects (such as moon face and buffalo hump, increased susceptibility to infection, etc.) associated with excessive levels of these substances. Glucocorticoids are used to treat the following disorders:

(1) <u>Treatment of inflammatory diseases such as rheumatoid arthritis, osteoarthritis (degenerative joint disease), and rheumatic carditis</u>.

NOTE: Pharmacologic doses of glucocorticoids are not curative, but rather they help improve the symptoms associated with these various diseases.

(a) Rheumatoid arthritis. Optimal therapy for patients who have only one or two joints afflicted with rheumatoid arthritis is 20 to 25 milligrams of hydrocortisone administered by intra-articular injection. More advanced cases of this disease require 5 to 20 milligrams of triamcinolone or 10 milligrams of prednisone orally in divided doses.

(b) Osteoarthritis (degenerative joint disease). Patients with osteoarthritis are sometimes administered 20 to 25 milligrams of hydro-cortisone by intra-articular injection. This administration should be done infrequently because of dissolvement of joints.

(c) Rheumatic joints. The administration of glucocorticoids in patients who have rheumatic carditis is reserved for patients who fail to respond to salicylates in life-threatening situations. Prednisone, 40 milligrams, is given orally in divided daily doses as treatment in these instances.

(2) <u>Treatment of inflamed joints, tendons, bursae, and soft tissues</u>. These conditions are treated locally with hydrocortisone injections.

(3) <u>Treatment of renal disease</u>. Prednisone, 80 to 120 milligrams, is given daily in oral doses to people who have nephrotic syndrome due to primary renal disease. Prednisone has little or no effect in acute or chronic glomerulonephritis.

(4) Treatment of collagen disease. An example of a collagen disease is systemic lupus erythematosus. Manifestations of collagen disease are well controlled by glucocorticoids that help to decrease morbidity and prolong survival time. Prednisone, 80 to 120 milligrams, is given orally for two to three weeks in the treatment of these conditions.

(5) Treatment of allergic disease. Glucocorticoids suppress manifestations of allergic disease, they inhibit inflammation and antibody production.

(6) Treatment of bronchial asthma. Hydrocortisone may be administered to patients with bronchial asthma in order to provide them with dramatic relief. However, the use of hydrocortisone is usually reserved for patients who have not been responsive to other anti-asthmatic drugs due to the side effects associated with glucocorticoid therapy.

(7) Treatment of various skin disorders. Many patients with noninfective skin disorders (such as allergic, inflammatory, or pruritic dermatosis) experience remarkable relief of symptoms with topical use of steroids. Topical use of these drugs is of benefit in severe sunburn, nonvenomous insect bites, and self-limiting cutaneous conditions such as eczema.

(8) Treatment of malignancies. Glucocorticoids are used in conjunction with other chemotherapeutic agents in the treatment of acute lymphocytic leukemia and lumphomas because of their anti-lymphocytic effect.

(9) Treatment of septic shock. The use of corticosteroids in septic shock has been adopted by most physicians and is used in very large doses early in the treatment of shock. Their beneficial effect appears to be related primarily to their action on cellular membranes. That is, they decrease the patient's reaction to septic, endotoxin, or hemorrhagic shock.

9-10. ADVERSE EFFECTS ASSOCIATED WITH GLUCOCORTICOID THERAPY

As with any medication, patients taking glucocorticoids should anticipate certain adverse effects. The likelihood of such adverse effects correlates with the dose of the drug and the duration of therapy, the age and condition of the patient, and the underlying disease. This paragraph will focus on the common adverse effects associated with glucocorticoid therapy.

a. **Peptic Ulceration.** The glucocorticoids are said to produce peptic ulceration by interfering with tissue repair, decreasing the protection provided by the gastric mucus barrier, and increasing gastric acid and pepsinogen production. Physicians do not all agree that glucocorticoid therapy causes peptic ulcers. However, they do agree that glucocorticoid therapy can hide the symptoms of peptic ulcers so that ulceration or bleeding can occur without warning pains. Some physicians prescribe antacids in hopes of reducing the likelihood of peptic ulcers in patients on glucocorticoid therapy. It is known that antacids can decrease the amount of glucocorticoids absorbed, especially if small doses of the glucocorticoids are administered.

b. **Hypokalemic Alkalosis and Edema.** As you will recall, mineralocorticoids increase the absorption of sodium into the blood (thus less sodium leaves the body in the urine) and decrease the reabsorption of potassium into the blood (thus more potassium leaves the body in the urine). Thus, the patient who continues to ingest his normal amount of sodium per day may find himself with edema (where sodium goes, it takes water) and hypokalemia (more sodium stays in and makes more potassium leave the body) if he is taking glucocorticoids.

c. **Iatrogenic Cushing's Syndrome.** As you will recall, Cushing's disease results from hypersecretion of the adrenal glands. With iatrogenic Cushing's syndrome, the excessive amounts of glucocorticoids present in the body can be attributed to the medications the patient is taking. As you might expect, the same signs will be seen in both types of patients, moon face, buffalo hump, edema, hypertension, etc.

d. **Diabetes Mellitus.** Persons taking glucocorticoids may find that their diabetes is aggravated because of the glucocorticoid therapy. Also, the glucocorticoids may make patients with latent diabetes into diabetics.

e. **Moon Face and Buffalo Hump.** These conditions, which are also found in persons who suffer from hypersecretion of the adrenal glands, are also found in some people who are administered glucocorticoids. See paragraph 9-6b for a review of this topic,

f. **Osteoporosis.** This adverse effect is associated with the long-term administration of large doses of these agents. Essentially, the gluco-corticoids suppress the formation of bone and inhibit the absorption of calcium from the gastrointestinal tract.

g. **Adrenal Insufficiency.** When therapeutic amounts of glucocorticoids are given for long periods of time, adrenocortical suppression occurs because therapeutic levels of glucocorticoids tend to suppress the release of adrenocorticotropin (ACTH) from the pituitary gland through negative feedback. See paragraph 9-9 for further discussion.

h. **Increased Susceptibility to Infection.** Persons taking glucocorticoids find themselves to be susceptible to infection, especially tuberculosis, bacterial infections of the skin, and fungal or yeast infections. Of real concern is the fact that glucocorticoids tend to mask infections. Thus, infections can become severe before they are recognized.

i. **Central Nervous System Effects.** Persons taking large doses of glucocorticoids can undergo personality and behavioral changes that are usually manifested by euphoria. These persons may also be unable to sleep (insomnia), have increased appetite, be nervous or irritable, and be hyperactive.

j. **Growth Suppression.** Growth is suppressed in children who receive long-term administration of glucocorticoids in daily, divided doses. Hence, such therapy should be restricted to children who must receive that type of therapy.

k. **Posterior Subcapsular Cataract Formation.** This type of cataract formation is associated with prolonged systemic glucocorticoid therapy and it appears to be dose-related (e.g., 20 milligrams of Prednisone taken orally for several years). Children are more frequently affected with this adverse effect than are adults.

9-11. CAUTIONS AND WARNINGS ASSOCIATED WITH GLUCOCORTICOID THERAPY

The following cautions and warnings are associated with glucocorticoid therapy:

a. Glucocorticoid therapy should be used with the greatest caution in patients who have the following disorders:

  (1) Peptic ulcers.

  (2) Diabetes mellitus.

  (3) Osteoporosis.

  (4) Active infections.

b. Glucocorticoid therapy should be used with caution in patients who have inactive tuberculosis. (It has been shown that reactivation of tuberculosis can occur in patients who take glucocorticoids.)

c. Adrenocortical insufficiency can be avoided in patients who are on long-term glucocorticoid therapy by keeping the dosage as low as possible and by using intermittent dosage (i.e., taking the drug every other day) when possible.

d. Abruptly stopping prolonged glucocorticoid therapy should be avoided since this may precipitate acute adrenal insufficiency.

e. All patients who have been on glucocorticoid therapy within four to six months prior to surgery should be given supplemental doses of glucocorticoids (e.g., 200 milligrams of hydrocortisone a day before surgery and 100 milligrams of hydrocortisone intravenously at the time of surgery).

f. The prolonged administration of glucocorticoids in children should be restricted to the most urgent indications due to the adverse effects associated with these agents.

g. Topical glucocorticoids should not be applied to open cuts or wounds because of possible systemic absorption of the drugs.

h. Viral vaccinations should be avoided by patients who are on glucocorticoid therapy.

9-12. GLUCOCORTICOID PREPARATIONS

a. **Hydrocortisone (HC, Solu-Cortef®).** Hydrocortisone has a high level glucocorticoid activity and a moderate level of mineralocorticoid activity. It is the drug preferred for replacement therapy in acute or chronic adrenocortical insufficiency and in forms of congenital adrenal hyperplasia. This drug is available in oral, parenteral, and topical dosage (e.g., dental paste).

b. **Prednisone (Deltasone®).** Prednisone is a form of cortisone that is available in parenteral and oral dosage forms. This agent is used primarily in the treatment of inflammatory conditions, stress, or trauma. Prednisone has a high level of glucocorticoid activity and a low level of mineralocorticoid activity. Hence, this agent is not suitable to use as the only agent in treating patients who need drugs with sufficient mineralocorticoid activity.

c. **Methylprednisolone Sodium Succinate (Solu-Medrol®).** This agent has a high level of glucocorticoid activity and a low level of mineralocorticoid activity. It is used in inflammatory and allergic conditions. Methylprednisolone is available in oral and parenteral forms for systemic effects and in cream form for the local effects.

d. **Dexamethasone (Decadron®, Hexadrol®).** Dexamethasone is a derivative of methylprednisolone (a substance similar to prednisone) which is used primarily in inflammatory or allergic conditions. Dexamethasone is available in inhalation, oral, and injectable dosage forms. This drug has a high level of glucocorticoid activity and a low level of mineralocorticoid activity.

e. **Triamcinolone (Aristocortv, Kenalog®).** Triamcinolone has a high level of glucocorticoid activity and a slight level of mineralocorticoid activity. This product is available in oral and parenteral dosage forms for systemic effects and in various types of topical dosage forms for local effects.

9-13. TOPICAL PREPARATIONS

a. **Bethamethasone (Valisone®).** This product has a high level of glucocorticoid activity and a slight level of mineralocorticoid activity. It is available in cream, lotion, gel, and ointment dosage forms for topical administration. This drug is used in the treatment of various skin disorders (not open wounds).

b. **Flucinolone (Synalar®).** This product is available in cream, ointment, and solution topical dosage forms.

c. **Fluocinonide (Lidex®).** This product is available in cream, ointment, and tape dosage forms.

d. **Flurandrenolide (Cordran®).** This product is available in cream, lotion, ointment, and tape dosage forms for topical application.

e. **Halcinonide (Halog®).** This product is available in cream, ointment, and solution dosage forms for topical application.

9-14. RELATIVE POTENCIES OF SYSTEMIC ADRENOCORTICAL STERIODS

Table 9-1 below compares some of the systemic adrenocortical steroids in the areas of anti-inflammatory potency, sodium retaining potency, and equivalent dose. This chart allows you to compare some of the most commonly used adrenocortical steroids in these important areas.

Compound	Anti-Inflammatory Potency	Sodium Retaining Potency	Equivalent Dose
Hydrocortisone (Cortisol)	1	1	20.0 mg
Cortisone	0.8	0.8	25.0 mg
Deoxycorticosterone	0.0	100	-
Aldosterone	0.0	3000	-
Prednisone	4	0.8	5.0 mg
Methylprednisolone	5	0.8	4.0 mg
Triamcinolone	5	0.0	4.0 mg
Dexamethasone	30	0.0	0.75 mg

Table 9-1. Comparison of systemic adrenocortical steroids.

Continue with Exercises

EXERCISES, LESSON 9

INSTRUCTIONS: The following exercises are to be answered by marking the lettered response that best answers the question or best completes the incomplete statement or by writing the answer in the space provided.

   After you have completed all the exercises, turn to "Solutions to Exercises" at the end of the lesson and check your answers.

1.   Which of the following hormones are produced by the cortex of the adrenal gland?

   a.   Androgens, mineralocorticoids, and glucocorticoids.

   b.   Estrogen, aldosterone, and insulin.

   c.   Testosterone, aldosterone, and cortisone.

   d.   Aldosterone, cortisone, and insulin.

2.   The principle glucocorticoid is:

   a.   Aldosterone.

   b.   Insulin.

   c.   Thyroid.

   d.   Hydrocortisone.

3.   What is the predominant physiological function of hydrocortisone (cortisol)?

   a.   Forming glucose from nonglucose factors.

   b.   Increasing the reabsorption of sodium in the kidney.

   c.   Increasing the concentration of potassium in perspiration.

   d.   Decreasing the reabsorption of sodium in the kidney.

4. A decrease in the amount of mineralocorticoids in the blood can result in:

   a. Hypertension.

   b. Diabetes mellitus.

   c. Hypotension.

   d. Cushing's disease.

5. Cushing's disease is caused by:

   a. Hypersecretion of hormones by the adrenal glands.

   b. Hyposecretion of hormones by the adrenal glands.

   c. Hyposecretion of glucocorticoids.

   d. Hyposecretion of mineralocorticoids.

6. What is the condition associated with the long-term administration of therapeutic amounts of glucocorticoids?

   a. Hypothyroidism.

   b. Adrenocortical suppression.

   c. Hypertension.

   d. Diabetes mellitus.

7. Betamethasone is used in the treatment of:

   a. Systemic bacterial infections.

   b. Skin disorders (not open wounds).

   c. Systemic mycotic (fungal) infections.

   d. Tuberculosis.

8. One of the side effects associated with the use of glucocorticoids is:

   a. Weight loss.

   b. Buffalo face.

   c. Severe diarrhea.

   d. Edema (swelling of the feet or lower legs).

9. Deltasone® is used in the treatment of:

   a. Inflammatory conditions.

   b. Peptic ulcers.

   c. Acne.

   d. Cushing's disease.

SPECIAL INSTRUCTIONS FOR EXERCISES 10 THROUGH 13. In exercises 10 through 13, match the trade name listed in Column B with its corresponding generic name listed in Column A.

Column A	Column B
10. ___ Flurandrenolide	a. Kenalog®
11. ___ Prednisone	b. Deltasone®
12. ___ Triamcinolone	c. Cordran®
13. ___ Hydrocortisone	d. Solu-Cortef®

Check Your Answers on Next Page

SOLUTIONS TO EXERCISES, LESSON 9

1. a   (para 9-3)

2. d   (para 9-5a)

3. a   (para 9-5a)

4. c   (paras 9-4a, b)

5. a   (para 9-6b)

6. b   (para 9-8)

7. b   (para 9-13a)

8. d   (para 9-10b)

9. a   (para 9-12b)

10. c   (para 9-13d)

11. b   (para 9-12b)

12. a   (para 9-12e)

13. d   (para 9-12a)

End of Lesson 9

LESSON ASSIGNMENT

LESSON 10	Insulin and Oral Hypoglycemic Agents.
LESSON ASSIGNMENT	Paragraphs 10-1 through 10-22.
LESSON OBJECTIVES	After completing this lesson, you should be able to:

10-1. From a group of statements, select the statement that best describes why insulin is not therapeutically effective when it is administered orally.

10-2. From a group of statements, select the statement that describes the role of insulin in the physiological processes of the body.

10-3. Given the names of particular sites in the body, select the site at which insulin is produced.

10-4. From a group of statements, select the statement that describes how the level of insulin in the blood is regulated.

10-5. Given a group of statements, select the statement that describes diabetes mellitus.

10-6. From a group of conditions, select the condition(s) that are complications associated with diabetes mellitus.

10-7. From a list of signs and/or symptoms, select the sign(s) and/or symptom(s) that can indicate the presence of diabetes mellitus.

10-8. Given the name of a clinical test for discovering/ monitoring diabetes mellitus and a group of statements, select the statement that describes that clinical test.

10-9. Given the name of a basic type of diabetes mellitus, select the statement that describes that type or its treatment.

10-10. Given a group of concentrations, select the concentrations in which insulin is typically available.

10-11. From a group of statements, select the statement that best describes the use or storage of insulin preparations.

10-12. Given the trade, generic, or commonly used name of an insulin product and a group of use(s), onsets of action, duration of action, or precautionary statements, select the use(s), onset of action, duration of action, or precautionary statement associated with the given agent.

10-13. Given one of the following conditions: hypoglycemia or hyperglycemia and a group of statements, select the statement that describes the cause, signs and/or symptoms, or treatment for the given condition.

10-14. From a group of statements, select the statement that describes the mechanism of action of the oral hypoglycemics.

10-15. Given the names of several chemical substances, select the substance(s) likely to interact with oral hypoglycemics.

10-16. Given the trade and/or generic name of an oral hypoglycemic agent and a group of uses, side effects, and cautions and warnings, select the use(s), side effect(s), or caution(s) and warning(s) associated with the given agent.

10-17. Given the trade, generic, or commonly used name of an insulin product or hypoglycemic agent and a group of trade, generic, or commonly used names of drugs, select the trade, generic, or commonly used name that corresponds to the given drug name.

SUGGESTION

After completing the assignment, complete the exercises at the end of this lesson. These exercises will help you to achieve the lesson objectives.

LESSON 10

INSULIN AND THE ORAL HYPOGLYCEMIC AGENTS

Section I. PHYSIOLOGY OF INSULIN

10-1. INTRODUCTION

There are an estimated 11 million individuals in the United States who have diabetes mellitus. Many of these persons are authorized care in Army medical treatment facilities. Because of this, you will be dispensing insulin or oral hypoglycemic agents to these patients. The medications you dispense will not "cure" diabetes, but the medications will make it possible for these diabetics to live a more normal life.

10-2. HISTORY OF INSULIN

The existence of insulin has been known for many years. As early as 1889, scientists were aware of the fact that the surgical removal of an animal's pancreas resulted in that animal's having signs similar to those associated with human diabetes mellitus. In 1922, a human suffering from diabetes mellitus was successfully treated with a hormonal product known as insulin. Since that time, insulin has been obtained from the pancreases of slaughtered animals. Such insulin has allowed the millions of persons who use insulin to continue living. Today, breakthroughs in genetic engineering have resulted in an insulin exactly like that of humans. This new insulin is called Humulin®.

10-3. THE CHEMICAL INSULIN

Insulin is a chemical substance. It consists of 51 amino acids connected in two chains. Because of its chemical composition, insulin is inactivated by digestive enzymes. Therefore, it cannot be taken orally, it must be administered by injection.

10-4. ACTIONS OF INSULIN

Insulin is an enzyme. That is, it is a chemical catalyst that enhances the processes by which the tissues of the body use glucose. Insulin impacts both the use of glucose as fuel for the tissues and the storage of glucose (with as glycogen or as fat). Therefore, the key word is <u>energy</u>. Specifically, insulin affects metabolism by increasing the use and decreasing the production of glucose, increasing the storage and decreasing the production and oxidation of fatty acids, and increasing the formation of protein.

10-5. PRODUCTION OF INSULIN IN THE BODY

a. Insulin is produced and stored in the beta cells of the Islets of Langerhans of the pancreas. Insulin is released from storage in the pancreas into the bloodstream.

b. The level of glucose in the blood is the primary regulator of the secretion of insulin into the bloodstream. When an individual has not eaten in a long while, the level of insulin in the blood is at a minimum. Also, some gastrointestinal hormones (i.e., cholecystokinin, gastrin, and secretin) and amino acids stimulate insulin secretion. After the person ingests food, a combination of the presence of amino acids, glucose, and gastrointestinal hormones acts to stimulate insulin secretion and raise the level of insulin in the blood. While the level of insulin in the blood is high, the body uses the glucose in the blood for energy and it converts excess glucose to fat for future energy needs.

10-6. CONDITIONS DUE TO ABNORMAL AMOUNTS OF INSULIN IN THE BLOODSTREAM

The body requires a certain amount of insulin to be present in the blood when the insulin is needed. Although the level of insulin in the blood does not remain the same over a 24-hour period, insulin must be present in the blood at all times. The individual whose pancreas produces and releases insulin in the required amount at the time it is needed is fortunate indeed. However, not all persons are this fortunate. Diabetes mellitus is a disorder resulting from inadequate production or use of insulin. If, on the other hand, a patient has too high a level of insulin--due to the administration of too much insulin or lack of food after the administration of insulin--the patient's life can be in danger. These two conditions are discussed in the following section.

Section II. CONDITIONS DUE TO ABNORMAL AMOUNTS OF INSULIN IN THE BLOODSTREAM

10-7. DIABETES MELLITUS

a. **Description.** Diabetes mellitus is a disorder characterized by hyperglycemia (high levels of glucose In the blood) and glycosuria (glucose in the urine) resulting from inadequate production or use of insulin.

b. **Significance.** Over 10 million persons in the United States have diabetes mellitus. Diabetes mellitus affects both young and old alike. Insulin and oral hypoglycemic agents have helped prolong the life of persons who have diabetes mellitus. However, persons who have diabetes mellitus, even though it is successfully treated, sometimes have complications. Remember, diabetes mellitus can be treated, but it cannot be cured with the administration of either insulin or oral hypoglycemics. The complications most often associated with diabetes mellitus include blindness. Such blindness can result from several causes. Diabetic retinopathy, one of those causes of blindness, occurs because of the deterioration of the blood vessels in the eye.

Cataract formation is another complication associated with diabetes mellitus. It is theorized that such cataract formation occurs because of increased levels of sorbital in the lens of the eye.

c. **Signs of Diabetes Mellitus.** Fortunately, there are some signs that can indicate the presence of diabetes mellitus. Some of these signs are listed and discussed below. Remember, if you believe that you or any person you know has diabetes, you should contact a physician as soon as possible for professional evaluation.

(1) Polyuria. Polyuria means increased urine output. In diabetics, polyuria is caused by high level of glucose present in the blood. Since the glucose cannot be transferred into the cells of the body, the glucose increases in concentration in the blood. The glucose produces diuresis because it acts as an osmotic diuretic. Hence, output of urine is increased.

(2) Polydipsia. Polydipsia means increased thirst. The thirst is produced by the excessive level of glucose in the blood and the movement of fluids from the cells into the blood in an attempt to dilute the glucose concentration.

(3) Polyphagia. Polyphagia means increased appetite. This polyphagia is caused by the cell's need for glucose. Although the concentration of glucose in the blood might be extremely high, the lack of insulin means that the cells cannot use that glucose.

(4) Hyperglycemia. Hyperglycemia refers to higher than normal levels of glucose in the blood. The normal level of glucose in the blood is 60 to 100 milligrams per 100 milliliters. Of course, the level of glucose will increase after the ingestion of food.

(5) Glucosuria. Glucosuria refers to the presence of glucose in the urine. Glucose is in the urine because it is in high levels in the blood and is removed from the blood in the kidneys (see para 10-7c(1) above).

d. **Clinical Tests for Discovering and Monitoring Diabetes.** Suppose you think you have diabetes mellitus. Perhaps you have been drinking more fluids than usual. Perhaps you have more urine output than in the past. How can a person determine if he/she has diabetes mellitus? Fortunately, tests are available that can help the physician to determine whether or not a person has diabetes. The glucose tolerance test is given under controlled conditions under the direction of a physician to determine if a person has diabetes. After the diagnosis of diabetes mellitus has been confirmed, the physician will prescribe insulin or some oral hypoglycemic agent as a treatment for the condition. Even then, the level of glucose in the blood must be monitored periodically. The methods below can be used by the diabetic in the home to monitor glucose levels in the patient's body.

(1) Tes-Tape® (Glucose Enzymatic Test Strip). Tes-Tape® measures the presence of glucose in the urine. Shades in the color of the strip after it has been dipped in urine can be compared with colors printed on the package. Each color corresponds to a known concentration of glucose in urine. Although Tes-Tape® results are not as precise as those which can be obtained in a laboratory, the tester can obtain a general idea of how much glucose is present in the urine. Such information can be valuable to the physician.

(2) Dextrostix® (reagent strips). Dextrostix® is a product that is used to determine the level of glucose in the blood. Fingertip or venous blood is applied to the strip. Later, the color of the strip is compared to colors on the package label. Each color corresponds to a particular level of glucose in the blood.

(3) N-Multistix® (reagent strips). N-Multistix® is a product used for the determination of protein, glucose, ketones, bilirubin, occult blood, urobilinogen, and nitrite in the urine.

(4) Diastix® (reagent strips). Diastrix® is a product that is used in the determination of glucose in the urine. Color comparison charts show the level of glucose.

(5) Keto-Diastix® (reagent strips). Keto-Diastix® is a product used in the determination of ketones and glucose in the urine. Color comparison charts show the level of glucose and ketones in the urine.

(6) Dextrometer™ (reflectance colorimeter with digital display). This product is a machine that can be used with Dextrostix® reagent strips to determine precisely the level of glucose in the blood. The readings from the machine help the person to monitor their diet and insulin intake to a greater degree.

10-8. TYPES OF DIABETES MELLITUS

There are two basic types of diabetes mellitus: juvenile-onset and maturity-onset. Both these types of diabetes are thought to occur in persons who have inherited a predisposition to the condition. It is thought, also, that juvenile-onset diabetes is initiated by viral infections of a certain kind (like German measles and mumps). Remember, the type of diabetes does not depend on the age of the patient.

a. **Type I Diabetes Mellitus (Juvenile-Onset Diabetes) (Acute-Onset Diabetes).** Juvenile-onset diabetes results from an insufficient secretion of insulin from the pancreas. This type of diabetes begins suddenly (i.e., acute onset). Furthermore, the symptoms associated with diabetes mellitus appear quite suddenly in juvenile-onset diabetes. Persons who have juvenile-onset diabetes mellitus must use insulin injections to control the diabetes.

b. **Type II Diabetes Mellitus (Maturity-Onset Diabetes).** Maturity-onset diabetes mellitus results from an individual's reduced sensitivity to the effects produced by insulin. Maturity-onset diabetes is characterized by the slow onset of symptoms and signs associated with diabetes. Maturity-onset diabetes can often be controlled by requiring the patient to follow a strict diet plan. Oral hypoglycemic agents are also used in the treatment of this condition.

Section III. TREATMENT OF DIABETES MELLITUS BY INSULIN THERAPY

10-9. INTRODUCTION

As previously mentioned (see para 10-8), insulin is essential in the treatment of juvenile-onset diabetes mellitus. Insulin has been successfully used in the treatment of juvenile-onset diabetes since 1922. Typically, a person with juvenile-onset diabetes mellitus must remain on insulin therapy for the remainder of the lifespan. As a person who works in the pharmacy, you must be familiar with the different types of insulin and topics of interest associated with insulin therapy.

10-10. SOURCES OF INSULIN

a. Insulin is primarily obtained from the pancreases of slaughtered beef cattle and pigs. Hence, it is labeled "beef" or "pork" depending on the source of the pancreases. Insulin you have in the pharmacy consists of either a mixture of pork or beef insulin or single-source products (i.e., insulin prepared either from beef or pork pancreases). The information specific to the source of the insulin is contained on the product label. The mixture products are usually dispensed. However, when a patient has been taking either pork or beef insulin, the source should not be switched.

b. A new type of insulin, Humulin®, has begun being used by some diabetics. This new product is made by bacteria and by chemical alteration of pork insulin. Interestingly, this type of insulin is very similar to human insulin.

10-11. MEASUREMENT OF INSULIN

a. You know that many medications have their concentrations expressed in terms of milligrams per milliliter or milligrams per tablet. Insulin is expressed in terms of units per milliliter. These units refer to the activity of the insulin.

b. Insulin preparations are most commonly supplied in two concentrations, 40 units per milliliter and 100 units per milliliter.

10-12. USE OF INSULIN PREPARATIONS

Most insulin preparations are suspensions. Therefore, the patient must ensure that the insulin is thoroughly mixed before the syringe and needle is used to remove it from the bottle. THE INSULIN BOTTLE MUST NOT BE SHAKEN BEFORE THE DOSE

IS EXTRACTED. If the bottle is shaken, air bubbles may be introduced into the product and the measured dose may be inaccurate (i.e., air bubbles are measured instead of insulin). To properly mix the insulin, the patient should roll the bottle slowly between the palms of the hands. Insulin bottles should be discarded when they contain lumps or visible grains of insulin or if the contents of the vial are discolored.

10-13. STORAGE OF INSULIN PREPARATIONS

Insulin preparations should be refrigerated, but they should not be frozen. Specifically, insulin preparations should be stored between two and 8°C (36° to 46° F). Expiration dates should be examined to insure the product is in date when it is dispensed and used.

10-14. INSULIN SYRINGES

The patient should use only one brand or type of syringe to either mix or administer the insulin. Differences in brands or types of syringes (even those made by the same manufacturer) can mean the patient is receiving too little or too much insulin. This occurs because of the unmeasured volume of fluid between the bottom calibration on the syringe and the tip of the needle.

10-15. MIXING OF INSULIN TYPES

Depending on patient needs, some types of insulin may be mixed. Such mixing would, of course, be directed by the physician who deals with the patient. References (like the United States Pharmacopeia Dispensing Information) should be consulted to determine if such mixing is possible.

10-16. TYPES OF INSULIN

The various types of insulin you will encounter in your pharmacy are listed and discussed below:

a. **Insulin Injection (Regular Insulin, Crystalline Zinc Insulin).** Insulin injections may be given subcutaneously in the treatment of diabetic hyperglycemia and intravenously in the treatment of diabetic ketoacidosis. This product is available in the 40 and 100 unit strengths in a mixture of beef and pork insulin. The 100 unit strength is available as either beef or pork source. The onset of action of this product is from 30 minutes to one hour. The time required to reach the peak effect is from two to four hours. The duration of action of this product ranges from five to seven hours.

b. **Protamine Zinc Insulin Suspension (PZI Insulin).** This product is administered subcutaneously only. It is typically administered once a day, from 30 to 60 minutes before breakfast. The onset of action of this product is from four to six hours. The peak effect of PZI insulin is reached within four to six hours after administration. The duration of action of the preparation is approximately 36 hours.

c. **Insulin Zinc Suspension (Lente Insulin®).** This product is usually administered subcutaneously once a day. Most patients administer lente insulin approximately 30 to 60 minutes before breakfast. The onset of action of this preparation ranges from one to three hours. The time required for peak effect ranges from 8 to 12 hours. The duration of action of this product is from 24 to 28 hours.

d. **Prompt Insulin Zinc Suspension (Semilente®).** This product is administered subcutaneously. Typically, it is given once a day, 30 to 60 minutes before breakfast. The onset of action of Semilente® is from one to three hours. The time required for peak effect is from two to eight hours. The duration of action of this preparation is from 12 to 16 hours.

e. **Extended Insulin Zinc Suspension (Ultralente®).** This product is usually administered subcutaneously. It is usually given 30 to 60 minutes before breakfast. The onset of action of this product is from four to six hours. The time required to reach the peak effect is from 18 to 24 hours. The duration of action of Ultralente® is approximately 36 hours.

f. **Isophane Insulin Suspension (NPH Insulin®).** This product is usually administered subcutaneously once a day. It is typically given 30 to 60 minutes before breakfast. The onset of action of NPH Insulin is from three to four hours. The time required to obtain the peak effect ranges from 6 to 12 hours. The duration of action of NPH Insulin ranges from 24 to 28 hours.

g. **Globin Zinc Insulin Injection (Globin Insulin®).** This product is administered subcutaneously. It is usually administered once a day, from 30 to 60 minutes before breakfast. THIS PRODUCT IS NOT MIXED WITH OTHER INSULIN TYPES BECAUSE OF ITS pH. The onset of action of globin insulin is two hours. The time required for peak effect ranges from eight to 16 hours. The duration of action of this product is 24 hours.

h. **Isophane Insulin Suspension and Insulin Injection.** This product consists of 70 percent of isophane insulin suspension and 30 percent of insulin injection. The pork source is the only one available. This product is administered subcutaneously. Typically, it is administered once a day, 15 to 30 minutes before breakfast.

10-17. IRREGULARITIES OF INSULIN THERAPY

Theoretically, a person who has been prescribed insulin should have few problems with diabetes mellitus if food intake is controlled and if insulin administration is properly maintained. However, such control is easier said than done. Periods of stress (physical or mental in nature) can interfere with the delicate balance a diabetic has to maintain in order to function properly. If the diabetic ingests too much food (e.g., eats several pieces of candy at a holiday celebration), this delicate balance can be upset. Diabetics and their friends must be aware of potential difficulties associated with diabetes mellitus. Hypoglycemia and hyperglycemia are two of these potential difficulties.

a. **Hypoglycemia ("Low Blood Sugar").** Hypoglycemia (also known as "low blood sugar" or "insulin reaction") results from an overdose of insulin or an oral hypoglycemic agent, from the too frequently administered insulin, from unaccustomed exercise, or from a delayed or skimpy meal. In other words, there is insufficient glucose present in the patient's blood. In this condition the diabetic speech becomes slurred and the patient appears to be intoxicated. It is critical that this condition be properly diagnosed by medical personnel. Hypoglycemia can be quickly treated. One, the diabetic can be given a source of energy (e.g., a teaspoonful of sugar or a candy bar) by mouth. Two, medical treatment personnel can administer glucagon injection, a product that acts on liver glycogen in order to convert the glycogen to glucose.

b. **Hyperglycemia ("Diabetic Coma").** Hyperglycemia ("diabetic coma" or acidosis) results from the patient's neglecting to maintain proper dieting habits, the patient's missing of required insulin doses, the patient's taking an underdose of insulin, or from the patient's taking the insulin in doses that are too far apart. Hyperglycemia can be treated with the administration of insulin. It is best that the patient's physician be made aware of the patient's condition as soon as possible. This is necessary because the patient's dosage of insulin might have to be changed.

Section IV. ORAL HYPOGLYCEMIC AGENTS

10-18. INTRODUCTION

In individuals with maturity-onset diabetes mellitus, it is sometimes not necessary to require the administration of insulin. Diet, in some instances can control the diabetes. In other cases, the patient might have to take oral hypoglycemic agents to control the diabetes mellitus. Oral hypoglycemic agents are not effective in the treatment of juvenile-onset diabetes mellitus.

10-19. MECHANISM OF ACTION OF ORAL HYPOGLYCEMIC AGENTS

The oral hypoglycemic agents are sulfonylurea derivatives. These agents do not increase the production of insulin in the beta cells of Islet of Langerhans. Instead, they increase the secretion of insulin from the beta cells. The mechanism of this effect is not known. Overall, the effect of these agents is to reduce the concentration of glucose in the patient's blood.

10-20. POSSIBLE DRUG INTERACTIONS

A person who is taking an oral hypoglycemic agent may experience nausea, vomiting, and abdominal pain (similar to that seen in disulfiram therapy) when alcohol is consumed. Furthermore, patients who are on oral hypoglycemic therapy should be evaluated by their physicians when the patients are also taking propranolol, oxytetracycline, or coumarin-type anticoagulants.

10-21. DOSING INFORMATION

A person who is taking an oral hypoglycemic agent should maintain a diet suggested by the attending physician. Specifically, the patient should avoid "cheating" (eating too much food, eating sweets, etc.). Such "cheating" can interfere with the effectiveness of the treatment approach.

10-22. SPECIFIC ORAL HYPOGLYCEMIC AGENTS

a. **Acetohexamide (Dymelor®).** Acetohexamide is an oral hypoglycemic agent. Typically, the patient is given 250 milligrams a day initially and the dosage is gradually increased until the diabetes is controlled. Side effects associated with this agent include drowsiness, photosensitivity reactions, gastrointestinal upset, muscle cramps, and diarrhea. Patients taking this drug should be cautioned not to consume alcohol or to take other medications without the knowledge of the attending physician.

b. **Chlorpropamide (Diabinese®).** Chlorpropamide is an oral hypoglycemic agent that is sometimes used in other patients because of its antidiuretic effect. As with acetohexamide, the initial dosage of this drug (100 to 250 milligrams) is gradually increased until the desired effects are achieved. Side effects associated with this agent include drowsiness, gastrointestinal upset, muscle cramps, and water retention (antidiuretic effect). Patients taking this product should be cautioned not to consume alcohol or to take other medications without the knowledge of the attending physician.

c. **Tolazamide (Tolinase®).** Tolazamide is used as an oral hypoglycemic agent. Side effects associated with tolazamide include drowsiness, muscle cramps, and diarrhea. Patients taking this drug should be cautioned not to consume alcohol or to take other medications without the knowledge of the attending physician.

d. **Tolbutamide (Orinase®).** Tolbutamide is used as an oral hypoglycemic agent. Side effects associated with tolbutamide include drowsiness, muscle cramps, and diarrhea. Patients taking tolbutamide should be cautioned not to consume alcohol or to take other medications without the knowledge of the attending physician.

Continue with Exercises

EXERCISES, LESSON 10

INSTRUCTIONS: The following exercises are to be answered by marking the lettered response that best answers the question or best completes the incomplete statement or by writing the answer in the space provided.

After you have completed all the exercises, turn to "Solutions to Exercises" at the end of the lesson and check your answers.

1. Insulin is not therapeutically effective when it is taken orally because:

   a. It is not absorbed because of its pH.

   b. It is changed to glycogen by the hydrochloric acid in the stomach.

   c. It is metabolized into fatty acids before it is absorbed.

   d. It is inactivated by digestive enzymes.

2. Which of the following are signs associated with diabetes mellitus?

   a. Decreased appetite and excessive thirst.

   b. The presence of glucose in the urine and excessive thirst.

   c. Lower than normal blood glucose levels and increased urine output.

   d. Increased appetite and lower than normal blood glucose levels.

3. Insulin is produced and stored in the beta cells of the:

   a. Gallbladder.

   b. Islets of Langerhans in the liver.

   c. Posterior ventrolateral nucleus of the thalamus.

   d. Islets of Langerhans in the pancreas.

4. The level of insulin in the blood is regulated by:

   a. The level of glucose in the blood.

   b. The level of cholecystokinin in the blood.

   c. The glucose-fatty acid feedback mechanism.

   d. The level of sucrose or glucose in the digestive system.

5. Diabetes mellitus is:

   a. A disease in which there is excessive production of insulin by the pancreas.

   b. A chronic condition caused by inadequate absorption of carbohydrates by the intestines.

   c. A disorder resulting from inadequate production or use of insulin.

   d. An illness characterized by hypoglycemia and glycosuria.

6. Which of the following are complications associated with diabetes mellitus?

   a. Decreased levels of sorbital in the lens of the eye.

   b. Hypertension.

   c. Diabetic retinopathy.

   d. Hypoglycemia.

7. A Dextrometer® can be used to:

   a. Determine the level of glucose in a person's blood.

   b. Determine the levels of glucose and ketones in the patient's urine.

   c. Determine the levels of protein, glucose, ketones, and biliruben in a patient's blood.

   d. Determine the level of occult blood present in a sample of urine.

8.   Maturity-onset diabetes mellitus is described as:

   a.   A condition caused by viral infections (like German measles and mumps) and characterized by hyperglycemia and polyuria.

   b.   A condition which results from an individual's reduced sensitivity to the effects produced by insulin.

   c.   A type of diabetes characterized by rapid onset of the signs of diabetes.

   d.   A type of diabetes in which insulin is no longer produced in the body.

9.   Juvenile-onset diabetes mellitus is treated by:

   a.   Oral hypoglycemic agents.

   b.   Strict diet plans.

   c.   Surgery and strict diet plans.

   d.   Injections of insulin.

10.   Insulin is commonly available in the following concentrations.

   a.   10 units per milliliter and 50 units per milliliter.

   b.   40 units per milliliter and 100 units per milliliter.

   c.   50 units per milliliter and 100 units per milliliter.

   d.   100 units per milliliter and 250 units per milliliter.

11.   The duration of action of PZI Insulin® is:

   a.   18 hours.

   b.   24 hours.

   c.   36 hours.

   d.   48 hours.

12. Hypoglycemia in a person who is taking insulin for diabetes mellitus can be treated by:

    a. Having the person eat a candy bar.

    b. Administering insulin to the person.

    c. Giving the person an oral hypoglycemic agent.

    d. Administering diphenhydramine (Benadryl®).

13. One side effect associated with Diabinese® is:

    a. Water retention.

    b. Hyperglycemia.

    c. Polyuria.

    d. Cataracts.

SPECIAL INSTRUCTIONS FOR EXERCISES 14 THROUGH 17. In exercises 14 through 17, match the trade (or commonly used) name listed in Column B with its corresponding generic name listed in Column A.

	Column A		Column B
14. _____	Chlorpropamide	a.	NPH insulin®
15. _____	Prompt Insulin Zinc Suspension	b.	Dymelor®
16. _____	Acetohexamide	c.	Diabinesev
17. _____	Isophane Insulin Suspension	d.	Semilente®

Check Your Answers on Next Page

SOLUTIONS TO EXERCISES, LESSON 10

1. d (para 10-3)

2. b (para 10-7c(2)(5))

3. d (para 10-5)

4. a (para 10-5b)

5. c (para 10-7a)

6. c (para 10-7b)

7. a (para l0-7d(6))

8. b (para 10-8b)

9. d (para 10-8a)

10. b (para 10-11b)

11. c (para 10-16b)

12. a (para 10-17a)

13. a (para 10-22b)

14. c (para 10-22b)

15. d (para 10-16b)

16. b (para l0-22a)

17. a (para 10-16f)

End of Lesson 10

LESSON ASSIGNMENT

LESSON 11   Oxytocics and Ergot Alkaloids.

LESSON ASSIGNMENT   Paragraphs 11-1 through 11-13.

LESSON OBJECTIVES   After completing this lesson, you should be able to:

11-1. Given a group of statements, select the statement that describes the role of oxytocin in the birth process.

11-2. Given a group of statements and the name of one of the stages of labor, select the statement that describes that stage.

11-3. From a list of uses, select the use(s) of oxytocin.

11-4. Given the trade and/or generic name of an oxytocic agent and a group of uses, side effects, or cautions and warnings, select the use(s), side effect(s), or caution(s) and warning(s) associated with the given agent.

11-5. From a list of uses, select the use(s) of ergot alkaloids.

11-6. From a group of statements, select the statement that describes ergotism.

11-7. Given the trade and/or generic name of an ergot agent and a list of uses, side effects, cautions and warnings, or patient information statements, select the use(s), side effect(s), caution(s) and warning(s), or patient information statement(s) associated with the given drug.

11-8. From a list of conditions, select the condition(s) in which the use of ergot alkaloids and/or oxytocics is/are contraindicated.

11-9. Given the trade or generic name of an oxytocic or ergot alkaloid agent and a list of trade and/or generic names of medications, select the trade or generic name that corresponds to the given drug name.

SUGGESTION

After completing the assignment, complete the exercises at the end of this lesson. These exercises will help you to achieve the lesson objectives.

LESSON 11

OXYTOCICS AND ERGOT ALKALOIDS

Section I. OXYTOCICS

11-1. INTRODUCTION

In previous lessons, the female reproductive system was discussed. Usually females have little difficulty delivering the offspring. In some instances, however, the physician may need to intervene in the birthing process. In these cases, the physician may choose to use an oxytocic to speed up the birth process.

11-2. THE PROCESS OF BIRTH

During gestation (the time the fetus is in the uterus), the uterus is relatively quiet in terms of muscle contraction. However, as the time draws near for the process of birth to begin, the uterus begins to contract. These forceful contractions are necessary for the fetus to be expelled from the uterus. Oxytocin is a hormone that causes the uterus to contract.

11-3. ACTION OF OXYTOCIN

Oxytocin directly stimulates contractions of the muscles of the uterus. In general, the gravid uterus is much more responsive to oxytocic action than is the nongravid uterus. In other words, the closer a woman is to giving birth to the child, the more responsive her uterus will be to the effects of oxytocin.

11-4. ROLE OF OXYTOCIN IN THE BIRTH PROCESS

Oxytocin is produced in the neurohypophysis. Oxytocin is a substance that causes the uterus to contract. Another hormone, relaxin, helps to relax some of the ligaments attached to the pubic area. Together, these hormones act to produce conditions favorable to the birth of the fetus. If it were not for the actions of relaxin, the forceful uterine contractions produced by oxytocin would harm the fetus and the mother. Oxytocin, therefore, serves to begin labor and to expel the afterbirth (placenta, etc.) after the delivery of the infant.

11-5. THE STAGES OF LABOR

To understand the role of oxytocics in the delivery of a baby, the three stages of labor must be understood (See figure 11-1). These stages and what happens in them are presented below:

a. **Stage I.** Stage I of labor is characterized by regular contractions of the uterus as well as other physical changes. The contractions become increasingly more intense as labor proceeds. Oxytocin, a hormone produced in the neurohypophysis, is usually released to cause the onset of uterine contractions.

b. **Stage II.** Stage II of labor is characterized by the actual delivery of the infant(s).

c. **Stage III.** Stage III of labor is characterized by the expulsion of the afterbirth (placenta, amniotic sac, and membranous tissue contained in the uterus).

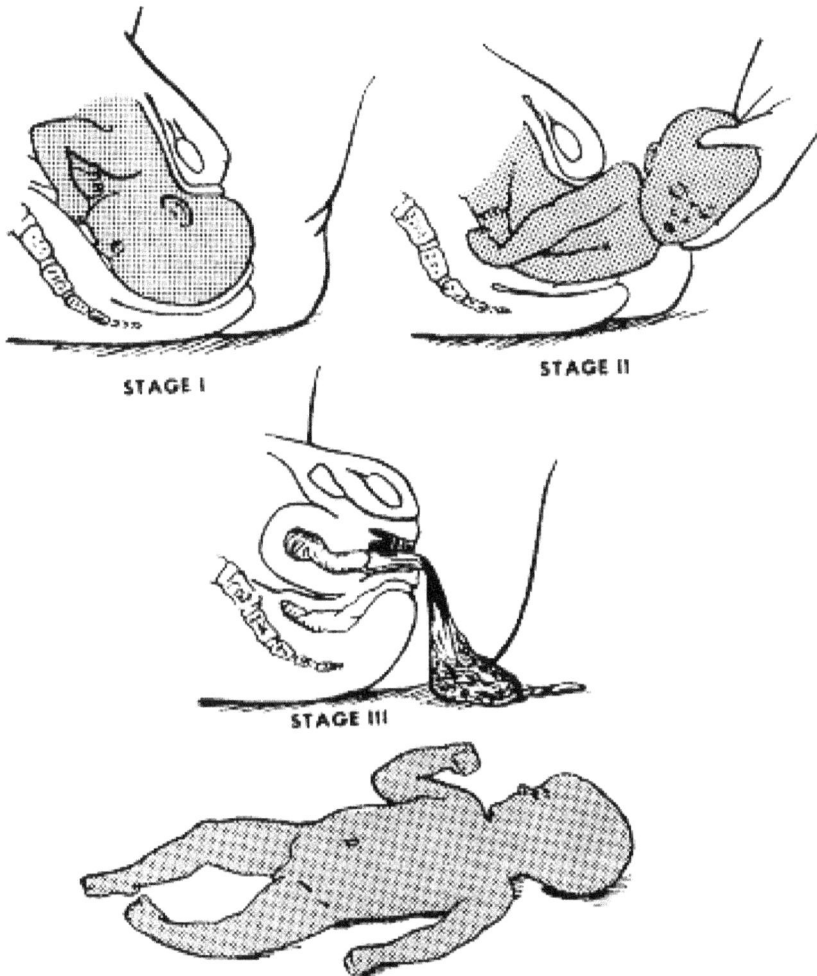

Figure 11-1. The stages of labor.

11-6. USES OF OXYTOCIN

Oxytocin has many uses in medicine. A few of these uses will be discussed here.

a. **Induce Labor at Term.** If the physician believes it is required, oxytocin may be administered intravenously to the pregnant woman at term in order to induce contractions of the uterus.

b. **Control Postpartum Hemorrhage.** Oxytocin can also be used to reduce uterine bleeding after the infant has been born. Remember, oxytocin causes contractions of the uterus.

c. **Relieve Postpartum Breast Engorgement.** Oxytocin is used to relieve postpartum breast engorgement in women who are going to breastfeed their infants in that it causes "milk let-down." "Milk let-down" is a situation in which the milk in the breasts travels from alveoli to the nipples where it can be suckled by the infant. If the milk does not travel from the alveoli to the nipples, the breasts can become swollen and sore. In addition to relieving postpartum breast engorgement, oxytocin can also aid in milk ejection from the breasts by having the milk move toward the nipples.

d. **Prevent Uterine Atony.** After delivery, the uterus must return to its normal size and position. Oxytocin can help in this process by causing the uterine muscle to contract back to its original position. Thus, ocytocin can prevent uterine atony (i.e., when the uterus loses its proper muscle tone).

e. **Aid in Placental Transfer.** Placental expulsion can be aided by the administration of oxytocin.

11-7. NOTE CONCERNING USE OF MORE THAN ONE OXYTOCIC AGENT AT A TIME

The physician should never administer more than one oxytocic at any one time due to the synergistic effect produced. See MD0804, Pharmacology I, for a discussion of synergism.

11-8. UTERINE STIMULANTS

The following products are used as uterine stimulants.

a. **Oxytocin (Pitocin®, Synthocinon®).** Oxytocin can be used on either an inpatient or an outpatient basis. On an inpatient basis, the drug is used to induce labor and/or to aid in contro1ling postpartum hemorrhage. For these uses, the physician can use either the injection or the buccal tablet dosage form. The dosage of either dosage form is adjusted based on the uterine response of the patient. On an outpatient basis, oxytocin is used to aid in breast milk ejection. The physician uses the nasal spray dosage form for this use. The usual dose of the nasal spray dosage form is one spray in each nostril two to three minutes before nursing. Side effects associated with the use of oxytocin include increased blood pressure, nausea and vomiting, and labored breathing.

b. **Ergonovine Maleate (Ergotrate®).** Ergonovine maleate is used to control postpartum hemorrhage. It is not used to induce labor. The dosage of this product is adjusted based on the uterine responses. Ergonovine maleate is supplied in both injection and tablet dosage forms. Side effects associated with this agent include increased blood pressure, nausea and vomiting, and labored breathing. Both the tablet and injection dosage forms are used on an inpatient basis; however, on rare occasions the tablets may be dispensed for outpatient use.

c. **Methylergonovine Maleate (Methergine®).** Methylergonovine maleate is used to control postpartum hemorrhage and to prevent uterine atony. It is supplied in both injection and tablet dosage forms. The usual dosage for the injection is 0.2 milligram every two to four hours as needed. The usual dosage for the tablet is one tablet three or four times daily for a maximum of one week during puerperium. (NOTE: Puerperium is the period of hospital confinement after a woman has given birth to the child.) The side effects associated with this agent include increased blood pressure, nausea, vomiting, and labored breathing.

Section II. ERGOT ALKALOIDS

11-9. INTRODUCTION

Ergot alkaloids are agents which are derivatives of <u>Claviceps purpurea</u>, the ergot fungus. This fungus naturally attacks wheat and rye. Some of the effects of ergot alkaloids were discovered when grain with the ergot fungus was ingested by people many years ago. Specifically, some persons who ate the contaminated grain developed gangrene due to the vasoconstriction caused by the ergot alkaloids. Furthermore, pregnant women who ate the contaminated grain aborted the fetuses because the ergot alkaloids produce effects similar to oxytocin (i.e., uterine contractions).

11-10. USES OF THE ERGOT ALKALOIDS

Ergot alkaloids are mainly used in the <u>management of migraine headaches</u>, but they can also be used to <u>control postpartum hemorrhage</u>.

11-11. ERGOTISM

The primary problem associated with ergot alkaloids is the possibility of the patient suffering from ergotism. Ergotism is an intoxication or poisoning due to an overdose of the ergot alkaloids. Ergotism is characterized by hot and cold sensations in the hands and feet (sometimes called St. Anthony's Fire), numbness, tingling, vasoconstriction leading to gangrene, vomiting, and convulsions with a possible loss of consciousness and death.

11-12. SPECIFIC ERGOT AGENTS

The following ergot agents are commonly dispensed to patients.

a. **Ergotamine Tartrate (Gynergen®, Ergomar®).** Ergotamine tartrate is used in the management of migraine headaches. This product is available in both an injection and in a tablet dosage form. The usual dosage for injection is 0.5 to 1.0 milliliter given intramuscularly (IM). The usual dosage of the tablets is two to six tablets per attack given at one-half hour intervals. The main concern associated with ergot therapy is ergotism (see para 11-11). In order to prevent ergotism, the maximum dose for the injection is two milliliters per week, while the maximum dosage for the tablets is six tablets per day, 10 tablets per week, or 30 tablets per month. It is imperative that the patient be informed of the dosage restrictions for the tablet form. Ergomar® is available only in buccal tablet form. The usual dose of this product is one tablet administered buccally every 30 minutes as needed. The dosage is not to exceed three per day or five per week.

b. **Ergotamine Tartrate with Caffeine (Cafergot®).** Cafergot® is commonly used in the treatment of migraine headaches. It is useful in the management of migraine headaches because the caffeine enhances the effect of the ergotamine tartrate in constricting the blood vessels of the brain. The usual dosage is two tablets at the onset of a headache and one tablet every 30 minutes after until, if necessary, a maximum of six tablets are taken. If the patient is using the suppository form of the product, the usual dose is one suppository at the onset of a headache and another suppository after one hour, if necessary, until a maximum of two suppositories are inserted. Ergotism is seen in patients who take high doses of this medication. With the tablet dosage form, the maximum number of tablets to be taken per day is 6, per week is 10, and per month is 30. With the suppository dosage form, the maximum number per day is two and per week is five.

c. **Ergotamine Tartrate with Caffeine and Pentobarbital (Cafergot P-B®).** This product is used in the treatment of migraine headaches. The pentobarbital is added for its sedative effect. The product is supplied in both tablet and suppository dosage forms. The usual dose of the tablet form is two tablets at the onset of a migraine headache and one tablet every one-half hour. The maximum number of tablets which can be taken per day is 6, per week is 10, and per month is 30. The dosage of the suppository form is one suppository at the onset of a migraine headache and one suppository after one hour. The maximum number of suppositories is two per day and five per week. This preparation may cause drowsiness because of the sedative effect produced by pentobarbital. The patient should be cautioned not to drink alcohol while under the influence of this medication.

d. **Methysergide Maleate (Sansert®).** Methysergide maleate is used to prevent the occurrence of migraine headaches. Hence, this product is taken on a daily basis by the patient. This product is available in a 2.0 milligram tablet. The usual dosage of the product is 4 to 8 milligrams per day. Methysergide maleate can be used for persons who are not responsive to other types of ergot alkaloids. Furthermore, this drug is used by people who are disabled by their migraine headaches. Sansert® is usually taken with meals. Typically, a patient who takes this product is told by the physician not to take the medication for three to four weeks of every six months in order to allow the body to deplete some of the ergot alkaloids. This helps to prevent ergotism.

e. **Ergotamine Tartrate, Phenobarbital, and Belladonna Alkaloids (Bellergal®, Bellergal-S®).** This product is not typically used in the management of migraine headaches, although it is an ergot alkaloid preparation. Instead, it is used in the management of nervous disorders and disorders characterized by exaggerated autonomic response. Some menopausal, cardiovascular, gastrointestinal, and genitourinary disorders fall into these categories. Bellergal® is available in tablet form with the usual dosage being one tablet in the morning, one tablet at noon, and two tablets at bedtime. Bellergal-S®, an extended action tablet dosage form, has a usual dosage of one tablet in the morning and one tablet in the evening. Bellergal® and Bellergal-S® may cause drowsiness as a side effect. You should caution the patient receiving this medication that alcohol should not be consumed when taking this medication.

11-13. CONTRAINDICATIONS FOR OXYTOCICS AND ERGOT ALKALOID PRODUCTS

Both the oxytocics and the products containing ergot alkaloids produce vasoconstriction. Consequently, these categories of drugs are contraindicated in patients who have peripheral vascular disease (PVD), cardiac or pulmonary disease, impaired renal or hepatic function, hypertension, or are in the third trimester of pregnancy. The contraindication is especially true for ergot alkaloids taken by pregnant women in the management of migraine headaches.

Continue with Exercises

EXERCISES, LESSON 11

INSTRUCTIONS: The following exercises are to be answered by marking the lettered response that best answers the question or best completes the incomplete statement or by writing the answer in the space provided.

After you have completed all the exercises, turn to "Solutions to Exercises" at the end of the lesson and check your answers.

1. Which of the following statements describes the role of oxytocin in the birth process?

    a. Oxytocin causes the uterus to contract in order to expel the fetus.

    b. Oxytocin causes some of the ligaments attached to the pubic area to relax in order that the baby can be expelled from the uterus without injury.

    c. Oxytocin causes the uterus to undergo atony in order to protect the fetus during the birth process.

    d. Oxytocin causes the uterine muscles to relax during the birth process in order that the fetus can move from the uterus without injury.

2. Which of the following are uses of oxytocin?

    a. Control postpartum hemorrhage and prevent milk ejection.

    b. Prevent uterine atony and prevent placental expulsion.

    c. Induce uterine atony and relieve postpartum breast engorgement.

    d. Prevent uterine atony and induce labor at term.

3. Ergonovine maleate is used to:

    a. Treat hypertension.

    b. Control postpartum hemorrhage.

    c. Prevent morning sickness.

    d. Prevent uterine atony.

4. Ergot alkaloids are used to:

   a. Treat gangrene and to prevent vasoconstriction.

   b. To manage migraine headaches and to induce uterine contractions.

   c. Control postpartum hemorrhage and to manage migraine headaches.

   d. Treat St. Anthony's Fire and to prevent uterine atony.

5. Ergotism is described as:

   a. A serious condition caused by ergot alkaloids in which the patient experiences numbness due to intense vasodilation.

   b. An intoxication due to overdose of the ergot alkaloids which is characterized by hot and cold sensations in the hands and feet.

   c. A problem associated with the therapeutic use of ergot alkaloids in which the patient experiences hot and cold sensations in the lower abdomen.

   d. A condition characterized by hot and cold sensations in the hands and feet which is caused by oxytocin intoxication.

6. Ergomar® is used in the:

   a. Treatment of insomnia.

   b. Treatment of alcoholism.

   c. Management of migraine headaches.

   d. Inducement of labor.

7. One side effect associated with the use of Cafergot® is:

   a. Ergotism (with high doses).

   b. Drowsiness.

   c. Hypertension.

   d. Postpartum breast engorgement.

8. Both oxytocics and ergot alkaloid products are contraindicated in patients who have:

    a. Hypotension.

    b. Migraine headaches.

    c. Diabetes mellitus.

    d. Peripheral vascular disease (PVD).

SPECIAL INSTRUCTIONS FOR EXERCISES 9 THROUGH 12. In exercises 9 through 12, match the generic name listed in Column A with its corresponding trade name in Column B.

Column A	Column B
9. ___ Ergotamine tartrate with caffeine	a. Cafergot®
10. ___ Methylergonovine maleate	b. Sansert®
11. ___ Methysergide maleate	c. Ergotrate®
12. ___ Ergonovine maleate	d. Methergine®

Check Your Answers on Next Page

SOLUTIONS TO EXERCISES, LESSON 11

1. a (para 11-4)

2. d (para 11-6)

3. b (para 11-8b)

4. c (para 11-10)

5. b (para 11-11)

6. c (para 11-12a)

7. a (para   11-12b)

8. d (para 11-13)

9. a (para 11-12b)

10. d (para 11-8c)

11. b (para 11-12d)

12. c (para 11-8b)

End of Lesson 11

www.ingramcontent.com/pod-product-compliance
Lightning Source LLC
Chambersburg PA
CBHW080335220326
41598CB00030B/4512

* 9 7 8 0 9 8 3 0 7 1 9 5 2 *